practice management and EHR

A TOTAL PATIENT ENCOUNTER FOR MEDISOFT® CLINICAL

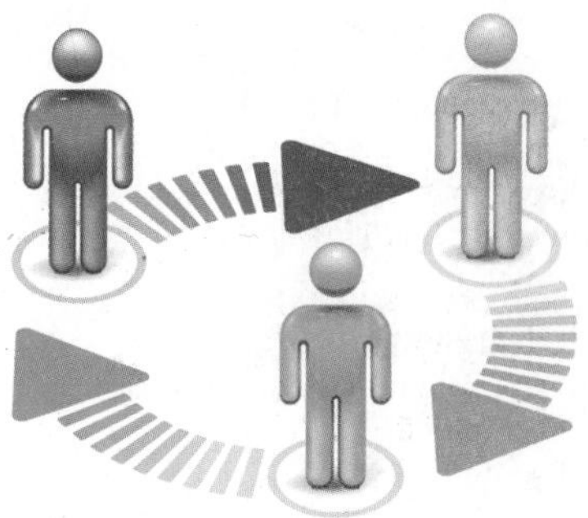

Susan M. Sanderson, CPEHR

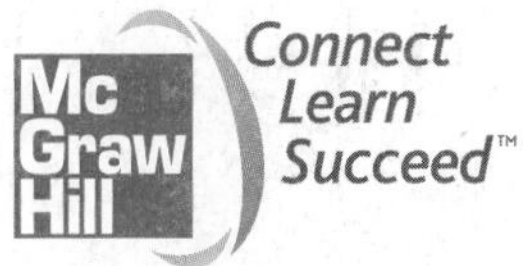

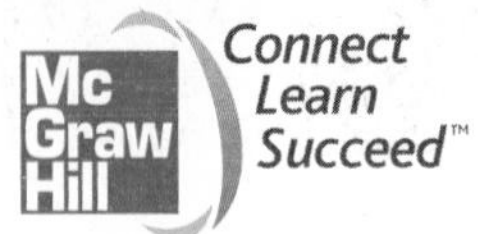

PRACTICE MANAGEMENT AND EHR: A TOTAL PATIENT ENCOUNTER FOR MEDISOFT® CLINICAL

Published by McGraw-Hill, a business unit of The McGraw-Hill Companies, Inc., 1221 Avenue of the Americas, New York, NY, 10020.

This book is printed on acid-free paper.
Printed in the United States of America.
2 3 4 5 6 7 8 9 0 QDB/QDB 1 0 9 8 7 6 5 4 3 2 1

ISBN 978-0-07-337494-9
MHID 0-07-337494-6

Vice president/Editor in chief: *Elizabeth Haefele*
Vice president/Director of marketing: *Alice Harra*
Publisher: *Kenneth S. Kasee Jr.*
Senior sponsoring editor: *Natalie J. Ruffatto*
Managing developmental editor: *Michelle L. Flomenhoft*
Executive marketing manager: *Roxan Kinsey*
Lead digital product manager: *Damian Moshak*
Director, Editing/Design/Production: *Jess Ann Kosic*
Project manager: *Marlena Pechan*
Buyer II: *Louis Swaim*
Senior designer: *Marianna Kinigakis*
Senior photo research coordinator: *Lori Hancock*
Media project manager: *Brent dela Cruz*
Cover design: *Pam Verros, pv design*
Interior design: *Pam Verros, pv design*
Typeface: *11/13.5 Palatino*
Compositor: *Aptara, Inc.*
Printer: *Quad/Graphics*
Cover credit: © *Dan Tero/iStockphoto*

Photo Credits:
CO1: © iStock/Getty RF
CO2: © Digital Vision/Getty RF
CO3: Getty RF
CO4: Getty RF
CO5: © Brad Wilson/Getty Images
CO6: © Thinkstock/Getty RF
CO7: © Jupiter Images/Getty Images
CO8: © iStock RF
CO9: © Corbis RF
CO10: © Blend Images/Getty RF
CO11: © Getty RF
CO12: © Bambu Productions/Getty Images
CO13: © Getty RF

CPT codes are based on CPT 2011.
ICD-9-CM codes are based on ICD-9-CM 2011.

All names, situations, and anecdotes are fictitious. They do not represent any person, event, or medical record.

Library of Congress Cataloging-in-Publication Data

Sanderson, Susan M.
Practice management and EHR : a total patient encounter for Medisoft clinical / Susan M. Sanderson.
p. ; cm.
Includes index.
ISBN-13: 978-0-07-337494-9 (alk. paper)
ISBN-10: 0-07-337494-6 (alk. paper)
1. MediSoft. 2. Medical records—Data processing. 3. Medical offices—Automation. I. Title.
[DNLM: 1. MediSoft. 2. Practice Management. 3. Fees and Charges. 4. Medical Records Systems, Computerized. 5. Software. W 80]
R864.S264 2012
610.285—dc22

2010051750

www.mhhe.com

brief contents

contents

part 2 Documenting Patient Encounters 151

chapter 7

part 3 Charge Capture and Billing Patient Encounters 385

preface

Practice Management and EHR Without the Hassles of Software Installation!

Welcome to *Practice Management and EHR: A Total Patient Encounter for Medisoft Clinical (PMEHR)*! This is an exciting time to be participating in the health professions. Employment opportunities in health care are plentiful, and taking steps toward diplomas, degrees, and certifications in this field is commendable.

For many years, McGraw-Hill has led the way in providing market-leading products in practice management and medical billing with Susan M. Sanderson's *Computers in the Medical Office (CiMO)*. In the past few years, however, technology has begun to change. Today electronic health records (EHRs) are important. *PMEHR* provides the experience students need to understand the medical billing cycle and become familiar with the seamless integration of patient clinical records in that cycle. By completing the activities in *Connect Plus*, students will learn transferable skills that will prepare them for success in the medical office, regardless of what program their practice uses.

Electronic health records programs are getting so much attention in part because of the federal American Reinvestment and Recovery Act (ARRA). The ARRA has dedicated more than $19 billion to the implementation and support of health information technology over the next three to five years. Physicians are eligible to obtain financial assistance to implement EHR by 2014, making patient records available electronically. In addition to moving away from paper records, many EHRs will give patients access to their personal health records (PHRs), helping them become educated consumers.

EHR implementation will create an increased need for qualified health information technology workers. Every health care professional who comes in contact with patient records—from medical coders to billers, from medical assistants to doctors—must have an understanding of EHR. With a highly skilled workforce, EHR will help improve the quality of health care for everyone.

PMEHR provides a comprehensive introduction to integrated practice management and EHR, providing hands-on experience to clinical health care workers as well as to their administrative and financial colleagues. Congratulations on embarking on this exciting new adventure!

Here's What Instructors and Students Can Expect from *PMEHR*

- A book by Susan M. Sanderson, CPEHR, an experienced and accredited author of numerous texts, including the market-leading *Computers in the Medical Office (CiMO)*
- One completely integrated solution with instruction on how practice management software works with EHR software, illustrating the complete patient encounter
- The opportunity to learn not only how to use a combined practice management and EHR solution, but also the why behind learning those skills
- The opportunity to learn a transferable skill
- No need for software installation—all Medisoft Clinical applications will be completed within McGraw-Hill *Connect Plus*
- The opportunity to complete Medisoft Clinical exercises in *Connect Plus* via the **Watch It, Try It, Apply It** system, which is explained later in this preface

Here's How Instructors Have Described *PMEHR*

"*This is the BEST book on the market. I love its content and ease of use for the students. Finally, an accurate, up-to-date book that covers what the students can expect in the field.*"

Deborah Eid, MHA, CBCS, DiHOM, Carrington College

"*I've been an educator for over 16 years teaching Medisoft with Susan Sanderson's leadership through her textbooks. The first edition of this textbook takes Medisoft to new heights.*"

Janis A. Klawitter, AS, CMA (AAMA), CPC, San Joaquin Valley College

"*This is a great book for teaching about practice management and the electronic medical record. It integrates all steps of a patient encounter in relationship to use of this software. It puts so much information into a realistic occurrence at the medical office. The text will be very useful in teaching the concepts associated with the patient encounter including insurance, legal aspects of using electronic media, documentation, and billing.*"

Nikki Marhefka, MEd, MT (ASCP), CMA (AAMA), Central Penn College

The flow of the content works very well with the explanation of medical office flow. It provides a bridge between the two software entities. Overall, this text provides the essential materials and information needed for understanding the PMEHR computer component and the medical insurance, billing, and clinical nature of a patient's electronic information. I also find strength in the framework provided by the LOs for each chapter but still providing a story-like reading experience. Trying to locate an answer to a question within the content of a text when a student needs a full description for understanding a concept is like an answer to this teacher's prayers!

Jane W. Dumas, MSN, CCMA, CET, CPT, CHI (NHA), Remington College

I love it! This text will be beneficial because students can receive training on both the practice management program and the electronic health records at the same time. Students enjoy working hands-on, and the exercises in the text helps the student navigate step by step through the PMEHR program while providing important information about topics such as documentation guidelines, HIPAA rules, and reimbursement issues. This text is the total package. It provides training in the two essential programs that students will need to know how to use to work in the health care industry, practice management and electronic health records.

Nikita Carr, CPC, CMBS, Centura College

Ms. Sanderson has done a spectacular job on this book, as always. The two software pieces have been blended together so well. I am astonished! This book will work so well in the classroom and is the answer to our prayers of how to integrate an electronic heath record course into our existing curriculum. It will be a smooth transition for those of us who now teach Medisoft to integrate the clinical piece into our classroom. The introduction of concepts and flow of material and exercises makes learning easy. The screenshots are particularly helpful for both students and instructors. The style of writing is superb; simplistic, yet thorough. Integration of the billing software with the electronic health record makes perfect sense! This format will give the student an overall experience of a day in the life of an office.

Robin Maddalena, CMT, Branford Hall Career Institute

Organization of *PMEHR*

PMEHR is divided into five parts:

Part	Coverage
1. Managing the Revenue Cycle	Part 1 sets the stage for understanding the uses of an integrated practice management and electronic health record program in the medical practice.
2. Documenting Patient Encounters	Part 2 presents the use of the PM/EHR during the patient encounter, covering scheduling, check-in, intake, exam documentation, and coding. Medisoft Clinical software is introduced.
3. Charge Capture and Billing Patient Encounters	Part 3 presents the use of the PM/EHR to capture the charges resulting from the patient encounter and then collect time-of-service (TOS) payments, create and follow up on claims, post payments from payers and patients, and create statements.
4. Producing Reports and Following Up	Part 4 covers the final steps in the PM/EHR cycle, focusing on financial and clinical reports as well as patient collections.
5. Source Documents	Part 5 provides the source documents—patient information forms, electronic encounter forms, and remittance advice forms—needed to complete the exercises throughout the book.

Content Highlights of *PMEHR* by Chapter

(Information about the book's pedagogical elements appears in the Walkthrough starting on page xxv.)

- Chapter 1 explains the improvements to health care that are based on health information technology (HIT). The chapter covers key government initiatives, defines the clinical encounter and the billing cycle, and discusses the benefits of integrated practice management and electronic health record programs. The chapter also explains the roles of professional health care and administrative staff in implementing HIT in physician practices.

Medical Documentation and Billing Cycle

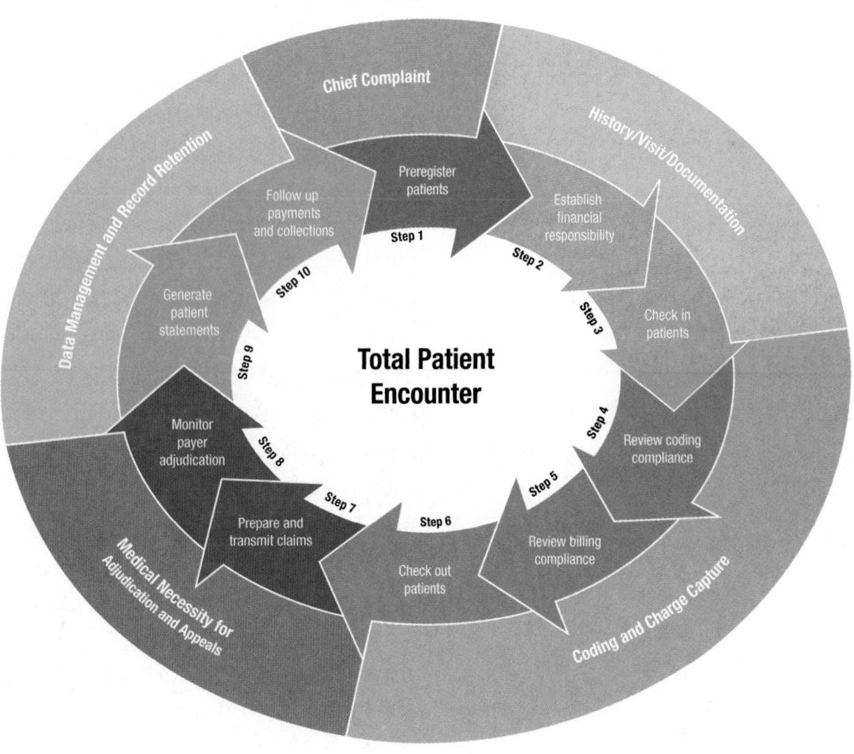

- Chapter 2 defines the legal medical record and provides an overview of key health care regulation, including HIPAA and HITECH. It explores privacy and security concerns associated with electronic health information. The chapter also covers fraud and abuse in order to help office staff complete tasks in a PM/EHR in compliance with regulatory obligations.
- Chapter 3 introduces Medisoft Clinical, a program that combines practice management and electronic health record functions. The chapter opens with a description of the security features of the program that ensure compliance with HIPAA/HITECH regulations. Students are then introduced to the major features of the program, and learn how the program is used during each step of the office visit, from scheduling and pre-registration, to documenting patient care, all the way to collections and account follow-up.
- Chapter 4 presents the knowledge and skills needed to use a PM/EHR to create appointments for new and established patients and to reschedule appointments, as well as to add provider breaks, create recall lists, and print providers' schedules. The chapter also describes how Medisoft Clinical is used to verify insurance eligibility.
- Chapter 5 explains the patient registration process and describes how patient data are organized in Medisoft Clinical. The chapter also covers the skills needed to use a PM/EHR to check patient balances and create chart numbers and cases.
- Chapter 6 introduces the stages of patient flow, and then describes the main sections of a patient chart in Medisoft Clinical. The student learns how to use an EHR to record a patient's history, allergies, medications, vital signs, and chief complaint. Students also practice sending and receiving intra-office messages and creating patient reminder letters.
- Chapter 7 describes methods used to enter documentation in an EHR, including the use of dictation and transcription, voice recognition software, and templates. Students practice entering progress notes with and without the use of a template. The e-prescribing and electronic order entry features of an EHR are also presented. The chapter then introduces the basics of coding, including ICD-9-CM and ICD-10-CM, CPT, and E/M, and explains both paper and electronic encounter forms.
- Chapter 8 provides essential background knowledge on insurance plans, policies, and methods of payment, and the skills required to maintain insurance plan information in Medisoft Clinical.
- Chapter 9 introduces students to the charge capture process in an office using an integrated PM/EHR. This is followed by a discussion of coding and billing compliance, with a focus on strategies to avoid common coding and billing problems. Students then review and post charges that have been electronically transmitted and record time-of-service payments.

Finally, students practice using Medisoft Clinical to locate and print patient education materials to be given to the patient at checkout.

› Chapter 10 provides an overview of the content and format of electronic and paper claims, and then illustrates the flow of claims from the PM/EHR to a clearinghouse and on to the payer. Students gain the skills required to create, submit, and monitor insurance claims through the claim adjudication process.

› Chapter 11 describes how to interpret a remittance advice (RA) from a health plan and to enter and apply insurance payments in a PM/EHR. The process of appealing claims and postpayment audits are discussed. Students also learn how to create patient statements and process a check returned for nonsufficient funds.

› Chapter 12 explains the content of standard reports and how they are used to help generate and monitor practice revenue as well as to improve the delivery of health care, including the use of reports in PM/EHR to demonstrate meaningful use.

› Chapter 13 provides an overview of the accounts receivable follow-up process, including the use of aging reports. The correct procedures for collections, including payment plans and the write-offs of uncollectible balances, are described.

How to Complete the Medisoft Clinical Exercises in Chapters 3–13 Using Watch It, Try It, Apply It!

Using *Connect Plus*, an online assignment, assessment, and e-book solution, students complete key tasks in Medisoft Clinical. No software installation is required! (McGraw-Hill can help you with the access details for *Connect Plus* when you are ready.)

Step 1. Students read the steps of the exercise listed in the text.

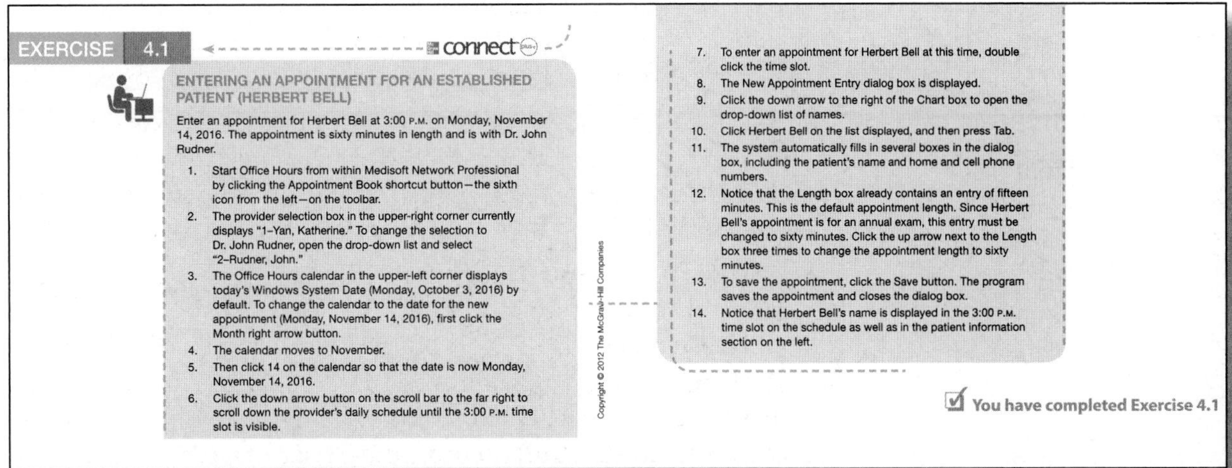

EXERCISE 4.1 connect plus+

ENTERING AN APPOINTMENT FOR AN ESTABLISHED PATIENT (HERBERT BELL)

Enter an appointment for Herbert Bell at 3:00 P.M. on Monday, November 14, 2016. The appointment is sixty minutes in length and is with Dr. John Rudner.

1. Start Office Hours from within Medisoft Network Professional by clicking the Appointment Book shortcut button—the sixth icon from the left—on the toolbar.
2. The provider selection box in the upper-right corner currently displays "1–Yan, Katherine." To change the selection to Dr. John Rudner, open the drop-down list and select "2–Rudner, John."
3. The Office Hours calendar in the upper-left corner displays today's Windows System Date (Monday, October 3, 2016) by default. To change the calendar to the date for the new appointment (Monday, November 14, 2016), first click the Month right arrow button.
4. The calendar moves to November.
5. Then click 14 on the calendar so that the date is now Monday, November 14, 2016.
6. Click the down arrow button on the scroll bar to the far right to scroll down the provider's daily schedule until the 3:00 P.M. time slot is visible.
7. To enter an appointment for Herbert Bell at this time, double click the time slot.
8. The New Appointment Entry dialog box is displayed.
9. Click the down arrow to the right of the Chart box to open the drop-down list of names.
10. Click Herbert Bell on the list displayed, and then press Tab.
11. The system automatically fills in several boxes in the dialog box, including the patient's name and home and cell phone numbers.
12. Notice that the Length box already contains an entry of fifteen minutes. This is the default appointment length. Since Herbert Bell's appointment is for an annual exam, this entry must be changed to sixty minutes. Click the up arrow next to the Length box three times to change the appointment length to sixty minutes.
13. To save the appointment, click the Save button. The program saves the appointment and closes the dialog box.
14. Notice that Herbert Bell's name is displayed in the 3:00 P.M. time slot on the schedule as well as in the patient information section on the left.

You have completed Exercise 4.1

Step 2. Students go online to *Connect Plus* to watch a demonstration of the exercise being completed in Medisoft Clinical—**Watch It.**

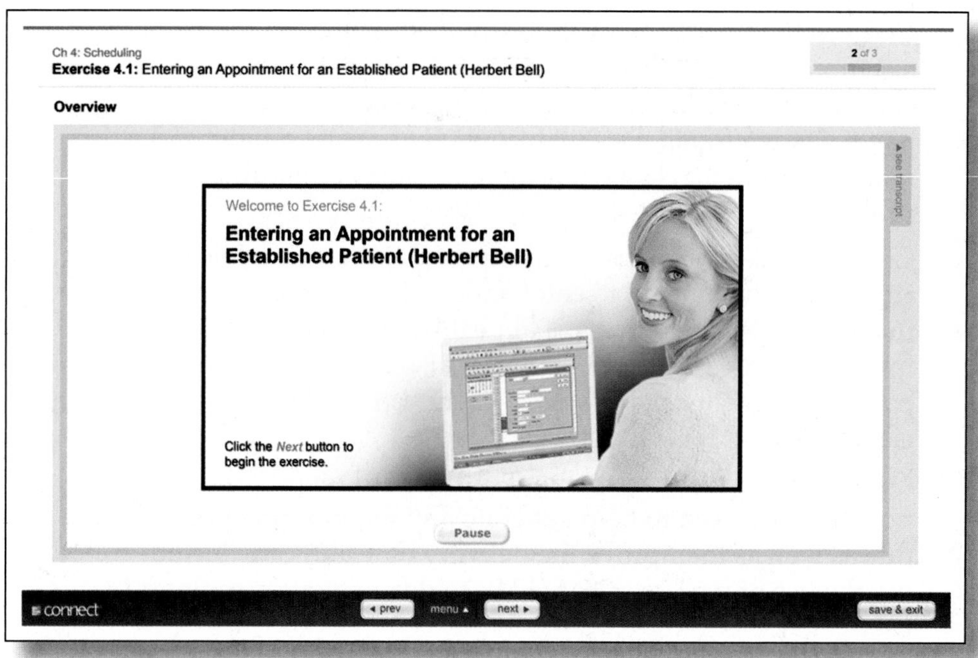

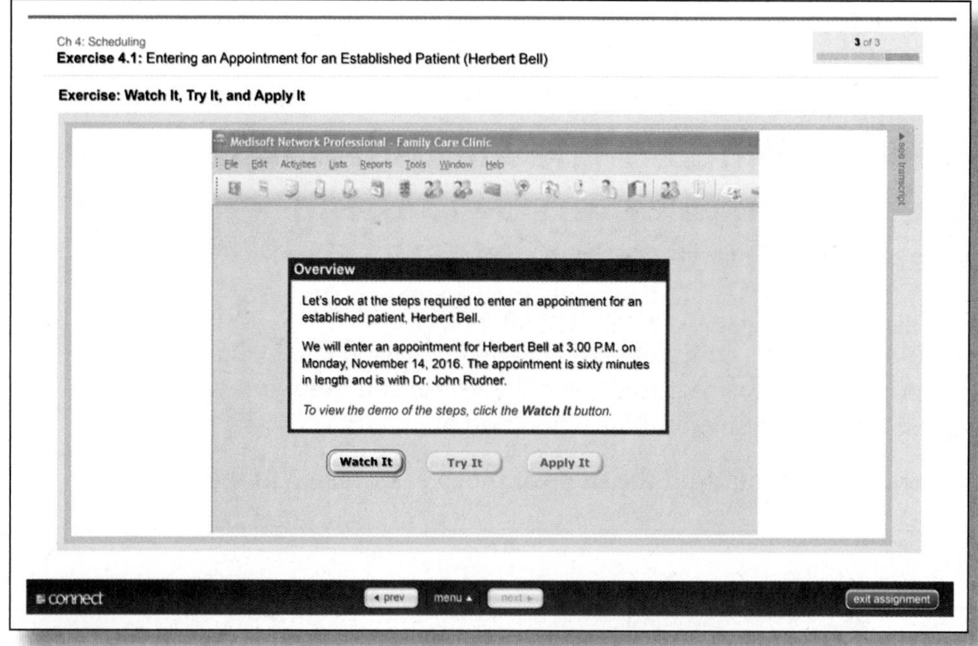

Step 3. Students then complete the same exercise themselves, with hints given when an incorrect click or entry is made—**Try It.**

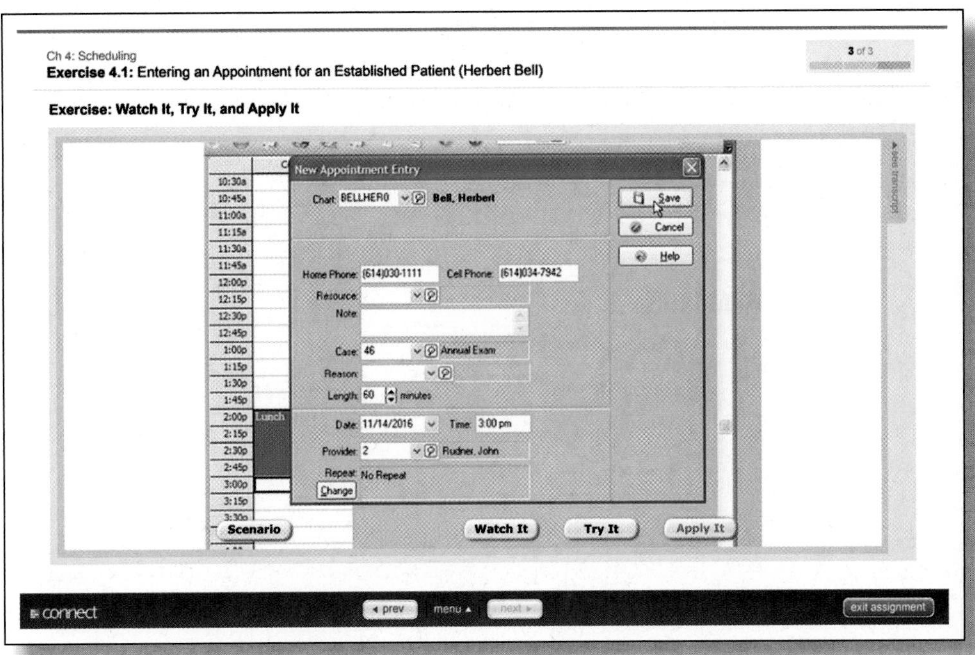

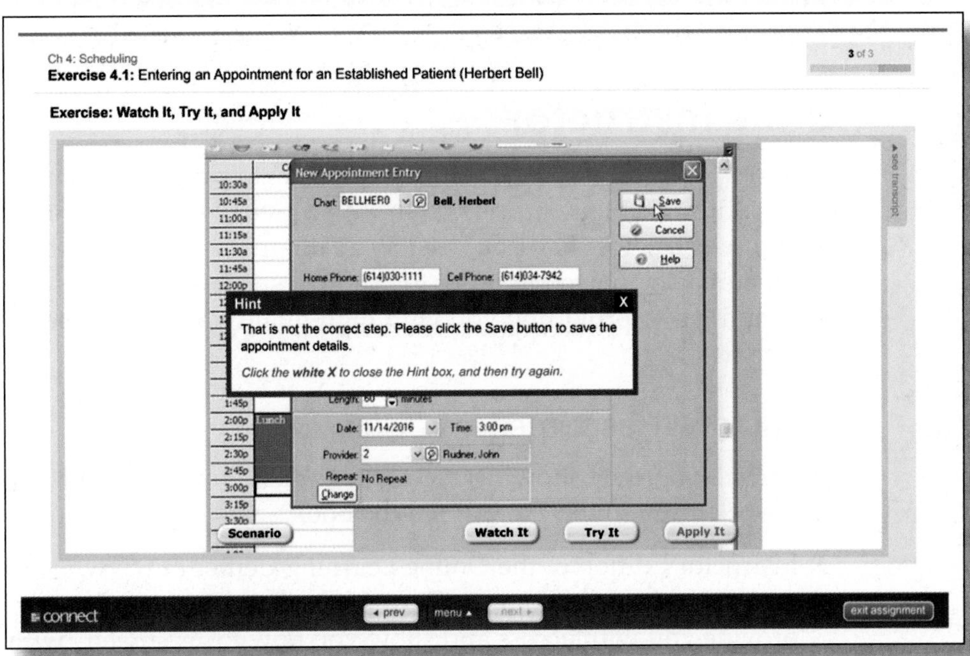

Step 4. Finally, students answer several related assessment questions to confirm their understanding of the task they just completed. Feedback is provided once the answers are submitted, and then the assessment can be reported to the gradebook—**Apply It.**

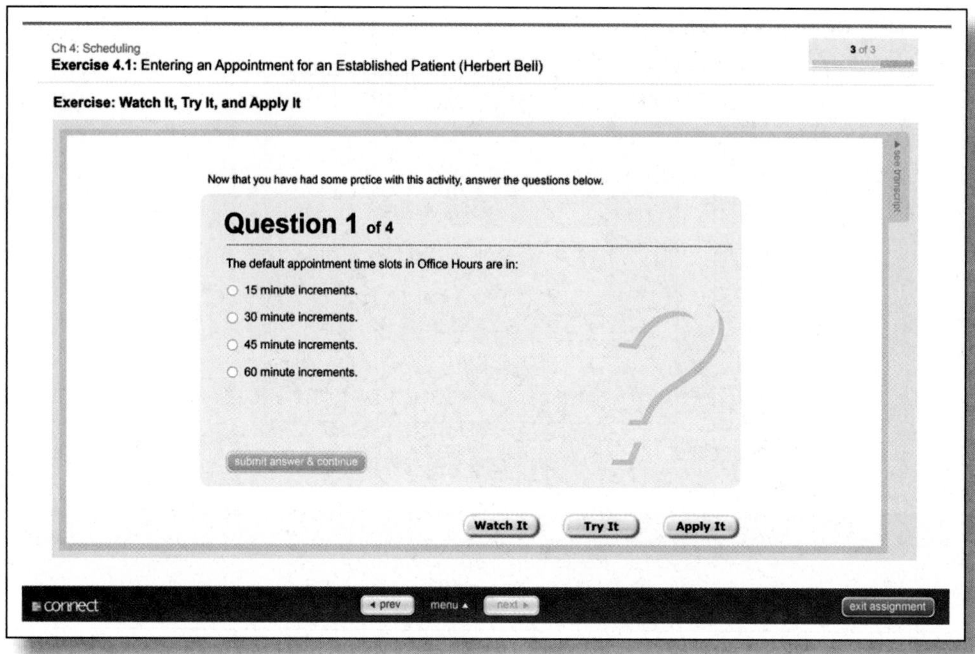

To the Instructor

McGraw-Hill knows how much effort it takes to prepare for a new course. Through focus groups, symposia, reviews, and conversations with instructors like you, we have gathered information about what materials you need in order to facilitate successful courses. We are committed to providing you with high-quality, accurate instructor support.

Instructors' Resources

You can rely on the following materials to help you and your students work through the exercises in the book:

- Instructor Edition of the Online Learning Center at www.mhhe.com/pmehr. Your McGraw-Hill sales representative can provide you with access and show you how to "go green" with our online instructor support.
- Instructor's Manual with course overview, lesson plans, sample syllabi, transition guides, answer keys for end-of-chapter questions, and correlations to competencies from several organizations such as ABHES, CAAHEP, and CAHIIM. More details can be found in the Instructor's Manual at the book's website at www.mhhe.com/pmehr.

- A PowerPoint slide presentation for each chapter, containing teaching notes keyed to Learning Outcomes. Each presentation seeks to reinforce key concepts and provide a visual for students. The slides are excellent for in-class lectures.
- Test bank and answer key for use in classroom assessment. The comprehensive test bank includes a variety of question types, with each question linked directly to its Learning Outcome, Bloom's Taxonomy, and difficulty level. Both a Microsoft Word version and a computerized version (EZ Test) of the test bank are provided.
- Instructor Asset Map to help you find the teaching material you need with a click of the mouse. These online chapter tables are organized by Learning Outcomes, and allow you to find instructor notes, PowerPoint slides, and even test bank suggestions with ease. The Asset Map is a completely integrated tool designed to help you plan and instruct your courses efficiently and comprehensively. It labels and organizes course material for use in a multitude of learning applications.
- McGraw-Hill *Connect Plus* is a revolutionary online assignment and assessment solution that provides instructors and students with tools and resources to maximize their success. Through *Connect Plus*, instructors enjoy simplified course setup and assignment creation. Robust, media-rich tools and activities tied to the textbook Learning Outcomes ensure that you'll create classes geared toward achievement. You'll have more time with your students and spend less time agonizing over course planning.

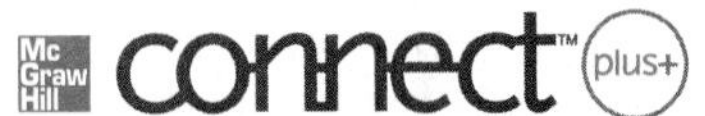

Need Help? Contact the Digital CARE Support Team

Visit our Digital CARE Support website at www.mhhe.com/support. Browse the FAQs (frequently asked questions) and product documentation, and/or contact a CARE support representative. The Digital CARE Support Team is available Sunday through Friday.

McGraw-Hill and Blackboard

McGraw-Hill Higher Education and Blackboard have teamed up. What does this mean for you?

1. **Your life, simplified.** Now you and your students can access McGraw-Hill's *Connect Plus* and Create from within your Blackboard course with a single sign-on. Say goodbye to the days of logging in to multiple applications.
2. **Deep integration of content and tools.** Not only does a single sign-on get you to *Connect Plus* and Create, but it also gets you deep integration of McGraw-Hill content and content engines in Blackboard. Whether you're choosing a book for your course or building *Connect Plus* assignments, all the tools you need are right where you want them—inside Blackboard.

3. **Seamless gradebooks.** Are you tired of keeping multiple gradebooks and manually synchronizing grades into Blackboard? When a student completes an integrated *Connect Plus* assignment, the grade for that assignment automatically (and instantly) feeds to your Blackboard grade center.

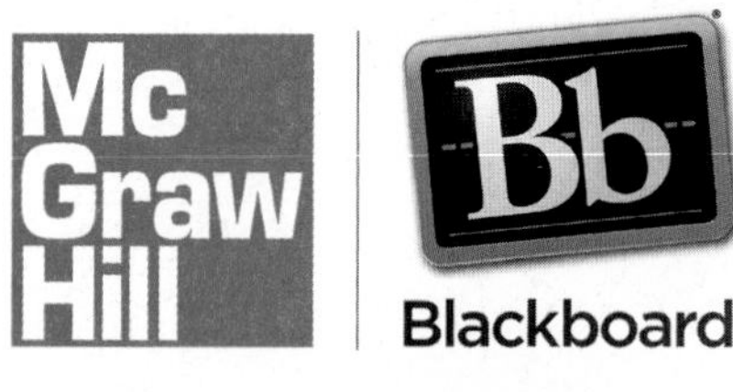

4. **A solution for everyone.** Whether your institution is already using Blackboard or you just want to try Blackboard on your own, we have a solution for you. McGraw-Hill and Blackboard can now offer easy access to industry-leading technology and content, whether your campus hosts it or we do. Be sure to ask your local McGraw-Hill representative for details.

about the author

Susan M. Sanderson, Senior Technical Writer for Chestnut Hill Enterprises, Inc., has authored all Windows-based editions of *Computers in the Medical Office*. She has also written *Case Studies for Use with Computers in the Medical Office* and *Electronic Health Records for Allied Health Careers. PMEHR* is her latest title.

In her more than ten years' experience with Medisoft (and now Medisoft Clinical), Susan has participated in alpha and beta testing, has worked with instructors to site test materials, and has provided technical support to McGraw-Hill customers.

In 2009 Susan earned CPEHR (Certified Professional in Electronic Health Records) certification. In addition, she is a member of the Healthcare Information and Management Systems Society (HIMSS). Susan is a graduate of Drew University with further study at Columbia University.

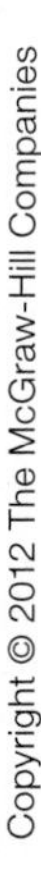

Many pedagogical tools have been incorporated throughout the book to help students learn.

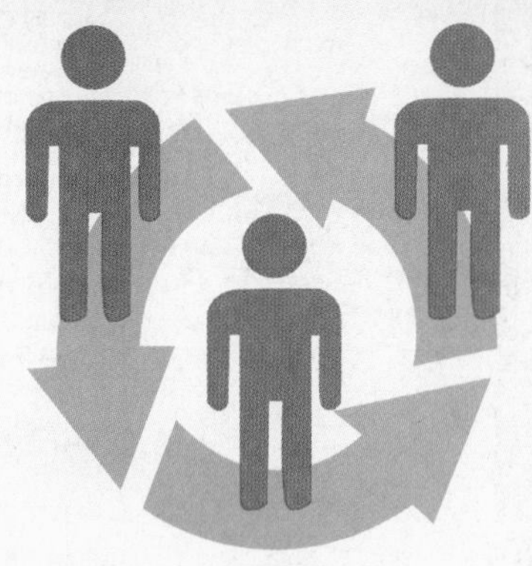

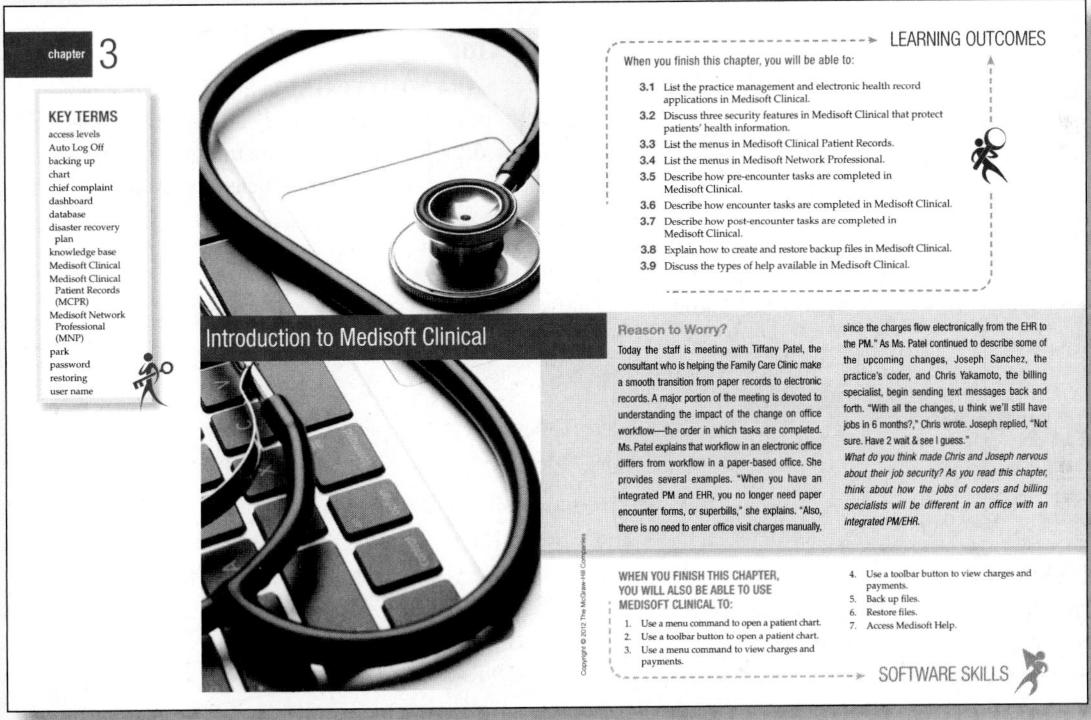

chapter 3

KEY TERMS
access levels
Auto Log Off
backing up
chart
chief complaint
dashboard
database
disaster recovery plan
knowledge base
Medisoft Clinical
Medisoft Clinical Patient Records (MCPR)
Medisoft Network Professional (MNP)
park
password
restoring
user name

Introduction to Medisoft Clinical

LEARNING OUTCOMES

When you finish this chapter, you will be able to:

3.1 List the practice management and electronic health record applications in Medisoft Clinical.
3.2 Discuss three security features in Medisoft Clinical that protect patients' health information.
3.3 List the menus in Medisoft Clinical Patient Records.
3.4 List the menus in Medisoft Network Professional.
3.5 Describe how pre-encounter tasks are completed in Medisoft Clinical.
3.6 Describe how encounter tasks are completed in Medisoft Clinical.
3.7 Describe how post-encounter tasks are completed in Medisoft Clinical.
3.8 Explain how to create and restore backup files in Medisoft Clinical.
3.9 Discuss the types of help available in Medisoft Clinical.

Reason to Worry?

Today the staff is meeting with Tiffany Patel, the consultant who is helping the Family Care Clinic make a smooth transition from paper records to electronic records. A major portion of the meeting is devoted to understanding the impact of the change on office workflow—the order in which tasks are completed. Ms. Patel explains that workflow in an electronic office differs from workflow in a paper-based office. She provides several examples. "When you have an integrated PM and EHR, you no longer need paper encounter forms, or superbills," she explains. "Also, there is no need to enter office visit charges manually, since the charges flow electronically from the EHR to the PM." As Ms. Patel continued to describe some of the upcoming changes, Joseph Sanchez, the practice's coder, and Chris Yakamoto, the billing specialist, begin sending text messages back and forth. "With all the changes, u think we'll still have jobs in 6 months?," Chris wrote. Joseph replied, "Not sure. Have 2 wait & see I guess."

What do you think made Chris and Joseph nervous about their job security? As you read this chapter, think about how the jobs of coders and billing specialists will be different in an office with an integrated PM/EHR.

WHEN YOU FINISH THIS CHAPTER, YOU WILL ALSO BE ABLE TO USE MEDISOFT CLINICAL TO:

1. Use a menu command to open a patient chart.
2. Use a toolbar button to open a patient chart.
3. Use a menu command to view charges and payments.
4. Use a toolbar button to view charges and payments.
5. Back up files.
6. Restore files.
7. Access Medisoft Help.

SOFTWARE SKILLS

Copyright © 2012 The McGraw-Hill Companies

Chapter Opener

The **chapter opener** sets the stage for what will be learned in the chapter.

Learning Outcomes

Learning Outcomes are written to reflect the revised version of Bloom's Taxonomy and to establish the key points the student should focus on in the chapter. In addition, major chapter heads are structured to reflect the Learning Outcomes and are numbered accordingly.

Key Terms

Key terms are first introduced in the chapter opener so the student can see them all in one place.

Case Opener

A brief case study is presented so students can better understand how the content will apply to their future experiences in the health care profession.

Software Skills

The **Software Skills** objectives provide students with a checklist of the software skills they should have by the completion of the chapter (starting with Chapter 3). Mastery of the information listed here is necessary to complete the next chapter.

5.1 Patient Registration

Preregistration, as explained in Chapter 4, is the process of obtaining basic patient information and setting up an appointment time that suits the patient's needs. When patients arrive at the front desk for their appointments, registration staff follow the process of **registration** to obtain more detailed information about patients and their particular health plans before their encounters with providers.

registration process of gathering personal and insurance information about a patient before an encounter with a provider

patient information form form that includes a patient's personal, employment, and insurance data needed to complete a health care claim; also known as a registration form

Information for New Patients

If the patient is new to the practice, these six types of information are gathered:

1. Medical history
2. Detailed patient and insurance information
3. Identification verification
4. Financial agreement and authorization for treatment
5. Assignment of benefits statement

Learning Aids

Key Terms

Key terms are defined in the margin so that students will become familiar with the language needed to perform medical billing and documentation tasks.

Glossary

The **Glossary** at the back of the book also makes it easy to find a term's definition.

HIPAA/HITECH TIP

Who Is Requesting PHI?

Although the HIPAA Privacy Rule permits sharing PHI for treatment, payment, and operations (TPO) purposes without authorization, it also requires verification of the identity of the person who is asking for the information. The person's authority to access PHI must also be verified. If the requestor's right to the information is not certain, the best practice is to have the patient authorize the release of PHI.

Tips

HIPAA/HITECH Tips highlight this important information for students. **Medisoft Clinical Tips** in the margin suggest ways to be a more efficient user of the software.

MEDISOFT TIP

SHORTCUT

The Copy Address button saves time when entering patients with the same address, such as family members. Clicking on the Copy Address button provides an option to copy demographic information from a patient already in the database.

work phone, cell phone, fax, and other. To make data entry faster, phone and fax numbers are entered without parentheses or hyphens. The program adds the parentheses and hyphens automatically.

Birth Date The patient's birth date is entered in the Birth Date box using the pop-up calendar or by keying in the date using the MMDDCCYY format. In the MMDDCCYY format, *MM* stands for the month, *DD* stands for the day, *CC* represents the century, and *YY* stands for the year. Each month, day, century, and year entry must contain two digits, and no punctuation can be used. For example, March 5, 1958, would be keyed ***03051958***. Alternatively, the date can be entered using one or two digits for the day and month, four digits for the year, and separating each entry with a slash. Using this method, March 5, 1958, would be keyed ***3/5/1958***. Medisoft

Exercises

Thinking It Through

Thinking It Through exercises at major points in the chapter challenge students to stop and think through the information that has been presented.

Chapter Exercises

Exercises within the chapter provide students with hands-on practice using Medisoft Clinical through *Connect Plus* and the Watch It, Try It, Apply It system.

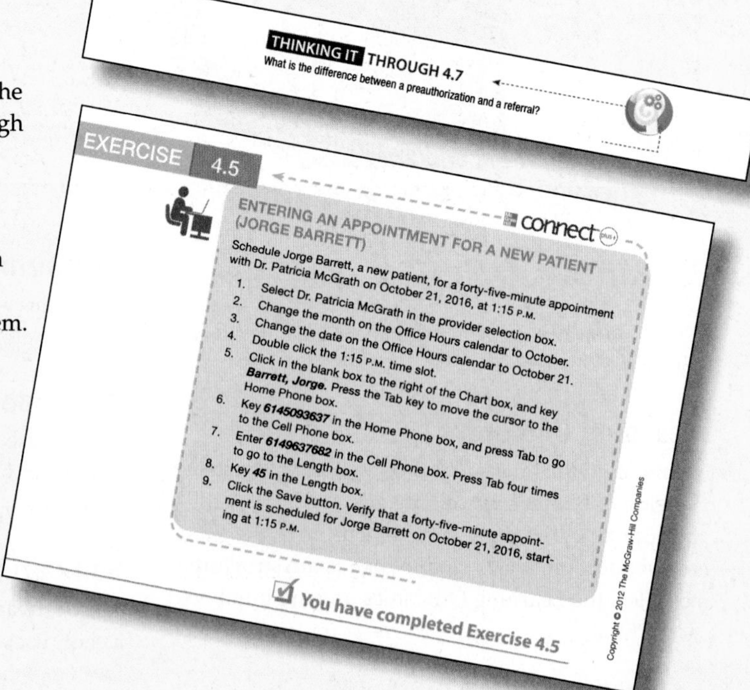

THINKING IT THROUGH 4.7

What is the difference between a preauthorization and a referral?

EXERCISE 4.5

ENTERING AN APPOINTMENT FOR A NEW PATIENT (JORGE BARRETT)

connect

Schedule Jorge Barrett, a new patient, for a forty-five-minute appointment with Dr. Patricia McGrath on October 21, 2016, at 1:15 P.M.

1. Select Dr. Patricia McGrath in the provider selection box.
2. Change the month on the Office Hours calendar to October.
3. Change the date on the Office Hours calendar to October 21.
4. Double click the 1:15 P.M. time slot.
5. Click in the blank box to the right of the Chart box, and key ***Barrett, Jorge***. Press the Tab key to move the cursor to the Home Phone box.
6. Key ***6145093637*** in the Home Phone box, and press Tab to go to the Cell Phone box.
7. Enter ***6149637682*** in the Cell Phone box. Press Tab four times to go to the Length box.
8. Key ***45*** in the Length box.
9. Click the Save button. Verify that a forty-five-minute appointment is scheduled for Jorge Barrett on October 21, 2016, starting at 1:15 P.M.

You have completed Exercise 4.5

End-of-Chapter Resources

Chapter Summary

The **Chapter Summary** is in a tabular, step-by-step format organized by learning outcomes, with page references to help students review the material.

Chapter Review

The **Chapter Review** contains the following exercises, all tagged with Learning Outcomes: terminology exercises; true-false, multiple-choice, and short-answer questions; and Applying Your Knowledge exercises.

chapter 8 summary

LEARNING OUTCOME	KEY CONCEPTS/EXAMPLES
8.1 Compare the major features of PPO, HMO, and POS health plans. Pages 388–390	A PPO offers patients lower fees in exchange for receiving services from plan providers, but does not usually require care coordination or referrals. An HMO locks patients into receiving services from providers with whom it has contracts; sometimes a primary care physician coordinates care and makes required referrals to specialists. A POS offers more flexibility to choose providers, but at an increased cost to the patient.
8.2 Identify the two parts of CDHPs. Pages 390–393	A consumer-driven health plan combines a high-deductible health plan (HDHP) that is usually a PPO for catastrophic coverage with one or more employer or employee funding options for out-of-pocket medical expenses.
8.3 Discuss the organization and regulation of employer-sponsored group health plans and self-insured plans. Pages 393–396	Employer-sponsored group health plans are organized by employers to provide heath care benefits to employees. The insurance coverage is purchased from an insurance carrier or managed care organization. Group health plans are subject to state laws for coverage and payment. Self-insured plans are also organized by employers, but the employers insure the plan's members themselves rather than
8.4 Expla... of Medicare... C, and D. Pages 396–	

CHAPTER 8 REVIEW CHAPTER REVIEW

chapter review

MATCHING QUESTIONS

Match the key terms with their definitions.

_____ 1. *[LO 8.6]* allowed charge
_____ 2. *[LO 8.1]* third-party payer
_____ 3. *[LO 8.2]* consumer-driven health plan (CDHP)
_____ 4. *[LO 8.4]* Medicare
_____ 5. *[LO 8.5]* fee schedule
_____ 6. *[LO 8.1]* point-of-service (POS) plan
_____ 7. *[LO 8.4]* Medicaid

a. Managed health care system in which providers offer health care to members for fixed periodic payments.
b. Managed care network of health care providers who agree to perform services for plan members at discounted fees.
c. Maximum charge a plan pays for a service or procedure.
d. Federal and state assistance program that pays for health care services for people who cannot afford them.

CHAPTER 8 REVIEW CHAPTER REVIEW

10. *[LO 8.3]* The largest employer-sponsored health program in the United States is the _____.
   a. Blue Cross and Blue Shield Association (BCBS)
   b. Medicare program
   c. Federal Employees Health Benefits (FEHB) program
   d. Medicaid program

SHORT-ANSWER QUESTIONS

Define the following abbreviations.

1. *[LO 8.2]* FSA _______________
2. *[LO 8.4]* CMS _______________
3. *[LO 8.3]* ERISA _______________
4. *[LO 8.2]* HDHP _______________
5. *[LO 8.5]* MPFS _______________
6. *[LO 8.4]* CHAMPVA _______________
7. *[LO 8.1]* PCP _______________
8. *[LO 8.3]* BCBS _______________
9. *[LO 8.3]* FEHB _______________
10. *[LO 8.5]* UCR _______________

APPLYING YOUR KNOWLEDGE

8.1 *[LO 8.1, 8.2]* An out-of-state vacationer with a broken ankle has a high-deductible consumer-driven health plan. The patient has already met half of the $1,000 annual deductible. The PPO is a 80-20 plan in network and a 60-40 plan out-of-network. The out-of-network physician's bill is $4,500. How much does the patient owe? How much should the PPO pay?

____

____

connect Enhance your learning at mcgrawhillconnect.com!
• Practice Exercises • Activities
• Worksheets • Integrated eBook

acknowledgments

Suggestions have been received from faculty and students throughout the country. We rely on this vital feedback with all of our books. Each person who has offered comments and suggestions has our thanks.

The efforts of many people are needed to develop and improve a product. Among these people are the reviewers and consultants who point out areas of concern, cite areas of strength, and make recommendations for change. In this regard, the following instructors provided feedback that was enormously helpful in preparing the first edition of *PMEHR*.

Special thanks to Beth Rich and Ursula Cole for working on the patient records, as well as to those instructors who reviewed the exercises for *Connect Plus.*

Symposia

An enthusiastic group of trusted faculty members active in this course area attended symposia to provide crucial feedback.

Amelia Island, Florida

Stacey Ashford
CPC, Remington College

Bonnie J. Crist
MEd, CMA (AAMA), Harrison College

Jill Ferrari
MA, MT, MLT (ASCP), Sullivan University

Cindy Glewwe
MEd, RHIA, Rasmussen College

Shelly Halper
AAS, NCMA, RMA, NCPT, NCICS, Fox College

Jennifer L. Holmes
Concorde Career Colleges, Inc.

Michelle Knighton
MBA, RHIA, Herzing University Online

Angela Massengill
RMA (AMT), Institute of Business and Medical Careers

Michelle R. McClatchey
BS, Westwood College

Debra L. Soucy
CPC, The Salter School

Stacey Wilson
CMA (AAMA), MT/PBT (ASCP), MHA, Cabarrus College of Health Sciences

Tucson, Arizona

Amy L. Blochowiak
MBA, ACS, AIAA, AIRC, ARA, FLHC, FLMI, HCSA, HIA, HIPAA, MHP, PCS, SILA-F, Northeast Wisconsin Technical College

Nikita Carr
CPC, CMBS, Centura College

Robin Maddalena
CMT, Branford Hall Career Institute

Cheryl Miller
MBA/HCM, Westmoreland County Community College

Tammy L. Shick
Great Lakes Institute of Technology

Lynn A. Skafte
CMA, Rasmussen College

Heidi Weber
BS, CMA (AAMA), RMA, Globe Education Network

Workshops

In 2009 and 2010, McGraw-Hill conducted fifteen allied health workshops, providing an opportunity for more than six hundred faculty members to gain continuing education credits as well as to provide feedback on our products.

Book Reviews and Surveys

Many instructors participated in surveys and manuscript reviews throughout the development of the book.

Gail Albert
CMA (AAMA), Berks Technical Institute

Stacey Ashford
CCA, CPC, Remington College

Amy L. Blochowiak
MBA, ACS, AIAA, AIRC, ARA, FLHC, FLMI, HCSA, HIA, HIPAA, MHP, PCS, SILA-F, Northeast Wisconsin Technical College

Nikita Carr
CPC, CMBS, Centura College

Molly Cohen
BA, CPC, Carrington College

Ursula Cole
CMA (AAMA), CCS-P, Harrison College

Michelle Cranney
MBA, RHIT, CCS-P, Virginia College Online

Bonnie J. Crist
MEd, CMA (AAMA), Harrison College

Amanda Davis-Smith
NCMA, Sanford-Brown College

Marsha Dolan
MBA, RHIA, FAHIMA, Missouri Western State University

Jane W. Dumas
MSN, CCMA, CET, CPT, CHI (NHA), Remington College

Deborah Eid
MHA, CBCS, DiHOM, Carrington College

Jill Ferrari
MA, MT, MLT (ASCP), Sullivan University

W. Howard Gunning
MSEd, CMA (AAMA), Southwestern Illinois College

Paula Refus-Hagstrom
RHIA, RHIT, Ferris State University

Ellen Halibozek
MS, CPC, CLAD, CCMA, Corinthian Colleges

Karli A. Harris
CMA, LPN, Harris School of Business

Gregory Hartnett
BS, CPC, HIA, MHA, Sanford-Brown Institute

Lynn Hightower
RHIT, CCS, Panola College

Elizabeth Hoffman
MAEd, CMA (AAMA), CPT (ASPT), Baker College of Clinton Township

Susan Holler
MSEd, CMRS, Bryant and Stratton College

Diana Hollwedel
LPN, CMA, CPT, Career Institute of Florida

Deborah C. Kenney
CMA, CBCS, Harris School of Business

Janis A. Klawitter
AS, CMA (AAMA), CPC, San Joaquin Valley College

Michelle Knighton
MBA, RHIA, Herzing University Online

Mary Koloski
CBCS, CHI, Florida Career College

Loreen W. MacNichol
CMRS, RMC, CCS-P, Kaplan University

Robin Maddalena
CMT, Branford Hall Career Institute

Sheniqua Maefau
LVN, CMA, ICDC College

Nikki Marhefka
MEd, MT (ASCP), CMA (AAMA), Central Penn College

Gregory Martinez
BS, MS, Wichita Technical Institute

Angela Massengill
RMA, Institute of Business and Medical Careers

Ethel Matney
Polytech Adult Education

Danielle Mbadu
MA, MEd, Kaplan Higher Education Campuses

Michelle McClatchey
BS, Westwood College

Kathleen Meskunas
LPN, RMA, CHI, CPT, MTS, McCann School of Business and Technology

Cheryl A. Miller
MBA/HCM, Westmoreland County Community College

Lane Miller
MBA/HCM, Medical Careers Institute

Ana Orabona Ocasio
EdD, RHIA, CCS, University of Puerto Rico

Julie Pepper
CMA (AAMA), BS, Chippewa Valley Technical College

Sandi Petro
Laurel Business Institute

Cassandra Pinnell
Rasmussen College–Ocala Campus

Linda Reynolds
CMA, South University Montgomery

Beth A. Rich
CPC-H, Pittsburgh Technical Institute

Diane Roche Benson
CMA (AAMA), BSHCA, MSA, CFP, ASE, NSC-SCFAT, CDE, CMRS, CPC, AHA BLS-I, FA-I, PALS, ACLS, CAAM-I, Wake Technical Community College, University of Phoenix

Joni Schlatz
MS, RHIT, Central Community College

Carol Schneider-Turek
RHIT, Midstate College

Nena Scott
MSEd, RHIA, CCS, CCS-P, Itawamba Community College

Amy Shay
BS, RHIT, Tidewater Community College

Tammy Shick
Great Lakes Institute of Technology

Betty Shingle
NR-CMA, CCS, PHT, MT (ASCP), H (ASCP), Penn Commercial Business and Technical School

Lisa Smith
RMA, BMO/LXMO, Keiser University

Debra L. Soucy
CPC, The Salter School

Tammy Stone
CPC, Anthem Education Group

Kelly Titus
CPC, San Joaquin Valley College

Heidi Weber
BS, CMA (AAMA), RMA, Globe Education Network

Thomas Wesley
MA, BS, AS, EMT, Minnesota School of Business

Stacey Wilson
CMA (AAMA), MT/PBT (ASCP), MHA, Cabarrus College of Health Sciences

Shelley Wingness
Duluth Business University

Susan Zolvinski
RMA, AHI, Brown Mackie College

Acknowledgments from the Author

To the students and instructors who will use this book, your feedback and suggestions will be greatly appreciated.

I especially want to thank the editorial team at McGraw-Hill—Liz Haefele, Natalie Ruffatto, Raisa Kreek, and Michelle Flomenhoft—for their enthusiastic support and their willingness to go the extra mile to get a first edition published!

Thank you to the outstanding EDP staff: senior designer Anna Kinigakis created a terrific new design, which was implemented through the production process by Marlena Pechan, project manager; Louis Swaim, buyer; Lori Hancock, senior photo research coordinator; and Cathy Tepper, media project manager.

Thank you to the digital team for your many efforts with *Connect Plus:* Damian Moshak, Thuan Vinh, Crystal Szewczyk, Brent dela Cruz, and Janean Utley.

This book would not be available were it not for the tireless efforts of Roxan Kinsey, executive marketing manager, who believed in *PMEHR* from day one.

Finally, a great big thank you to my coworkers at Chestnut Hill Enterprises, Inc.—Cynthia Newby, Susan Magovern, Myrna Breskin, and Derek Noland—for their wisdom, dedication, and patience. This book is truly the result of a group effort.

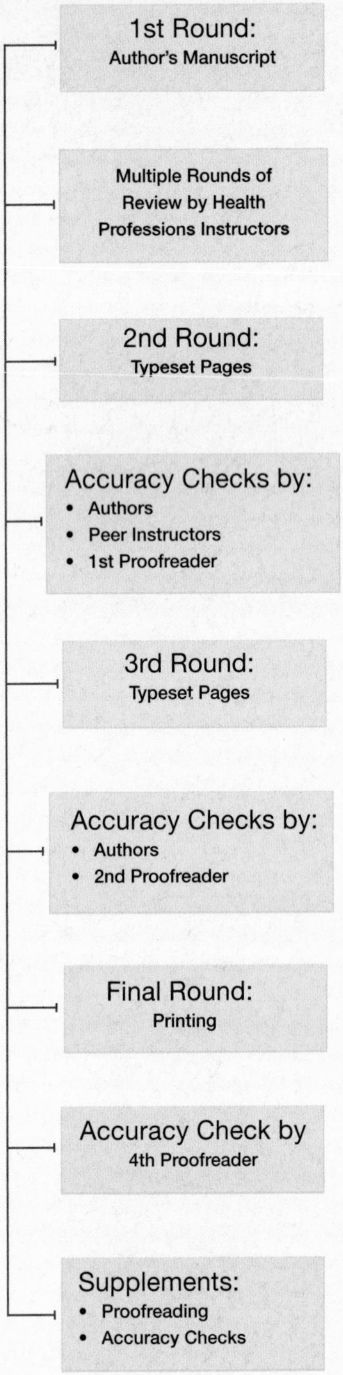

1st Round:
Author's Manuscript

Multiple Rounds of
Review by Health
Professions Instructors

2nd Round:
Typeset Pages

Accuracy Checks by:
- Authors
- Peer Instructors
- 1st Proofreader

3rd Round:
Typeset Pages

Accuracy Checks by:
- Authors
- 2nd Proofreader

Final Round:
Printing

Accuracy Check by
4th Proofreader

Supplements:
- Proofreading
- Accuracy Checks

A COMMITMENT TO ACCURACY

You have a right to expect an accurate textbook, and McGraw-Hill invests considerable time and effort to make sure that we deliver one. Listed below are the many steps we take to make sure this happens.

OUR ACCURACY VERIFICATION PROCESS

First Round—Development Reviews

STEP 1: Numerous **health professions instructors** review the draft manuscript and report on any errors that they may find. The authors make these corrections in their final manuscript.

Second Round—Page Proofs

STEP 2: Once the manuscript has been typeset, the **authors** check their manuscript against the page proofs to ensure that all illustrations, graphs, examples, and exercises have been correctly laid out on the pages, and that all codes have been updated correctly.

STEP 3: An outside panel of **peer instructors** completes a review of content in the page proofs to verify its accuracy. The authors add these corrections to their review of the page proofs.

STEP 4: A **proofreader** adds a triple layer of accuracy assurance in pages by looking for errors; then a confirming, corrected round of page proofs is produced.

Third Round—Confirming Page Proofs

STEP 5: The **author team** reviews the confirming round of page proofs to make certain that any previous corrections were properly made and to look for any errors they might have missed on the first round.

STEP 6: The **project manager,** who has overseen the book from the beginning, performs **another proofread** to make sure that no new errors have been introduced during the production process.

Final Round—Printer's Proofs

STEP 7: The **project manager** performs a **final proofread** of the book during the printing process, providing a final accuracy review.

In concert with the main text, all supplements undergo a proofreading and technical editing stage to ensure their accuracy.

RESULTS

What results is a textbook that is as accurate and error-free as is humanly possible. Our authors and publishing staff are confident that the many layers of quality assurance have produced books that are leaders in the industry for their integrity and correctness. *Please view the Acknowledgments section for more details on the many people involved in this process.*

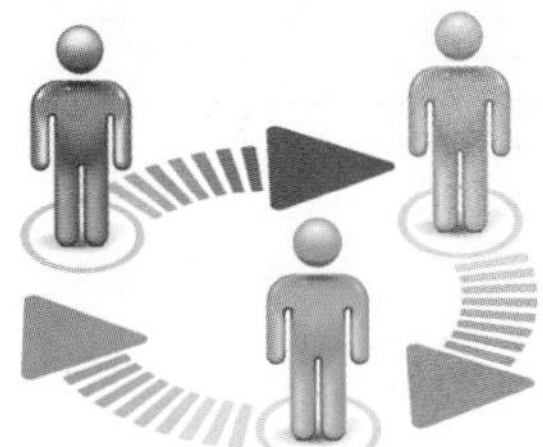

part one

Managing the Revenue Cycle

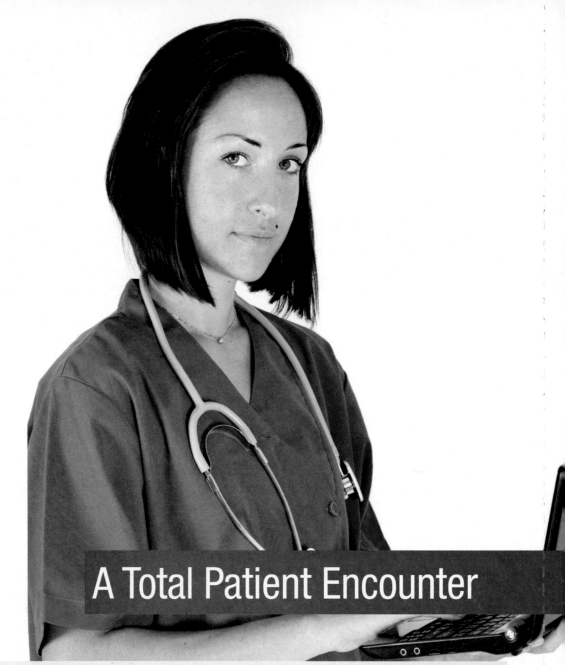

chapter 1

A Total Patient Encounter

KEY TERMS

accounts receivable (A/R)
American Recovery and Reinvestment Act of 2009 (ARRA)
cash flow
certification
continuity of care
data mining
data warehouse
diagnosis code
documentation
electronic health record (EHR)
electronic medical record (EMR)
electronic prescribing
encounter
health informatics
health information exchange (HIE)
Health Insurance Portability and Accountability Act of 1996 (HIPAA)
health information technology (HIT)
integrated PM/EHR program
meaningful use
medical assistant (MA)
medical biller
medical coder
medical documentation and billing cycle
medical malpractice
medical necessity
medical record
National Health Information Network (NHIN)
patient examination
pay for performance (P4P)
personal health record (PHR)
Physician Quality Reporting Initiative (PQRI)
practice management (PM) program
procedure code
records retention schedule
regional extension centers (RECs)
revenue cycle management (RCM)
standards

LEARNING OUTCOMES

When you finish this chapter, you will be able to:

1.1 Compare practice management (PM) programs and electronic health records (EHRs).

1.2 Discuss the government health information technology (HIT) initiatives that have led to integrated PM/EHR programs.

1.3 List the eight facts that are documented in the medical record for an ambulatory patient encounter.

1.4 Identify the additional uses of clinical information gathered in patient encounters.

1.5 Compare electronic medical records, electronic health records, and personal health records.

1.6 Describe the four functions of a practice management program that relate to managing claims.

1.7 List the steps in the medical documentation and billing cycle.

1.8 Compare the roles and responsibilities of clinical and administrative personnel on the physician practice health care team.

1.9 Explain how professional certification and lifelong learning contribute to career advancement in medical administration.

The New Program . . .

On his way out of the office Friday afternoon, Dr. Rudner stuck his head in Dr. McGrath's office. "Are you ready? Monday is the big day." "Yes, I'm actually looking forward to Tiffany's visit," Dr. McGrath replied. Tiffany Patel is a certified RHIA and an EHR implementation specialist with Physician's Total Programs. She will be spending several days in the office to set up the practice's EHR and to train staff members.

"I think once the staff is trained and gets some hands-on experience, we'll be good to go," said Dr. McGrath.

Dr. Rudner responded, "I'm wondering how it's going to impact our cash flow and patient flow . . . and workflow. But since our staff had a part in selecting Medisoft Clinical, we have everyone on board. And you know our staff is top notch. Alex is a terrific medical assistant, Chris knows billing inside and out, and Joseph is a coding pro."

"I'm sure it will be challenging, but in the end, we'll be able to provide better care to our patients," Dr. McGrath replied.

"That's the bottom line. See you Monday," Dr. Rudner said as he left Dr. McGrath's office and headed down the hall.

1.1 Health Information Technology: Tools for a Total Patient Encounter

Do you remember what it was like to make a call from a pay phone or to wait for the bank to open to withdraw cash or make a deposit? If you needed cash when the bank was closed, you were out of luck. This is almost unimaginable today; we are used to having access to our money twenty-four hours a day, seven days a week. Perhaps you are too young to remember life before cell phones, ATM machines, and the Internet. Look at Table 1.1. How many of the activities listed in the "Then" column do you remember doing?

We have become accustomed to using technology in our daily lives, and most of us would not want to go back to the old way of doing things. Technology saves time, gives us more choices, and generally makes life easier.

Technology has also become a part of daily life in the medical office. Innovations are changing the way medicine is practiced. Diabetes patients measure their blood glucose levels at home and wirelessly transmit readings to their physician. X-rays no longer require film, and they are available for almost instant reading with digital imaging. A paramedic performs an ECG on an incoming patient in the back of an ambulance and wirelessly transmits the images to the emergency room before the patient arrives. When a boy on vacation in Florida experiences unusual shortness of breath, the doctor at the walk-in clinic in Florida is able to view his medical record on the computer, even though the boy's pediatrician is in a different state. These are just a few examples of the ways in which technology is changing the delivery of health care.

TABLE 1.1 Activities Then and Now

What Do You Want to Do?	Then	Now
Get your mail	Wait for the post office to deliver it	Check your e-mail online
Pay some bills	Write a check and mail it	Pay over the Internet
Make a phone call away from home	Look for a pay phone booth	Use a cell phone
See a movie	Go to a theater	Download and watch it on your computer or TV
Buy some music	Go to a store that sells CDs	Download music files
Find out how to get to a restaurant	Call the restaurant and ask for directions, making sure to write them down	Enter the restaurant's address in your GPS
Get in touch with a friend	Make a phone call from home or a pay phone	Send a text message
Take some photographs	Buy film, load your camera, take pictures, unload film, bring film to a store to have it developed	Use a digital camera

Practice Management Programs and Electronic Health Records

The use of computers and electronic communications to manage medical information and its secure exchange is known as **health information technology (HIT).** Physicians and facilities use HIT to help them accomplish many of the tasks they do each day. To receive payment for their services, physicians use software known as **practice management (PM) programs.** These programs perform administrative and financial functions, such as scheduling patients' appointments, billing patients and health plans, receiving and recording payments, and managing collections. Since the software transmits data electronically, physicians receive payment in less time than when they send in paper claims and wait for checks to arrive in the mail. As they recognized some of the benefits that PMs could provide, they made the transition from paper to computer. Today, most practices no longer write patients' names in an appointment book and fill in paper claim forms. Figure 1.1 displays a sample appointment entry screen from a practice management program.

health information technology (HIT) the use of computers and electronic communications to manage medical information and its secure exchange

practice management (PM) program program used to perform administrative and financial functions in a medical office

electronic health record (EHR) a computerized lifelong health care record for an individual that incorporates data from all sources that provide treatment for the individual

So while patients' financial records have been electronic for over a decade, clinical records—the information about a patient's health entered by doctors, nurses, and other health care professionals—are still primarily stored in paper charts. In the last several years, however, more and more physicians are converting paper charts to computerized records. An **electronic health record (EHR)** is a computerized lifelong health care record for an individual that incorporates data from all sources that provide treatment for the individual.

While EHRs are intended to replace paper records, their capabilities go beyond that of their paper equivalent. Since EHRs include information entered by all health care professionals who treat the patient, the programs make it easier to access and share patient information. Doctors, nurses, therapists, and other health care professionals can access the patient record via computer, regardless of whether they are in the same office, several miles away, or across the country. Figure 1.2 is a sample screen from an electronic health program.

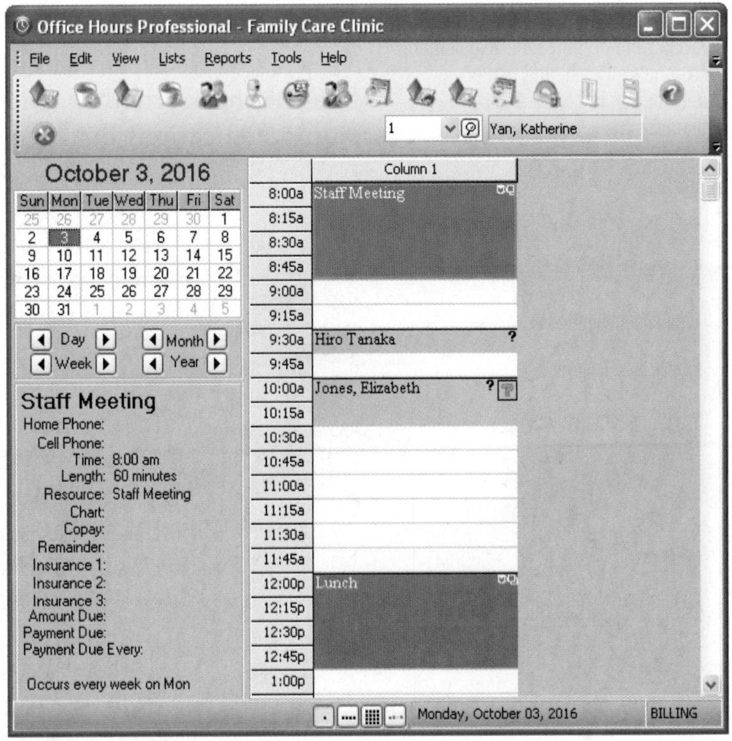

Figure 1.1 Sample Appointment Entry Screen from Practice Management Program

Health Informatics

Although access to information is a major advantage, EHRs provide even more benefits. With the push of

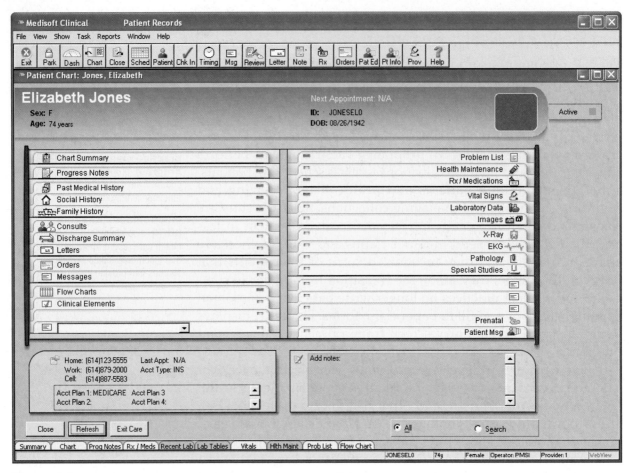

Figure 1.2 Sample Patient Chart Folders in an Electronic Health Program

health informatics knowledge required to optimize the acquisition, storage, retrieval, and use of information in health and biomedicine

a button, a physician can access the most recent treatment guidelines or check whether a new prescription might interact with existing medications before electronically sending it to the patient's pharmacy. Many people in government positions, as well as leaders in health care, believe that EHRs have the potential to improve the quality of health care, prevent many medical errors, and reduce health care costs.

It is for this reason that the Bureau of Labor Statistics predicts that the field of **health informatics** (also known as *medical informatics*) will grow by 20 percent through 2018. A vast array of health organizations—from physician practices, clinics, hospitals, and other institutions to insurance companies and public health education groups—will require knowledgeable employees to help transition to and make the most of new health technology. As shown in Figure 1.3, these new employees need health care skill, computer skill, and knowledge of health care reform for the greatest career opportunities for advancement.

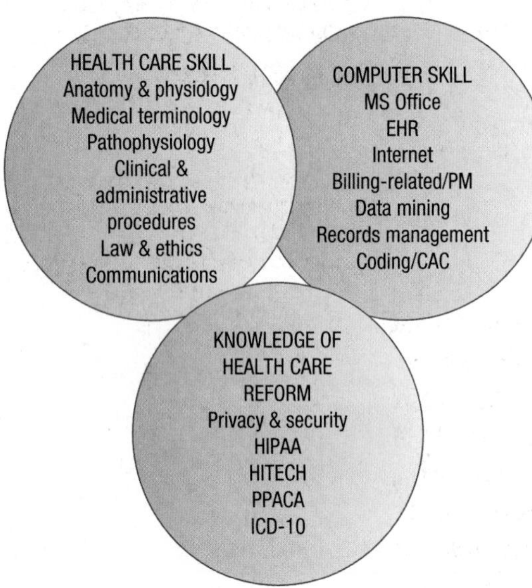

Figure 1.3 Health Informatics Skills

THINKING IT THROUGH 1.1

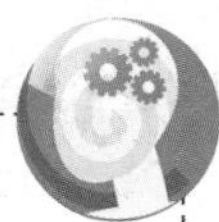

A seventy-six-year-old man with a history of heart disease experiences chest pain while on vacation. He calls 911 and is transported to the nearest hospital. When he arrives in the emergency room, he is conscious and able to communicate with doctors. He tells the staff that he had prior heart attacks and that he had his six-month checkup with his cardiologist just before he left for vacation.

- How would an EHR enable doctors to determine a course of action in less time than was possible in a paper record-keeping environment?
- What information might the emergency room doctors be able to access from the cardiologist's EHR?

1.2 Major Government HIT Initiatives

Since the 1990s, the government has taken an active role in promoting the use of health information technology. Major government HIT initiatives in the last twenty years include:

- Electronic exchange and protection of health information
- Electronic prescribing of medications
- Medical treatment plans based on clinical evidence of effectiveness
- Electronic health records

Electronic Exchange and Protection of Health Information: HIPAA

The **Health Insurance Portability and Accountability Act of 1996 (HIPAA)** protects patients' private health information, ensures health care coverage when workers change or lose jobs, and uncovers fraud and abuse in the health care system. HIPAA helps keep people's health information safe by means of **standards**—required technical specifications—for the electronic exchange of administrative and financial health information, such as requiring the use of electronic rather than paper insurance claims. (HIPAA is covered in depth in Chapter 2.)

Health Insurance Portability and Accountability Act of 1996 (HIPAA) legislation that protects patients' private health information, ensures health care coverage when workers change or lose jobs, and uncovers fraud and abuse in the health care system

standards technical specifications for the electronic exchange of information

electronic prescribing a technology that enables a physician to transmit a prescription electronically to a patient's pharmacy

The Medicare Improvements for Patients and Providers Act: MIPPA

The Medicare Improvements for Patients and Providers Act of 2008 (MIPPA) provides financial incentives for practitioners who use **electronic prescribing** (e-prescribing), a technology that enables a physician to transmit a prescription electronically to a patient's pharmacy. The system electronically checks for drug interactions and allergies and eliminates prescription errors caused by illegible handwriting. MIPPA requires the use of e-prescribing starting in 2011 and reduces payments to providers who fail to e-prescribe.

Medical Treatment Plans Based on Clinical Evidence of Effectiveness: PQRI

Physician Quality Reporting Initiative (PQRI) a Medicare program that gives bonuses to physicians when they use treatment plans and clinical guidelines that are based on scientific evidence

American Recovery and Reinvestment Act of 2009 (ARRA) a $787 billion economic stimulus bill passed in 2009 that allocates $19.2 billion to promote the use of HIT

The 2006 Tax Relief and Health Care Act requires the Centers for Medicare and Medicaid Services (CMS) to set up the **Physician Quality Reporting Initiative (PQRI).** This program gives bonuses to physicians when they use treatment plans and clinical guidelines that are based on scientific evidence. For example, patients aged five through forty years with a diagnosis of mild, moderate, or severe persistent asthma should be prescribed either the preferred long-term control medication (inhaled corticosteroid) or an acceptable alternative treatment.

Electronic Health Records: HITECH

In his 2004 State of the Union address, President George W. Bush recommended greater use of information technology in health care and set the goal of establishing electronic health records for all Americans within ten years. Funding was limited, however, and the technology was not widely adopted. In 2009 the Obama administration led Congress in passage of the **American Recovery and Reinvestment Act of 2009 (ARRA),** a $787 billion economic stimulus bill. The main health care provision in ARRA is the Health Information Technology for Economic and Clinical Health (HITECH) Act. This legislation advances the use of health information technology by:

- Requiring the government to develop standards for health information to be exchanged electronically and to use health information to improve the quality and coordination of care
- Investing $20 billion in health information technology infrastructure and Medicare and Medicaid incentives to facilitate the adoption of electronic health records by doctors and hospitals
- Generating a minimum of $10 billion in savings for the government and additional savings in the health care sector through improvements in quality of care and care coordination and reductions in medical errors and duplicate care
- Strengthening federal privacy and security laws to protect patients' health information

As a result of the HITECH Act, the Congressional Budget Office estimates that approximately 90 percent of doctors and 70 percent of hospitals will be using electronic health records within the next ten years.

Meaningful Use

The portion of the HITECH Act that has received the most attention is the provision that provides financial incentives to physicians, hospitals, and other health care providers. Under the HITECH Act, physicians who adopt and use EHRs are eligible for annual payments of up to $44,000 from Medicare and Medicaid. Physicians who derive at least 30 percent or more of their income from Medicaid are eligible

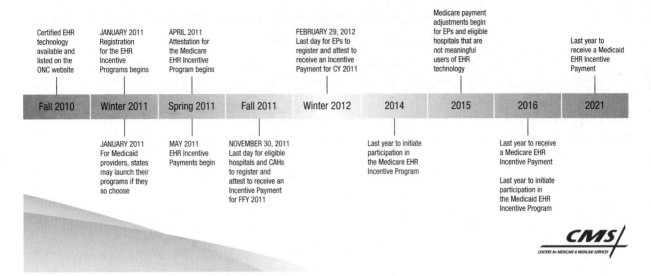

Figure 1.4 Medicare and Medicaid Incentive Timeline for EHRs

for up to $64,000, and doctors who practice in underserved areas are eligible for an extra 10 percent from Medicare. Figure 1.4 shows an implementation timeline for the financial incentives.

To be eligible for the financial incentives, providers must do more than simply purchase EHRs; they must demonstrate meaningful use of the technology. **Meaningful use** is the utilization of certified EHR technology to improve quality, efficiency, and patient safety in the health care system. The government has specified a series of objectives that determine whether meaningful use requirements have been met. In the first two years of the program (2011–2012), these objectives consist of a core set and a menu set. The objectives differ for physicians and hospitals. Physicians must meet fifteen core objectives and five of ten objectives from the menu set. The objectives for 2011–2012 are listed in Table 1.2.

meaningful use the utilization of certified EHR technology to improve quality, efficiency, and patient safety in the health care system

regional extension centers (RECs) centers that offer information, guidance, training, and support services to primary care providers who are in the process of making the transition to an EHR system

health information exchange (HIE) a network that enables the sharing of health-related information among provider organizations according to nationally recognized standards

Regional Extension Centers

Even with government financial incentives, successful implementation of EHRs is not expected to be quick or easy. Small practices, where most primary care is delivered, may lack the expertise and resources required to purchase, install, and use the new technology. Recognizing the challenges associated with implementing HIT, the HITECH Act called for the creation of **regional extension centers (RECs).** Patterned after the agriculture extension service the government created almost a century ago, the RECs offer information, guidance, training, and support services to primary care providers who are in the process of making the transition to an EHR system.

Health Information Exchange

To meet meaningful use criteria, providers must be able to exchange clinical information outside the organization. One of the ways that providers share information is through the use of local, state, and regional health information networks. A **health information exchange (HIE)** enables the sharing of health-related information among provider

TABLE 1.2 Eligible Providers' Meaningful Use Core and Menu Objectives		
Core Objectives		
Improve quality, safety, and efficiency, and reduce health disparities	Computerized physician order entry (CPOE)	More than 30% of unique patients with at least one medication in their medication list have at least one medication order entered using CPOE
	Implement drug-drug and drug-allergy interaction checks	Functionality enabled for entire EHR reporting period
	E-prescribing (eRx)	More than 40% of all permissible prescriptions are transmitted electronically
	Record demographics	More than 50% of all unique patients have demographics recorded as structured data
	Maintain an up-to-date problem list of current and active diagnoses	More than 80% of all unique patients have at least one entry or an indication that no problems are known for the patient recorded as structured data
	Maintain active medication list	More than 80% of all unique patients have at least one entry (or an indication that no medications are prescribed) recorded as structured data
	Maintain active medication allergy list	More than 80% of all unique patients have at least one entry (or an indication that the patient has no known medication allergies) recorded as structured data
	Record and chart changes in vital signs	For more than 50% of all unique patients age 2 and over, height, weight, and blood pressure are recorded as structured data
	Record smoking status for patients 13 years or older	More than 50% of all unique patients age 13 and over have smoking status recorded as structured data
	Implement one clinical decision support rule	Implement one clinical decision support rule
	Report ambulatory clinical quality measures to CMS/states	For 2011, provide aggregate numerator, denominator, and exclusions through attestation as discussed in section II(A)(3) of the final rule. For 2012, electronically submit the clinical quality measures discussed in section II(A)(3) of the final rule
Engage patients and families in their health care	Provide patients with an electronic copy of their health information, upon request	More than 50% of all patients who request an electronic copy of their health information are provided it within 3 business days
	Provide clinical summaries for patients for each office visit	Clinical summaries are provided to patients for more than 50% of all office visits within 3 business days
Improve care coordination	Capability to exchange key clinical information among providers of care and patient-authorized entities electronically	Performed at least one test of certified EHR technology's capacity to electronically exchange key clinical information
Ensure adequate privacy and security protections for personal health information	Protect electronic health information	Conduct or review a security risk analysis per 45 CFR 164.308 (a)(1) and implement security updates as necessary and correct identified security deficiencies as part of a risk management process

(continued)

TABLE 1.2 *(continued)*		
Menu Set		
Improve quality, safety, and efficiency, and reduce health disparities	Implement drug-formulary checks	Functionality enables and has access to at least one internal or external drug formulary for the entire EHR reporting period
	Incorporate clinical lab test results as structured data	More than 40% of all clinical lab test results of patients whose results are in a positive/negative or numerical format are incorporated as structured data
	Generate lists of patients by specific conditions	Generate at least one report listing patients with a specific condition
	Send reminders to patients per patient preference for preventive/follow-up care	More than 20% of all unique patients 65 years or older or 5 years old or younger were sent an appropriate reminder
Engage patients and families in their health care	Provide patients with timely electronic access to their health information	More than 10% of all unique patients are provided timely (within 4 business days) electronic access to their health information subject to the provider's discretion to withhold certain information
	Use certified EHR technology to identify patient-specific education resources and provide to patient, if appropriate	More than 10% of all unique patients are provided patient-specific education resources
Improve care coordination	Medication reconciliation	The provider performs medication reconciliation for more than 50% of transitions into the care of the provider
	Summary of care record for each transition of care/referrals	The provider who transitions or refers their patient to another setting or care or provider provides a summary of care record for more than 50% of transitions of care and referrals
Improve population and public health	Capability to submit electronic data to immunization registries/systems	Performed at least one test of certified EHR technology's capacity to submit electronic data to immunization registries and follow-up submission of the test is successful
	Capability to provide electronic syndromic surveillance data to public health agencies	Performed at least one test of certified EHR technology's capacity to provide electronic syndromic surveillance data to public health agencies and follow-up submission is the test is successful

Source: www.cms.gov/ehrincentiveprograms/.

organizations according to nationally recognized standards. Examples of the use of an HIE include sharing patient records with physicians outside the physician's own medical group, transmitting prescriptions to pharmacies, and ordering tests from an outside lab. The goal of an HIE is to facilitate access to clinical information for the purpose of providing quality care to patients. The HITECH Act created the State Health Information Exchange Cooperative Agreement, which provides funding to increase connectivity and information sharing both within and between states, including the development of health information exchanges (HIEs).

National Health Information Network (NHIN) a common platform for health information exchange across the country

integrated PM/EHR programs programs that share and exchange demographic information, appointment schedules, and clinical data

The **National Health Information Network (NHIN)** is a key component of the government's HIT strategy that will provide a common platform for health information exchange across the country. The NHIN is a set of standards, services, and policies that enable the secure exchange of health information over the Internet. To build a national network of interoperable health records, HIE networks must be developed at the local, state, and regional levels. Once connected, these networks will form the basis for the NHIN. Encouraging the use of electronic health record (EHR) systems is the first step in the creation of a nationwide interoperable electronic health information system.

Integrated PM/EHR Programs

As a result of the government initiative, physician offices began to purchase EHRs and make the transition to computerized patient records. Most practices already had practice management programs in place for billing and scheduling. The addition of an EHR meant that two separate programs required a lot of the same information. Patient names, addresses, and insurance identification numbers all had to be entered twice—once in the EHR that contained clinical information, and again in the PM that managed billing. When an appointment was scheduled, it also had to be entered in both programs. It soon became evident that this was not efficient and might lead to errors.

To solve this problem, practices now use **integrated PM/EHR programs** that can share and exchange demographic information, appointment schedules, and clinical data. The use of integrated programs increases patient safety, improves the quality of patient care, and reduces operating costs. Clinical and financial data are accessed from any computer, enabling the health care team to easily perform important tasks such as:

- Entering and locating information in a patient record
- Monitoring the flow of patients in the practice
- Recording documentation electronically
- Submitting orders for inpatient or outpatient tests and procedures
- Transmitting prescriptions and renewals to pharmacies
- Receiving laboratory and imaging results electronically
- Creating electronic encounter forms that are populated with diagnosis and procedure codes
- Posting charges from the electronic encounter form
- Creating, reviewing, and submitting electronic claims
- Recording payments from payers and patients
- Using data to take advantage of government and private payer financial incentives

Introduction to Medisoft Clinical

Medisoft Clinical, the name of the software you will use throughout this text/workbook, is an integrated practice management program and electronic health record (PM/EHR). The program

THINKING IT THROUGH 1.2

The federal government continues to take an active role in promoting the use of health information technology. The government is offering financial incentives to physicians who use e-prescribing and electronic health record systems, in part because of physicians' slow adoption of the technologies. Assuming that the physicians understand the benefits of both technologies, why do you think they have not been quick to send prescriptions electronically and enter their visit notes in an EHR?

combines the practice management features of Medisoft Advanced Accounting with a fully functional electronic health record. In this course, you will acquire the knowledge and skills to work effectively in today's technology-driven health care environment, including hands-on practice with an integrated program used by physicians throughout the country. Billers and medical assistants who have these competencies will be well prepared to secure positions and succeed in their careers.

1.3 Documenting the Patient Encounter

An **encounter,** also known as a visit, is the meeting of a patient with a physician or other medical professional for the purpose of providing health care. At the heart of the encounter is the **patient examination.** After the patient is escorted to the exam room, the medical assistant gathers information such as the patient's current medications and allergies and the reason for the visit. The patient's vital signs—blood pressure, temperature, oxygen level, and pulse—are measured and recorded, as are other data such as height and weight. The medical assistant then notifies the provider that the patient is ready to be seen. After reviewing the patient's record, the provider enters the room, discusses the patient's reason for the visit and medical history, and completes a physical examination.

encounter the meeting of a patient with a physician or other medical professional for the purpose of providing health care (also known as a visit)

patient examination an examination of a person's body in order to determine his or her state of health

If the visit is for routine preventive services such as an annual physical examination, the provider makes an assessment of the patient's condition. If symptoms are present that must be managed, the provider develops a differential diagnosis—a mental list of all the possible causes of the patient's condition or symptoms. The provider may write orders for lab work, diagnostic tests, medications, or further visits with specialists to confirm or rule out particular diagnoses. Based on the suspected or confirmed diagnosis, a treatment plan is determined by the provider.

Types of Clinical Encounters

Health care providers supply preventive and acute care to patients, as well as ongoing treatment for chronic illnesses. Care to keep diseases from occurring or to enable early detection and treatment is known as *preventive care;* it includes routine annual physical examinations, immunizations, screening tests, and behavioral counseling. *Acute care* is provided for illnesses with a sudden onset that are

Figure 1.5 Rising Number of Americans with Chronic Conditions

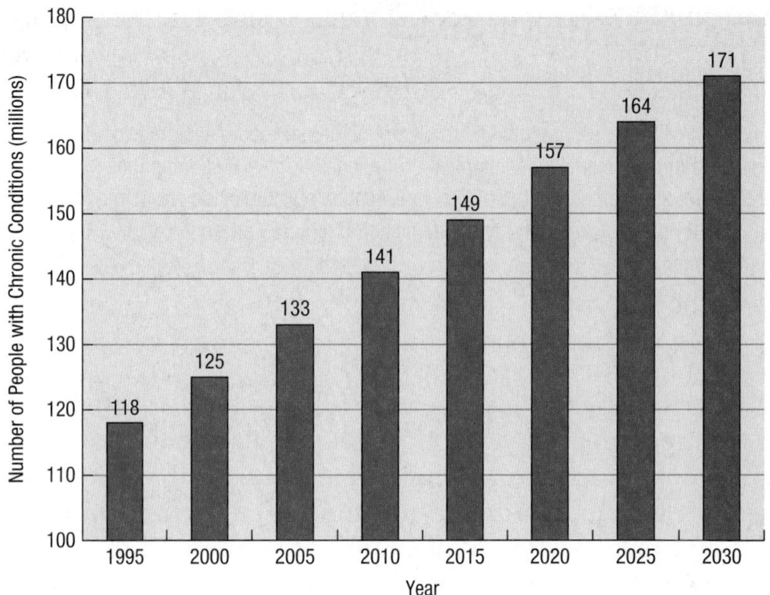

time limited—not expected to continue more than a few days or weeks, such as a recovery from a broken bone. *Chronic* illnesses, on the other hand, must be treated over the long term. A patient with a chronic illness requires some level of ongoing medical treatment for a lengthy period of time, in some cases for a lifetime. Chronic diseases, such as heart disease, diabetes, asthma, and AIDS, are the leading causes of death and disability in the United States. Consider these facts:

- Seventy-five percent of the $2.3 trillion—over $7,000 per person—that the United States spends on health care goes toward treating chronic conditions like diabetes, heart disease, and cancer.
- Two-thirds of elderly patients have five or more chronic conditions, so the number of patients with chronic conditions will increase dramatically in proportion to the aging population of the United States.
- In particular, diabetes is gaining; it is estimated that by 2034, nearly twice as many Americans as today will suffer from diabetes, and spending on the disease will triple.

Figure 1.5 illustrates the past, present, and projected future incidence of chronic disease.

The Medical Record

documentation the record created when a physician provides treatment to a patient

medical record a chronological health care record that includes information that the patient provides, such as medical history, as well as the physician's assessment, diagnosis, and treatment plan

Patient encounters, whether for acute, chronic, or preventive health care, generate clinical information about the patients' conditions and courses of treatment. Clinical information is used by health care professionals and patients to make judgments and decisions about patients' health care. For this reason, every time a health care provider treats a patient, a record, known as **documentation,** is made of the encounter. This chronological **medical record,** or chart, includes information that the patient provides, such as medical history, as well as the physician's assessment, diagnosis, and treatment plan. Records also contain laboratory test results, X-rays and other diagnostic images, lists of medications prescribed, and reports that indicate the results of operations and other medical procedures.

The contents of medical records vary depending on the setting in which they are created and used, such as whether they are for acute care or ambulatory care. Acute care is most often provided in a hospital, which treats patients with urgent problems that cannot be handled in another setting. A patient in this setting is expected to require an overnight stay, and so is called an inpatient. *Ambulatory care* refers to treatment that is provided without admission to a hospital in settings such as physician practices, hospital emergency rooms, and clinics for outpatients.

Physicians' office charts tend to track the ongoing health and wellness needs of the individual. Eight data points are included in an ambulatory care medical record:

1. Patient's name
2. Encounter date and reason
3. Appropriate history and physical examination
4. Review of all tests that were ordered
5. Diagnosis
6. Plan of care, or notes on procedures or treatments that were given
7. Instructions or recommendations that were given to the patient
8. Signature of the provider who saw the patient

In addition, a patient's medical record contains:

- Biographical and personal information, including the patient's full name, Social Security number, date of birth, full address, marital status, home and work telephone numbers, and employer information as applicable
- Copies of all communications with the patient, including letters, telephone calls, faxes, and e-mail messages; the patient's responses; and a note of the time, date, topic, and physician's response to each communication
- Copies of prescriptions and instructions given to the patient, including refills
- Original documents that the patient has signed, such as an authorization to release information and an advance directive about end-of-life care
- Medical allergies and reactions, or their absence
- Up-to-date immunization record and history if appropriate, such as for a child
- Previous and current diagnoses, test results, health risks, and progress
- Copies of referral or consultation letters

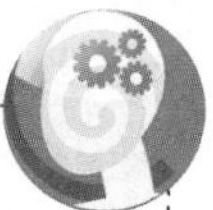

THINKING IT THROUGH 1.3

Jane Mendoza is a fifty-four-year-old woman with hypertension and asthma. She visits her primary care physician for monitoring of her hypertension and a pulmonary specialist for her asthma. While shopping for groceries recently, she fell on the ice and broke her ankle. She was taken to the hospital, admitted, and had surgery on the ankle the next day. She is taking medication for all three conditions, prescribed by the three different physicians. Is her ankle break a chronic or acute condition? How many chronic conditions does Jane have?

- Hospital admissions and release documents
- Records of any missed or canceled appointments
- Requests for information about the patient (from a health plan or an attorney, for example), and a detailed log listing to whom information was released

Whether created in a physician practice or in a hospital, the medical record allows health care professionals involved in the patient's care to provide continuity of care to individual patients. **Continuity of care** refers to coordination of care received by a patient over time and across multiple health care providers.

continuity of care coordination of care received by a patient over time and across multiple health care providers

medical malpractice the provision of medical services at a less than an acceptable level of professional skill that results in injury or harm to a patient

1.4 Other Uses of Clinical Information

Although the primary use of clinical information is to provide effective health care to the patient, clinical information also has several important secondary uses. These uses involve legal issues, quality review, research, education, public health and homeland security, and billing and reimbursement.

Legal Issues

Clinical information may be used as evidence in a legal matter involving a patient or a provider. For example, an individual may bring a lawsuit against another driver's automobile insurance plan as a result of back injuries sustained in an accident. The automobile insurance plan would require access to the clinical information to determine whether the individual was being treated for back problems before the accident.

Clinical information is also important in protecting the physician from accusations of **medical malpractice,** the provision of medical services at a less than acceptable level of professional skill that results in injury or harm to a patient. A patient who feels that a physician has made an error in diagnosis or treatment may bring a lawsuit known as a malpractice claim. Such claims include alleging that the wrong medication was prescribed and accusing physicians of failing to follow up on ordered tests. Accurate and complete documentation is an important part of a defense against the accusation that a patient was not treated appropriately, as it shows that the physician followed the medical standards of care that apply in the state. The standard of care is the actions or measures that a reasonable health care professional in the same location would take in similar circumstances. Health care providers are liable (that is, legally responsible) for providing this level of care to their patients.

Quality Review

Individuals and institutions in the health care field must regularly evaluate the adequacy and appropriateness of the care they deliver. Clinical data are analyzed to obtain a measure of the quality of the services provided to the patient. Increasingly, data on quality are being linked to physician reimbursement. The Medicare PQRI program is an example of **pay for performance (P4P)** that provides financial incentives to physicians who provide evidence-based treatments to their patients. Evidence-based medicine is medical care that uses the latest and most accurate clinical research in making decisions about the care of patients. For example, a hospital that is in the top 10 percent of statistics on the fewest post-surgery infections could receive additional compensation from a payer. In the physician office, a provider might be financially rewarded for significantly increasing the number of women over the age of sixty-five who are screened for osteoporosis.

pay for performance (P4P) provision of financial incentives to physicians who provide evidence-based treatments to their patients

Research

Clinical information collected during a patient visit is used by medical researchers to develop new methods of treatment and to compare the effectiveness of existing treatments. For example, researchers who are conducting clinical trials of a new medication need access to clinical information to validate that patients meet the criteria for the study.

Education

Case studies that are used to train a wide range of health professionals are developed with information from patient encounters. For example, medical students are presented with cases during their training. In these cases, the patient's identity is removed from the record, so patient confidentiality is not at risk.

Public Health and Homeland Security

The records of physicians and hospitals are also important in determining the incidence of disease and in developing methods to improve the health of the population. The incidence and spread of disease can be followed closely using health records. For example, in the event of an influenza pandemic, data from physician visits would be critical in detecting the outbreak early and in containing its effects.

Billing and Reimbursement

It is important to understand that physician practices are businesses as well as centers for patient care. In addition to the uses already described, the medical record is also the main source of information for physician reimbursement. Most patients have some form of medical insurance to help them pay for medical services. In order for the

THINKING IT THROUGH 1.4

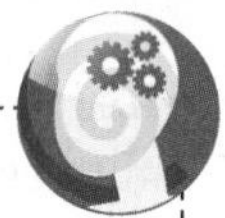

Pay for performance rewards physicians who follow the latest medical evidence when providing care to patients. This evidence often is in the form of generally agreed upon guidelines written by experts in the field. For example, physicians may be rewarded if a certain percentage of their patients have LDL cholesterol readings below 100. Scientific evidence indicates that individuals with LDL levels below 100 are less likely to develop coronary artery disease.

- Can you think of any reasons why physicians may not be in favor of pay for performance programs?
- How might pay for performance programs affect the physician–patient relationship?

insurer to make payment, the physician's documentation in the medical record must show that the service provided was warranted given the patient's condition. Reimbursement may be denied if this clinical information is incomplete or inaccurate.

1.5 Functions of an Electronic Health Record Program

Just as PMs are used to manage the claims and billing in a medical practice, the electronic health record (EHR) automates the management of clinical information about the practice's patients.

What's in a Name?

Since the idea of computer-based medical records came about, the records have been referred to by a number of different names. In the 1990s, they were known as electronic patient records (EPRs), computerized patient records (CPRs), and computerized medical records (CMRs). These terms gave way to the current usage, which includes electronic health records (EHRs), electronic medical records (EMRs), and personal health records (PHRs).

Although there is not universal agreement on definitions, the consensus is that **electronic medical records (EMRs)** are computerized records of one physician's encounters with a patient over time. They serve as the physician's legal record of patient care. While EMRs may contain information from external sources including pharmacies and laboratories, the information in the EMR reflects treatment of a patient by a single physician.

electronic medical record (EMR) computerized record of one physician's encounters with a patient over time

personal health records (PHRs) private, secure electronic health care files that are created, maintained, and owned by the patient

Electronic health records, on the other hand, can include information from the EMRs of a number of different physicians as well as from pharmacies, laboratories, hospitals, insurance carriers, and so on. Information is added to the record by health care professionals working in a variety of settings, and the record can be accessed by professionals when needed.

Personal health records (PHRs) are private, secure electronic files that are created, maintained, and owned by the patient. The patient decides whether to share the contents with doctors or other health professionals. PHRs typically include current medications and dosages, health insurance information, immunization records, allergies, medical test results, past surgeries, family medical history, and more. Personal health records are created and stored on the Internet, but the files can easily be downloaded to a storage device such as a flash drive for portability.

Contents of EHRs in Ambulatory Care Settings

As shown in Table 1.3, the content of an EHR in the physician practice is similar to the content of the paper medical record, or chart.

Functions and Uses

While paper and electronic health records serve many of the same purposes, the electronic record is much more than a computerized version of a paper record. The Institute of Medicine suggested that an EHR should include eight core functions (*Key Capabilities of an Electronic Health Record System,* 2003):

1. **Health information and data elements** This includes demographic information about the patient, such as address and phone number, as well as clinical information about the patient's past and present health concerns. An electronic health record must include information that enables health care providers to provide effective care to patients, such as

TABLE 1.3	Electronic Health Record Content
Patient identifying information	This demographic and insurance information is obtained when the patient first comes to the practice, and it is updated as needed.
History and physical	This section of the record contains information about the patient's past medical history, family medical problems, prior hospitalizations, current medications, and past surgeries. It also includes information from a physical examination.
Office visit notes	Office visit notes document the physician's findings during an examination, including observations of the patient's current medical problem, a diagnosis of the condition, and a plan for treatment. The notes also list physician orders. During each subsequent visit with the physician, notes about the patient's condition and response to treatment are added to the chart.
Laboratory tests and results	This portion of the patient record contains the results of all diagnostic procedures such as laboratory test results and pathology reports, including blood tests, X-rays, and biopsies.
Miscellaneous consents and releases	A number of miscellaneous forms are saved in the patient chart, such as release of information requests, Acknowledgment of Receipt of Notice of Privacy Practices, and consents for certain procedures.
Prescriptions	The patient chart contains a record of all medications prescribed by the physician as well as patient requests for refills.
External correspondence about patients	Correspondence to and from the patient or a third party, such as a consulting physician, is part of a patient record. Physicians receive requests to sign forms for patients, such as applications for disability benefits and proof of immunizations.

signs and symptoms, a problem list, procedures, diagnoses, a medication list, allergies, diagnostic test and radiology results, and health maintenance.

2. **Results management** Providers must have access to current and past laboratory, radiology, and other test results performed by anyone involved in the treatment of the patient. These computerized results can be accessed by multiple providers, when and where they are needed, which allows diagnosis and treatment decisions to be made more quickly.
3. **Order management** EHR programs must be able to send, receive, and store orders for medications, tests, and other services by any provider involved in treating the patient. Orders are then transmitted directly to the appropriate department for completion of the test or fulfillment of a prescription, which eliminates unnecessary delays and duplicate testing. The process of entering orders electronically is known as computerized physician order entry, or CPOE. CPOE has had an enormous impact on medication safety. Most medication errors occur during the process of prescribing and/or administering medication. Through computerized physician order entry of prescriptions, many medication errors can be eliminated. Many systems automatically alert the physician to potential errors in dosages, drug interactions, drug diagnosis interactions, and drug-allergy problems.
4. **Decision support** As the practice of medicine becomes more complex, the amount of information available to physicians continues to grow. Hundreds of new studies are published on a daily basis. It is not possible for a physician to remember all this information or to be aware of all the latest, most effective treatments. The latest medical evidence is incorporated into care only 50 percent of the time.

   Electronic health records allow computer-based access to the latest clinical research while the physician is still in the examination room with the patient. The physician can also view the latest information on medications, including suggested doses, common side effects, and possible interactions.

   In addition, electronic record systems provide a variety of alerts and reminders that physicians can use to improve a patient's health. A physician can, for example, see a list of all women patients over forty years of age who have not had mammograms in the past year and can send them letters reminding them that they are due for this preventive screening.
5. **Electronic communication and connectivity** Today a patient is typically treated by more than one provider in more than one facility. Physicians, nurses, medical assistants, referring doctors, testing facilities, and hospitals all need to communicate with one another to provide the safest and most effective care to patients. Health plans also need information

from the health record to process claims for reimbursement. Electronic health record systems offer a number of mechanisms to facilitate these communications, including e-mail and the Internet.

6. **Patient support** Electronic health records should offer patients access to appropriate educational materials on health topics and instructions for preparing for common medical tests. Patients on home health care should be able to use the EHRs to report to their physicians. Some EHR programs also offer tools that allow patients to access their medical records and to request appointments electronically.
7. **Administrative processes** The administrative area of health care also benefits from the use of EHRs. While most physician practices already use computers for billing and scheduling, an EHR streamlines the processes. Procedure and diagnosis codes entered by the physician in the EHR are transmitted electronically to the practice management program, where a coding specialist reviews them.
8. **Reporting and population management** Electronic health record programs also enhance reporting capabilities both for internal practice use and for external reporting requirements. This makes it easier for physician offices and health care organizations to comply with federal, state, and private reporting requirements.

Advantages of Electronic Health Records

EHR programs offer a number of advantages when compared to paper record-keeping systems. The most frequently cited advantages are increased patient safety, improved quality of care, and greater efficiency.

Safety

There is growing evidence that electronic record keeping can reduce medical errors and improve patient safety. Some of the factors that contribute to greater safety include the following:

- Medication and physician order errors due to illegible handwriting are eliminated.
- Providers receive instant electronic alerts about patient allergies and possible drug interactions.
- Physicians receive alerts when medications deemed unsafe have been pulled from the market.
- Medical records are not lost in the event of a natural disaster, such as a hurricane, or an intentional attack such as a terrorist bombing, provided that an electronic backup copy of the records is stored at a secure off-site location.
- Information is communicated in a timely manner in the event of an act of bioterrorism or the widespread outbreak of disease.

Quality

A 2001 report titled *Crossing the Quality Chasm: A New Health System for the 21st Century* (Institute of Medicine, 2001) found that only 55 percent of Americans receive recommended medical care that is consistent with guidelines based on scientific knowledge. Electronic health records make it possible for providers to deliver more effective care to patients based on a complete picture of their past and present condition. Effective care is defined as "providing services based on scientific knowledge to those who could benefit and at the same time refraining from providing services to those not likely to benefit." With EHRs, physicians have access to evidence-based guidelines for diagnosing and treating conditions and to the latest clinical research and best practice guidelines.

Electronic health records also enhance the quality of health care in the following ways:

- Patients are contacted with reminders for preventive care screenings.
- Patients suffering from chronic diseases, such as diabetes, are able to monitor their conditions at home and report results via the Internet, saving them numerous visits to the doctor.
- Health care consumers can review data about the quality and performance of providers and facilities and can choose facilities and providers accordingly.

Efficiency

The retrieval of information from an EHR is immediate, which greatly improves efficiency and can be critical in emergency situations. Compared to sorting through papers in a folder, an electronic search saves critical time when vital patient information is needed. Electronic health records also save valuable time by reducing the time it takes health care providers to enter information about patients. Currently, physicians spend almost 40 percent of their time documenting their encounters with patients. With EHRs, physicians are finished entering notes when the patient leaves the examination room or shortly after. Nurses and medical assistants also record information directly into the computer, so there is no need to copy information to a paper chart.

Implementation Issues

Despite offering a number of significant advantages, the migration from paper to electronic records has been slowed by a number of barriers, including cost, lack of standards, training and workflow issues, and privacy and security concerns.

- **Cost** An electronic health record system is estimated to cost approximately $33,000 per physician to install and roughly $8,400 per physician per year to maintain. These estimates include one-time costs associated with switching from paper to electronic records, such as scanning existing paper

THINKING IT THROUGH 1.5

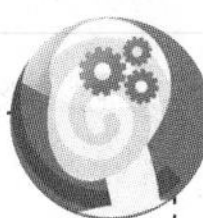

Grace Melillo has been working in Dr. Snyder's office for over twenty years. Soon after her children left home to attend college, she went back to school and obtained her certification as a medical assistant. When she started working in the 1980s, most physicians did not use computers. About ten years ago, the office installed a practice management program for billing and scheduling. This did not affect Grace, since she was in a large office that divided administrative and clinical duties among the medical assistants. Grace had always worked as a clinical assistant, escorting patients to exam rooms, measuring vital signs, and asking patients about their medications.

Next month, the practice is going to begin using an electronic health record program. Both clinical and administrative medical assistants will be trained on the system and will be expected to use it. Since finding this out, Grace has been telling her coworkers that once the EHR is in place, some of them will be let go, since the technology eliminates the need for a large staff.

- Does Grace have a valid point? Do you think that technology such as a PM or EHR eliminates the need for office staff?
- What could be done to change Grace's attitude toward the new technology?

records into the new system and purchasing updated computers.

- **Lack of standards** A lack of standards for sharing digital information has been a major obstacle to EHR adoption. Without common standards, EHRs cannot share clinical information in a meaningful way, whether from one physician office to another or from a physician office to an inpatient facility such as a hospital. Major efforts are underway to create such standards.
- **Training and workflow issues** It often takes a significant amount of time for staff members to become proficient with new technology. Technology also alters the workflow in a physician office, which can require staff members to make adjustments. For example, in a practice using an EHR, there is no need to pull charts of patients with upcoming appointments. Papers such as referral letters, lab reports, and copies of prescriptions are not filed in folders, and charts do not have to be filed at the end of the day. While these improve efficiency, the job responsibilities and tasks of staff members must be analyzed and altered as necessary. This is a time-consuming process, and individuals may be resistant to change.
- **Privacy and security risks** One of the greatest challenges to EHR implementation is protecting private information about a patient's past and present health. By its nature, information contained in an electronic health record is stored on a computer and exchanged with other providers and facilities. There is always a risk that hackers may break into computers or that security may be unintentionally breached. The frequent transfer of patient health information from one computer to another over a network, along with the number of people who have access to the record, increases the likelihood of the information's

being obtained by an unauthorized party. While the HIPAA and ARRA laws address the issue of patient privacy and the security of electronic patient information, there is more work to be done in this area, as discussed in greater detail in Chapter 2.

1.6 Functions of a Practice Management Program

Practice management programs are the HIT applications that facilitate the day-to-day financial operations of a medical practice. PMs automate the medical billing cycle, so staff members can record patient demographics, schedule appointments, maintain lists of payers, perform billing tasks, and generate reports.

Initial Setup

Not all medical offices use the same PM, but most programs operate in a similar manner. Initially, the program is prepared for use by entering basic facts about the practice. Often a computer consultant or an accountant helps set up these records. Information about many aspects of the business is entered, including:

- **Patient data** Information about each patient, such as name, address, contact numbers, insurance coverage, and more
- **Provider data** Information about each provider, including facts about providers, referring providers, and outside providers such as labs
- **Health plan data** Details about the health plans used by the practice's patients
- **Transaction data** The dates of visits, the location of treatment, diagnosis and procedure codes, and payments made at the time of office visits

In addition, the program's security feature is set up to accommodate the requirements of the staff.

Daily Activities

Once the initial setup and data entry are complete, the PM is used to complete many of the daily tasks of a medical practice, including:

- Verifying insurance eligibility and benefits
- Organizing patient and payer information
- Generating and transmitting insurance claims
- Monitoring the status of claims
- Recording payments from payers
- Generating patients' statements, posting payments, and updating accounts
- Managing collections activities
- Creating financial and productivity reports

THINKING IT THROUGH 1.6

Autoposting—in which payments from health plans are automatically posted to patient accounts in a practice management program—takes less time than posting payments manually. However, some practices prefer to have a person post payments. Why do you think this is the case?

Focus on Health Care Claim Processing

One of the most important uses of a PM is to process health care claims, from creation to transmission, payer payment decisions, and payment posting.

Creating Electronic Claims

The PM collects required digital information from its various databases to create a claim file. This file can be printed, but in most cases it is sent electronically, using an Internet connection. This replaces the previous task of filling out paper claim forms and sending them in the mail.

Electronic Monitoring of Claim Status

The PM is used to follow up on the status of claims being adjudicated by health plans. If payer response is slow, the PM can be used to transmit electronic queries to locate the claim in the health plan's processing system and ensure prompt payment.

Receiving Electronic Payment Notification

When the payer has adjudicated the claims, the PM receives a remittance advice (RA), which lists the amount that has been paid on each claim as well as codes that represent the reasons for nonpayment or partial payment. PMs are designed to receive RAs as electronic documents sent over the Internet. Such a document is sometimes called an electronic remittance advice (ERA).

Once the payment information has been reviewed and determined to be as expected, the data on the RA are entered in the PM and applied to each patient's account. While this process may be done manually by matching payments with individual patient transactions and then entering the payments in the program, many practices with PMs use a process called *autoposting*. In autoposting, the payment data are automatically posted to the correct patient accounts in the PM, and the medical biller performs an audit function, verifying that the payments are correct, rather than manually entering the information. Every date and procedure has to be carefully checked to uncover any errors or underpayments and to follow up with the health plan.

Handling Electronic Payments

Also contributing to improved cash flow is the PM's ability to handle electronic payments that are sent directly to the practice's bank accounts. This transaction is called an EFT, for electronic funds transfer, and it puts revenue in the bank much faster than does receiving and depositing manual checks.

1.7 The Medical Documentation and Billing Cycle

A physician practice's main focus is to care for patients, but to provide this care, the practice must be successful from a business perspective. Practices incur a number of expenses on a recurring basis, such as salaries, supplies, utilities, insurance, and equipment leasing. To meet its expenses, a practice needs a steady flow of income, known as revenue. This income comes from billing and collecting for services provided to patients. To maintain a regular **cash flow**—the movement of monies into or out of a business—specific tasks must be completed on a regular schedule before, during, and after a patient visit.

cash flow the movement of monies into and out of a business

medical documentation and billing cycle a ten-step process that results in timely payment for medical services

The **medical documentation and billing cycle** consists of ten steps that are required to maintain accurate patient records and to receive timely payment for services. This cycle is illustrated in Figure 1.6. The inner circle represents the billing cycle; the outer

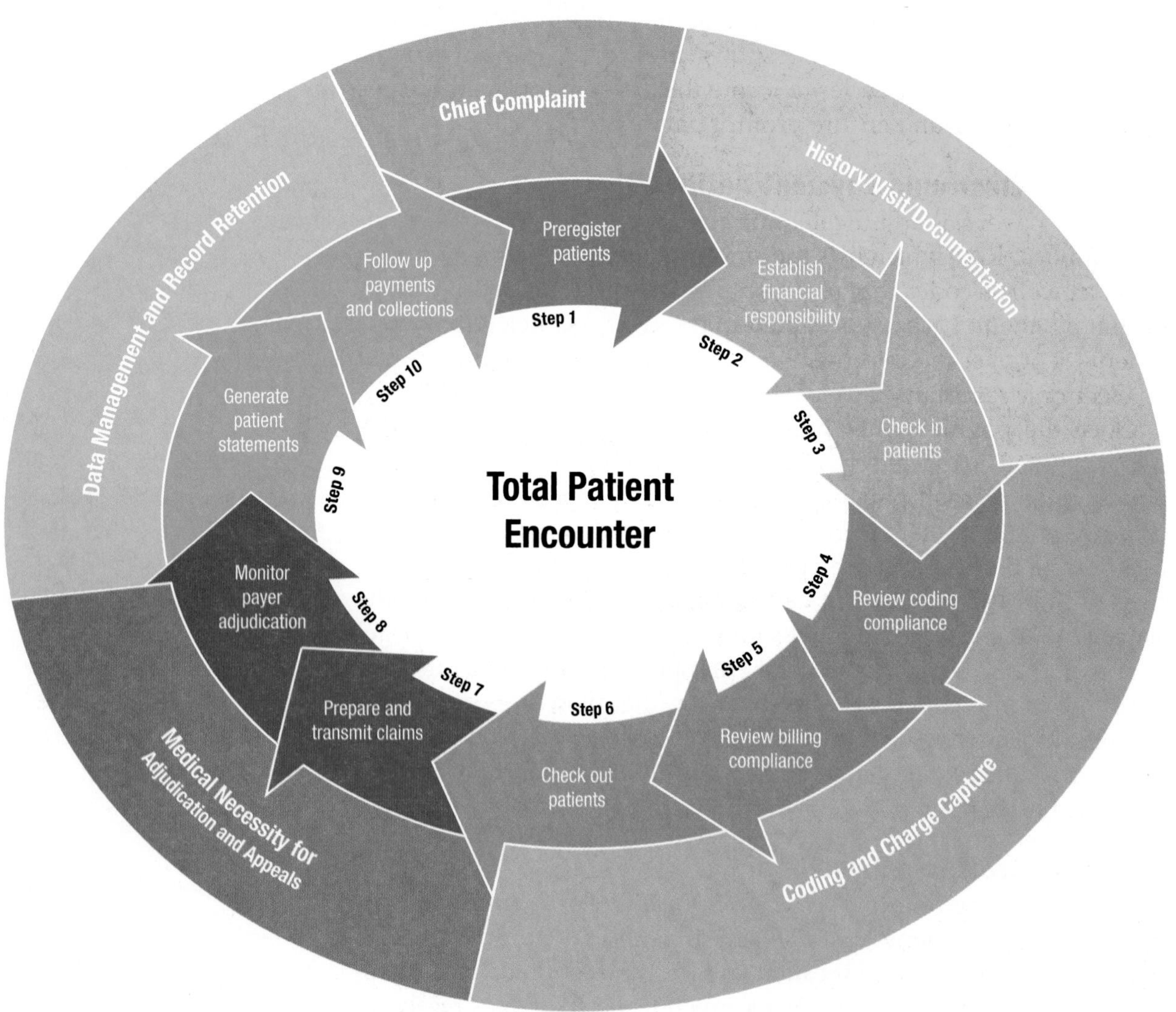

Figure 1.6 The Medical Documentation and Billing Cycle

TABLE 1.4	Steps in the Medical Documentation and Billing Cycle
Before the encounter	Step 1: Preregister patients
During the encounter	Step 2: Establish financial responsibility Step 3: Check in patients Step 4: Review coding compliance Step 5: Review billing compliance Step 6: Check out patients
After the encounter	Step 7: Prepare and transmit claims Step 8: Monitor payer adjudication Step 9: Generate patient statements Step 10: Follow up payments and collections

circle contains the medical documentation cycle. As you can see in the illustration, the two cycles are interrelated. For example, during Step 1, Preregistration, a new patient phones for an appointment. Both billing and clinical information must be collected during the phone call. From a billing perspective, the office wants to know whether the patient has insurance that will cover some or all of the cost of the visit, or whether the patient will pay for the visit. From a health or medical perspective, the staff wants to know the reason the person needs to see the doctor, known as the chief complaint. As the medical documentation and billing cycle continues, so does the interaction between the two types of information.

Steps in the Medical Documentation and Billing Cycle

Step 1: Preregister Patients

The first step in the cycle is to gather information so patients can be preregistered before their office visit. This information includes the patient's name, contact information, the chief complaint, and whether the patient is new to the practice. The information is obtained over the telephone or via the Internet, if the practice has a website.

Step 2: Establish Financial Responsibility for Visit

Most patients are covered by some type of health plan. While scheduling the appointment, it is important to determine whether the patient has insurance and, if so, to obtain the identification number, plan name, and name of the person who is the policyholder. Once the insurance information is obtained, the patient's current eligibility and benefits are verified with the payer. Verification may be done by telephone, but most often it is done via the Internet and takes a matter of seconds.

It is also important to make sure that the health plan's conditions for payment, such as advance approval requirements for particular treatments or procedures, are met before treatment is provided. In addition, physicians usually participate in some health plans and not in others. If the physician does not participate in the plan, the patient may be liable for all charges. All of this must be determined and communicated to the patient before the appointment.

Step 3: Check In Patients

When patients arrive in the office, they are asked to complete or update patient information forms that have the personal, employment, and medical insurance data needed to collect payment for services. Most offices ask all patients to update this information periodically to ensure that it is current and accurate. As practices move from paper to electronic documents, a patient information form may be electronic. Electronic forms can be completed online before an office visit. Some offices provide a computer in a private area near the waiting room where patients can complete the electronic form if they do not have access to a computer at home. During check-in, it is also common practice to photocopy or scan the patient's insurance identification card and photo ID.

Patient coinsurance or copayments, as required under the policy of the patient's health plan, may be paid during check-in or checkout, depending on the medical practice's procedures. In addition, if a patient owes a balance from a previous visit, this amount may also be also collected. Coinsurance is a partial payment of the office visit charges; the amount of the partial payment is the estimated patient responsibility for the procedure or service provided. For example, if the fee for the anticipated procedure is $80 and the patient is responsible for 20 percent of charges, the patient may be asked to pay $16 at check-in. Copayments are fixed fees, also under the policy of the patient's health plan, and are always collected at the time of service (check-in or checkout).

New patients receive information about the practice's financial policy at the time of their first visit, so they understand that they are responsible for payment of charges that are not paid by their health plans. Most practices accept checks, cash, and debit and credit cards for payment. Some practices also offer payment plans to patients.

During the office visit, a physician evaluates, treats, and documents a patient's condition. The visit documentation varies depending on a number of factors, including whether the patient is new or established. A provider who sees a patient for the first time obtains the patient's medical history. Once the patient is established, the visit documentation focuses more on the current medical needs of the patient.

Step 4: Review Coding Compliance

The physician records the procedures performed and/or treatments provided, as well as the determination of the patient's diagnoses. Then the physician (or medical assistant/coder) converts these written diagnoses and procedures to medical codes for reporting to health plans for payment.

diagnosis code a code that represents the physician's determination of a patient's primary illness

The patient's primary compliant (the illness or condition that is the reason for the visit) is assigned a **diagnosis code** from the *International Classification of Diseases,* Ninth Revision, *Clinical Modification* (ICD-9-CM) (this process is explained in Chapter 7).

EXAMPLES

The ICD-9-CM code for Alzheimer's disease is 331.0.
The ICD-9-CM code for influenza with other respiratory manifestations is 487.1.

Similarly, each procedure the physician performs is assigned a **procedure code** that stands for the particular service, treatment, or test. This code is selected from the *Current Procedural Terminology* (CPT) (see Chapter 7). A large group of codes covers the physician's evaluation and management of a patient's condition during office visits or visits at other locations, such as nursing homes. Other codes cover groups of specific procedures, such as surgery, pathology, and radiology. Yet another group of codes covers supplies and other services.

procedure code a code that represents the particular service, treatment, or test provided by a physician

medical necessity treatment that is in accordance with generally accepted medical practice

EXAMPLES

99460 is the CPT code for the physician's examination of a normal newborn infant in a hospital or birthing center.
27130 is the CPT code for a total hip replacement operation.

These codes are stored and before the practice submits them to an insurance plan for payment, they must be reviewed for compliance. In the area of coding, compliance requires checking that the codes are up to date and follow the official guidelines of the American Hospital Association and the American Medical Association (AMA). Also, the diagnosis and the medical services that are documented in the patient's medical record should be logically connected, so that the **medical necessity** of the charges is clear to the health plan. The AMA has defined medical necessity as "services or products that a prudent physician would provide to a patient for the purpose of preventing, diagnosing, or treating an illness, injury, or its symptoms in a manner that is:

1. In accordance with generally accepted standards of medical practice
2. Clinically appropriate in terms of type, frequency, extent, site, and duration
3. Not primarily for the convenience of the patient, physician, or other health care provider."

If medical necessity is not met, the physician will not receive payment from the health plan.

Step 5: Review Billing Compliance

Medical practices bill numerous health plans and government payers. The provider's fees for services are listed on the medical practice's fee schedule. Most medical practices have standard fee schedules listing their usual fees. Each charge, or fee, is related to a specific procedure code.

However, the fees listed on the master fee schedule are not necessarily the amount the provider will be paid. Instead, each of the health plans and government payers reimburses the practice according to its own negotiated or government-mandated fee schedule. Many providers enter into contracts with health plans that require a discount from standard fees. In addition, although there is a separate fee associated with each code, each code is not necessarily billable. Whether it can be billed depends on the payer's particular rules. Following these rules when preparing claims results in billing compliance.

Step 6: Check Out Patients

Checkout is the last step that occurs when the patient is still in the office. The medical codes have been assigned and checked, and the amounts to be billed have also been verified according to payers' rules.

The PM/EHR then is used to calculate the charges for the visit, and to ask for payment for the types of charges usually collected at time of service:

- Previous balances
- Copayments or coinsurance
- Noncovered or overlimit fees
- Charges of nonparticipating providers
- Charges for self-pay patients
- Deductibles

(Each of these charges is explained in Chapter 9.) A receipt is prepared for the payments made by the patients, and follow-up work is scheduled as ordered by the physician.

Step 7: Prepare and Transmit Claims

To receive payment, medical practices must produce documents for health plans and patients. One kind of document is an insurance claim. For a health plan to pay a claim, certain information about the patient must be shared. For example, a health plan needs to know the procedures the provider performed while the patient was in the office, the patient's diagnosis, and the date and location of the encounter.

Health plans also require basic information about the provider who is treating the patient, including the provider's name and identification number. Beyond the basic information requirements that are common to all payers, there are differences in what information is required on an insurance claim. A payer lists the required information in a provider's manual that is available to the medical office. In general, the information needed to create a claim is found on two documents—the patient information form and the encounter form. These documents are increasingly electronic rather than paper-based. The majority of health care claims are transmitted electronically.

Step 8: Monitor Payer Adjudication

When the payer receives the claim, it goes through a series of steps designed to determine whether the claim should be paid, a process called *adjudication*. Claims may be paid in full, partially paid, or denied. The results of the claim review, including an explanation of why charges were not paid in full or were denied entirely, are sent to the provider along with the payment. This information is reviewed for accuracy by a member of the billing staff, such as a medical insurance specialist, who compares each payment and explanation with the claim to check that:

- All procedures that were listed on the claim also appear on the payment transaction
- Any unpaid charges are explained
- The codes on the payment transactions match those on the claim
- The payment listed for each procedure is as expected

If any discrepancies are found, a request for a review of the claim is filed with the payer. If no issues are discovered, the amount of the payment is recorded. The payment may be in the form of a paper check, or it may be sent electronically to the practice's bank. Depending on the rules of the health plan, the patient may be billed for an outstanding balance. In other circumstances, an adjustment is made and the patient is not billed. Occasionally, an overpayment may be received, and a refund check is issued by the medical practice.

Step 9: Generate Patient Statements

If charges are billed to the patient, a statement is created and sent to the patient. The statement lists all services performed, along with the charges for each. The statement lists the amount paid by the health plan and the remaining balance that is the responsibility of the patient. Some practices send statements electronically, but the majority still create and mail paper documents.

Most medical practices have a regular schedule, referred to as a billing cycle, for sending statements to patients. For example, some practices bill half the patients on the fifteenth of the month and the other half on the thirtieth.

Step 10: Follow Up Payments and Collections

A practice must track **accounts receivable (A/R)**—monies that are coming into the practice—and produce financial reports that provide information about its financial health. Some reports are produced on a daily basis, while others are created on a monthly or an annual basis. This financial information also helps a practice decide whether to buy or lease new equipment, adopt new technology, expand to a larger office, add staff members, and so on. Financial reports can tell a practice which payers are denying more claims than others or are paying less than the expected amount. This information can be used in deciding whether to renew a contract with a payer, or renegotiate the contract, or adjust fees.

accounts receivable (A/R) monies that are coming into a practice

Increasing Patient Financial Responsibility

In the past, physicians received the majority of their revenue from health plans, so collecting payments from patients was not a high priority. If the patient owed a balance after the insurance paid, the amount was likely to be small. For a number of reasons, this has begun to change. The ever-rising cost of health insurance has forced many employers to change the plans they offer to their employees. The new plans require employees to carry a greater share of the cost burden than in the past.

The average family pays approximately $1,000 a year in out-of-pocket expenses, those that the patient pays before the health plan contributes, and this amount is expected to rise. When health plans pay less, patients pay more. Accordingly, the amount of revenue that physicians receive from health plans is shrinking, and the amount that they receive from patients is growing. For this reason, physicians are seeking new ways to ensure that they receive payments from their patients.

It is much more difficult (and expensive) to try to obtain payment after a patient has left the office than to do so while the patient is in the office, so some practices estimate a patient's portion of visit charges during check-in and collect payment at that time. Managing the activities associated with a patient encounter to ensure that the provider receives full payment for services is known as **revenue cycle management (RCM).** RCM is not just concerned with collecting payment from patients; it also focuses on improving cash flow from health plans.

revenue cycle management (RCM) management of the activities associated with a patient encounter to ensure that the provider receives full payment for services

Activities associated with managing the revenue cycle to improve cash flow include:

- Gathering complete and accurate information at registration
- Verifying insurance eligibility before the patient sees the provider
- Educating patients about the practice's financial policy and their own insurance benefits
- Increasing the number of payments collected at check-in
- Ensuring that all services performed by the provider are included on a claim
- Improving the accuracy of procedural and diagnostic coding
- Minimizing the time between submission of claims and receipt of payment
- Reducing the number of claims that are not paid or are not paid in full
- Reducing the number of overdue patient accounts

Data Management and Records Retention

The information collected throughout the medical documentation and billing cycle must be managed and retained. The data stored by a medical practice come from a variety of different databases, including practice management programs, electronic health record programs, and financial systems that process payroll and manage

THINKING IT THROUGH 1.7

Alan Berger is checking in at the front desk for his appointment. The medical practice recently instituted a new financial policy that requires patients to make an estimated payment upon check-in. The receptionist checks his eligibility and benefits and sees that he is responsible for 20 percent of covered charges under his Blue Cross and Blue Shield plan. After checking the appointment schedule and determining that the estimated charge for today's visit is $160, she asks Mr. Berger for a payment of $32. Mr. Berger replies that he did not know he was expected to pay up-front, and asks the receptionist to mail him a bill.

- What should have been done before implementing the new financial policy?
- How should the receptionist handle Mr. Berger's request to mail the bill?

accounts receivable and payable. Information from all the databases is loaded into a **data warehouse,** a collection of data that includes all areas of an organization's operations. It does not replace the individual databases, which are still used for the day-to-day operations of the practice. Rather, it facilitates the storage, maintenance, and analysis of large amounts of data by creating a single source of stored data.

Data mining is the process of analyzing large amounts of data to discover patterns or knowledge. The results are used in many areas of the health care organization, from choosing the best course of treatment for a patient to identifying insurance plans that reimburse at below-average rates. Health information management professionals perform data warehousing and data mining activities. You will read about careers in health information management later in this chapter.

A physician practice must also establish a records retention schedule to ensure that patients' medical information is available for medical, legal, research, and other uses. A **records retention schedule** is a plan for the management of records, listing types of records and how long they should be kept. Retention schedules must comply with state and federal laws. While many states require physicians to maintain medical records for seven years, some states, including Hawaii, require records to be retained for twenty-five years after the last entry. The federal government specifies retention limits for some types of information. For example, laboratory pathology tests must be maintained for ten years, and other lab records for just two years.

data warehouse a collection of data that includes all areas of an organization's operations

data mining the process of analyzing large amounts of data to discover patterns or knowledge

records retention schedule a plan for the management of records that lists types of records and indicates how long they should be kept

1.8 The Physician Practice Health Care Team: Roles and Responsibilities

It takes a talented, dedicated group of health care professionals to care for patients and to run a successful health care business. Staff members who provide treatment to patients are known as clinicians, while those who manage the business aspects of health care are called administrative staff. Administrative staff, including medical billers and coders, receptionists, practice managers, compliance officers, and anyone else who works behind the scenes in a medical office, do not provide medical treatment or testing. Some administrative workers, such as schedulers, do interact with patients, but they do not provide medical care.

In large practices, administrative roles are likely to be specialized. For example, one person schedules appointments, another processes Medicare claims, and another follows up on patient accounts. Small offices usually combine several of these tasks into one staff role. The person who processes claims may also be required to collect on patient accounts. The best preparation for medical office work is to gain a broad understanding of the different clinical and administrative staff roles.

Physicians

Physicians (MDs and DOs) are the primary clinicians in the practice. They diagnose illness and injury, prescribe and administer treatment, and advise patients about how to prevent and manage disease.

Physician Assistants

Physician assistants (PAs) are formally trained to provide diagnostic, therapeutic, and preventive health care services under the supervision of a physician. They take medical histories, examine and treat patients, order and interpret laboratory tests and X-rays, make diagnoses, and prescribe medications. They also treat minor injuries by suturing, splinting, and casting. In most states, PAs may prescribe medications.

Nurses

Nurses perform a wide range of clinical and nonclinical duties. When caring for patients, nurses develop care plans or contribute to existing plans. Plans may include numerous activities, such as administering medication; starting, maintaining, and discontinuing intravenous (IV) lines for fluid, medication, blood, and blood products; administering therapies and treatments; observing patients and recording their observations; and consulting with physicians and other health care clinicians.

Medical Assistants

medical assistant (MA) health care professional who performs both administrative and certain clinical tasks in physician offices

Medical assistants (MAs) are trained to perform both administrative and certain clinical tasks in physician offices. MAs assist physicians by taking patient medical histories and vital signs, providing patient education, collecting specimens and performing basic medical laboratory tests, and administering medications. They prepare for and assist with examinations and procedures.

The range and scope of their tasks depends on the amount and type of training as well as the location, size, and specialty of the practice. In small practices, medical assistants perform many different clinical and administrative tasks. In large practices, they tend to specialize in particular areas. Some MAs may focus on the clinical areas, while others pursue certification as medical coders or billers, as explained below.

The scope of clinical practice also depends upon state laws that regulate the duties of medical assistants. For example, tasks such as drawing blood, giving injections, and starting or disconnecting IVs are permissible in some states and not in others.

According to the U.S. Department of Labor, the clinical tasks that medical assistants may perform include:

- Taking medical histories and recording vital signs
- Preparing patients for examinations
- Assisting physicians during examinations
- Collecting and preparing laboratory specimens
- Performing basic laboratory tests
- Explaining treatment procedures to patients
- Instructing patients about medications and special diets
- Preparing and administering medications as directed
- Correctly disposing of contaminated supplies
- Sterilizing medical instruments

The administrative duties of medical assistants include:

- Scheduling and managing appointments
- Scheduling inpatient and outpatient admissions and procedures
- Performing bookkeeping duties such as preparing bank deposits and posting payments and adjustments
- Processing insurance claims

Medical Billers and Coders

The term **medical biller** describes all the tasks that are completed by administrative staff members during the medical billing cycle. Typically, front office staff members handle duties such as reception (registration) and scheduling. Back office staff duties are related to billing, insurance, and collections. Job titles in common use are billing clerk, insurance specialist, reimbursement specialist, and claims specialist.

medical biller health care professional who performs administrative tasks throughout the medical billing cycle

Common tasks are:

- Verifying patient insurance information and eligibility before medical services are provided
- Collecting payments that are due, such as copayments, at the time of service
- Maintaining up-to-date information about health plans' billing guidelines
- Following federal, state, and local regulations on maintaining the confidentiality of information about patients
- Abstracting information from patients' records for accurate billing

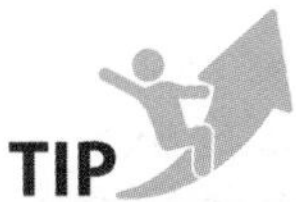

TIP

Medical billing tasks may be handled by a medical billing specialist, a medical insurance specialist, a medical coder, or an administrative medical assistant. This text/workbook uses the term *medical biller* to include any administrative tasks.

- Billing health plans and patients, maintaining effective communication to avoid problems or delayed payments
- Assisting patients with insurance information and required documents
- Processing payments and requests for further information about claims and bills
- Maintaining financial records
- Updating the forms and computer systems the practice uses for patient information and health care claims processing

medical coder medical office staff member with specialized training who handles the diagnostic and procedural coding of medical records

Medical coders are trained in the correct use of standard medical code sets (covered in Chapter 7). In larger practices, a medical coder or a coding team handles coding, while the medical biller or billing group handles billing and claims processing.

Practice or Office Manager

Practice managers or office managers are responsible for directing the successful business operation of physician practices. A large practice may employ a practice manager who has graduate education in business and sometimes a clinical background as well. Smaller offices are commonly managed by an office manager well versed in running a practice with fewer clinicians.

The practice manager's duties include budgeting office revenues and expenses; monitoring performance against budgets; performing payroll and accounting tasks; space planning; determining office and clinical policies, procedures, and guidelines; and hiring and managing office employees. Individuals wishing to pursue a career in health care management must be knowledgeable about all aspects of practice operations. Although many practice managers have backgrounds in a clinical specialty or training in health care administration, some enter these jobs with a general business education.

Compliance Officer

Federal regulations also require the designation of a team member to serve as the practice compliance officer. This person is often either a physician or the practice manager. The compliance officer in a physician practice investigates and resolves all compliance issues relating to coding, billing, documentation, and reimbursement. Compliance officers' duties are based on HIPAA/ARRA rules, as covered in Chapter 2.

Working as a Team

Collecting payment for services is not the sole responsibility of the administrative staff. All personnel—both administrative and clinical—play key roles in the process, and each must communicate critical information to other staff members for reimbursement to occur. Without complete information, health claims created after the office visit will not be paid by health plans.

Staff members who schedule patient appointments start the reimbursement process by collecting necessary information from patients, such as current phone numbers and insurance identification numbers. Before the appointment, a staff member checks the patient's eligibility and benefits.

Data collected during the scheduling phone call is confirmed once the patient arrives in the office. The front desk collects payment from the patient, based on the information obtained in the eligibility and benefits check.

The physician, physician assistant, nurse, and medical assistant also have responsibilities for ensuring that the practice receives reimbursement for services. Documenting the patient encounter is primary among these responsibilities. The documentation must be complete and must demonstrate medical necessity to the health plan. The appropriate procedure and diagnosis codes must be assigned and recorded on an encounter form, which may be paper or electronic.

Referring to the information on the encounter form, staff working the checkout desk determine whether the patient owes any additional payment, even if payment was collected during check-in. The patient is responsible for charges if the services are not covered by his or her health plan. If the encounter form does not contain the appropriate diagnosis and procedure codes, payment cannot be collected at checkout.

The billing and coding staff are responsible for generating and transmitting insurance claims, but first they must review the information on the encounter form. In addition, they must use their knowledge of each health plan's rules and regulations to determine whether all necessary information has been captured on the claim. Once the claim has been submitted, they are responsible for following up to ensure the claim is paid. If a claim is rejected, they review the reason for the rejection and follow up with the relevant staff member.

When payments arrive, a medical biller reviews the amounts to make sure they are as expected, and then posts the payments in the practice management program. Next, patient statements must be created and mailed. Finally, staff must follow up on unpaid accounts and initiate collections activities when appropriate.

Everyone working in the medical office plays a key role in the billing cycle. Successful reimbursement requires a team effort. If one team member does not do a good job, there is a chance that the practice will not be paid as expected. In addition, team members need to share information. The front office, back office, and clinical staff all need to communicate if the practice is to receive timely payment for services in situations such as the following:

- A claim is rejected because the patient's identification number is incorrect; the biller must talk to the scheduler or front desk person who collected that information.
- An encounter form is missing a diagnosis code; the biller needs to speak with the physician.
- The billing staff notices that information a payer requires is missing from a claim; the biller needs to obtain the missing information from the appropriate staff member.

THINKING IT THROUGH 1.8

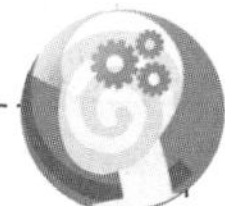

John Guastella is a medical biller responsible for analyzing why claims are not paid as expected. He spends his days researching each claim and determining the cause of the partial payment. A few weeks ago, the practice manager asked him to begin creating weekly reports that list each claim, the dollar amount not collected, and the source of the problem. He e-mails the report to the practice manager, who reviews the contents and follows up with office staff. Last week, John noticed that some staff members avoided him in the lunchroom. He feels uncomfortable preparing a report that pinpoints which staff members have made mistakes—even if their errors resulted in the practice not receiving payment.

- Why is John being avoided?
- What could be done to change the way unpaid claims are handled in the office?

- An eligibility check reveals that the patient is not covered by the health plan; the scheduler needs to contact the patient to review the information on file.
- A claim is not paid because the patient's plan does not cover the treatment provided; the biller needs to check with the staff member who performed the eligibility and verification check to determine what went wrong.

1.9 Administrative Careers Working with Integrated PM/EHR Programs

Health care is information-intensive. Every encounter an individual has with the health care system—from seeing a physician, to having blood drawn at a lab, to picking up a prescription at a pharmacy—is documented and stored. The accuracy and availability of this information plays a major role in determining the outcome of a patient's health care experience.

On its own, health information technology does little to ensure a positive outcome for the patient. The usefulness and value of the information depend on a workforce of skilled professionals capable of creating, managing, and analyzing the data. To manage the information effectively, health care workers, regardless of their specific job roles, need information technology skills. The knowledge required extends beyond basic computer literacy to:

- Using word processing and presentation software
- Searching, retrieving, and managing data from internal sources, external databases, and the Internet
- Communicating using e-mail, instant messaging, listservs, and file transfers
- Understanding and following security measures such as access control and data security

An office that has made the transition to an integrated practice management program and electronic health record program also requires a staff that is familiar with health information technology. Two major curricula, Registered Health Information Technician and Registered Health Information Manager, are available under the guidance of the American Health Information Management Association (AHIMA) to provide a strong foundation in health information management (HIM).

The technician level is an associate degree program intended to prepare students to examine medical records for accuracy, report patient data for reimbursement, and help provide information for medical research and statistical data. The manager level is a baccalaureate degree program that produces graduates skilled in the collection, interpretation, and analysis of patient data who can interact with all levels of an organization—clinical, financial, and administrative—that employ patient data in decision making. The graduate is trained to assume managerial positions related to these functions.

Whether or not students choose to specialize in HIT, every graduate of an allied health program will be required to use health information technology on the job. As the United States moves toward the adoption of electronic health records, the demand for allied health graduates with skills in information technology and familiarity with computers exceeds the supply.

Gaining Certification in Your Field

As in other medical fields, individuals with certification generally have an easier time finding employment and advancing on the job than do those without certification. **Certification** acknowledges that an individual has mastered a standard body of knowledge and meets certain competencies. Employers look for certification when filling open positions, and certified individuals usually earn higher salaries than those who are not certified. Certification is offered in most allied health specialties. The field of health information technology offers a number of certifications, including the following:

certification a nationally recognized designation that acknowledges that an individual has mastered a standard body of knowledge and meets certain competencies

- Registered Health Information Technician (RHIT) certification is offered by the American Health Information Management Association (AHIMA; www.ahima.org).
- Registered Health Information Administrator (RHIA) certification is also offered by AHIMA.
- The American Association of Medical Assistants (AAMA) offers a Certified Medical Assistant (CMA) designation to individuals who pass an examination after earning a diploma in medical assisting from an accredited school (AAMA; www.aama-natl.org).
- Medical assistants may, alternatively, acquire the Registered Medical Assistant (RMA) designation from the American Medical Technologists (AMT; www.amt1.com).
- The Certified Professional in Healthcare Information and Management Systems (CPHIMS) designation is offered by the Healthcare Information and Management Systems Society

(HIMSS; www.himss.org). It is intended for health care information and management systems professionals who possess a combination of educational and work experience.

- Certification in Healthcare Privacy and Security (CHPS) is offered by AHIMA and signifies competence in designing, implementing, and administering privacy and security measures. A minimum of a baccalaureate degree is required to be considered for the certification.
- Health IT Certification (www.healthitcertification.com) offers a Certified Professional in Electronic Health Records (CPEHR) credential. Individuals who pass the certification examination demonstrate competency in the planning, implementation, and operation of electronic health record systems.
- A Certified Professional in Health Information Technology (CPHIT) credential offered by Health IT Certification indicates mastery in planning, selecting, implementing, using, and managing health information technology (HIT) and electronic health record (EHR) applications.
- The Certified Professional in Health Information Exchange (CPHIE) credential, also offered by Health IT Certification is awarded to individuals who have mastered a body of knowledge about exchanges of electronic information among organizations.
- A number of certifications in medical coding are available from AHIMA and from the American Academy of Professional Coders (AAPC; www.aapc.com). A coder who completes an education program may become an apprentice coder, but full certification is reserved for individuals with additional education and on-the-job experience.
- The American Association of Professional Coders (AAPC) in conjunction with the National Alliance of Medical Auditing Specialists (NAMAS) offers a Certified Professional Medical Auditor (CPMA) credential related to EHRs. This certification focuses on federal regulations as they pertain to physician practices (www.healthitcertification.com).
- The Certified Tumor Registrar (CTR) certification in tumor registry is available from the National Cancer Registrars Association (NCRA; www.ncra-usa.org).

A Commitment to Lifelong Learning

The field of health care is always changing. This makes it an exciting area for employment, but it also presents challenges. To keep pace with rapid change, professionals must keep their knowledge and skills current. Education does not end with the awarding of a certificate or a degree; in the health care field, it is a lifelong commitment. Most professional organizations require certified members to keep

THINKING IT THROUGH 1.9

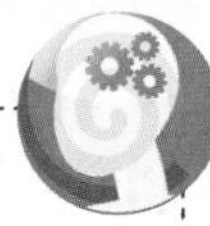

Read the following help wanted advertisement:

We are a large, multispecialty physician practice seeking an enthusiastic, self-motivated college graduate looking for an administrative position. We prefer a candidate who was involved in extracurricular school activities or held a leadership role in a club or an organization. The individual selected for this position will work with the physicians, medical assistants, the accounts receivable department, and scheduling staff. The position requires computer proficiency, outstanding communication skills (both verbal and written), health care experience, and a professional image. Flexibility and the ability to multitask are essential components for success in this role.

- Why is the practice interested in whether the person participated in extracurricular activities?
- Do you think participation in extracurricular activities is relevant to the position?

up to date by taking annual training courses to refresh or extend their knowledge. Continuing education sessions are assigned course credits by the credentialing organizations, and satisfactory completion of a test on the material is often required. Employers often approve attendance at seminars that apply to the practice's goals and ask the person who attends to update other staff members.

Technology makes it easy to access information from many different sources. A wide range of information is available on the Internet, including up-to-date professional information. Sources of information include:

- **Websites** Locations on the Internet that contain a collection of linked documents, images, and files.
- **Blogs** Websites with regular entries of commentary, descriptions of events, or other materials such as videos.
- **Newsfeeds** Listings of news headlines and excerpts that are sent automatically to subscribers.
- **Webinars and podcasts** Educational sessions delivered via the Internet. A podcast is an audio recording in digital format that can be played back on a computer or a mobile device.
- **e-Books** Digital versions of books that can be viewed using a computer, an e-book reader, or a mobile device.
- **Videos** A wide range of videos can be viewed online or downloaded and viewed, many with educational content.
- **Listservs** Electronic mailing lists for groups interested in a common topic. E-mails sent to the list are automatically delivered to individuals who sign up to receive them.
- **Social networking sites** Online communities of people who share common interests and/or activities. In health care and other businesses, these networks can be used to share knowledge, exchange ideas, and find job opportunities, among other things.

chapter 1 summary

LEARNING OUTCOME	KEY CONCEPTS/EXAMPLES
1.1 Compare practice management (PM) programs and electronic health records (EHRs). Pages 5–7	- A practice management program performs administrative and financial functions, such as scheduling patients' appointments, billing patients and health plans, receiving and recording payments, and managing collections. An electronic health record is a computerized lifelong health care record for an individual that incorporates data from all sources that provide treatment for the individual.
1.2 Discuss the government health information technology (HIT) initiatives that have led to integrated PM/EHR programs. Pages 5–7	- The Health Insurance Portability and Accountability Act of 1996 (HIPAA) helps keep people's health information safe by means of required technical specifications for the electronic exchange of administrative and financial health information. - The Medicare Improvements for Patients and Providers Act provides financial incentives for practitioners who use electronic prescribing. - The 2006 Tax Relief and Health Care Act requires the Centers for Medicare and Medicaid Services (CMS) to set up the Physician Quality Reporting Initiative (PQRI), which gives bonuses to physicians when they use treatment plans and clinical guidelines that are based on scientific evidence. - The American Recovery and Reinvestment Act of 2009 (ARRA) includes the Health Information Technology for Economic and Clinical Health (HITECH) Act, which requires the government to develop standards for health information to be exchanged electronically and to use health information to improve the quality and coordination of care, provides Medicare and Medicaid incentives to facilitate the adoption of electronic health records by doctors and hospitals, and strengthens federal privacy and security laws to protect patients' health information. - The National Health Information Network (NHIN) is a set of standards, services, and policies that enable the secure exchange of health information over the Internet to build a national network of interoperable health records.

LEARNING OUTCOME	KEY CONCEPTS/EXAMPLES
1.3 List the eight facts that are documented in the medical record for an ambulatory patient encounter. Pages 13–16	- The eight facts are: 1. Patient's name 2. Encounter date and reason 3. Appropriate history and physical examination 4. Review of all tests that were ordered 5. Diagnosis 6. Plan of care, or notes on procedures or treatments that were given 7. Instructions or recommendations that were given to the patient 8. Signature of the provider who saw the patient
1.4 Identify the additional uses of clinical information gathered in patient encounters. Pages 16–18	- Additional uses of clinical information include legal issues, quality review, research, education, public health and homeland security, and billing and reimbursement.
1.5 Compare electronic medical records, electronic health records, and personal health records. Pages 18–24	- Electronic medical records (EMRs) are computerized records of one physician's encounters with a patient over time. They serve as the physician's legal record of patient care. Electronic health records (EHRs) can include information from the EMRs of a number of different physicians as well as from pharmacies, laboratories, hospitals, insurance carriers, and so on. Personal health records (PHRs) are private, secure electronic files that are created, maintained, and owned by the patient. PHRs typically include current medications and dosages, health insurance information, immunization records, allergies, medical test results, past surgeries, family medical history, and more.
1.6 Describe the four functions of a practice management program that relate to managing claims. Pages 24–25	- The four functions of a practice management program that relate to managing claims are creating electronic claims, monitoring claim status electronically, receiving notification of electronic payments, and handling electronic payments.

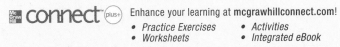

LEARNING OUTCOME	KEY CONCEPTS/EXAMPLES
1.7 List the steps in the medical documentation and billing cycle. Pages 26–33	- The steps in the medical documentation and billing cycle are: 1. Preregistering patients 2. Establishing financial responsibility 3. Checking in patients 4. Reviewing coding compliance 5. Reviewing billing compliance 6. Checking out patients 7. Preparing and transmitting claims 8. Monitoring payer adjudication 9. Generating patient statements 10. Following up on patient payments and collections
1.8 Compare the roles and responsibilities of clinical and administrative personnel on the physician practice health care team. Pages 33–38	- Clinical personnel provide treatment to patients, while administrative personnel manage the business aspects of health care. Administrative staff work behind the scenes in a medical office and do not provide medical treatment or testing. Some administrative workers, such as schedulers, do interact with patients.
1.9 Explain how professional certification and lifelong learning contribute to career advancement in medical administration. Pages 38–41	- Individuals with certification generally have an easier time finding employment and advancing on the job than do those without certification. Certification acknowledges that an individual has mastered a standard body of knowledge and meets certain competencies. Employers look for certification when filling open positions, and certified individuals usually earn higher salaries than those who are not certified. - Most professional organizations require certified members to keep up to date by taking annual training courses to refresh or extend their knowledge. Continuing education sessions are assigned course credits by the credentialing organizations, and satisfactory completion of a test on the material is often required.

chapter review

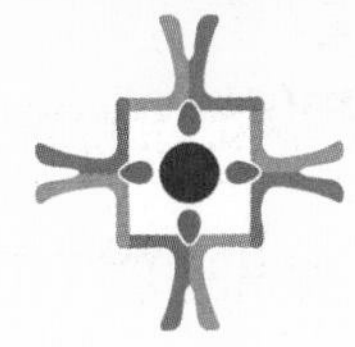

MATCHING QUESTIONS

Match the key terms with their definitions.

_____ 1. ***[LO 1.7]*** medical necessity

_____ 2. ***[LO 1.5]*** electronic medical record

_____ 3. ***[LO 1.1]*** health information technology

_____ 4. ***[LO 1.7]*** revenue cycle management

_____ 5. ***[LO 1.9]*** certification

_____ 6. ***[LO 1.3]*** patient examination

_____ 7. ***[LO 1.4]*** pay for performance (P4P)

_____ 8. ***[LO 1.2]*** ARRA

_____ 9. ***[LO 1.1]*** practice management program

_____ 10. ***[LO 1.1]*** electronic health record

a. Oversight of the activities associated with a patient encounter to ensure that the provider receives full payment for services.

b. An examination of a person's body in order to determine his or her state of health.

c. Computerized record of one physician's encounters with a patient over time.

d. Treatment that is in accordance with generally accepted medical practice.

e. Provision of financial incentives to physicians who provide evidence-based treatments to their patients.

f. Using computers and electronic communications to manage medical information.

g. Computerized lifelong health care record with data from all sources.

h. Federal act that provides financial incentives for adoption of electronic health records.

i. Program used to perform administrative and financial functions in a medical office.

j. Nationally recognized designation that acknowledges that an individual has mastered a standard body of knowledge and meets certain competencies.

TRUE-FALSE QUESTIONS

Decide whether each statement is true or false.

_____ 1. ***[LO 1.1]*** Practice management programs are designed to manage patients' clinical records.

_____ 2. ***[LO 1.2]*** Integrated PM/EHR programs increase patient safety, improve quality of care, and reduce operating costs.

_____ 3. ***[LO 1.3]*** The ambulatory care medical record is a log of a patient's hospitalizations.

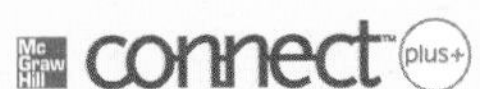

_____ 4. ***[LO 1.3]*** The medical assistant determines the patient's diagnosis during a physical examination.

_____ 5. ***[LO 1.4]*** Medical records may be used to protect physicians from accusations of medical malpractice.

_____ 6. ***[LO 1.7]*** During the second step of the medical documentation and billing cycle, the patient's eligibility for insurance benefits is verified.

_____ 7. ***[LO 1.6]*** Practice management programs are used to monitor the status of claims that have been sent to health plans.

_____ 8. ***[LO 1.5]*** Personal health records and electronic health records are both maintained by the physician.

_____ 9. ***[LO 1.8]*** Clinical personnel treat patients.

_____ 10. ***[LO 1.9]*** Certification is considered helpful for securing an administrative position in a medical practice.

MULTIPLE-CHOICE QUESTIONS

Select the letter that best completes the statement or answers the question.

1. ***[LO 1.1]*** Specialized programs that help process patients' appointments, billing, payments, and collections are called _________.
   a. electronic health records
   b. clinical encounters
   c. practice management programs
   d. pay-for-performance programs

2. ***[LO 1.2]*** The federal law that protects patients' private health information, ensures coverage during job changes, and uncovers fraud and abuse is the _________.
   a. Health Insurance Portability and Accountability Act of 1996
   b. Medicare Prescription Drug, Improvement, and Modernization Act of 2003
   c. Physician Quality Reporting Initiative
   d. American Recovery and Reinvestment Act of 2009

3. ***[LO 1.3]*** Which of the following must be included in medical office records for patients?
   a. parent's name
   b. country of birth
   c. diagnosis
   d. educational history

4. ***[LO 1.5]*** Which of the following is not a concern when a physician practice is implementing an EHR?
   a. changes to the practice workflow
   b. the inability to share information due to a lack of clinical standards
   c. cost
   d. revenue management

5. ***[LO 1.4]*** Tying financial incentives to evidence-based clinical treatments is known as ________.
   a. medical malpractice
   b. the medical documentation and billing cycle
   c. revenue cycle management
   d. pay for performance
6. ***[LO 1.7]*** The purpose of managing the revenue cycle is to generate ________.
   a. cash flow
   b. patient encounters
   c. coding
   d. medical records
7. ***[LO 1.1]*** Practice management programs are used to ________.
   a. create electronic prescriptions
   b. provide continuity of care
   c. manage payments from payers electronically
   d. exchange health information
8. ***[LO 1.1]*** Electronic health records contain information that ________.
   a. is maintained by the patient
   b. may be entered by a number of physicians and other providers
   c. is entered only by the patient's primary care physician
   d. states the amount the patient owes from previous visits
9. ***[LO 1.8]*** Administrative personnel on the health care team ________.
   a. are considered clinical staff
   b. may include physician assistants and nurses
   c. may include medical clinical assistants
   d. may include medical administration assistants and billers
10. ***[LO 1.9]*** Professional certification is maintained over time by requirements for ________.
    a. graduate-level education
    b. ongoing continuing education
    c. international conferences
    d. none of the above

SHORT-ANSWER QUESTIONS

Define the following abbreviations.

1. ***[LO 1.7]*** A/R ______________________
2. ***[LO 1.1]*** EHR ______________________
3. ***[LO 1.5]*** EMR ______________________
4. ***[LO 1.2]*** HIE ______________________

CHAPTER 1 REVIEW CHAPTER REVIEW

5. *[LO 1.1]* HIT ____________________

6. *[LO 1.2]* NHIN ____________________

7. *[LO 1.4]* P4P ____________________

8. *[LO 1.5]* PHR ____________________

9. *[LO 1.1]* PM ____________________

10. *[LO 1.7]* RCM ____________________

APPLYING YOUR KNOWLEDGE

Working with Documentation

1.1 *[LO 1.3]* Label the eight data points that are included in an ambulatory care medical record.

a. Georgina Warez ____________

b. Saw this 27-year-old female patient on 10-1-2016 for a complaint of urinary tract problem. ____________

c. Patient complains of frequency of urination, urgency, and burning sensation for about 3–5 days. She denies hematuria. She has slight suprapubic discomfort. She has been treated for bladder infection in the past. Her last menstrual period was 4 days ago. Upon examination, I confirmed a very vague tenderness over the suprapubic area. Flanks are clear. ____________

d. Her laboratory results are: WBC 11,200. Urinalysis shows yellow, cloudy urine; specific gravity 1.015; 3–5 RBCs; 80–100 WBCs; and many bacteria. ____________

e. Urinary tract infection. ____________

f. Septra DS 1 b.i.d. was ordered X 10 days. ____________

g. Repeat urinalysis after the 10-day medication regimen. ____________

h. Grace Marotta, MD____________

Managing the Revenue Cycle

1.2 *[LO 1.7]* List the ten steps in the medical documentation and billing cycle.

Step 1: ____

Step 2: ____

Step 3: ____

Step 4: ____

Step 5: ____

Step 6: ____________________

Step 7: ____________________

Step 8: ____________________

Step 9: ____________________

Step 10: ____________________

1.3 ***[LO 1.7]*** Which documentation or billing step do you think each of the following tasks is related to?

_____ a. calculating what patients owe the practice after claims are paid

_____ b. checking off procedure codes on a form following the patient's examination

_____ c. calling the representative of a health plan to learn the patient's eligibility and benefits for an immunization to prevent swine flu

_____ d. calling a patient about an overdue bill

_____ e. sending an e-mail message to a health plan concerning a claim that seems to be missing

_____ f. electronically transmitting a claim to a health plan

_____ g. reviewing a new patient's name and contact information before the visit

_____ h. scanning a patient's driver's license

_____ i. sending an e-mail query to a physician who has entered a prostate cancer screening code on the encounter form for a female patient

_____ j. calculating the amount to be billed a health plan whose contract stipulates that it will pay 10 percent less than the amount customarily charged to patients

Working with Integrated PM/EHR Programs

1.4 ***[LO 1.1, 1.2]*** Which program, a PM or an EHR, do you think would handle each of the following tasks?

_____ a. The medical assistant verifies and documents a patient's medications and allergies during an examination.

_____ b. A patient's payment of coinsurance is entered.

_____ c. A physician enters needed prescriptions and orders tests following a patient's examination.

_____ d. A biller sends a claim for the encounter to the patient's health plan.

_____ e. A payment from the health plan is received via EFT and checked.

chapter 2

KEY TERMS

abuse
Acknowledgment of Receipt of Notice of Privacy Practices
ASC X12 Version 5010
audit
breach
breach notification
business associate
Centers for Medicare and Medicaid Services (CMS)
clearinghouse
code set
covered entity
electronic data interchange (EDI)
electronic protected health information (ePHI)
encryption
fraud
Health Care Fraud and Abuse Control Program
Health Information Technology for Economic and Clinical Health (HITECH) Act
HIPAA Electronic Health Care Transactions and Code Sets (TCS)
HIPAA National Identifiers
HIPAA Privacy Rule
HIPAA Security Rule
National Provider Identifier (NPI)
Notice of Privacy Practices (NPP)
protected health information (PHI)
release of information (ROI)
treatment, payment, and health care operations (TPO)

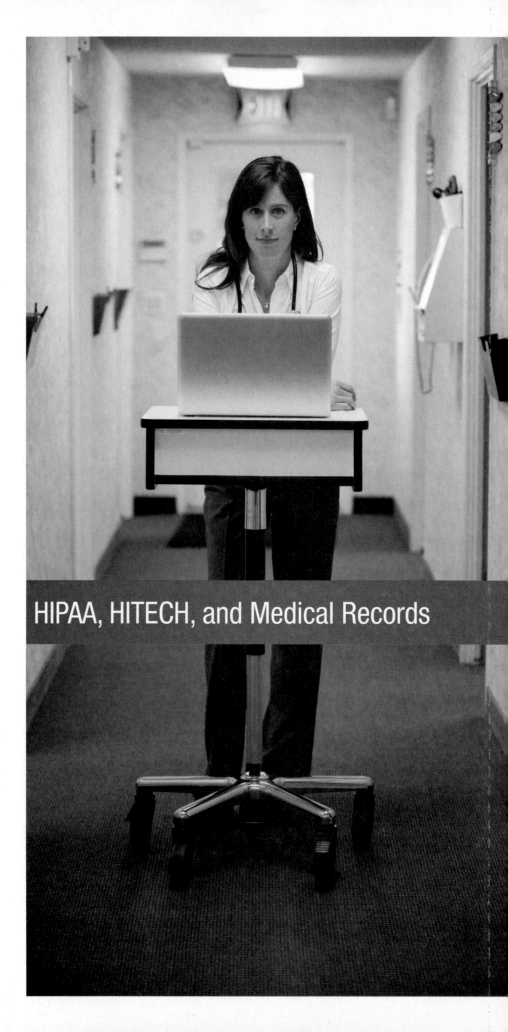

HIPAA, HITECH, and Medical Records

LEARNING OUTCOMES

When you finish this chapter, you will be able to:

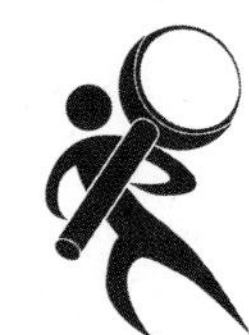

- **2.1** List several legal uses of a patient's medical record.
- **2.2** Define HIPAA and HITECH, and name the three types of covered entities that must comply with them.
- **2.3** Discuss how the HIPAA Privacy Rule protects patients' protected health information (PHI).
- **2.4** Discuss how the HIPAA Security Rule protects electronic protected health information (ePHI).
- **2.5** Explain the purpose of the HITECH breach notification rule.
- **2.6** State the goal of the HIPAA Electronic Health Care Transactions and Code Sets (TCS) standards and list the HIPAA transactions and code sets standards that will be required in the future.
- **2.7** Discuss some of the most common threats to the privacy and security of electronic information and ways in which the HITECH Act addresses them.
- **2.8** Define fraud and abuse in health care and cite an example of each.
- **2.9** Describe the various government agencies that are responsible for enforcing HIPAA.
- **2.10** Identify the parts of a compliance plan and the types of documentation used to demonstrate compliance.

Should We Release This Record?

Chris Yakamoto took the call from Anthony Battistuta's insurance company. Chris is aware that Anthony is a patient at Family Care Clinic who is being followed for his diabetes, which is well controlled at this point. The insurance company representative asks, "Would you please transmit data from of all of Mr. Battistuta's records concerning his history of diabetes and Dr. McGrath's treatment plan? We are examining an insurance claim from his last visit and need this information." Chris wonders, "Is this permissible under the patient privacy rules that are stated in our compliance plan?"

Studying this chapter will give you the knowledge to correctly answer this question, which is similar to situations that administrative medical staff must often handle properly under the HIPAA/HITECH laws.

2.1 The Legal Medical Record

Medical records, or charts, are created by physicians and other providers in physician practices, hospitals, surgery centers, clinics, and other health care facilities. They are created and shared to help make accurate diagnoses of patients' conditions and to trace the course of care.

A patient's medical record contains facts, findings, and observations about that patient's health history. It also contains communications with and about the patient in the health care setting. The medical record in the medical office begins with a patient's first contact and continues through all treatments and services. The record provides continuity and communication among physicians and other health care professionals who are involved in the patient's care. Patient medical records are also used in research and for education.

Patient medical records are legal documents. Physicians own the physical record (although patients own the information about themselves), and properly documented patient care is part of the physician's defense against accusations that patients were not treated correctly. Medical records should clearly state who performed what service and describe why, where, when, and how it was done. Physicians document the rationale behind their treatment decisions. This rationale is the basis for the concept of medical necessity—a clinically logical link between a patient's condition and the treatment provided.

Documentation means organizing a patient's health record in chronological order, using a systematic, logical, and consistent method. The patient's health history, examinations, tests, and results of treatments are all documented. Complete and comprehensive documentation is important to show that physicians have followed the medical standards of care that apply in their state.

Medical standards of care are state-specified performance measures for the delivery of health care by medical professionals. Health care providers are liable (legally responsible) for providing this level of care to their patients. The term *medical professional liability* describes this responsibility of licensed health care professionals. Medical malpractice can result when a provider injures or harms a patient due to failure to follow the standards.

Regardless of whether providers are using paper or electronic health records, they follow generally recognized guidelines to document patient encounters. The initial examinations and assessments show the treatment plan for the patient. Progress reports document the patient's progress and response to the treatment plan. Discharge summaries are prepared during the patient's final visit for a particular treatment plan. If either the patient or the physician ends the relationship, the physician must still maintain the patient's medical record. The physician also sends the patient a letter that documents the situation and provides for continuity of care with the next provider.

The documentation of diagnoses and treatments is also used as proof of billed services. An unwritten law of medical insurance is

THINKING IT THROUGH 2.1

Sally Darfure is sixty-four years old and has severe diabetes and high blood pressure. She requires regular blood tests to monitor the diabetes. Both her primary care physician and her endocrinologist (diabetes specialist) draw blood regularly. Neither office uses an electronic health record system.

- In your opinion, how could an EHR system help ensure continuity of care in this situation?
- Do you think Sally's insurance carrier will agree to pay regularly for separate blood work for both physicians?

that if it was not documented, it was not done, and if it was not done, it cannot be billed. Payers use documentation to decide whether reported services should be reimbursed.

2.2 Health Care Regulation

To protect consumers' health, both the federal and state governments pass laws that affect the medical services offered to patients. To protect the privacy of patients' health information, additional laws cover the way health care plans and providers exchange this information as they conduct business. The increased use of information technology in health care creates an increased need for privacy. Allied health personnel must know how to protect patients' personal health information, how to respond to requests for this information from other parties, and how to safeguard the electronic exchange of information on behalf of patients.

Federal Regulation

The main federal government agency responsible for health care is the **Centers for Medicare and Medicaid Services,** known as **CMS.** An agency of the Department of Health and Human Services (HHS), CMS administers the Medicare and Medicaid programs to more than 90 million Americans. It implements annual federal budget acts and laws such as the Medicare Prescription Drug, Improvement, and Modernization Act that helps Medicare beneficiaries pay for medicine and for annual physical examinations.

Centers for Medicare and Medicaid Services (CMS) federal agency in the Department of Health and Human Services that runs Medicare, Medicaid, clinical laboratories, and other government health programs; responsible for enforcing all HIPAA standards other than the privacy and security standards

CMS also performs activities to ensure the quality of health care, such as:

- Regulating all laboratory testing other than research performed on humans
- Preventing discrimination based on health status for people buying health insurance
- Researching the effectiveness of various methods of health care management, treatment, and financing
- Evaluating the quality of health care facilities and services

The rest of the health care industry often models its practices on CMS policy. When a change is made in Medicare rules, for example, private payers often adopt a similar rule.

A critical piece of legislation is called the Health Insurance Portability and Accountability Act (HIPAA) of 1996. This law is designed to:

- Ensure the security and privacy of health information
- Ensure the portability of employer-provided health insurance coverage for workers and their families when they change or lose their jobs
- Increase accountability and decrease fraud and abuse in health care
- Improve the efficiency of health care delivery by creating standards for electronic transmission of health care transactions

State Regulation

States are also major regulators of the health care industry. Operating an insurance company without a license is illegal in all states. State commissioners of insurance investigate consumer complaints about the quality and financial aspects of health care. State laws ensure the solvency of insurance companies and managed care organizations, so that they will be able to pay enrollees' claims. States may restrict price increases on premiums and other charges to patients, require that policies include a guaranteed renewal provision, and control the situations in which an insurer can cancel a patient's coverage. State laws also contain a patchwork of privacy protections and protections related to information security.

HIPAA Rules

Patients' medical records—progress notes, reports, and other clinical materials—are legal documents that belong to the provider who created them, but the information belongs to the patient. A provider cannot refuse to give a patient the information in the records unless providing it would be detrimental to the patient's health.

Patients control the amount and type of information that is released to other parties, except for the use of the data to treat them or to conduct the normal business transactions of the practice. In most cases, only patients and their legally appointed representatives have the authority to authorize the release of information to anyone not directly involved in their care. There are exceptions for certain situations involving criminal acts and public health matters.

All members of the physician practice health care team handle issues such as requests for information from patients' medical records. They need to know what information can be released about patients' conditions and treatments. What information can be legally shared with other providers and health plans? What information must the patient specifically authorize to be released? The answers to these questions are based on the HIPAA Administrative Simplification provisions.

Congress passed the Administrative Simplification provisions partly because of rising health care costs. A significant portion of every health care dollar is spent on administrative and financial tasks. These costs can be controlled if the business transactions of health care are standardized and handled electronically.

Electronic Data Interchange

The Administrative Simplification provisions encourage the use of **electronic data interchange (EDI).** EDI is the computer-to-computer exchange of routine business information using publicly available electronic standards. Practice staff members use EDI to exchange health information about their practices' patients with payers and clearinghouses. Each electronic exchange is a transaction, which is the electronic equivalent of a business document.

EDI transactions are not visible in the way that an exchange of paperwork, such as a letter, is. An example of a nonmedical transaction is the process of getting cash from an ATM. In an ATM transaction, the computer-to-computer exchange is made up of computer language that is sent and answered by the machines. This exchange happens behind the scenes. It is documented on the customer's end with the transaction receipt that is printed; the bank also has a record at its location.

electronic data interchange (EDI) computer-to-computer exchange of routine business information using publicly available electronic standards

Health Information Technology for Economic and Clinical Health (HITECH) Act provisions in the American Recovery and Reinvestment Act (ARRA) of 2009 that extend and reinforce HIPAA and contain new breach notification requirements for covered entities and business associates, guidance on ways to encrypt or destroy PHI to prevent a breach, requirements for informing individuals when a breach occurs, higher monetary penalties for HIPAA violations, and stronger enforcement of the Privacy and Security Rules

The Administrative Simplification Provisions

There are three parts to HIPAA's Administrative Simplification provisions:

1. **HIPAA Privacy Rule** The privacy requirements cover patients' health information, whether paper, electronic, or otherwise.
2. **HIPAA Security Rule** The security requirements state the administrative, technical, and physical safeguards that are required to protect patients' electronic health information.
3. **HIPAA Electronic Transactions and Code Sets standards** The standards require every provider who does business electronically to use the same health care transactions, code sets, and identifiers.

HITECH Act

A number of the provisions of the American Recovery and Reinvestment Act (ARRA) of 2009, enacted February 17, 2009, and also known as Public Law 111-5, extend and reinforce HIPAA. The major provision relating to the privacy and security standards is Title XIII—the **Health Information Technology for Economic and Clinical Health (HITECH) Act.** As the health care industry in the United States moves toward widespread use of EHRs and the electronic transmission of health information, the HITECH Act increases protection for patients' privacy by implementing new breach notification requirements, higher monetary penalties for HIPAA violations, and greater enforcement of the Privacy and Security Rules.

To prevent breaches of health information, the HITECH Act requires keeping patients' protected health information secure by making it "unusable, unreadable, or indecipherable to unauthorized individuals" using specified technologies and methods. The Department of Health and Human Services has released guidance on specific technologies and methods that can make it impossible for unauthorized individuals to use, read, or decipher this information.

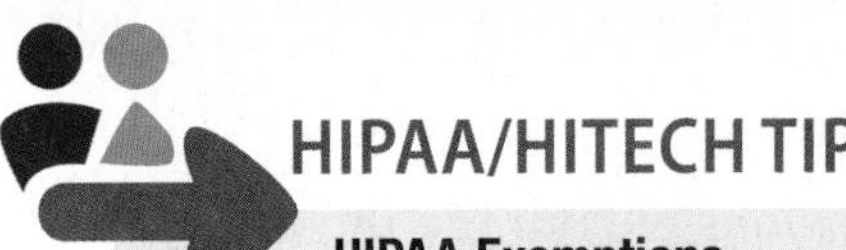

HIPAA/HITECH TIP

HIPAA Exemptions

Certain benefits are always exempt from the HIPAA standards even when provided by health plans, including coverage for accidents only, disability income coverage, liability insurance, workers' compensation, automobile medical payment and liability insurance, credit-only insurance (such as mortgage insurance), and coverage for on-site medical clinics.

In the case of breaches of unsecured health information by covered entities or their business associates, HITECH requires health care providers, health plans, and other entities covered by HIPAA to notify individuals that their health information has been compromised.

The act also calls for an increase in monetary penalties for privacy and security violations and for greater enforcement of the Privacy and Security Rules, including regular compliance checks and the assignment of a new chief privacy officer under the Office of the National Coordinator for Health Information Technology. The chief privacy officer is appointed by the secretary of the HHS. The compliance date for the HITECH provisions connected with HIPAA was February 2010.

Covered Entities: Complying with HIPAA and HITECH

covered entity under HIPAA, health plan, clearinghouse, or provider who transmits any health information in electronic form in connection with a HIPAA transaction

clearinghouse company that processes electronic health information and executes electronic transactions such as insurance verification and claim submission for providers

Health care organizations that are required by law to obey the HIPAA regulations are called covered entities. A **covered entity** is an organization that electronically transmits any information that is protected under HIPAA. Other organizations that work for the covered entities must also agree to follow the HIPAA rules.

Covered Entities

Under HIPAA, three types of covered entities must follow the regulations:

1. **Health plans** The individual or group plan that provides or pays for medical care. Health plans include government and private-payer plans.
2. **Health care providers** People or organizations that furnish, bill, or are paid for health care in the normal course of business, including physicians, nurses, hospitals, home health agencies, outpatient clinics, laboratories, pharmacies, dentists, long-term care facilities, and others.
3. **Health care clearinghouses** A **clearinghouse** is a company that helps providers process health information and execute electronic transactions, such as the submission of insurance claims. Clearinghouses process health information by converting it into a format that meets HIPAA standards.

Business Associates

HIPAA also affects many others in the health care field. For instance, outside medical billers are not covered entities. However, they must follow HIPAA's rules in order to do business with covered entities.

THINKING IT THROUGH 2.2

Under the Privacy Rule, not all individuals and businesses who perform outside services for covered entities are considered business associates. For example, under the Privacy Rule, outside legal and financial services are considered business associates, but delivery companies and management consultants are not. Why is this the case? What distinguishes a business associate from other outside vendors?

In HIPAA terms, they are **business associates**—individuals or businesses whose services involve the use or disclosure of personal health information (PHI) to perform a function or activity on behalf of a covered entity but who are not a part of the covered entity's workforce. Business associates include the following:

- Law firms
- Accountants
- Benefits management companies
- Information technology (IT) contractors
- Medical transcription companies
- Compliance consultants
- Collection agencies
- Credit bureaus
- Temporary office personnel
- Pharmacy chains

Enforcement was slack prior to ARRA, because covered entities could only encourage a business associate to abide by HIPAA rules as part of their contractual agreement. Under the HITECH Act, HIPAA's Privacy and Security Rules extend directly to business associates. This means that business associates will be subject to the same penalties as covered entities—for example, hospitals and physician groups—for privacy and security violations.

business associate person or organization that requires access to PHI to perform a function or activity on behalf of a covered entity but is not part of its workforce

HIPAA Privacy Rule law that regulates the use and disclosure of patients' protected health information

2.3 HIPAA Privacy Rule

The first part of the Administrative Simplification provisions includes the HIPAA Standards for Privacy of Individually Identifiable Health Information rule, known as the **HIPAA Privacy Rule.** Enacted on April 14, 2003, it provides protection for individually identifiable health information and grants certain rights to individuals in regard to their medical records. It was the first comprehensive federal protection for the privacy of health information. Before that, an individual's personal health information and medical records were governed by a patchwork of federal and state laws. Some state laws were strict, but others were not.

The Privacy Rule says that a covered entity must:

- Have a set of privacy practices that are appropriate for its health care services

- Notify patients about their privacy rights and how their information can be used or disclosed
- Train employees so that they understand the privacy practices
- Appoint a privacy official responsible for seeing that the privacy practices are adopted and followed
- Safeguard patients' records

protected health information (PHI) individually identifiable health information transmitted or maintained by electronic media or in any other form or medium

The HIPAA Privacy Rule covers the use and disclosure of patients' **protected health information (PHI).** PHI is defined as individually identifiable health information that is transmitted or maintained by electronic media, such as over the Internet, or that is transmitted or maintained in any other form or medium. Covered entities must follow HIPAA regulations for the protection of health information. However, not all of a patient's information is subject to the law. Table 2.1 lists the information that meets the definition of PHI.

The Privacy Rule applies to PHI in any form, whether it is communicated verbally, written or printed on paper, or maintained in an electronic format.

Minimum Necessary Standard

When using or disclosing health information, a covered entity must try to limit the information to the minimum amount of PHI necessary for the intended purpose. The *minimum necessary standard* means using reasonable safeguards to protect PHI from being accidentally released to those not needing the information during an appropriate use or disclosure. For example, a medical insurance specialist would not disclose a patient's history of cancer on a workers' compensation claim for a broken wrist. Only the information the recipient needs to know is given. Similarly, a medical assistant would not hand over medical supplies and a prescription to someone who was not a family member or a legally appointed representative of the patient.

TABLE 2.1 Information Considered Protected Health Information (PHI)
Name
Address (including street address, city, county, ZIP code)
Names of relatives and employers
Birth date
Telephone numbers
Fax number
E-mail address
Social Security number
Medical record number
Health plan beneficiary number
Account number
Certificate or license number
Serial number of any vehicle or other device
Website address
Fingerprints or voiceprints
Photographic images

HIPAA/HITECH TIP

NPPs on the Website

If a covered entity has a website that describes its services and benefits, it must also put its NPP on the site.

Designated Record Set

The covered entity must release a designated record set only, not all information. For purposes of the HIPAA Privacy Rule, a *record* is any item, collection, or grouping of information that includes PHI and is maintained by a covered entity. The HIPAA term for a group of records is *designated record set (DRS)*. For a provider, the designated record set is the medical and billing records the provider maintains. It does not include appointment and surgery schedules, requests for lab tests, and birth and death records. It also does not include mental health information, psychotherapy notes, and genetic information, which are protected by more stringent release guidelines. For a health plan, the designated record set includes enrollment information, payment information, claim decisions, and the medical management systems of the plan.

Notice of Privacy Practices and Acknowledgment

To comply with the Privacy Rule, covered entities, including medical offices as well as other providers and health plans, must give each patient an explanation of privacy practices at the patient's first contact or encounter. To satisfy this requirement, a medical office gives the patient a copy of the office's **Notice of Privacy Practices (NPP)** (see Figure 2.1). The notice explains how patients' PHI may be used and describes the patients' rights. The NPP is usually a paper form that is handed to the patient; in the case of a provider conducting business electronically, this information may be received as an electronic file. A patient must be given a copy of the NPP at the time of the first encounter and at least once every three years thereafter.

For compliance purposes, covered entities keep track of when patients receive the form. The office must make a good-faith effort to obtain a patient's acknowledgment of having received and read the NPP. This is accomplished through a form known as the **Acknowledgment of Receipt of Notice of Privacy Practices** (see Figure 2.2). This form states that the patient has read the privacy practices and understands how the provider intends to protect the patient's rights to privacy under HIPAA. Like the NPP, the acknowledgment can be a paper form or an electronic file.

Notice of Privacy Practices (NPP) a HIPAA-mandated document stating the privacy policies and procedures of a covered entity

Acknowledgment of Receipt of Notice of Privacy Practices form accompanying a covered entity's Notice of Privacy Practices; covered entities must make a good-faith effort to have patients sign it

release of information (ROI) process followed by employees of covered entities when releasing patient information

Disclosure for Treatment, Payment, and Health Care Operations (TPO)

Members of the physician practice health care team follow a **release of information (ROI)** process to access PHI, prepare it for transmission, and send it to an individual or entity that has permission under HIPAA to obtain it. The Privacy Rule recognizes that medical offices and

Family Care Clinic

NOTICE OF PRIVACY PRACTICE

THIS NOTICE DESCRIBES HOW MEDICAL INFORMATION ABOUT YOU MAY BE USED AND DISCLOSED AND HOW YOU CAN GET ACCESS TO THIS INFORMATION. PLEASE REVIEW CAREFULLY.

WHY ARE YOU GETTING THIS NOTICE?

Family Care Clinic is required by federal and state law to maintain the privacy of your health information. The use and disclosure of your health information is governed by regulations under the Health Insurance Portability and Accountability Act of 1996 (HIPAA) and the requirements of applicable state law. For health information covered by HIPAA, we are required to provide you with this notice and will abide by this notice with respect to such health information. If you have questions about this notice, please contact out Privacy Officer at 877-555-1313. We will ask you to sign an "acknowledgment" indicating that you have been provided with this notice.

WHAT HEALTH INFORMATION IS PROTECTED?

We are committed to protecting the privacy of Information we gather about you while providing health-related services. Some examples of protected health information are:

- Information indicating that you are a patient receiving treatment or other health-related services from our physicians or staff;
- Information about your health condition (such as a disease you may have);
- Information about health care products or services you have received or may receive in the future (such as an operation); or
- Information about your health care benefits under an insurance plan (such as whether a prescription is covered);

When combined with:

- Demographic information (such as your name, address, or insurance status);
- Unique numbers that may identify you (such as your Social Security number, your phone number, or your driver's license number); and
- Other types of information that may identify who you are.

SUMMARY OF THIS NOTICE

This summary includes references to paragraphs throughout this notice that you may read for additional information.

1. Written Authorization Requirement

We may use your health information or share it with others in order to treat your condition, obtain payment for that treatment, and run our business operations. We generally need your written authorization for other uses and disclosures of your health information, unless an exception described in notice applies.

2. Authorizing Transfer of Your Records

Your may request that we transfer your records to another person or organization by completing a written authorization form. This form will specify what information is being released, to whom, and for what purpose. The authorization will have an expiration date.

3. Canceling Your Written Authorization

If you provide us with written authorization, you may revoke, or cancel, it at any time, except to the extent that we have already relied upon it. To revoke a written authorization, please write to the doctor's office where you initially gave your authorization.

4. Exception to Written Authorization Requirement

There are some situations in which we do not need your written authorization before using your health information or sharing it with others. They include:

Treatment, Payment, and Operations

As mentioned above, we may use your health information or share it with others in order to treat your condition, obtain payment for that treatment, and run our business operations.

Family and Friends

If you do not object, we will share information about your health with family and friends involved in your care.

Research

Although we will generally try to obtain your written authorization before using your health information for research purposes, there may be certain situations in which we are not required to obtain your written authorization.

De-identified Information

We may use or disclose your health information if we have removed any information that might identify you. When all identifying information is removed, we say that the health information is "completely de-identified." We may also use and disclose "partially de-identified" information if the person who will receive it agrees in writing to protect your privacy when using the information.

Incidental Disclosures

We may inadvertently use or disclose your health information despite having taken all reasonable precautions to protect the privacy and confidentiality of your health information.

Emergencies or Public Need

We may use or disclose your health information in an emergency or for important public health needs. For example, we may share your information with public health officials at the state or city health departments who are authorized to investigate and control the spread of diseases.

5. How to Access Your Health Information

You generally have the right to inspect and get copies of your health information.

6. How to Correct Your Health Information

You have the right to request that we amend your health information if you believe it is inaccurate or incomplete.

7. How to Identify Others Who Have Received Your Health Information

You have the right to receive an "accounting of disclosures." This is a report that identifies certain persons or organizations to which we have disclosed your health information. All disclosures are made according to the protections described in this Notice of Privacy Practices. Many routine disclosures we make (for treatment, payment, or business operations, among others) will not be included in this report. However, it will identify any nonroutine disclosures of your information.

8. How to Request Additional Privacy Protections

You have the right to request further restrictions on the way we use your health information or share it with others. However, we are not required to agree to the restriction you request. If we do agree with your request, we will be bound by our agreement.

9. How to Request Alternative Communications

You have the right to request that we contact you in a way that is more confidential for you, such as at home instead of at work. We will try to accommodate all reasonable requests.

10. How Someone May Act on Your Behalf

You have the right to name a personal representative who may act on your behalf to control the privacy of your health information. Parents and guardians will generally have the right to control the privacy of health information about minors unless the minors are permitted by law to act on their own behalf.

11. How to Learn About Special Protections for HIV, Alcohol and Substance Abuse, Mental Health, and Genetic Information

Special privacy protections apply to HIV-related information, alcohol and substance abuse treatment information, mental health information, psychotherapy notes, and genetic information.

12. How to Obtain a Copy of This Notice

If you have not already received one, you have the right to a paper copy of this notice. You may request a paper copy at any time, even if you have previously agreed to receive this notice electronically. You can request a copy of the privacy notice directly from your doctor's office. You may also obtain a copy of this notice from our website or by requesting a copy at your next visit.

13. How to Obtain a Copy of Revised Notice

We may change our privacy practices from time to time. If we do, we will revise this notice so you will have an accurate summary of our practices. You will be able to obtain your own copy of the revised notice by accessing our website or by calling your doctor's office. You may also ask for one at the time of your next visit. The effective date of the notice is noted in the top right corner of each page. We are required to abide by the terms of the notice that is currently in effect.

14. How to File a Complaint

If you believe your privacy rights have been violated, you may file a complaint with us or with the federal Office for Civil Rights. To file a complaint with us, please contact our Privacy Officer.

No one will retaliate or take action against you for filling a complaint.

Figure 2.1 Example of a Notice of Privacy Practices

Acknowledgment of Receipt of Notice of Privacy Practices

I understand that the providers of Family Care Clinic may share my health information for treatment, billing, and health care operations. I have been given a copy of the organization's Notice of Privacy Practices that describes how my health information is used and shared. I understand that Family Care Clinic has the right to change this notice at any time. I may obtain a current copy by contacting the practice's office or by visiting the website at www.xxx.com

My signature below constitutes my acknowledgment that I have been provided with a copy of the Notice of Privacy Practices.

____

Signature of Patient or Legal Representative Date

If signed by legal representative,
relationship to patient: ________________________

Figure 2.2 Example of an Acknowledgment of Receipt of Notice of Privacy Practices

payers must be able to exchange PHI in the normal course of business. *Use of PHI* means sharing or analysis within the entity that holds the information. *Disclosure* means the release, transfer, provision of access to, or divulging of PHI outside the entity holding the information.

The rule says that there are three everyday situations in which PHI can be used and disclosed by providers without the patient's permission. These situations are **treatment, payment, and health care operations (TPO):**

treatment, payment, and health care operations (TPO) under HIPAA, three conditions under which patients' protected health information may be released without their consent

- *Treatment* means providing and coordinating a patient's medical care. Physicians and other medical staff can discuss the patient's case in the office and with other physicians. Laboratory or X-ray technicians may call to obtain clarification of unreadable requests. This information can be provided by the physician or another medical staff member.
- *Payment* refers to the exchange of information with health plans. Medical office staff members can take the required information from patients' records and prepare health care claims that are transmitted to health plans.
- *Health care operations* are the general business management functions needed to run the office. They include such activities as tracking and measuring adherence to quality standards, staff training, and business planning.

Release by Any Method

Information for TPO can be released by using any method of communication, including in writing, orally, by fax, or by e-mail.

PHI Release to People Acting on a Patient's Behalf

A member of the physician practice health care team or another employee of a covered entity may release PHI to a family member, a relative, a friend, or another individual who asks for information on behalf of the patient. The covered entity must have reasonable assurance that the person has been identified by the patient as being involved in his or her care. The covered entity can release this information if the patient does not object. Informal permission can be obtained by asking the patient. If the patient is not present or is incapacitated, the covered entity can make the disclosure if doing so is in the best interests of the patient.

EXAMPLES

A health plan discloses relevant PHI to a beneficiary's daughter who has called to assist her hospitalized elderly mother with a payment issue.

A pharmacist dispenses filled prescriptions to a son who is picking up the items for his mother.

Release of Information for Purposes Other than TPO

For the provider to use or disclose PHI other than for treatment, payment, or operations (TPO), the patient must sign an authorization to release the information. For example, a patient who wishes a provider to disclose PHI to a life insurance company must authorize this action. This is an example of a general authorization. Information about alcohol or drug abuse, sexually transmitted diseases (STDs) (except in the case of public health issues in some states) or human immunodeficiency virus (HIV), and behavioral or mental health services may not be released without a specific authorization from the patient.

Authorization Document

The authorization document must be easy to understand and must include the following information:

- A description of the information to be used or disclosed
- The name or other specific identification of the persons authorized to use or disclose the information
- The name of the persons or group to whom the covered entity may make the use or disclosure
- A description of each purpose of the requested use or disclosure
- An expiration date
- The signature of the individual (or authorized representative) and the date

In addition, the rule states that a valid authorization must include:

- A statement of the individual's right to revoke the authorization in writing
- A statement about whether the covered entity is able to base treatment, payment, enrollment, or eligibility for benefits on the authorization

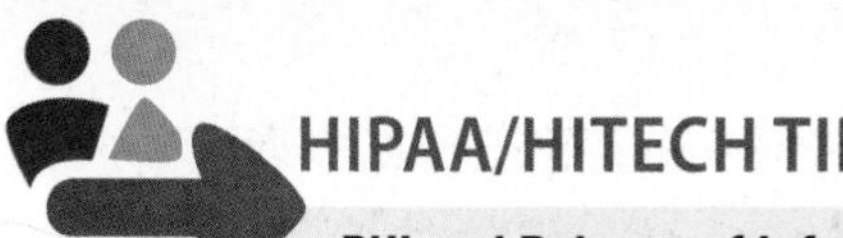

HIPAA/HITECH TIP

PHI and Release of Information Document

A patient release of information document is not needed when PHI is shared for TPO under HIPAA. However, state law may require authorization to release data, so many practices continue to ask patients to sign releases.

- A statement that information used or disclosed after the authorization may be disclosed again by the recipient and may no longer be protected by the rule

Uses or disclosures for which the covered entity has received specific authorization from the patient do not have to follow the minimum necessary standard. A sample authorization form is shown in Figure 2.3.

Accounting for Disclosures

Patients have the right to an accounting of disclosures of their PHI. The medical office keeps a disclosure log for each patient so that authorized disclosures can be listed. When a patient's PHI is accidentally disclosed, the disclosure should also be documented in the individual's medical record, since the individual did not authorize it and it was not a permitted disclosure. An example is faxing a discharge summary to the wrong physician's office.

Exceptions to Disclosure Standards

The rules for use and disclosure do not apply to the release of PHI in certain circumstances, including such public interest purposes as public health, law enforcement, research, workers' compensation cases, and national security situations. Even in such cases, however, other conditions may need to be met before PHI can be released. For example, if the provider receives a judicial order requiring a patient's PHI for use as evidence in a court of law, the provider may release it without the patient's approval.

De-identified Health Information There are no restrictions on the use or disclosure of de-identified health information. *De-identified health information* is information that neither identifies nor provides a reasonable basis for identifying an individual. For example, for information to be de-identified, the following identifiers must be removed from patient data: names, medical record numbers, health plan beneficiary numbers, device identifiers (such as pacemakers), and biometric identifiers, such as fingerprints and voiceprints.

State Statutes Some state statues are more stringent than HIPAA specifications with regard to the use and disclosure of PHI. Areas in which state statutes may differ from HIPAA include the following:

- Designated record set
- Psychotherapy notes

What specific information can be released

To whom

For what purpose

Patient Name: ______
Health Record Number: ______
Date of Birth: ______

1. I authorize the use or disclosure of the above named individual's health information as described below.

2. The following individual(s) or organization(s) are authorized to make the disclosure: ______

3. The type of information to be used or disclosed is as follows (check the appropriate boxes and include other information where indicated):

- ❑ problem list
- ❑ medication list
- ❑ list of allergies
- ❑ immunization records
- ❑ most recent history
- ❑ most recent discharge summary
- ❑ lab results (please describe the dates or types of lab tests you would like disclosed): ______
- ❑ x-ray and imaging reports (please describe the dates or types of x-rays or images you would like disclosed): ______
- ❑ consultation reports from (please supply doctors' names): ______
- ❑ entire record
- ❑ other (please describe): ______

4. I understand that the information in my health record may include information relating to sexually transmitted diseases, acquired immunodeficiency syndrome (AIDS), or human immunodeficiency virus (HIV). It may also include information about behavioral or mental health services, and treatment for alcohol and drug abuse.

5. The information identified above may be used by or disclosed to the following individuals or organization(s):
Name: ______
Address: ______

Name: ______
Address: ______

6. This information for which I'm authorizing disclosure will be used for the following purpose:
- ❑ my personal records
- ❑ sharing with other health care providers as needed/other (please describe): ______

7. I understand that I have a right to revoke this authorization at any time. I understand that if I revoke this authorization, I must do so in writing and present my written revocation to the health information management department. I understand that the revocation will not apply to information that has already been released in response to this authorization. I understand that the revocation will not apply to my insurance company when the law provides my insurer with the right to contest a claim under my policy.

8. This authorization will expire (insert date or event): ______

If I fail to specify an expiration date or event, this authorization will expire six months from the date on which it was signed.

9. I understand that once the above information is disclosed, it may be redisclosed by the recipient and the information may not be protected by federal privacy laws or regulations.

10. I understand authorizing the use or disclosure of the information identified above is voluntary. I need not sign this form to ensure health care treatment.

Signature of patient or legal representative: ______ Date: ______

If signed by legal representative, relationship to patient: ______

Signature of witness: ______ Date: ______

Distribution of copies: Original to provider; copy to patient; copy to accompany use or disclosure

Note: This sample form was developed by the American Health Information Management Association for discussion purposes. It should not be used without review by the issuing organization's legal counsel to ensure compliance with other federal and state laws and regulations.

Figure 2.3 Example of an Authorization to Use or Disclose Health Information

THINKING IT THROUGH 2.3

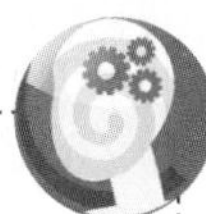

- A physician consults with another physician about a patient's condition by e-mail. Has the HIPAA Privacy Rule been followed?
- Two nurses are having a confidential conversation about a patient's condition in the hospital hallway directly outside the visitor waiting room for that floor. Someone visiting another patient accidentally overhears their conversation. Has the HIPAA Privacy Rule been followed?
- On July 13, 2010, Angelo Diaz requests City Medical, the office of his primary care physician, for an accounting of disclosures of his electronic PHI for the last year. The receptionist provides him with a printout. Angelo notices that the printout does not include TPO disclosures. The receptionist says that the office has never been responsible for tracking TPO disclosures. Is the receptionist correct? Should the office be able to provide Angelo Diaz with TPO disclosures for the last year?

- Rights of inmates
- Information compiled for civil, criminal, or administrative court cases

When a state law and the federal HIPAA provision both cover a particular situation, the law that is the strictest—the one with the toughest provisions—is followed. Each practice's privacy official reviews state laws and develops policies and procedures accordingly.

Patients' Rights

The HIPAA Privacy Rule also provides significant rights to patients, including the right to:

- Receive a written notice of information practices
- Ask to access, inspect, and obtain a copy of their PHI
- Request an accounting of most disclosures of their health information
- Request amendment of records (meaning to fix incorrect information, but not to change or delete items because the patient does not agree with the data)
- Receive communications from providers through an alternate means, such as in a closed envelope rather than on a postcard
- File a complaint about a violation with the organization or with the Office for Civil Rights (OCR) in the Department of Health and Human Services
- Request restrictions on uses or disclosures of their PHI

In addition, the HITECH Act contains these new provisions:

- **Accounting of disclosures** Individuals are permitted to ask for an accounting of the disclosures of their electronic PHI, including TPO, over the preceding three years. Previously, individuals could request an accounting over the preceding six years, but TPO was not part of the disclosures.

- **Restricting access to some PHI** When an individual asks a covered entity to not release PHI to a health plan for purposes of carrying out payment or health care operations (not for treatment purposes), and the individual has paid the provider in full for the out-of-pocket expenses associated with the service, the covered entity must comply with the patient's request to restrict release of the PHI. This is a change to the previous HIPAA rule, under which a covered entity was permitted to deny the patient's request.

2.4 HIPAA Security Rule

HIPAA Security Rule law that requires covered entities to establish administrative, physical, and technical safeguards to protect the confidentiality, integrity, and availability of health information

electronic protected health information (ePHI) PHI that is created, received, maintained, or transmitted in electronic form

The **HIPAA Security Rule,** the second part of the Administrative Simplification provisions, was enacted in 2005 specifically to protect health information on computer networks, the Internet, and electronic storage media. The security requirements indicate the administrative, technical, and physical safeguards that are required to protect the privacy of patients' electronic health information against unintended disclosure through breach of security.

While the HIPAA Privacy Rule requires covered entities to protect PHI in any form—paper, electronic, or otherwise—the HIPAA Security Rule focuses specifically on electronic health information. **Electronic protected health information (ePHI)** is PHI that is created, received, maintained, or transmitted in electronic form. The regulations apply to information stored on physical devices such as computers, USB flash drives, CDs, and magnetic tapes as well as to information located on computer networks or sent or received over the Internet.

The goals of the HIPAA security standards (see Figure 2.4) are to ensure:

- The confidentiality of ePHI, so that the information is shared only among authorized individuals or organizations
- The integrity of ePHI, so that the information is not changed in any way during storage or transmission and that it is authentic and complete and can be relied on to be sufficiently accurate for its purpose
- The availability of ePHI, so that the systems responsible for delivering, storing, and processing data are accessible when needed in both routine and emergency situations

Figure 2.4 Security Goals

The HIPAA security standards do not state specific actions that covered entities must take to protect ePHI. The rule is intentionally flexible, recognizing that security policies and procedures vary according to the size of the organization and the nature of the work performed. For example, the policies and procedures required in a two-physician practice are different from those needed in a large city hospital. Each covered entity must determine which security measures and specific technologies are reasonable and appropriate for implementation in its organization.

The security standards contain requirements for three types of safeguards to prevent security breaches: administrative, physical, and technical.

Administrative Safeguards

Administrative safeguards are the administrative actions that a covered entity must perform, or train staff to do, to carry out security requirements. These actions include implementing office policies and procedures to prevent, detect, contain, and correct security violations. The management of security is assigned to one individual who conducts a risk assessment of the current level of data security. Once that assessment is complete, security policies and procedures are developed or modified to meet current needs.

Examples of administrative safeguards include the creation of a sanction policy that states the consequences of violations of security policies and procedures by employees, agents, and contractors; a backup plan for recovering from a security incident that jeopardizes critical data; a disaster recovery plan; and an emergency mode operation plan. Security training is provided to educate staff members on the policies and to raise awareness of security and privacy issues.

Physical Safeguards

Physical safeguards are mechanisms to protect electronic systems, equipment, and data from threats, environmental hazards, and unauthorized intrusion. These include devices that limit physical access to facilities housing protected information, such as reinforced doors, locks, and identification badge readers. Physical security also includes maintaining appropriate controls of files that are retained, stored, or scheduled for destruction.

Technical Safeguards

Technical safeguards are the technology and related policies and procedures used to protect electronic data and control access to it. They include the use of firewalls, intrusion detection systems, access control, and antivirus software.

Firewalls

A firewall examines traffic entering and leaving a computer network, using defined rules to determine whether to allow it to continue toward its destination. Packet filtering is a process in which a firewall examines each piece of information traveling into or out of the network. The firewall acts as a gatekeeper, deciding who has legitimate access to a network and what data should be allowed in and out. Firewalls can log attempted intrusions and report them to appropriate security personnel.

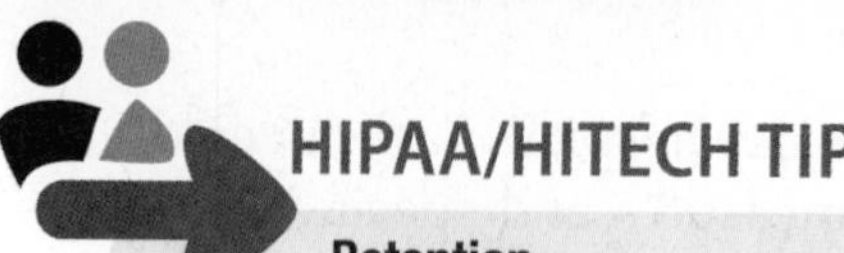

HIPAA/HITECH TIP

Retention

According to the American Health Information Management Association (AHIMA), transactional and billing records must be retained for at least ten years. Medical histories should be retained indefinitely.

Intrusion Detection Systems

An intrusion detection system (IDS) provides constant surveillance of the network. Unlike a firewall, an IDS monitors and analyzes packet data streams, searching for unauthorized activity. If such activity is suspected, the suspicious user's access to the network is immediately terminated.

Access Control

User authentication procedures are necessary to confirm the claimed identity of all users who access the data. In this context, authentication confirms that the user is the person he or she claims to be. In contrast, authorization is the process of determining whether an identified individual has been granted access rights to information. Authorization procedures are necessary to ensure that only appropriate users view the information.

Passwords are specific codes that are required for gaining access to information on a computer or network. The code is known by the user, but it is not known to others. This very basic user authentication system is used in most health care organizations, since it is easy to implement. Used successfully, a password utilization program can keep unauthorized users from successfully logging onto a system or network. Password logging programs can track all successful and failed log-in attempts, which can be useful in detecting possible break-in attempts.

Much more sophisticated systems, including biometric methods, are being used to identify individuals who gain entry to the information. Biometric devices use some measurable feature of an individual to authenticate the person's identity. They can use such physical characteristics as fingerprints, facial features, or retinal patterns to confirm identity. Because they are based on unique physical characteristics, they cannot be forged, stolen, or duplicated.

Role-based authorization limits access to patient information based on the user's role in an organization. Once access rights have been assigned, each user is given a key to the designated databases. The user must enter an ID and a key to see files to which he or she has been granted access rights. Role-based authorization meets the HIPAA standard of releasing only the minimum amount of information necessary to provide care. In a medical office, for example, a billing specialist requires access to more areas in an electronic health record than does a medical assistant. Technology permits the system to prevent the user from viewing or modifying any part of the record that is not directly related to his or her job.

THINKING IT THROUGH 2.4

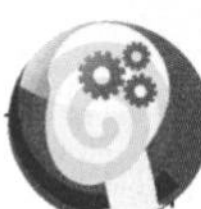

A medical assistant at a small medical practice took home an office laptop to work on one of the office's brochures over the weekend. The laptop, which contained clinical and billing information for the practice, was left unattended at a coffee shop and was stolen. Both the clinical data and the billing database were protected by passwords. An encryption program was also used to protect the data. What types of safeguards do these represent? Do you think these security methods will be enough to block a breach in the patients' information? Do you think it was a good idea for the medical assistant to take the laptop home?

Encryption is the process of converting data into an unreadable format before it is distributed. To read a message, the recipient must have a key that deciphers the information. For example, encryption can protect the privacy of restricted data that are stored on a laptop computer even if the computer is stolen. Similarly, it can protect data that are transmitted over a network even if that network is accessed by an unauthorized third party. These techniques also make it possible to determine whether the information has been altered in any way.

encryption process of converting electronic information into an unreadable format before it is distributed

breach under the HIPAA Privacy Rule, impermissible use or disclosure that compromises the security or privacy of PHI that could pose a significant risk of financial, reputational, or other harm to the affected person

Audit trails are records that show who has accessed a computer or a network and what operations were performed. At a minimum, an audit trail should contain the following information:

- Type of event
- Date and time of occurrence
- User ID associated with the event
- Program, command, or method used to initiate the event
- Patient and data elements that were changed

The log is reviewed on a regular basis to detect irregularities. If an error or a suspicious entry has been made, the program lists the name of the person and the date the information was entered.

Antivirus Software

Antivirus software scans a system for known viruses. After detection, the software attempts to remove the virus from the system and, in some cases, fix any problems the virus created. Antivirus tools cannot detect and eliminate all viruses. New viruses are continually being developed, and antivirus software must be regularly updated to maintain its effectiveness.

2.5 HITECH Breach Notification Rule

The HITECH Act includes new security breach notification requirements with regard to PHI. Previously, HIPAA did not require covered entities to inform individuals when a breach occurred. Under HITECH, HHS has directed health care providers, health plans, and other HIPAA-covered entities to notify affected individuals following the discovery of a breach of unsecured health information.

A **breach** is an impermissible use or disclosure under the Privacy Rule that compromises the security or privacy of PHI in a way that could pose a significant risk of financial, reputational, or other harm to the affected person. If such a breach occurs, the covered entity must follow breach notification procedures. Covered entities and their business associates are also responsible for determining whether a breach has occurred to which the notification obligations under the act and its implementing regulations apply. The enforcement date for the breach notification rule was February 2010.

Guidance on Securing PHI

The HITECH Act refers to unsecured PHI as unprotected health information that is not secured through the use of specified technologies or methods that make PHI unusable, unreadable, or indecipherable to unauthorized individuals. HHS has released guidance on technologies and methods that can be used to render PHI unusable, unreadable, or indecipherable, calling for methods that either encrypt or destroy the data and explaining which methods are acceptable. If PHI has not been secured through one or more of these methods and there is a breach, a covered entity is required to follow the provision's breach notification procedures.

If paper or electronic PHI is to be destroyed, proper methods used to destroy the information include the following:

- Shredding, burning, pulping, or pulverizing paper, film, or other hard-copy records so that PHI is rendered essentially unreadable and indecipherable and otherwise cannot be reconstructed
- Maintaining labeled prescription bottles and other PHI in opaque bags in a secure area and using a disposal vendor as a business associate to pick up and shred or otherwise destroy the PHI
- For PHI on electronic media, clearing (using software or hardware products to overwrite media with nonsensitive data), purging (degaussing: exposing the media to a strong magnetic field in order to disrupt the recorded magnetic domains), or destroying the media (disintegrating, pulverizing, melting, incinerating, or shredding)

Although covered entities are not required to follow the guidance on acceptable methods, if the encryption and destruction methods specified in the guidance are used to secure data, covered entities may be exempt from the breach notification requirements for breaches of the data. In addition, the rule notes several exceptions to the definition of *breach*, including certain good-faith uses and disclosures among a company's workforce members, as long as the private information is not further acquired, accessed, used, or disclosed without authorization.

Breach Notification Procedures

Following the discovery of a breach of unsecured PHI, a covered entity must notify each individual whose unsecured PHI has been, or is reasonably believed to have been, inappropriately accessed, acquired, or disclosed. Following the discovery of a breach by a

THINKING IT THROUGH 2.5

- The breach notification rule states "if there is no significant risk of harm to the individual, then no breach has occurred, and no notification is required." If PHI from a medical office is inadvertently disclosed to the wrong business associate (for instance, if a list of patients with overdue account information is sent to the wrong medical billing vendor) and the vendor informs you of the mistake, has a breach occurred?
- Review the HITECH specifications above regarding breaches and business associates. If a business associate causes a breach, who is responsible for notifying the individuals affected?

business associate, the business associate must notify the covered entity of the breach and of the identity of the individuals whose unsecured PHI has been, or is reasonably believed to have been, breached. The act requires the notifications to be made without unreasonable delay, but in no case later than sixty calendar days after discovery of the breach. An exception may be made to the deadline only when a law enforcement official determines that notification would impede a criminal investigation or cause damage to national security.

HITECH specifies the following:

- Notice to patients of breaches "without reasonable delay" within sixty days
- Notice to covered entities by business associates when the business associates discover a breach
- Notice to "prominent media outlets" on breaches involving more than five hundred individuals
- Notice to "next of kin" on breaches involving patients who are deceased
- Notice to the secretary of HHS about breaches involving five hundred or more individuals without reasonable delay
- Annual notice to the secretary of HHS about breaches of "unsecured PHI" involving fewer than five hundred individuals that pose a significant financial risk or other harm to the individuals, such as to their reputations

The document notifying an individual of a breach, called the **breach notification,** must include (1) a brief description of what happened, including the date of the breach and the date of the discovery of the breach, if known; (2) a description of the types of unsecured PHI that were involved in the breach (such as full name, Social Security number, date of birth, home address, account number, or disability code); (3) the steps individuals should take to protect themselves from potential harm resulting from the breach; (4) a brief description of what the covered entity is doing to investigate the breach, to mitigate losses, and to protect against further breaches; and (5) contact procedures for individuals who have questions or want additional information, including a toll-free telephone number, an e-mail address, a website, or a postal address.

breach notification document used by a covered entity to notify individuals of a breach in their PHI required under the new HITECH breach notification rules

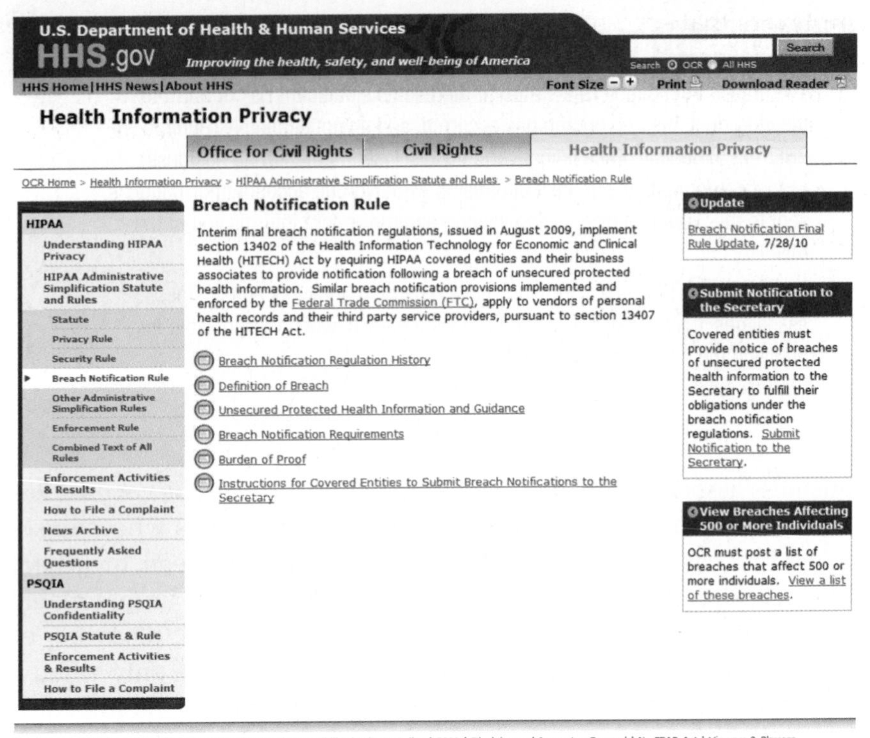

Figure 2.5 Breach Notification Rule Home Page

The prescribed forms for breach notification are available on the HHS website, as shown in Figure 2.5.

In addition, the rule requires the secretary of HHS to annually prepare and submit to Congress a report regarding the breaches about which the secretary was notified and all enforcement actions taken. This means that a covered entity must maintain a log of breaches involving fewer than five hundred individuals and submit it to HHS annually. HHS must post the report on the HHS public website. It is hoped that the negative publicity of public posting will act as a deterrent, offering greater incentives for covered entities and business associates to prevent breaches.

2.6 HIPAA Electronic Health Care Transactions, and Code Sets, and National Identifiers

HIPAA Electronic Health Care Transactions and Code Sets (TCS) the HIPAA rule governing the electronic exchange of health information

The **HIPAA Electronic Health Care Transactions and Code Sets (TCS)** standards, the third part of the Administrative Simplification provisions, went into effect in 2003. These standards apply to electronic formats, code sets, and identifiers.

All providers who do business electronically are required to use the same electronic formats for health care transactions and the same code sets for diagnoses, procedures, and supplies. Likewise, the HIPAA Employer Identifier and the National Provider Identifier standards mandate the use of certain identifying numbers by employers that sponsor health plans and by providers. The goal of the standards is to increase the efficiency of conducting business in health care. When these standards are fully implemented in the health care industry, exchange of information will be faster, more efficient, and more accurate.

Almost all members of the medical administrative team work with electronic transactions such as health care claims and insurance verification. They use the diagnosis and procedure codes to communicate the reason for patient services; these codes are studied to improve health care. An understanding of the different standards and of the changes to them over time is an important part of any allied health employee's job.

Standard Transactions

HIPAA transactions include the electronic data that are regularly sent back and forth between providers, health plans, and employers. Examples include electronic claims, payments, and the forms used to verify patients' insurance coverage. Each form is labeled with a number and a name. Either the number (such as "the 837") or the name (such as "the HIPAA Claim") may be used to refer to the particular electronic document format. Table 2.2 shows the complete list of transaction standards.

In addition to those listed in Table 2.2, HIPAA mandates two standards for use in the future: (1) Additional Information to Support a Health Care Claim or Encounter (to be used for claim attachments such as clinical reports and laboratory test results), and (2) First Report of Injury (for workers' compensation cases).

ASC X12 Version 4010

All electronic data interchanges use one of a number of electronic data standards for transmitting data. The data standard used for HIPAA transactions is known as ASC X12 Version 4010. The standard prescribes the character sets and data elements used in the exchange of documents and also provides the rules for the structure of the documents.

TABLE 2.2 HIPAA Electronic Transaction Standards

Number	Official Name
X12 837	Health Care Claims or Equivalent Encounter Information/Coordination of Benefits (*coordination of benefits* refers to an exchange of information between payers when a patient has more than one health plan)
X12 276/277	Health Care Claim Status Inquiry/Response
X12 270/271	Eligibility for a Health Plan Inquiry/Response
X12 278	Referral Certification and Authorization
X12 835	Health Care Payment and Remittance Advice
X12 820	Health Plan Premium Payments
X12 834	Health Plan Enrollment and Disenrollment

The American National Standards Institute (ANSI) is the organization that sets standards for electronic data interchange on a national level. The Accredited Standards Committee X12, Insurance Subcommittee (ASC X12N), is the ANSI-accredited organization that develops and maintains the administrative and financial electronic transactions standards adopted under HIPAA. The standards released by this subcommittee are referred to as the X12 standards. The current version of these standards mandated for HIPAA transactions is Version 4010 (Version 4, release 1).

ASC X12 Version 5010

When significant changes are required in data transactions—for example, in the way they are structured or in the data elements they contain—a new ASC X12 version is created. ASC X12 Version 4010 was created to accommodate the date changes from the year 1999 to 2000.

At present, ASC X12 Version 4010 is being replaced by **ASC X12 Version 5010** (Version 5, release 1). The compliance date for implementing Version 5010 is January 1, 2012. Version 5010 has structural, front matter, technical, and data content improvements. It includes updated standards for claims, remittance advices, eligibility inquiries, referral authorizations, and other administrative transactions. The updated standards are more specific in requiring the data that are needed, collected, and transmitted. Version 5010 also addresses changing requirements, such as providing an indicator for conditions that were "present on admission" on hospital claims. In addition, it accommodates the use of two new code sets for reporting health care diagnoses and inpatient procedures, discussed in the next section, that are not supported by Version 4010.

ASC X12 Version 5010 updated electronic data standard for transmitting HIPAA X12 documents, such as the HIPAA claim (X12 837), that replaces ASC X12 Version 4010 beginning in January 2012

code set alphabetic and/or numeric representations for data; a medical code set is a system of medical terms required for HIPAA transactions

BILLING TIP

Moving to Version 5010

IT vendors who support the practice's PM/EHR programs are responsible for verifying that all systems work properly under changing transmission requirements.

Standard Code Sets

HIPAA requires every provider who does business electronically to use the same code sets. Under HIPAA, a **code set** is a group of codes used for encoding data elements, such as tables of terms, medical concepts, medical diagnosis codes, and medical procedure codes. In the health care industry, there are medical code sets for diseases, for treatments and procedures, and for supplies or other items used to perform treatments and procedures. The standard code sets are listed in Table 2.3. Code sets are covered in detail in Chapter 7.

ICD-9-CM (Volumes 1 and 2): Codes for Diseases

Scientists and medical researchers have long gathered information from medical records about patients' illnesses and causes of death. To facilitate the data-gathering process, standardized codes have been developed to replace written descriptions of symptoms and conditions. The use of these standardized codes provides an accurate way to collect statistics to keep people healthy and to plan for needed health care resources as well as to record morbidity (disease) and mortality (death) data.

The diagnosis codes used in the United States are based on the *International Classification of Diseases* (ICD). The U.S. version of the

TABLE 2.3 HIPAA Standard Code Sets	
Purpose	**Standard**
Codes for diseases, injuries, impairments, and other health-related problems	*International Classification of Diseases*, Ninth Revision, *Clinical Modification* (ICD-9-CM), Volumes 1 and 2 (until ICD-10-CM mandate for October 1, 2013)
Codes for procedures or other actions taken to prevent, diagnose, treat, or manage diseases, injuries, and impairments	Physician services: *Current Procedural Terminology* (CPT) Inpatient hospital services: *International Classification of Diseases*, Ninth Revision, *Clinical Modification*, Volume 3: *Procedures* (until ICD-10-PCS mandate for October 1, 2013)
Codes for other medical services	Healthcare Common Procedures Coding System (HCPCS)
Codes for dental services	*Current Dental Terminology* (CDT-4)

ninth revision of ICD (ICD-9), published in 1979, is called *ICD-9 Clinical Modification, or ICD-9-CM*. An ICD-9-CM diagnosis code has three, four, or five digits plus a description. The system is built on categories for diseases, injuries, and symptoms.

EXAMPLE

415.1 Pulmonary embolism and infarction (four digits)

CPT Level 1: Codes for Physician Procedures and Services

CPT Level I codes, usually referred to simply as *CPT codes*, list the procedures and services that are commonly performed by physicians across the country. These codes, which are developed and maintained by the American Medical Association (AMA), provide a standard method of communicating treatment services among doctors, insurance companies, and patients. Medical procedures are grouped into six sections, and each section is assigned a numeric range. Procedures are then assigned five-digit codes within that range.

Sample CPT Sections	Code Range
Anesthesia	00100–01999
Radiology	70010–79999

Sample CPT Codes

00730	Anesthesia for procedures on upper posterior abdominal wall
70100	Radiologic examination of the mandible

HCPCS Level II

The Healthcare Common Procedure Coding System (HCPCS), Level II, was set up to describe specific products, supplies, and services that patients receive that are not in CPT. In the early 1980s, the use of

HCPCS codes for claims was optional. With the implementation of HIPAA in 1996, HCPCS became mandatory.

A HCPCS code has five characters; it begins with a letter and is followed by four numbers. Each of the more than twenty sections of codes covers a related group of items. For example, the E section covers durable medical equipment—reusable medical equipment ordered by physicians for patients' use at home, such as walkers and wheelchairs.

Sample HCPCS Sections	Code Range
Medical and Surgical Supplies	A4000–A8999
Durable Medical Equipment (DME)	E0100–E9999

Sample HCPCS Codes

A4215	Needle, sterile, any size, each
E1221	Wheelchair with fixed arm, footrests

ICD-10-CM and ICD-10-PCS

In January 2009, HHS issued the ICD-10 final rule to replace the ICD-9-CM code set now in use with the greatly expanded ICD-10 code set. On October 1, 2013, ICD-10-CM and ICD-10-PCS will replace the original HIPAA standards for reporting diagnoses (ICD-9-CM, Volumes 1 and 2) and inpatient hospital procedures (ICD-9-CM, Volume 3), which were developed nearly thirty years ago.

The ICD-10-CM code set is maintained by the National Center for Health Statistics (NCHS) of the Centers for Disease Control and Prevention (CDC) for use in the United States. It is based on ICD-10, which was developed by the World Health Organization (WHO) and is used internationally. The new code set for inpatient hospital procedures (ICD-10-PCS) is maintained by CMS.

HIPAA National Identifiers

HIPAA National Identifiers HIPAA-mandated identification systems for employers, health care providers, health plans, and patients; national provider system and employer system are in place; health plan and patient systems have not been created

The HIPAA National Identifier standards mandate using certain identifying numbers in HIPAA transactions. There are **HIPAA National Identifiers** for employers, health care providers, health plans, and patients.

Identifiers are numbers of predetermined length and structure, such as Social Security numbers. They are important because the unique numbers can be used in electronic transactions. The new unique numbers can replace the many numbers that are currently used. Two identifiers have been set up—for employers and for providers—and two are to be established in the future—for patients and for health plans.

Employer Identification Number

The *Employer Identification Number (EIN)* issued by the Internal Revenue Service has been the HIPAA standard for the identification of employers in electronic transactions since July 30, 2002. The EIN is used when employers enroll or disenroll employees in a health plan (X12 834) or make premium payments to plans on behalf of their employees (X12 820).

THINKING IT THROUGH 2.6

Review the HIPAA Electronic Transaction Standards in Table 2.2 on page 73. Notice that two of the transactions have two numbers in the transaction names. Which transactions are these? What is the purpose of the two numbers?

National Provider Identifier

The **National Provider Identifier (NPI)** is the standard for the identification of providers when filing claims and other transactions. The NPI replaced other identifying numbers that were in use, such as the UPIN for Medicare and the numbers assigned by each payer to the provider, on May 23, 2008. The older numbers are known as *legacy numbers*.

The NPI has nine numbers and a check digit, for a total of ten numbers. The numbers are assigned by the federal government to individual providers, such as physicians, nurses, and pharmacists, and also to provider organizations such as hospitals, clinics, and pharmacies. CMS maintains the NPIs as they are assigned in the NPPES (National Plan and Provider Enumerator System), a database of all assigned numbers. Once assigned, an NPI will not change; it remains with the provider regardless of job or location changes.

All health care providers who transmit health information electronically must obtain NPIs, even if they use business associates to prepare the transactions. Most health plans, including Medicare, Medicaid, and private payers, and all clearinghouses must accept and use NPIs in HIPAA transactions. This includes small plans as well as larger ones.

National Provider Identifier (NPI) under HIPAA, system for identifying all health care providers using unique ten-digit identifiers

BILLING TIP

Physician and Group NPIs

If a physician is in a group practice, both the individual doctor and the group have NPIs.

2.7 Threats to Privacy and Security

As health information migrates from paper systems to computer systems and electronic networks, the threats to protected health information multiply. Instead of limiting access to office personnel only, electronic networks provide hundreds or even thousands of access points. The threats to information security come from a number of sources, including natural disasters and insufficient security in computer systems, as well as individuals' intentions to cause harm. Common threats include:

- Utility failures such as electrical power outages
- Natural disasters such as hurricanes, floods, fires, and earthquakes
- Problems with computer systems and software, such as insufficient security in the hardware or software, programming errors, changes to existing software including upgrades, and the addition of new users to the system
- Malware—any program that harms information systems, which is often brought into an organization through e-mail attachments or programs that are downloaded from the Internet (see Table 2.4)

TABLE 2.4	Types of Malware
Viruses	A virus self-replicates by inserting copies of itself into host programs or data files. Viruses are often triggered through user interaction, such as opening a file or running a program.
Worms	A worm is a self-replicating, self-contained program that usually executes itself without user intervention.
Trojan Horses	A Trojan horse is a self-contained, nonreplicating program that, while appearing to be benign, actually has a hidden malicious purpose. Trojan horses either replace existing files with malicious versions or add new malicious files to systems. They often deliver other attacker tools to systems.
Malicious Mobile Code	Malicious mobile code is software with malicious intent that is transmitted from a remote system to a local system and then executed on the local system, typically without the user's explicit instruction.
Blended Attacks	A blended attack uses multiple infection or transmission methods. For example, a blended attack could combine the propagation methods of viruses and worms.
Tracking Cookies	A tracking cookie is a persistent cookie that is accessed by many websites, allowing a third party to create a profile of a user's behavior. Tracking cookies are often used in conjunction with web bugs, which are tiny graphics on websites that are referenced within the HTML content of a webpage or e-mail. The only purpose of the graphic is to collect information about the user viewing the content.
Attacker Tools	Various types of attacker tools might be delivered to a system as part of a malware infection or other system compromise. These tools allow attackers to have unauthorized access to or use of infected systems and their data, or to launch additional attacks.
Non-malware Threats	These are often associated with malware. Phishing uses computer-based means to trick users into revealing financial information and other sensitive data. Phishing attacks frequently place malware or attacker tools on systems.

- Identity theft
- Subversive employees or contractors
- Outsiders who try to damage or steal information, otherwise known as computer hackers

Threats in Connection with EHRs

While a nationwide health information network in which each person has an electronic health record would bring many benefits—such as the increased use of information technology to cut costs, improve patient safety, and provide the best possible care—a large network also places large amounts of protected health information at greater risk. The use of portable computing and storage devices for moving the data from place to place adds to this risk.

Sharing Clinical Data Through Networks

More personal health information is being created, accessed, and maintained on computers than ever before. In an electronic health record system, personal health information is entered and stored in a computer database. The database then connects to other databases in health information networks, making it possible to share information with authorized providers, hospitals, pharmacies, laboratories, and others. The larger the network, the greater the risk, so while a health information network brings the most benefits, it also presents the greatest privacy and security challenges.

Portable Computers and Storage Devices

In the past, personal health information did not commonly leave a physician office or hospital facility. Desktop computers, bulky paper files, and large backup tapes made it difficult to move data from one place to another. In large part, the locks on office doors were safeguards against intruders.

Today, hardware and data are portable and leave medical offices and hospital buildings regularly, increasing the possibility that they will be lost or stolen. One of the benefits of electronic health records is being able to access information when and where it is needed. Many health care professionals use laptop computers, personal digital assistants (PDAs), and smart cell phones to access and store data. Laptops are popular because they can be moved from one location to another, such as from a physician's desk to an examining room. It is not uncommon for employees to carry laptops to and from work.

USB flash drives and other removable storage devices are smaller and are increasingly less expensive. They function like hard drives, and people require little instruction in using them to store data. Such small storage devices, including CDs and DVDs, easily fit in a briefcase. Although the portability of electronic data offers many benefits, the widespread use of portable hardware and small storage devices makes it more difficult to control access to a person's health information.

HITECH Provisions: Addressing Inadequacies in Privacy Standards

HIPAA is not a universal law; that is, it does not apply to every person or organization. It was designed to provide protection for personal health information that was exchanged by certain groups and individuals in certain electronic transactions. Since HIPAA was enacted in 1996, the field of health information technology has changed dramatically. Increasingly, an individual's personal health information is accessed, maintained, and exchanged by groups that may not be covered under current HIPAA privacy laws. The HITECH Act, enacted as part of the American Recovery and Reinvestment Act of 2009, tries to address this inadequacy in a number of ways. One way is by making business associates subject to the same privacy and security requirements as covered entities. Before the HITECH Act, only covered entities could be penalized for violations of the Privacy and Security Rules. Under HITECH, a much wider range of businesses must comply.

Overseas Business Associates

Overseas companies in India and other countries currently provide services to health care providers and organizations in the United States, including coding, transcription processing, and claim management. Some of these tasks cannot be completed without access to protected health information. Some companies in developing countries lack security systems that protect sensitive health data. Previously, offshore vendors did not have to comply directly with HIPAA security and privacy legislation. However, under HITECH, an overseas vendor that signs a business associate agreement with a U.S. covered entity is now required to abide by HIPAA.

Personal Health Records

Many different organizations, including employers, health plans, and providers, offer personal health records (PHRs) to individuals. Companies including Walmart, Intel, BP, Pitney Bowes, and Allied Materials have joined together to provide personal health record systems for their 2.5 million employees. Commercial software vendors are offering PHRs to individuals at no charge or for a fee. Previously, as business associates, PHR vendors were not directly required to comply with HIPAA. As a result, many of the PHRs offered were not covered by the Privacy Rule, leaving protected health information subject to release without a patient's consent or authorization.

Under HITECH, as business associates, PHR vendors and third-party partners supporting PHR hosting or management are now required to comply with the HIPAA Privacy and Security Rules, as well as with the new breach notification rules. Vendors using PHRs must notify patients and the Federal Trade Commission (FTC) of any breach caused by their products and services. The FTC is required to publish notification requirements for PHR vendors and third-party providers and to inform HHS if it is notified of a breach.

Private Sector Electronic Networks

While the federal government continues its work on developing a strategy for the creation of a national health information network (NHIN), businesses and organizations in the private sector (not associated with the government) have created new models of health information networks for sharing information. For example, health information exchanges (HIEs) have been created at the state, regional, and community levels. A health information exchange enables health care information to be exchanged electronically across organizations and retain its meaning. A regional health information organization (RHIO) is a type of HIE in which a group of health care entities in a geographic area exchange health information over an electronic network for the purpose of improving the delivery of health care. Participants may include health care providers, clinics, hospitals, laboratories, pharmacies, health plans, mental health agencies, and local health departments.

Previously, while some of these providers, such as health care providers and health plans, were subject to HIPAA privacy laws, the overall organizations were not. Under HITECH, organizations such

THINKING IT THROUGH 2.7

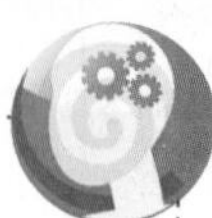

Health plans, employers, and the government are encouraging patients to create personal health records (PHRs). If a provider is using an EHR system, a patient can ask the provider to send data to his or her PHR. Because patients control the data in their PHRs, depending on the PHRs used, they may be able to add to or delete physician or hospital data. Why do you think physicians are advocating for safeguards to be added to PHRs so that patients cannot alter the information?

as HIEs and RHIOs that provide data transmission of PHI and require access to that information are now categorized as business associates and are therefore required to comply with HIPAA Privacy and Security Rules. Also, business agreements need to be executed between RHIO or HIE participants and the organization managing the RHIO or HIE.

2.8 Fraud and Abuse Regulations

Almost everyone involved in the delivery of health care is trustworthy and is devoted to patients' welfare. However, some people are not. Health care fraud and abuse laws help control cheating in the health care system. Are the laws really necessary? The evidence says that they are. During 2008, the federal government recovered an estimated $4.4 billion in fraud-related judgments and settlements. This loss directly affects patients, taxpayers, and government through higher health care costs, insurance premiums, and taxes. Health care fraud also may hurt patients, possibly subjecting some of them to unnecessary or unsafe procedures or making them victims of identity theft. Allied health employees are trained to be alert for health care fraud and abuse and to know which agencies are responsible for watching for them and acting when they are suspected.

The Health Care Fraud and Abuse Control Program

HIPAA created the **Health Care Fraud and Abuse Control Program** to uncover and prosecute fraud and abuse. The HHS Office of the Inspector General (OIG) has the task of detecting health care fraud and abuse and enforcing all laws relating to them. OIG works with the U.S. Department of Justice (DOJ), which includes the Federal Bureau of Investigation (FBI), under the direction of the U.S. attorney general to prosecute those suspected of medical fraud and abuse.

Health Care Fraud and Abuse Control Program government program to uncover misuse of funds in federal health care programs run by the Office of the Inspector General

Federal False Claims Act and State Laws

The federal False Claims Act (FCA, 31 USC § 3729) prohibits submitting a fraudulent claim or making a false statement or representation in connection with a claim. It also encourages reporting suspected fraud and abuse by protecting and rewarding people involved in *qui tam* (whistleblower) cases. The person who makes the accusation of suspected fraud is called the *relator*. Relators are generally current or former employees of insurance companies or

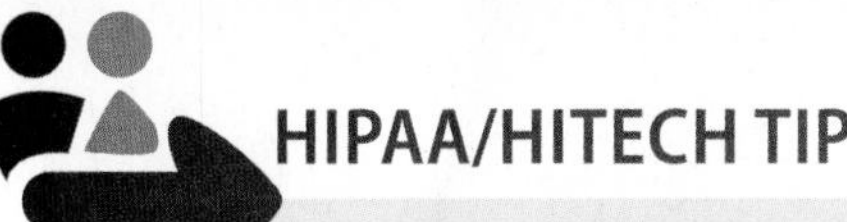

HIPAA/HITECH TIP

Extending Federal Laws to Private Payers

HIPAA created a new category of crimes that apply to billing transactions with private payers in addition to Medicare and Medicaid billing. These offenses include health care fraud, making false statements, theft and embezzlement, obstruction of criminal investigations, and money laundering.

medical practices, program beneficiaries, and independent contractors. Under the law, the relator is protected against employer retaliation. If the fraud investigation results in the payment of a fine to the federal government, the whistleblower may be entitled to 15 to 25 percent of the amount paid.

At present, twenty states also have passed versions of the federal False Claims Act. These laws allow private individuals to bring actions alone or to work with state attorneys general against any person who knowingly causes the state to pay a false claim. The state laws generally provide for civil penalties and damages related to the cost of any losses sustained because of the false claim.

OIG Enforcement Actions for Fraud, False Claims, and Substandard Care: Case Examples

Seven Miami-area residents were sentenced in a Medicare infusion fraud scheme. The employees, who worked at an infusion clinic, were ordered to pay $19.8 million in restitution and were sentenced to prison terms ranging from thirty-seven to ninety-seven months. In their guilty pleas, they admitted to activities including manipulating patients' blood samples to generate false medical records, ordering and administering medications to treat conditions that were falsely documented with fraudulent test results, and billing Medicare for services that were medically unnecessary or never provided.

Pfizer Inc. entered into a $1 billion civil False Claims Act settlement with the United States in connection with marketing and promotion practices associated with the anti-inflammatory drug Bextra and several other drugs. The settlement agreement includes a comprehensive five-year corporate integrity agreement between Pfizer and OIG. Pfizer and its subsidiary Pharmacia & Upjohn agreed to pay a total of $2.3 billion in this case, the largest health care fraud settlement in history, to resolve both the civil and criminal liability arising from the illegal promotion of certain pharmaceutical products.

Emmanuel Bernabe, the president and board chair of Pleasant Care Corporation, agreed to be permanently excluded from federal health care programs following an investigation of substandard care at nursing homes formerly operated by the corporation. OIG alleged that Bernabe, through his management and oversight of Pleasant Care, caused services to be furnished to Pleasant Care residents that substantially departed from the professional standard of care. For example, Pleasant Care failed to maintain adequate staffing levels, properly administer medication, provide adequate hydration and nutrition, and prevent accidents.

Additional Laws

Additional laws relating to health care fraud and abuse control include:

- An antikickback statute that makes it illegal to knowingly offer incentives to induce referrals for services that are paid for by government health care programs. Many financial actions are considered to be illegal incentives, including direct payments to other physicians and routine waivers of coinsurance and deductibles.
- Self-referral prohibitions (called Stark rules) that make it illegal for physicians or members of their immediate families to have financial relationships with clinics to which they refer their patients, such as radiology service clinics and clinical laboratories. (Note that there are many legal exceptions to this prohibition under various business structures.)
- The Sarbanes-Oxley Act of 2002 that requires publicly traded corporations to attest that their financial management is sound. These provisions apply to for-profit health care companies. The act includes whistleblower protection so that employees can report wrongdoing without fear of retaliation.

Definition of Fraud and Abuse

fraud intentional act of deception to take financial advantage of another person

abuse actions that improperly use another person's resources

Fraud is an act of deception undertaken with the intention of taking financial advantage of another person. Fraudulent acts are intentional; the individual expects an illegal or unauthorized benefit to result. For example, misrepresenting professional credentials and forging another person's signature on a check are fraudulent. Pretending to be a physician and treating patients without a valid medical license is also fraudulent.

Claims fraud occurs when health care providers or others falsely report charges to payers. A provider may bill for services that were not performed, overcharge for services, or fail to provide complete services under a contract. A patient may exaggerate an injury to get a settlement from an insurance company or may ask a medical insurance specialist to change a date on a chart so that a service is covered by a health plan.

In federal law, **abuse** is an action that misuses money that the government has allocated, such as Medicare funds. Abuse is illegal because taxpayers' dollars are misspent. An example of abuse is an ambulance service that billed Medicare for transporting a patient to the hospital when the patient did not need ambulance service. This abuse—billing for services that were not medically necessary—resulted in improper payment of the ambulance company. Abuse is not necessarily intentional. It may be the result of ignorance of a billing rule or of inaccurate coding.

Examples of Fraudulent and Abusive Acts

A number of billing practices are fraudulent or abusive. Investigators reviewing physicians' billing work look for patterns like these:

- Intentionally billing for services that were not performed or documented

EXAMPLES

A lab bills Medicare for two tests when only one was done.
A physician asks a coder to report a physical examination when the physician actually talked to the patient on the telephone.

- Reporting services at a higher level than was carried out

EXAMPLE

After a patient visit for a flu shot, the provider bills the encounter as a comprehensive physical examination plus a vaccination.

- Performing and billing for procedures that are not related to the patient's condition and therefore are not medically necessary

EXAMPLE

After reading an article about Lyme disease, a patient is worried about having worked in her garden over the summer, and she requests a Lyme disease diagnostic test. Although no symptoms or signs have been reported, the physician orders and bills for the *Borrelia burgdorferi* (Lyme disease) confirmatory immunoblot test.

Medicaid Fraud: A Case Example

Keven Wayne Louderback, a Springfield insurance broker, pleaded guilty to twelve felony counts related to Medicaid fraud. (Medicaid is the federal/state health insurance program for low-income beneficiaries.) According to Missouri Attorney General Chris Koster, Louderback misappropriated more than $700,000 from Medicaid by furnishing applications with false information to a Missouri Medicaid program that pays for private health insurance premiums for certain individuals with high medical costs. Louderback represented the monthly insurance premium rates as greater than they actually were and pocketed the overpayment. He also offered kickbacks to get people to enroll in an insurance program, fraudulently misstated an insurance company's rate, and forged documents to set out the false rate. Louderback pleaded guilty to five counts of Medicaid fraud, one count of offering a kickback to receive a Medicaid payment, four counts of insurance fraud, and two counts of forgery.

BILLING TIP

Fraud Versus Abuse

To bill when the task was not done is fraud; to bill when it was not necessary is abuse. Remember the rule: If a service was not documented, in the view of the payer it was not done and cannot be billed. To bill for undocumented services is fraudulent.

Excluded Parties

Employees, physicians, and contractors who have been found guilty of fraud may be excluded from being able to work for government

THINKING IT THROUGH 2.8

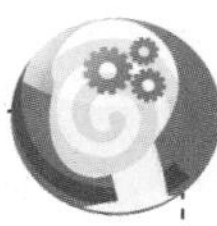

A cardiac clinic decided to bill regularly for two tests when one test was performed. Fearing the possibility of an OIG investigation, the clinic overbilled only patients who had insurance with private payers. It did not overbill Medicare or Medicaid patients. Do you think the clinic is liable for federal claim fraud under OIG?

programs. An OIG exclusion has national scope, and Congress has established a civil monetary penalty for institutions that knowingly hire excluded parties. OIG maintains the List of Excluded Individual/Entities (LEIE), a database that provides the public, health care providers, patients, and others with information about parties excluded from participation in Medicare, Medicaid, and federal health care programs. The list is available on OIG's website for the exclusion program.

2.9 Enforcement and Penalties

The HIPAA Final Enforcement Rule, implemented on March 16, 2006, imposed a single rule that reconciled the differences in the enforcement procedures of the privacy and the security standards. It makes clear that both acts (things that are done) and omissions (things that are not done, like failure to implement a particular provision) may be HIPAA violations. All the Administrative Simplification provisions legislated under the original HIPAA law (the Health Insurance Portability and Accountability Act of 1996) are covered under the Final Enforcement Rule. Members of the administrative medical team need to be aware of which agency is in charge of which law, the serious nature of penalties for violations of applicable laws, and the steps that can be taken to avoid even the suggestion of improper conduct.

HIPAA Enforcement Agencies

Enforcing HIPAA is the job of a number of government agencies. Which agency performs which task depends on the nature of the violation.

Office for Civil Rights

Civil violations (those that are based on civil law, such as trespassing, divorce cases, and breech of contract proceedings) of the HIPAA privacy and security standards are enforced by the Office for Civil Rights (OCR), an agency of HHS. OCR has the authority to receive and investigate complaints as well as to issue subpoenas for evidence in cases it is investigating. It is charged with enforcing the privacy standards because the privacy and security of one's health information is considered a civil right.

Previously, OCR enforced the privacy standards, and the Centers for Medicare and Medicaid (CMS) enforced the security standards. Because privacy and security are naturally intertwined, in July 2009, as part of the HITECH Act's goal of improved enforcement of the

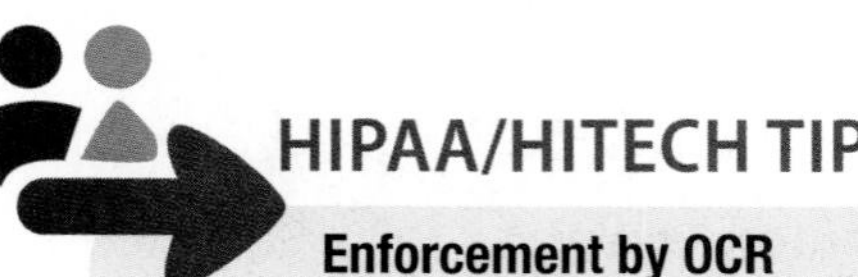

HIPAA/HITECH TIP

Enforcement by OCR

An individual does not have the right to sue a covered entity that may have disclosed his or her PHI inappropriately; action must be taken on the individual's behalf by OCR.

Privacy and Security Rules, HHS mandated combining the administration and enforcement of both rules under OCR. Figure 2.6 shows a page from the OCR website with information on filing a HIPAA privacy or security complaint.

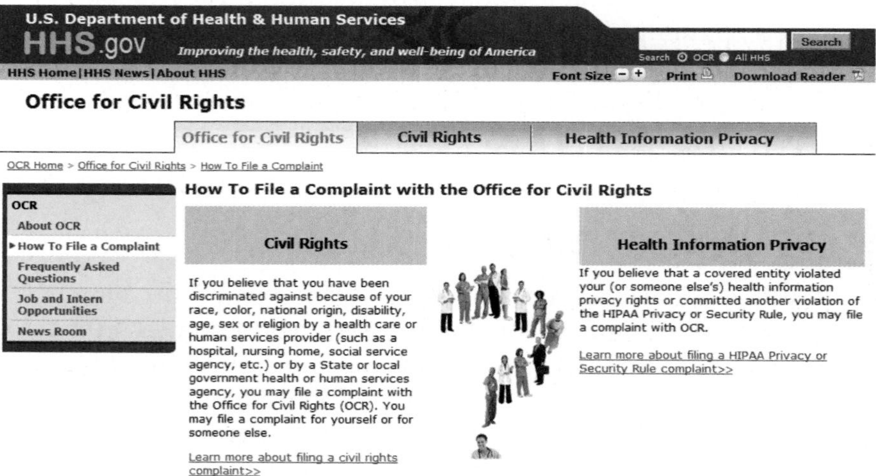

Figure 2.6 OCR Complaint Home Page

audit formal examination or review, such as a review to determine whether an entity is complying with regulations

OCR Audits Under HITECH Under HITECH, OCR is also required to conduct audits to ensure compliance with HIPAA rules. An **audit** is a formal examination or review. Income tax audits are performed to find out whether a firm's income or expenses were misreported. Similarly, compliance audits judge whether a health care organization's staff members comply with regulations.

An audit does not involve reviewing every document. Instead, a representative sample of the whole is studied to review whether erroneous or fraudulent behavior exists. Previously, audits were an allowable method of enforcement by OCR, but they were not required. Based on the HITECH Act, OCR is required to conduct audits—of both covered entities and business associates—to check for violations of HIPAA rules.

Department of Justice

Criminal violations (those that involve crimes, such as kidnapping, robbery, and arson) of the HIPAA privacy and security standards are prosecuted by the federal government's Department of Justice. DOJ is America's "law office" and the central agency for the enforcement of federal laws.

Centers for Medicare and Medicaid Services

The Centers for Medicare and Medicaid Services (CMS) is in charge of enforcing all the HIPAA standards other than the privacy and security

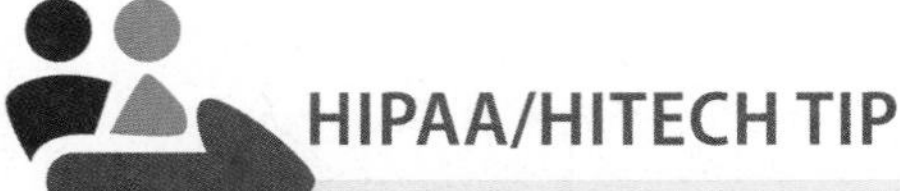

HIPAA/HITECH TIP

Ongoing Compliance Education

As explained in the next section, medical office staff members receive ongoing training and education in current rules so that they can avoid even the appearance of fraud.

standards. HHS authorized CMS—in addition to its major task of administering the Medicare and Medicaid programs—to investigate complaints of noncompliance and to enforce these HIPAA standards:

- The Electronic Health Care Transactions and Code Sets Rule
- The National Employer Identifier Number Rule
- The National Provider Identifier Rule
- The National Plan Identifier Rule (currently under development)

Figure 2.7 shows the CMS HIPAA enforcement home page.

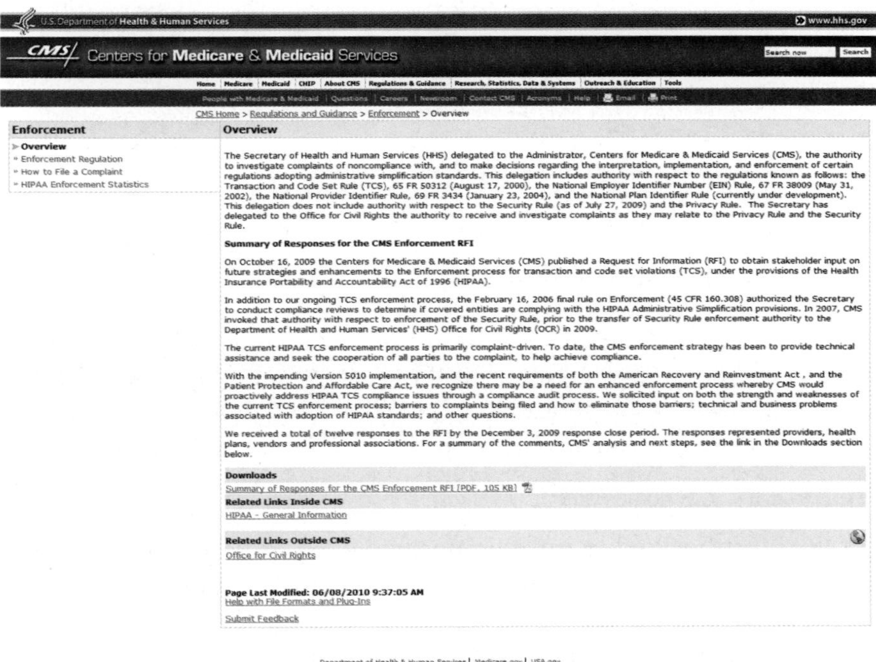

U.S. Department of Health & Human Services www.hhs.gov

CMS Centers for Medicare & Medicaid Services Search now Search

Home | Medicare | Medicaid | CHIP | About CMS | Regulations & Guidance | Research, Statistics, Data & Systems | Outreach & Education | Tools

People with Medicare & Medicaid | Questions | Careers | Newsroom | Contact CMS | Acronyms | Help | Email | Print

CMS Home > Regulations and Guidance > Enforcement > Overview

Enforcement

- **Overview**
- Enforcement Regulation
- How to File a Complaint
- HIPAA Enforcement Statistics

Overview

The Secretary of Health and Human Services (HHS) delegated to the Administrator, Centers for Medicare & Medicaid Services (CMS), the authority to investigate complaints of noncompliance with, and to make decisions regarding the interpretation, implementation, and enforcement of certain regulations adopting administrative simplification standards. This delegation includes authority with respect to the regulations known as follows: the Transaction and Code Set Rule (TCS), 65 FR 50312 (August 17, 2000), the National Employer Identifier Number (EIN) Rule, 67 FR 38009 (May 31, 2002), the National Provider Identifier Rule, 69 FR 3434 (January 23, 2004), and the National Plan Identifier Rule (currently under development). This delegation does not include authority with respect to the Security Rule (as of July 27, 2009) and the Privacy Rule. The Secretary has delegated to the Office for Civil Rights the authority to receive and investigate complaints as they may relate to the Privacy Rule and the Security Rule.

Summary of Responses for the CMS Enforcement RFI

On October 16, 2009 the Centers for Medicare & Medicaid Services (CMS) published a Request for Information (RFI) to obtain stakeholder input on future strategies and enhancements to the Enforcement process for transaction and code set violations (TCS), under the provisions of the Health Insurance Portability and Accountability Act of 1996 (HIPAA).

In addition to our ongoing TCS enforcement process, the February 16, 2006 final rule on Enforcement (45 CFR 160.308) authorized the Secretary to conduct compliance reviews to determine if covered entities are complying with the HIPAA Administrative Simplification provisions. In 2007, CMS invoked that authority with respect to enforcement of the Security Rule, prior to the transfer of Security Rule enforcement authority to the Department of Health and Human Services' (HHS) Office for Civil Rights (OCR) in 2009.

The current HIPAA TCS enforcement process is primarily complaint-driven. To date, the CMS enforcement strategy has been to provide technical assistance and seek the cooperation of all parties to the complaint, to help achieve compliance.

With the impending Version 5010 implementation, and the recent requirements of both the American Recovery and Reinvestment Act , and the Patient Protection and Affordable Care Act, we recognize there may be a need for an enhanced enforcement process whereby CMS would proactively address HIPAA TCS compliance issues through a compliance audit process. We solicited input on both the strength and weaknesses of the current TCS enforcement process; barriers to complaints being filed and how to eliminate those barriers; technical and business problems associated with adoption of HIPAA standards; and other questions.

We received a total of twelve responses to the RFI by the December 3, 2009 response close period. The responses represented providers, health plans, vendors and professional associations. For a summary of the comments, CMS' analysis and next steps, see the link in the Downloads section below.

Downloads

Summary of Responses for the CMS Enforcement RFI [PDF, 105 KB]

Related Links Inside CMS

HIPAA - General Information

Related Links Outside CMS

Office for Civil Rights

Page Last Modified: 06/08/2010 9:37:05 AM

Help with File Formats and Plug-Ins

Submit Feedback

Department of Health & Human Services | Medicare.gov | USA.gov

Web Policies & Important Links | Privacy Policy | Freedom of Information Act | No Fear Act

Centers for Medicare & Medicaid Services, 7500 Security Boulevard Baltimore, MD 21244

Figure 2.7 CMS Enforcement Home Page

Office of Inspector General

A fourth government group, OIG, a part of HHS, was directed under the 1996 HIPAA law to combat fraud and abuse in health insurance and health care delivery (Figure 2.8 shows the OIG home page). Most billing-related accusations under the False Claims Act are based on the guideline that providers who knew or should have known that a claim for service was false can be held liable. The intent to commit fraud does not have to be proved by the accuser in order for the provider to be found guilty. Actions that might be viewed as errors or occasional slips might also be seen as

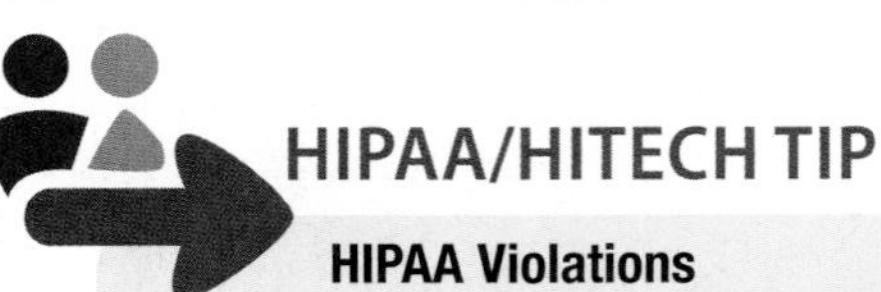

HIPAA Violations

Only covered entities and business associates—not their employees—can be charged with HIPAA violations. However, depending on the facts of the case, certain employees may be directly liable under other laws, like corporate criminal liability laws.

establishing a pattern of violations, which constitute the knowledge meant by "providers knew or should have known."

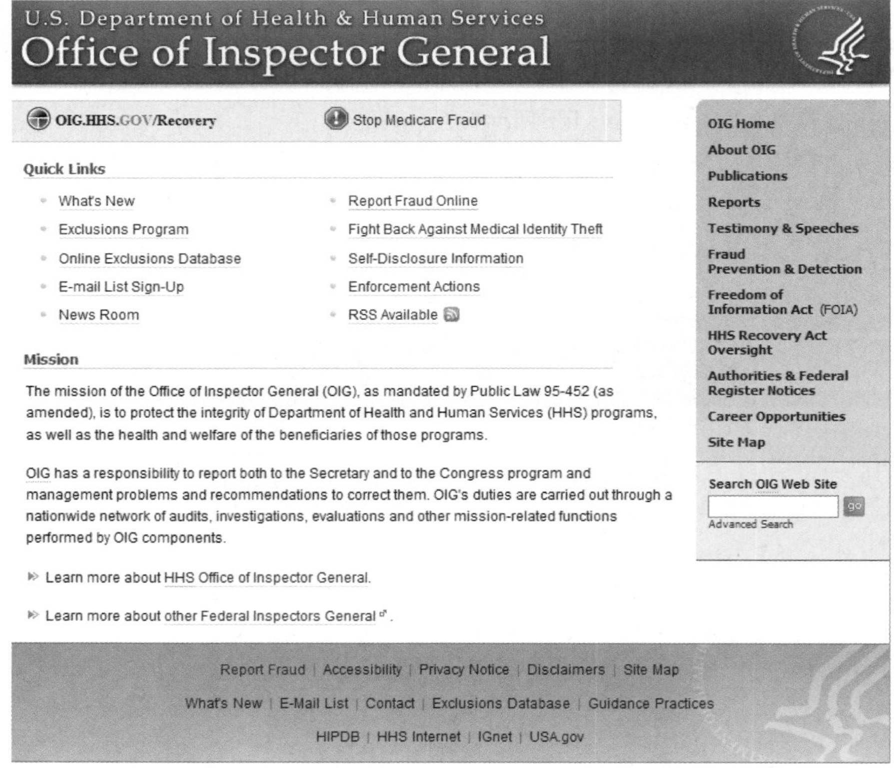

Figure 2.8 OIG Home Page

OIG is authorized to investigate suspected fraud cases and to audit the records of physicians and payers. Investigators review selected medical records to determine whether the documentation matches the billing. Accounting records are often reviewed as well. When problems are found, the investigation proceeds and may result in charges of fraud or abuse against the practice.

Although OIG says that "under the law, physicians are not subject to civil, administrative, or criminal penalties for innocent errors, or even negligence," decisions about whether there are clear patterns and inadequate internal procedures can be subjective at times, making the line between honest mistakes and fraud very thin. Medical practice staff members must avoid any actions that could be perceived as noncompliant.

Civil Money Penalties

Most privacy complaints are settled by voluntary compliance. But if the covered entity does not act to resolve the matter in a way that is

THINKING IT THROUGH 2.9

Alice, a new employee of City Medical, was asked for the Social Security numbers and health plan information of several patients over the phone. Without verifying the identity of the caller, Alice provided the information. After several months, it was evident that Alice had played into the hands of an organization involved in identity theft, resulting in financial damage to the patients whose data were compromised. City Medical trains its employees thoroughly with regard to protecting patients' health information. Alice admits that she received the training, but being new to the job, she did not think fast enough to apply what she had learned. Who is responsible—City Medical (the covered entity) or Alice (the employee)? What changes should City Medical think about making to avoid a recurrence?

satisfactory, the enforcing agency can impose civil money penalties (CMPs). HITECH increased HIPAA penalties and established a tiered system for deciding the level and penalty of each privacy violation. CMS and OCR can supersede the limits listed in Table 2.5, but with a cap of $50,000 per violation and $1.5 million for the calendar year for the same type of violation.

Criminal Case Procedures

If OCR or CMS receives a complaint that may lead to a criminal case, the agency will usually refer the complaint to DOJ for investigation. For criminal cases, such as for selling unique health identifiers for identity theft purposes, these penalties can be imposed:

	Fine	Prison
Knowingly obtaining PHI in violation of HIPAA	$50,000	1 year
Offenses done under false pretenses	$100,000	5 years
Using PHI for profit, gain, or harm	$250,000	10 years

TABLE 2.5 Monetary Penalties for HIPAA/HITECH Privacy Violations

Tier	Type of Cases	Minimum per Violation	Calendar-Year Maximum
A	Cases in which offenders did not realize they violated the act and would have handled the matter differently if they had known	$100	$25,000
B	Violations due to reasonable cause, and not to willful neglect	$1,000	$50,000
C	Infringements that the organization corrected, but were due to willful neglect	$10,000	$250,000
D	Violations due to willful neglect that the organization did not correct	$50,000	$1.5 million

2.10 Compliance Plans

Because of the risk of fraud and abuse liability, medical practices must be sure that billing rules are followed by all staff members. In addition to responsibility for their own actions, physicians are liable for the professional actions of employees they supervise. This responsibility is a result of the law of *respondeat superior,* which states that an employer is responsible for an employee's actions. Physicians are held to this doctrine, so they can be charged for the fraudulent behavior of any staff member.

A wise slogan is that "the best defense is a good offense." For this reason, medical practices write and implement compliance plans to uncover compliance problems and correct them to avoid risking liability. A compliance plan is a process for finding, correcting, and preventing illegal medical office practices. It is a written document prepared by a compliance officer and committee that sets up the steps needed to (1) audit and monitor compliance with government regulations, especially in the area of coding and billing, (2) have policies and procedures that are consistent, (3) provide for ongoing staff training and communication, and (4) respond to and correct errors.

The goals of the compliance plan are to:

- Prevent fraud and abuse through a formal process to identify, investigate, fix, and prevent repeat violations relating to reimbursement for health care services
- Ensure compliance with applicable federal, state, and local laws, including employment and environmental laws as well as antifraud laws
- Help defend the practice if it is investigated or prosecuted for fraud by substantiating the desire to behave compliantly and thus reduce any fines or criminal prosecution

Having a compliance plan demonstrates to outside investigators that the practice has made honest, ongoing attempts to find and fix weak areas.

Compliance plans cover more than just coding and billing. They also cover all areas of government regulation of medical practices, such as Equal Employment Opportunity (EEO) regulations (for example, hiring and promotion policies) and Occupational Safety and Health Administration (OSHA) regulations (for example, fire safety and handling of hazardous materials such as blood-borne pathogens).

Parts of a Compliance Plan

Generally, according to OIG, a voluntary plan should contain seven elements:

1. Consistent written policies and procedures
2. Appointment of a compliance officer and committee
3. Training plans
4. Communication guidelines

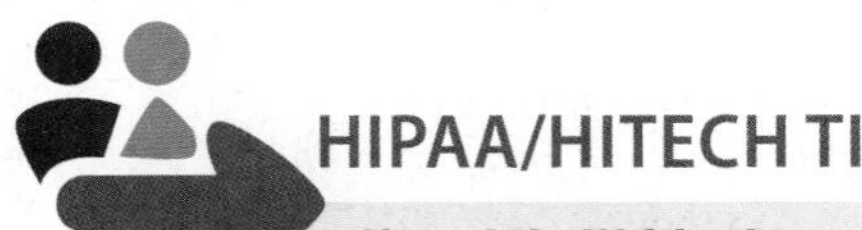

HIPAA/HITECH TIP

Have It in Writing!

Do not code or bill services that are not supported by documentation, even if instructed to do so by a physician. Instead, report this kind of situation to the practice's compliance officer.

5. Disciplinary systems
6. Auditing and monitoring
7. Responding to and correcting errors

Following OIG's guidance can help in the defense against a false claims accusation. Having a plan in place shows that efforts are made to understand the rules and correct errors. This indicates to OIG that the problems may not add up to a pattern or practice of abuse, but may simply be errors.

Compliance Officer and Committee

To establish the plan and follow up on its provisions, most medical practices appoint a compliance officer who is in charge of the ongoing work. The compliance officer may be one of the practice's physicians, the practice manager, or the billing manager. A compliance committee is also usually established to oversee the program.

Ongoing Training

Physician Training

Part of the compliance plan is a commitment to keep physicians trained in pertinent coding and regulatory matters. Often the medical insurance specialist or medical coder is assigned the task of briefing physicians on changed codes or medical necessity regulations. The following guidelines are helpful in conducting physician training classes:

- Keep the presentation as brief and straightforward as possible.
- In a multispecialty practice, issues should be discussed by specialty; all physicians do not need to know changed rules on dermatology, for example.
- Use actual examples, and stick to the facts when presenting material.
- Explain the benefits of coding compliance to the physicians, and listen to their feedback to improve job performance.
- Set up a way to address additional changes during the year, such as in an office newsletter or at compliance meetings.

Staff Training

An important part of the compliance plan is a commitment to train medical office staff members who are involved with coding and

THINKING IT THROUGH 2.10

As a member of the administrative staff for the practice, why would ongoing training be important to you?

billing. Ongoing training also requires having the current annual updates, reading health plans' bulletins and periodicals, and researching changed regulations. Compliance officers often conduct refresher classes in proper coding and billing techniques.

Code of Conduct

The practice's compliance plan emphasizes the procedures that are to be followed to meet existing documentation, coding, and medical necessity requirements. It also has a code of conduct for the members of the practice, which covers:

- Procedures for ensuring compliance with laws relating to referral arrangements
- Provisions for discussing compliance during employees' performance reviews and for disciplinary action against employees, if needed
- Mechanisms to encourage employees to report compliance concerns directly to the compliance officer to reduce the risk of whistleblower actions

Promoting ethical behavior in the practice's daily operations can also reduce employee dissatisfaction and turnover by showing employees that the practice has a strong commitment to honest, ethical conduct.

Audits

The HIPAA Security Rule requires covered entities to conduct four types of audits. Three are periodic, and one is annual. The three periodic audits are an information systems activity review, user log-in monitoring, and an audit log review (from computer systems and databases to review the storage, use, and disclosure of PHI). The annual audit, called an *evaluation,* is more commonly known as a compliance audit.

Documentation

Documentation is a primary requirement for demonstrating HIPAA compliance. Common documentation includes:

- Retaining written or electronic results of risk analysis
- Documenting the results of an audit
- Developing and implementing comprehensive privacy and security policies and procedures
- Documenting staff training and security incident threats

chapter 2 summary

LEARNING OUTCOME	KEY CONCEPTS/EXAMPLES
2.1 List several legal uses of a patient's medical record. Pages 52–53	Legal uses of patients' medical records, which contain the complete, chronological, and comprehensive documentation of their health history and status, include the following: - Documenting the rationale behind treatment decisions - Providing continuity and communication among physicians and other health care professionals involved in the patient's care - Verifying billing - Preparing and supporting health care claims - Conducting research - Furthering education
2.2 Define HIPAA and HITECH, and name the three types of covered entities that must comply with them. Pages 53–57	HIPAA is the Health Insurance Portability and Accountability Act of 1996. Its Administrative Simplifications standard includes the Privacy Rule, the Security Rule, and the Electronic Health Care Transactions and Code Sets standards. HITECH is the Health Information Technology for Economic and Clinical Health Act, part of the American Recovery and Reinvestment Act (ARRA) of 2009, which extends and reinforces HIPAA. Its breach notification rule is aimed at preventing breaches of protected health information. Health care providers, health plans, and business associates must comply with the provisions in HIPAA and HITECH.
2.3 Discuss how the HIPAA Privacy Rule protects patients' protected health information (PHI). Pages 57–66	Protected health information (PHI) is individually identifiable health information—such as a patient's name, address, Social Security number, and e-mail address—that is transmitted or maintained in any form or medium. The HIPAA Privacy Rule regulates the use and disclosure of patients' PHI. To release PHI for other than treatment, payment, or health care operations (TPO), a covered entity must have an authorization signed by the patient. The authorization document must be in plain language and have a description of the information to be used, who can disclose it and for what purpose, who will receive it, an authorization date, and the patient's signature.

LEARNING OUTCOME	KEY CONCEPTS/EXAMPLES
2.4 Discuss how the HIPAA Security Rule protects electronic protected health information (ePHI). Pages 66–69	PHI that is created, received, maintained, or transmitted in electronic form is known as ePHI. The HIPAA Security Rule requires covered entities to establish three types of safeguards to protect the confidentiality, integrity, and availability of ePHI: administrative safeguards (office policies and procedures); physical safeguards (mechanisms to protect electronic systems, equipment, and data from threats, environmental hazards, and unauthorized intrusion); and technical safeguards (technology and related policies and procedures used to protect electronic data and control access to it).
2.5 Explain the purpose of the HITECH breach notification rule. Pages 69–72	The breach notification rule of the HITECH Act is aimed at preventing breaches of protected health information. It requires patients' PHI to be made secure by making it "unusable, unreadable, or indecipherable to unauthorized individuals" using specified technologies and methods. In the case of breaches of unsecured health information by covered entities or their business associates, HITECH requires covered entities to notify individuals that their health information has been compromised through a breach notification letter.
2.6 State the goal of the HIPAA Electronic Health Care Transactions and Code Sets standards, and list the HIPAA transactions and code sets standards that will be required in the future. Pages 72–77	The HIPAA Electronic Health Care Transactions and Code Sets standards require all providers who do business electronically to use the same electronic formats for health care transactions and the same code sets for diagnoses, procedures, and supplies. The goal of the standards is to increase the efficiency of conducting business in health care. When the standards are fully implemented in the health care industry, exchange of information will be faster, more efficient, and more accurate. Future transaction standards are Additional Information to Support a Health Care Claim or Encounter and First Report of Injury. For electronic data interchange, ASC X12 Version 5010 will be required as of January 1, 2012. The ICD-10-CM and ICD-10-PCS code sets become mandatory on October 1, 2013. Identifiers for patients and for health plans will be developed in the future.

LEARNING OUTCOME	KEY CONCEPTS/EXAMPLES
2.7 Discuss some of the most common threats to the privacy and security of electronic information and ways in which the HITECH Act addresses them. Pages 77–81	Some of the most common threats to the privacy and security of electronic information are natural disasters, insufficient security in computer systems, and individuals' intentions to cause harm. The increased use of information technology in health care means that a greater volume of confidential clinical patient information is available in electronic form and that there are many more points of access to that information. In addition, the use of portable computing and storage devices increases the possibility of lost data or stolen devices. The HITECH Act addresses the increased security risk to ePHI by making business associates subject to the same privacy and security requirements as covered entities. Before the HITECH Act, only covered entities bore the burden of penalties for violations of the Privacy and Security Rules. Under HITECH, a much wider range of businesses must comply, including overseas vendors, personal health record vendors, health information exchanges, and regional health information organizations.
2.8 Define fraud and abuse in health care, and cite an example of each. Pages 81–85	Fraud is an intentional act of deception for the purpose of taking financial advantage of another person. Pretending to be a physician and treating patients without a valid medical license is an example of fraud. Abuse in this context is an action that misuses money that the government has allocated, such as Medicare funds. Abuse is not necessarily intentional. It may be the result of ignorance of a billing rule or of inaccurate coding. Abuse has taken place when an ambulance service bills Medicare for transporting a patient to the hospital when the patient did not need ambulance service.
2.9 Describe the various government agencies that are responsible for enforcing HIPAA. Pages 85–89	A number of government agencies are responsible for enforcing HIPAA. - The Office for Civil Rights administers and enforces the HIPAA Privacy and Security Rules and conducts audits of covered entities and business associates to ensure compliance. - Criminal violations of the privacy standards are prosecuted by the federal government's Department of Justice. - The Centers for Medicare and Medicaid Services enforces all HIPAA standards other than the privacy and security standards. - The Office of Inspector General is in charge of combating fraud and abuse in health insurance and health care delivery, and conducts regular audits of physician and payer records.

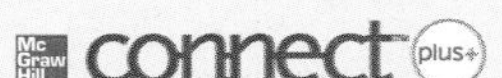

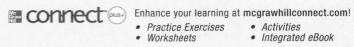

Enhance your learning at **mcgrawhillconnect.com**!

- *Practice Exercises*
- *Worksheets*
- *Activities*
- *Integrated eBook*

LEARNING OUTCOME	KEY CONCEPTS/EXAMPLES
2.10 Identify the parts of a compliance plan and the types of documentation used to demonstrate compliance. Pages 90–92	A medical practice compliance plan includes consistent written policies and procedures, appointment of a compliance officer and committee, training plans, communication guidelines, disciplinary systems, ongoing auditing and monitoring of claim preparation, and responding to and correcting errors. Having a formal process in place is a sign that the practice has made a good-faith effort to achieve compliance. Under the HIPAA Security Rule, covered entities must conduct three periodic audits and one annual audit. Documentation is a primary requirement for demonstrating HIPAA compliance, including risk analysis results, audit reports, and reports of security incident threats.

chapter review

MATCHING QUESTIONS

Match the key terms with their definitions.

_____ 1. ***[LO 2.6]*** ASC X12 Version 5010

_____ 2. ***[LO 2.3]*** electronic data interchange (EDI)

_____ 3. ***[LO 2.4]*** electronic protected health information (ePHI)

_____ 4. ***[LO 2.8]*** abuse

_____ 5. ***[LO 2.5]*** breach

_____ 6. ***[LO 2.9]*** audit

_____ 7. ***[LO 2.3]*** HIPAA Privacy Rule

_____ 8. ***[LO 2.5]*** breach notification

_____ 9. ***[LO 2.4]*** HIPAA Security Rule

_____ 10. ***[LO 2.2]*** Centers for Medicare and Medicaid Services (CMS)

a. Actions that improperly use another person's resources.

b. PHI that is created, received, maintained, or transmitted in electronic form.

c. The impermissible use or disclosure of a patient's PHI under the Privacy Rule due to a compromise in privacy or security that could pose a significant risk to the individual involved.

d. Law that requires covered entities to establish safeguards to protect the confidentiality, integrity, and availability of health information.

e. The computer-to-computer exchange of routine business information using publicly available electronic standards.

f. The federal agency in the Department of Health and Human Services that runs Medicare, Medicaid, clinical laboratories, and other government health programs.

g. The updated electronic data standard for transmitting HIPAA X12 documents.

h. A formal examination or review.

i. A document used by a covered entity to notify individuals of a breach in their PHI.

j. Law that regulates the use and disclosure of patients' protected health information.

TRUE-FALSE QUESTIONS

Decide whether each statement is true or false.

_____ 1. ***[LO 2.1]*** Medical standards of care are state-specified performance measures for the delivery of health care by medical professionals.

_____ 2. ***[LO 2.1]*** Once the patient or the physician ends the relationship, the physician's responsibility for maintaining the patient's medical record also ends.

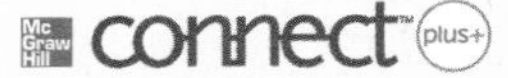

Enhance your learning at **mcgrawhillconnect.com!**

- *Practice Exercises*
- *Worksheets*
- *Activities*
- *Integrated eBook*

______ 3. ***[LO 2.2]*** The Administrative Simplification provisions passed by Congress encourage the use of electronic health care records.

______ 4. ***[LO 2.6]*** The HIPAA Electronic Health Care Transactions and Code Sets standards allow individual providers who agree to do business electronically to vary their standards of health care transactions under certain specified conditions.

______ 5. ***[LO 2.7]*** Under the HITECH Act, business associates of medical practices such as lawyers, pharmacists, and accountants are subject to the same HIPAA Privacy Rules as the medical practices with which they do business.

______ 6. ***[LO 2.3]*** For use or disclosure of protected health information other than for treatment, payment, or health care operations, the patient must sign an authorization to release the information.

______ 7. ***[LO 2.3]*** When a patient authorizes a release of his or her medical records, that release is irrevocable and carries no expiration date.

______ 8. ***[LO 2.5]*** If a medical practice experiences an unintentional breach of security in handling its electronic health records and the breach poses a significant financial risk to the patients, the practice must notify the patients involved within one year.

______ 9. ***[LO 2.6]*** Every health care provider who transmits health information electronically must obtain a National Provider Identifier, unless the provider uses outside business associates to prepare the transactions.

______ 10. ***[LO 2.10]*** Compliance officers and committees are created within a medical practice to update the staff on current HIPAA laws and their implications.

MULTIPLE-CHOICE QUESTIONS

Select the letter that best completes the statement or answers the question.

1. ***[LO 2.1]*** An unwritten law of medical insurance is that if it was not documented, it was not done, and if it was not done, it cannot be ________.
   a. adjusted
   b. breached
   c. billed
   d. safeguarded

2. ***[LO 2.2]*** The HIPAA Administrative Simplification provisions contain all of the following parts EXCEPT the ________.
   a. Privacy Rule
   b. Security Rule
   c. breach notification rule
   d. Electronic Health Care Transactions and Code Sets standards

3. ***[LO 2.5, 2.7]*** The HITECH Act provides all of the following EXCEPT ________.
   a. new breach notification requirements
   b. funding for experimental procedures
   c. higher monetary penalties for HIPAA violations
   d. greater privacy and security enforcement

4. ***[LO 2.3]*** The ________ is used to protect PHI from being accidentally released to those not needing the information during an appropriate use or disclosure.
   a. minimum necessary standard
   b. designated record set
   c. National Provider Identifier (NPI)
   d. maximum security standard
5. ***[LO 2.3]*** Individuals are permitted to ask for an accounting of the disclosures of their electronic protected health information including TPO disclosures over the preceding ________ years.
   a. two
   b. three
   c. five
   d. six
6. ***[LO 2.4]*** HIPAA security requirements state the administrative, technical, and ________ safeguards that are required to protect patients' electronic health information.
   a. personal
   b. clinical
   c. economic
   d. physical
7. ***[LO 2.4]*** According to the American Health Information Management Association (AHIMA), record retention requirements are at least ________ years for transactional and billing records.
   a. seven
   b. eight
   c. nine
   d. ten
8. ***[LO 2.4]*** Records that show who has accessed a computer or network and what operations were performed are known as ________ trails.
   a. user
   b. hacker
   c. audit
   d. compliance
9. ***[LO 2.6]*** The ________ codes used in the United States are based on the *International Classification of Diseases* (ICD).
   a. diagnosis
   b. treatment
   c. procedure
   d. transaction
10. ***[LO 2.9]*** The agency responsible for enforcing the Privacy and Security Rules is the ________.
   a. Office of Inspector General
   b. Office for Civil Rights
   c. Office of the Attorney General
   d. Federal Trade Commission

CHAPTER 2 REVIEW CHAPTER REVIEW

SHORT-ANSWER QUESTIONS

Define the following abbreviations.

1. ***[LO 2.2]*** EDI ____________________________
2. ***[LO 2.6]*** ICD ____________________________
3. ***[LO 2.3]*** PHI ____________________________
4. ***[LO 2.3]*** NPP ____________________________
5. ***[LO 2.3]*** TPO ____________________________
6. ***[LO 2.2]*** HIPAA ____________________________
7. ***[LO 2.6]*** NPI ____________________________
8. ***[LO 2.2]*** HITECH ____________________________
9. ***[LO 2.2]*** CMS ____________________________
10. ***[LO 2.6]*** HCPCS ____________________________

APPLYING YOUR KNOWLEDGE

Working with HIPAA

2.1 ***[LO 2.4, 2.5]*** How is the HITECH breach notification rule an extension of the HIPAA Security Rule?

2.2 ***[LO 2.3]*** Based on your knowledge of the HIPAA Privacy Rule, do you think each of the following actions is compliant?

a. A medical insurance specialist does not disclose a patient's history of an eating disorder on a workers' compensation claim for a broken leg. Only the information the recipient needs to know is given. ____________________________

b. A medical assistant faxes appropriate patient X-ray results before a scheduled surgery. ____________________________

c. Unsupervised maintenance and housekeeping personnel are allowed into record storage and processing areas. ____________________________

2.3 ***[LO 2.7]*** Identity theft occurs when a criminal uses another person's personal information to take on that person's identity. Any online transaction, such as online banking, increases an individual's risk of identity theft. In some cases, identity theft occurs when someone's medical information is stolen and misused. What are a number of ways in which a person's identity, such a Social Security number in a medical record, could be stolen?

____

____

2.4 ***[LO 2.4]*** Which technology safeguard—administrative, physical, or technical—is represented by each of the following policies?

a. Each individual authorized to work with patient records has a unique password. __________

b. Access to the hospital's record storage area requires electronic fingerprinting. __________

c. Medical claims sent from the provider to the clearinghouse are encrypted. __________

d. Paper files scheduled for destruction are kept securely in an offsite location. __________

e. A provider's sanction policy states the consequences for violations of security policies and procedures by employees. __________

f. A medical office revises the data backup procedure that is used as part of normal business activities. __________

2.5 ***[LO 2.5]*** A medical office recently changed locations. During the move, the medical records of 397 individuals (all beginning with the letter *P*) were inadvertently thrown into public dumpsters by the cleaning crew. The unsecured information includes complete medical histories dating back five years. The office manager decides that no notification to the patients or the HHS is required because the incident involves fewer than five hundred individuals. In what ways has the office manager misunderstood the breach notification rule?

____

____

Composing a Breach Notification Letter

2.6 ***[LO 2.5]*** The following case describes an incident in which an office laptop containing personal health information for two thousand patients was stolen.

Case

On November 18, 2016, City Medical discovers that a laptop is missing from its office. Officials suspect that at least one new employee is behind the theft and that it occurred sometime after office hours the previous night. The unsecured PHI involved in the breach includes partial medical records of approximately two thousand patients input over the past year, containing the patients' names, addresses, dates of birth, clinical data, and about nine hundred Social Security numbers. Although the data are encrypted, Britney Blackwell, the compliance officer at City Medical, expresses concern that the employee suspected of stealing the laptop may be able to obtain help in exposing the information. City Medical is therefore offering credit protection monitoring free of charge for one year to all patients involved. Corecheck, a company that provides identity-theft protection services, will provide the monitoring. The toll-free number for Corecheck is 800-707-1000. City Medical has reported the theft to authorities and is doing everything it can to track down the missing laptop and the suspected employee. City Medical has also hired a company to perform thorough background checks of all employees in the future and is reviewing its policies with regard to technical safeguards. City Medical's toll-free number for any questions or concerns regarding the loss of personal information is 800-888-2909.

Based on the template below, compose a breach notification letter to be sent to all patients of City Medical whose data have been compromised. City Medical's address is 5001 Avenue K, Oakland, CA 94601. The letter is sent two days after the breach is discovered. The slanted brackets indicate where you are to supply the missing information.

Assume that the first patient to whom the letter is sent is:
Beverly Abbington
667 Oak Street
Oakland, CA 94601

<LETTERHEAD OF THE ORGANIZATION, INCLUDING ADDRESS>

<Date of letter>

<Patient name>

<Patient address>

Dear <Patient name>:

This letter is to inform you that your personal health information on record with <Name of medical practice> was recently compromised. We first became aware of this breach on <Date>. We are notifying you and all others involved so that you can help ensure that this information is not used inappropriately.

<Provide the following details: (1) a brief description of what happened, including the date of the breach and the date of the discovery of the breach; (2) a description of the types of unsecured PHI that were involved in the breach; (3) the steps individuals should take to protect themselves from potential harm resulting from the breach; (4) a brief description of what the covered entity involved is doing to investigate the breach and to protect against any further breaches; (5) a toll-free telephone number or website for individuals to ask questions or learn additional information.>

<Name of medical practice> apologizes for any negative consequences this situation has brought about. We are hopeful that we can <name most likely solution to recovering the lost data>. Representatives are available twenty-four hours at our toll-free number to answer any questions you have. <Name of credit protection monitoring company> will help you in contacting the major credit bureaus to place a fraud alert on your credit report, order credit reports, and continue to monitor the reports. <Name of credit protection monitoring company> will also provide you with links to websites that offer information on what to do when personal information is compromised.

Sincerely,

<Name and title of appropriate contact person>

chapter 3

Introduction to Medisoft Clinical

KEY TERMS

access levels
Auto Log Off
backing up
chart
chief complaint
dashboard
database
disaster recovery plan
knowledge base
Medisoft Clinical
Medisoft Clinical Patient Records (MCPR)
Medisoft Network Professional (MNP)
park
password
restoring
user name

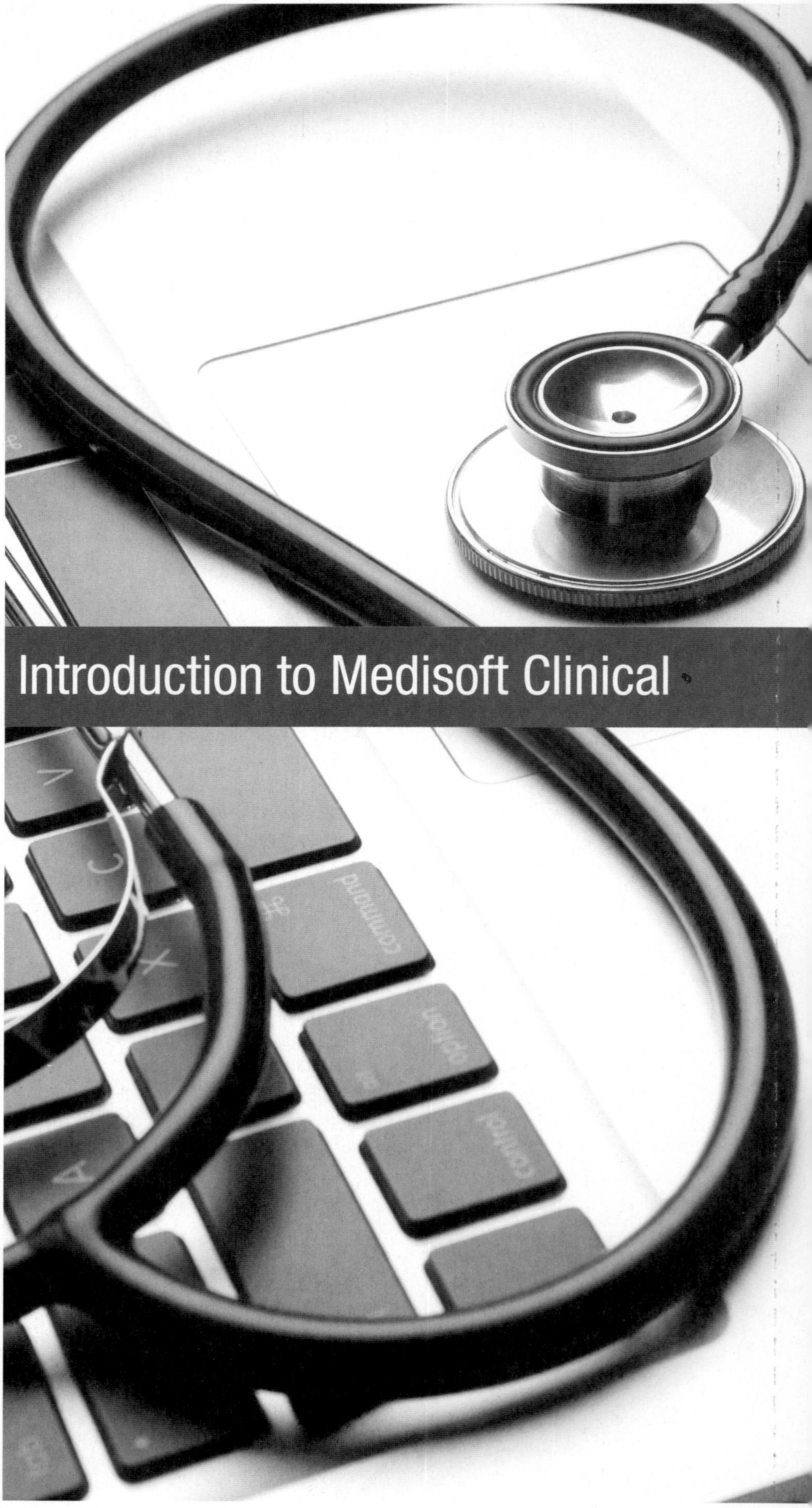

LEARNING OUTCOMES

When you finish this chapter, you will be able to:

3.1 List the practice management and electronic health record applications in Medisoft Clinical.

3.2 Discuss three security features in Medisoft Clinical that protect patients' health information.

3.3 List the menus in Medisoft Clinical Patient Records.

3.4 List the menus in Medisoft Network Professional.

3.5 Describe how pre-encounter tasks are completed in Medisoft Clinical.

3.6 Describe how encounter tasks are completed in Medisoft Clinical.

3.7 Describe how post-encounter tasks are completed in Medisoft Clinical.

3.8 Explain how to create and restore backup files in Medisoft Clinical.

3.9 Discuss the types of help available in Medisoft Clinical.

Reason to Worry?

Today the staff is meeting with Tiffany Patel, the consultant who is helping the Family Care Clinic make a smooth transition from paper records to electronic records. A major portion of the meeting is devoted to understanding the impact of the change on office workflow—the order in which tasks are completed. Ms. Patel explains that workflow in an electronic office differs from workflow in a paper-based office. She provides several examples. "When you have an integrated PM and EHR, you no longer need paper encounter forms, or superbills," she explains. "Also, there is no need to enter office visit charges manually, since the charges flow electronically from the EHR to the PM." As Ms. Patel continued to describe some of the upcoming changes, Joseph Sanchez, the practice's coder, and Chris Yakamoto, the billing specialist, begin sending text messages back and forth. "With all the changes, u think we'll still have jobs in 6 months?," Chris wrote. Joseph replied, "Not sure. Have 2 wait & see I guess."

What do you think made Chris and Joseph nervous about their job security? As you read this chapter, think about how the jobs of coders and billing specialists will be different in an office with an integrated PM/EHR.

WHEN YOU FINISH THIS CHAPTER, YOU WILL ALSO BE ABLE TO USE MEDISOFT CLINICAL TO:

1. Use a menu command to open a patient chart.
2. Use a toolbar button to open a patient chart.
3. Use a menu command to view charges and payments.
4. Use a toolbar button to view charges and payments.
5. Back up files.
6. Restore files.
7. Access Medisoft Help.

SOFTWARE SKILLS

3.1 Medisoft Clinical: A Practice Management/Electronic Health Record Program

Medisoft Clinical an integrated PM/EHR

Medisoft Network Professional (MNP) practice management application within Medisoft Clinical

Medisoft Clinical Patient Records (MCPR) electronic health record application within Medisoft Clinical

user name name that an individual uses for identification purposes when logging onto a computer or an application

password confidential authentication information

Medisoft Clinical is a practice management and electronic health record program for physician practices. The program is widely used in medical practices throughout the United States. Most of the concepts and techniques used in operating Medisoft Clinical are similar to those in other PM/EHR programs. Once you are familiar with Medisoft Clinical, you should be able to transfer many skills taught in this book to other programs. Throughout this text/workbook, we refer to the practice management application as **Medisoft Network Professional (MNP)** and to the electronic health record application as **Medisoft Clinical Patient Records (MCPR).**

This chapter begins with an overview of security features in Medisoft Clinical, and then introduces the practice management and electronic health record applications. Finally, the chapter describes how these applications are used to accomplish the tasks in the medical documentation and billing cycle, which you read about in Chapter 1.

3.2 Security Features in Medisoft Clinical

Medisoft Clinical has a number of built-in security features to ensure compliance with the HIPAA and HITECH privacy and security regulations.

User Names and Passwords

In order to log in to Medisoft Clinical, an individual must have a **user name** and a **password.** The use of user names and passwords prevents unauthorized access to the program, safeguards critical patient information, and protects patient confidentiality. As passwords are entered, the characters are replaced with asterisks (*) on the screen so there is no chance that someone will see the actual password characters. The system may be set up to limit the number of log-in attempts. If the number of unsuccessful attempts exceeds the number permitted, the user will not be allowed to access the system for a period of time, or in some cases, without a system administrator's intervention. The Medisoft Clinical Patient Records Sign In screen is illustrated in Figure 3.1.

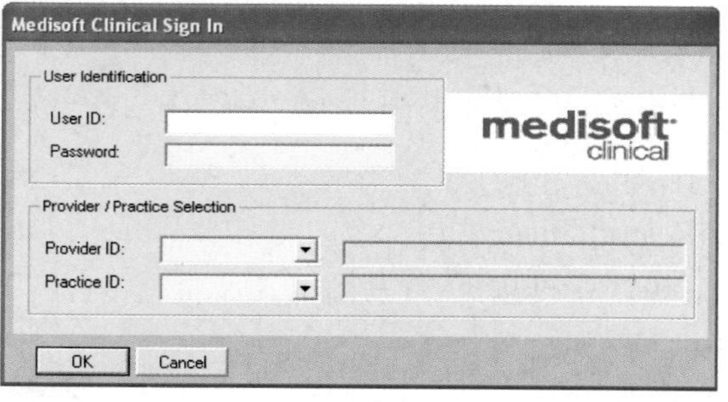

Figure 3.1 Medisoft Clinical Patient Records Sign In Screen

Requiring people to log in limits access to the program to those who have been assigned log-ins, and also allows the actions of users within the program to be tracked through an audit report. The audit function can be used to track changes made in the program as well as identify those who made the changes.

The Login/Password Management dialog box assists in the management of passwords and log-in attempts (see Figure 3.2). The program can be configured to control the following aspects of password management:

Renewal Interval Indicates how frequently users must change their passwords, in this case every ninety days.

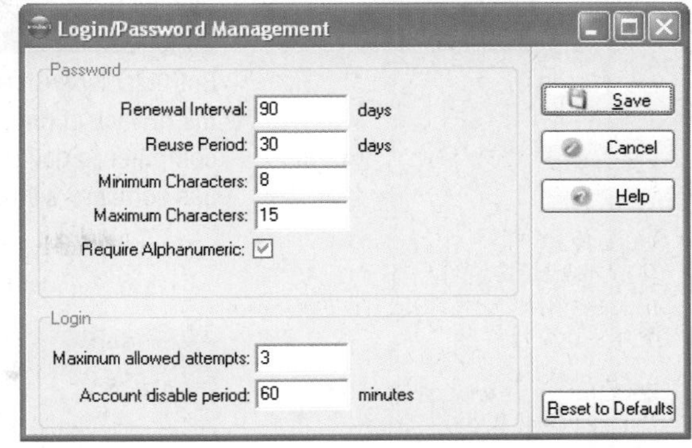

Figure 3.2 Medisoft Network Professional Login/Password Management Dialog Box

Reuse Period Indicates how long users must wait until they can reuse their last password. Here it is set so that they cannot select the same password for a period of thirty days.

Minimum Characters Indicates the minimum number of characters allowable for a password. In this case, passwords must be at least eight characters in length.

Maximum Characters Indicates the maximum number of characters allowable for a password. In this case, passwords must be no more than fifteen characters in length.

Require Alphanumeric When this box is checked, a password must contain at least one number and at least one letter.

Maximum Allowed Attempts Indicates how many unsuccessful log-in attempts may be made before a user is locked out of the program. Here a user is allowed three log-in attempts. After the third failed log-in attempt, the user is locked out of the program.

Account Disable Period Users are locked out of the program for a specified period of time when the maximum number of log-in attempts has been exceeded.

Access Levels

access levels security option that determines the areas of the program a user can access, and whether the user has rights to enter or edit data

Access levels define which areas of the program a user can view, and whether the user can only view the information or can also add, edit, or delete it. The program can be set up with a number of access levels for different positions in the office, such as receptionist, physician, nurse, medical assistant, and billing specialist. The program can also specify whether a user has to enter a password to access certain areas of the program. In most offices, access levels correspond to the user's job function on a need-to-know basis. If the user needs to know the information to perform tasks associated with the position, access is granted. If the information is not relevant to the user's job function, access may be denied. For example, a staff member responsible for scheduling may not be able to view a patient's laboratory test results. Likewise, a user responsible for following up on insurance claims may be able to view visit documentation in the patient chart, but not add, edit, or delete information. In Figure 3.3, the first column lists specific areas within the program, and the remaining columns represent the allowed actions for a user: Access, New, Edit, View, Del (delete), Pswd (password required). Access

THINKING IT THROUGH 3.1

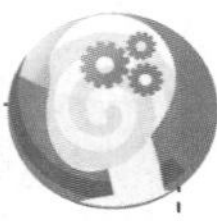

Both Medisoft Clinical applications contain features that are designed to protect the privacy of patient information. When would it be an advantage for a computer to go into Park? Auto Log Off? When would it be a disadvantage to use software with these features?

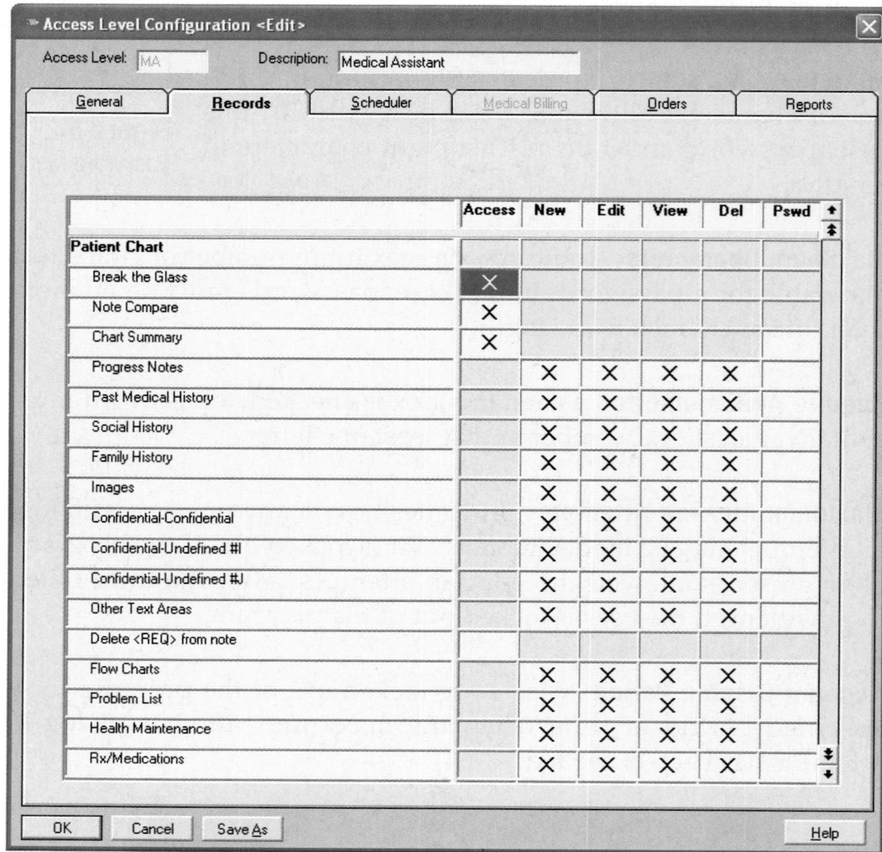

Access Level Configuration <Edit>

Access Level: MA   Description: Medical Assistant

General | Records | Scheduler | Medical Billing | Orders | Reports

	Access	New	Edit	View	Del	Pswd
Patient Chart						
Break the Glass	X					
Note Compare	X					
Chart Summary	X					
Progress Notes		X	X	X	X	
Past Medical History		X	X	X	X	
Social History		X	X	X	X	
Family History		X	X	X	X	
Images		X	X	X	X	
Confidential-Confidential		X	X	X	X	
Confidential-Undefined #I		X	X	X	X	
Confidential-Undefined #J		X	X	X	X	
Other Text Areas		X	X	X	X	
Delete <REQ> from note						
Flow Charts		X	X	X	X	
Problem List		X	X	X	X	
Health Maintenance		X	X	X	X	
Rx/Medications		X	X	X	X	

OK | Cancel | Save As | Help

Figure 3.3 Screen Showing the Areas of MCPR That a Medical Assistant Can Access, Edit, or View

levels play a major role in ensuring the security and confidentiality of patient records in a practice.

The Park Feature and Auto Log Off

park privacy and security feature in MCPR that allows a user to leave a workstation for a brief time without having to exit the program

Auto Log Off feature of MNP that automatically logs a user out of the program after a period of inactivity

The privacy and security feature in MCPR known as **park** allows a user to leave a workstation for a brief time without having to exit the program. When a workstation is parked, it cannot be accessed without reentering a valid operator's user name and password. If someone were to walk by and see the screen while the user was away from the computer, he or she would see the screen illustrated in Figure 3.4 rather than patient data.

The **Auto Log Off** feature in MNP performs a similar function. If no activity is detected for a specified number of minutes, the program automatically logs out the user.

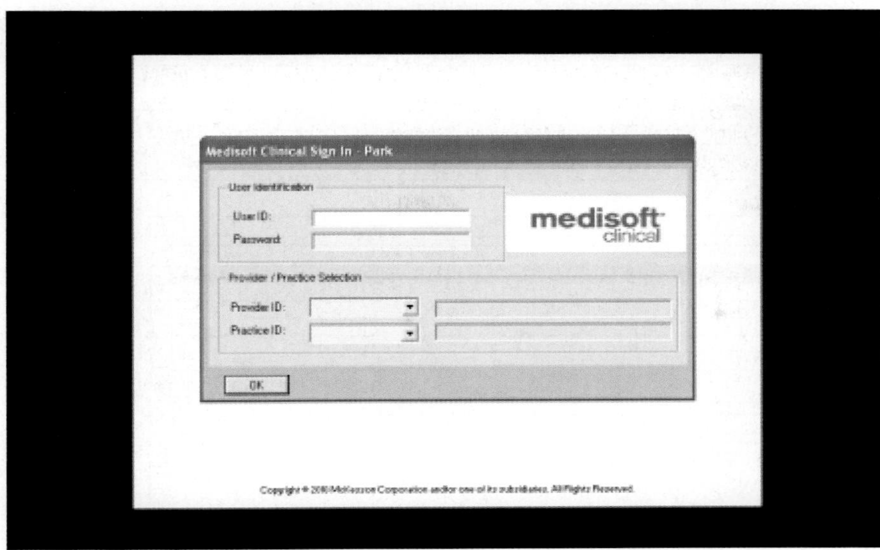

Figure 3.4 MCPR Screen in Park Mode

3.3 Medisoft Clinical Patient Records

Medisoft Clinical Patient Records (MCPR) is the electronic health record component of Medisoft Clinical. The program stores patient information in a number of databases. A **database** is a collection of related pieces of information. Each section of a patient chart is represented by a yellow folder, similar to folders used in a paper-based office. The term **chart** refers to a patient's medical record. Information about the patient is entered in the appropriate folder.

database a collection of related bits of information

chart folder that contains all records pertaining to a patient

Practices can customize the patient chart to include the folders that are relevant to their particular practice. Commonly used folders include:

- Progress notes
- Past medical history
- Social history
- Family history
- Consults
- Discharge summary
- Orders
- Messages
- Problem list (including diagnosis)
- Health maintenance
- Rx/medications
- Vital signs
- Laboratory data
- Images
- X-ray
- ECG
- Pathology

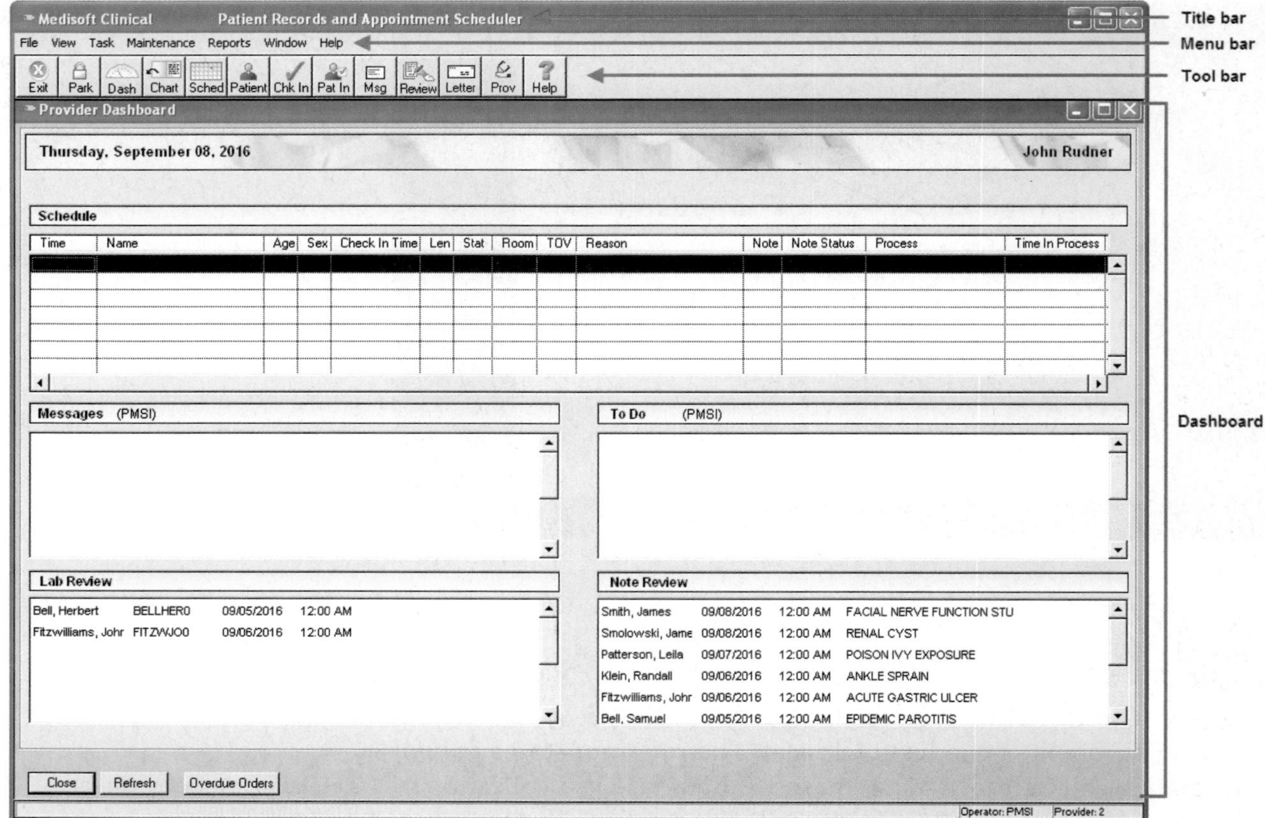

Figure 3.5 Main Medisoft Clinical Patient Records Window

Exploring the Main Medisoft Clinical Patient Records Window

The main screen, pictured in Figure 3.5, contains a number of different features.

Title Bar The title bar states the title of the program.

Menu Bar The menu bar contains the menus of MCPR commands. The names of the standard menu items are File, View, Task, Maintenance, Reports, Window, and Help. The menus and commands available may change depending on the task that is being performed. For example, the Maintenance menu will not appear when working in the patient chart because maintenance tasks cannot be performed while a patient chart is open.

Toolbar Located below the menu bar, the toolbar provides instant access to important MCPR functions (see Table 3.1). Clicking a button activates the related function in the program. The buttons on the toolbar vary depending on which function is in use.

dashboard a panel in MCPR that offers providers a convenient view of important information

The Dashboard

The main screen also displays the provider dashboard. The **dashboard** offers providers a convenient view of important information,

TABLE 3.1	Icons in the Medisoft Clinical Patient Records Toolbar	
Button	**Button Name**	**Activity**
Exit	Exit	Closes the charts and exits the program.
Park	Park	Protects the system from other viewers by locking the screen, requiring the next user to log in with a user name and password.
Dash	Dash	Opens the dashboard if it is not already open.
Chart	Chart	Opens a chart. More than one chart can be open at a time.
Sched	Sched	Opens the Appointment Scheduler program.
Patient	Patient	Opens a patient's registration screens for access to demographic information.
Chk In	Chk In	Checks in patients and tracks them through the visit.
Pat In	Pat In	Displays a patient's demographic information.
Msg	Msg	Enables staff to send messages (e-mail) to other staff members.
Review	Review	Displays the provider's review bin, which is similar to an in basket. All unsigned items go here automatically, including lab results, progress notes, and other incoming transmissions, to wait for the provider to review them.
Letter	Letter	Enables the writing of letters about specific patients and sends them to consulting physicians.
Prov	Prov	Changes the display to another provider or clinic.
Help	Help	Provides access to help features.

including messages, a to-do list, unsigned lab orders, notes, and more. Look at Figure 3.5 to view the provider dashboard in MCPR.

The main areas of the dashboard are Schedule, Messages, Lab Review, To Do. and Note Review. To access any of these features directly from the desktop, you would click the title of the section, such as Messages or To Do.

Schedule

The schedule area presents the provider's daily schedule with appointment time, patient name, length of visit, reasons for visit, whether the patient has checked in, and, if so, which room the patient is in.

Messages

The Messages section lists electronic messages for the provider. Unread messages appear in bold type. Information provided in this area includes the message priority (0 to 9), the sender of the message, the subject, and the date the message was received.

Lab Review

The Lab Review area presents lab results that the current provider needs to review. Information includes patient name, patient identification number, date of the lab work, and time the results were sent.

To Do

The To Do section of the dashboard lists action items for the provider, including the date the item was added to the list, the priority assigned to the task (1 to 9), the patient name, the patient identification number, and the subject of the item.

Note Review

This area presents notes for the provider to review, and contains a patient name, the date and time of the note, and the note's subject.

EXERCISE 3.1

connect plus+

STARTING MEDISOFT CLINICAL PATIENT RECORDS AND LOGGING IN

Start the Medisoft Clinical Patient Records application and log in.

1. Click Start > All Programs > Medisoft Clinical - Client > Medisoft Clinical Client. The Medisoft Clinical Sign In window appears.
2. Enter ***medasst*** in the User ID field. Notice that the Practice ID field was completed by the program.
3. Enter ***master1$*** in the Password field.
4. Click the drop-down triangle in the Provider ID field. The Provider Select dialog box opens.
5. Click the second line to select John Rudner, MD and click the OK button. You are returned to the Sign In screen.
6. Click OK. A Disclaimer screen appears. Click OK again.
7. The main Medisoft Clinical Patient Records window is displayed.

 **You have completed Exercise 3.1**

connect plus+

EXERCISE 3.2

USING A MENU COMMAND TO OPEN A PATIENT CHART

Practice selecting a menu command to open a patient chart.

1. Click the File menu, and select Open Chart. The Patient Lookup dialog box is displayed.
2. Click the Lookup button. A list of patients appears.
3. Click the line that contains the entry for Janine Bell. The line is blackened.
4. Click the OK button. Janine Bell's chart opens.
5. Click Close Chart on the File menu to close the patient's chart.

You have completed Exercise 3.2

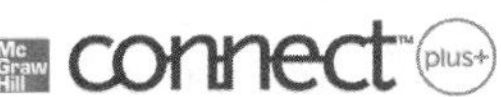

EXERCISE 3.3

USING A TOOLBAR BUTTON TO OPEN A PATIENT CHART

Practice using a toolbar button to open a patient chart.

1. Click the Chart button on the toolbar. The Patient Lookup dialog box is displayed.
2. Click the Lookup button. A list of patients appears.
3. Click the line that contains the entry for Janine Bell. The line is blackened.
4. Click the OK button. Janine Bell's chart opens.
5. Click the Close button on the toolbar to close the patient's chart.

You have completed Exercise 3.3

3.4 Medisoft Network Professional

Medisoft Network Professional (MNP) is the Medisoft Clinical application used for patient accounting. MNP also includes Office Hours, a scheduling program. Physician practices use MNP to:

- Schedule appointments
- Register patients
- Enter charges
- Create insurance claims
- Post payments

- Create statements
- Follow up on accounts
- Create reports

Exploring the Main Medisoft Network Professional Window

The main window in Medisoft Network Professional contains the title bar, menu bar, and toolbar (see Figure 3.6).

Title Bar The title bar states the title of the program.

Menu Bar Medisoft Network Professional offers choices of actions through a series of menus. Commands are issued by clicking options on the menus or by clicking shortcut buttons on the toolbar. The menu bar lists the names of the menus in Medisoft Network Professional: File, Edit, Activities, Lists, Reports, Tools, Window, and Help. Beneath each menu name is a pull-down menu with one or more options.

Toolbar Located below the menu bar, the toolbar contains twenty-six buttons with icons that represent the most common activities performed in MNP (refer to Figure 3.6). These buttons are shortcuts for frequently used menu commands. When you click a

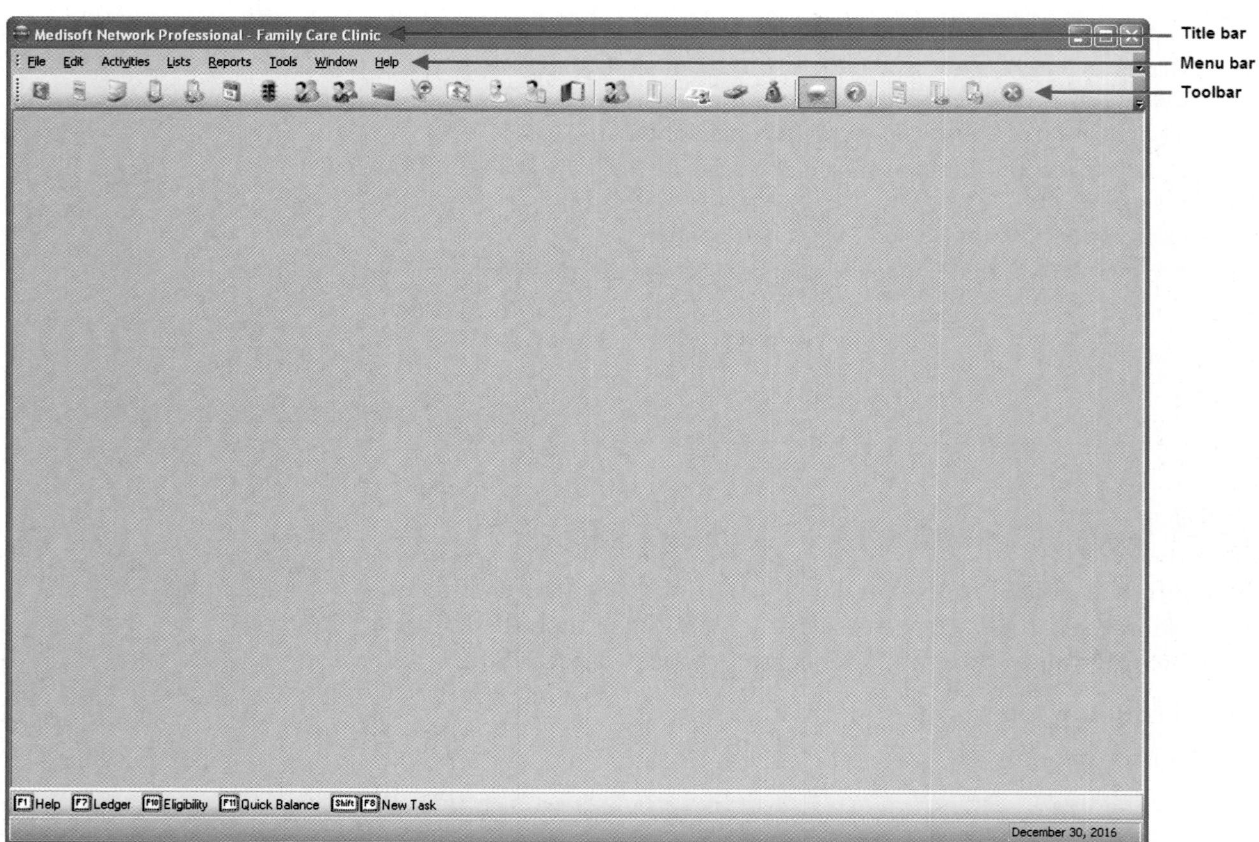

Figure 3.6 Main Medisoft Network Professional Window

button, the corresponding MNP dialog box opens. For example, clicking the Claim Management button opens the same dialog box as does selecting the Claim Management option on the Activities menu. When you move your cursor over an icon, a description of the icon is displayed. Throughout this text/workbook, the buttons can be used instead of the pull-down menus to perform common tasks. Table 3.2 lists the toolbar buttons and their associated activities.

connect plus+ **EXERCISE 3.4**

STARTING MEDISOFT NETWORK PROFESSIONAL AND LOGGING IN

Start the Medisoft Network Professional application and log in.

1. Click Start > All Programs > Medisoft > Medisoft Network Professional. The Medisoft User Login – Family Care Clinic window appears.
2. Enter ***billing*** in the Login Name field.
3. Enter ***master1$*** in the Password field and click OK. The main Medisoft Network professional window is displayed.

 **You have completed Exercise 3.4**

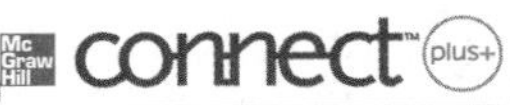

EXERCISE 3.5

USING A MENU COMMAND TO VIEW CHARGES AND PAYMENTS

Practice selecting a menu command to view a patient's charges and payments.

1. Click the Activities menu, and select Enter Transactions. The Transaction Entry dialog box is displayed.
2. Click the drop-down list button in the Chart field, and click Janine Bell. The charge and payment transactions for an office visit appear.
3. Review the two charges listed in the top section of the dialog box.
4. Review the payments entered by Herbert Bell (Janine's father) and the insurance plan, East Ohio PPO.
5. Click the Close button to close the dialog box.

 **You have completed Exercise 3.5**

TABLE 3.2	Medisoft Network Professional Toolbar Buttons	
Button	**Button Name**	**Activity**
	Transaction Entry	Enter, edit, or delete transactions.
	Claim Management	Create and transmit insurance claims.
	Statement Management	Create statements.
	Collection List	View, add, edit, or delete items on collection list.
	Add Collection List Item	Add items to the collection list.
	Appointment Book	Schedule appointments.
	View Eligibility Verification Results (F10)	Review results of eligibility verification inquiries.
	Patient Quick Entry	Use predefined templates to enter new patients.
	Patient List	Enter patient information.
	Insurance Carriers List	Enter insurance carriers.
	Procedure Code List	Enter procedure codes.
	Diagnosis Code List	Enter diagnosis codes.
	Provider List	Enter providers.
	Referring Provider List	Enter referring providers.
	Address List	Enter addresses.
	Patient Recall Entry	Enter patient recall data.
	Custom Reports List	Open a custom report.

(continued)

TABLE 3.2	(continued)	
	Quick Ledger	View a patient's ledger.
	Quick Balance	View a patient's balance.
	Enter Deposits and Apply Payments	Enter deposits and payments.
	Show/Hide Hints	Turn the Hints feature on and off.
	Medisoft Help	Access MNP's built-in help feature.
	Edit Patient Notes in Final Draft	Use the built-in word processor to create and edit patient notes.
	Launch Medisoft Reports	Obtain access to additional reports.
	Launch Work Administrator	Assign tasks to practice staff.
	Exit Program	Exit the MNP program.

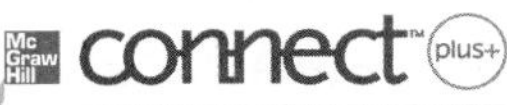

EXERCISE 3.6

USING A TOOLBAR BUTTON TO VIEW CHARGES AND PAYMENTS

Practice using a toolbar button to view a patient's charges and payments.

1. Click the Transaction Entry button on the toolbar. The Transaction Entry dialog box is displayed.
2. Click the drop-down list button in the Chart field, and click Janine Bell. The charge and payment transactions for an office visit appear.
3. Click the Close button to close the dialog box.

You have completed Exercise 3.6

3.5 Using Medisoft Clinical to Complete Pre-Encounter Tasks

In Chapter 1, you learned about the medical documentation and billing cycle. The tasks associated with each step in the cycle were originally performed using paper forms, without the assistance of computers. Computers were first used in the physician practice for scheduling and billing. Today, practices both large and small are shifting from paper medical records to electronic health records. The tasks formerly completed using paper are now performed electronically through the use of computers.

The remainder of this chapter explains how computer software—specifically Medisoft Clinical—is used to accomplish the tasks associated with each step in the cycle. In this section, the steps are grouped into three categories: pre-encounter, encounter, and post-encounter.

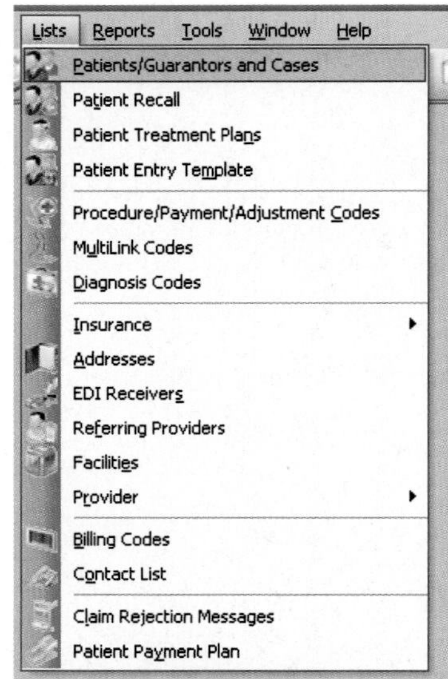

Figure 3.7 Patients/Guarantors and Cases Selection on the Lists Menu

Preregistration

The pre-encounter steps include preregistration and appointment scheduling. Preregistration consists of entering basic information about the patient in Medisoft Network Professional. The demographic information is entered in the Patient/Guarantor dialog box, which is accessed via the Lists menu (see Figure 3.7). When Patients/Guarantors and Cases is selected on the Lists menu, the Patient List dialog box is displayed (see Figure 3.8).

To enter preregistration information about a new patient, click the New Patient button. The Patient/Guarantor dialog box is displayed (see Figure 3.9). Basic information such as the patient's name, address, and telephone numbers are entered in the Name, Address tab. Additional information, including the assigned provider, are entered in the Other Information tab. The Payment Plan tab is usually not used during preregistration.

Entering the Chief Complaint/Reason for Visit

chief complaint patient's description of the symptoms or reasons for seeking medical care

If information about the patient's **chief complaint**—the patient's description of the symptoms or reasons for seeking medical care—is gathered during preregistration, a case must be created. Cases contain detailed information required to submit insurance claims. In MNP, the case folder consists of twelve tabs. During preregistration,

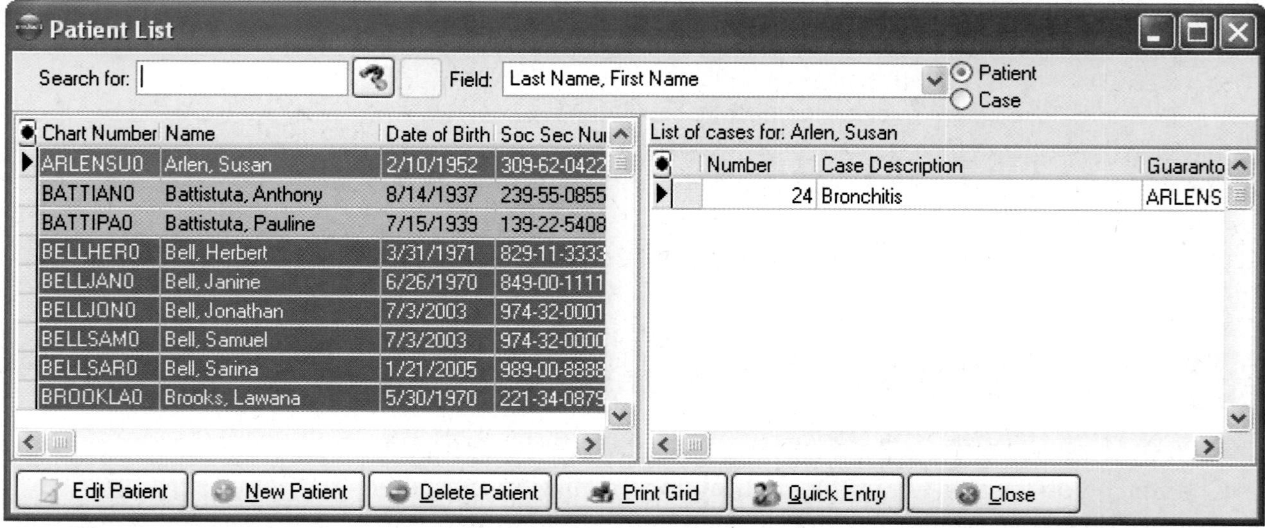

Figure 3.8 Patient List Dialog Box

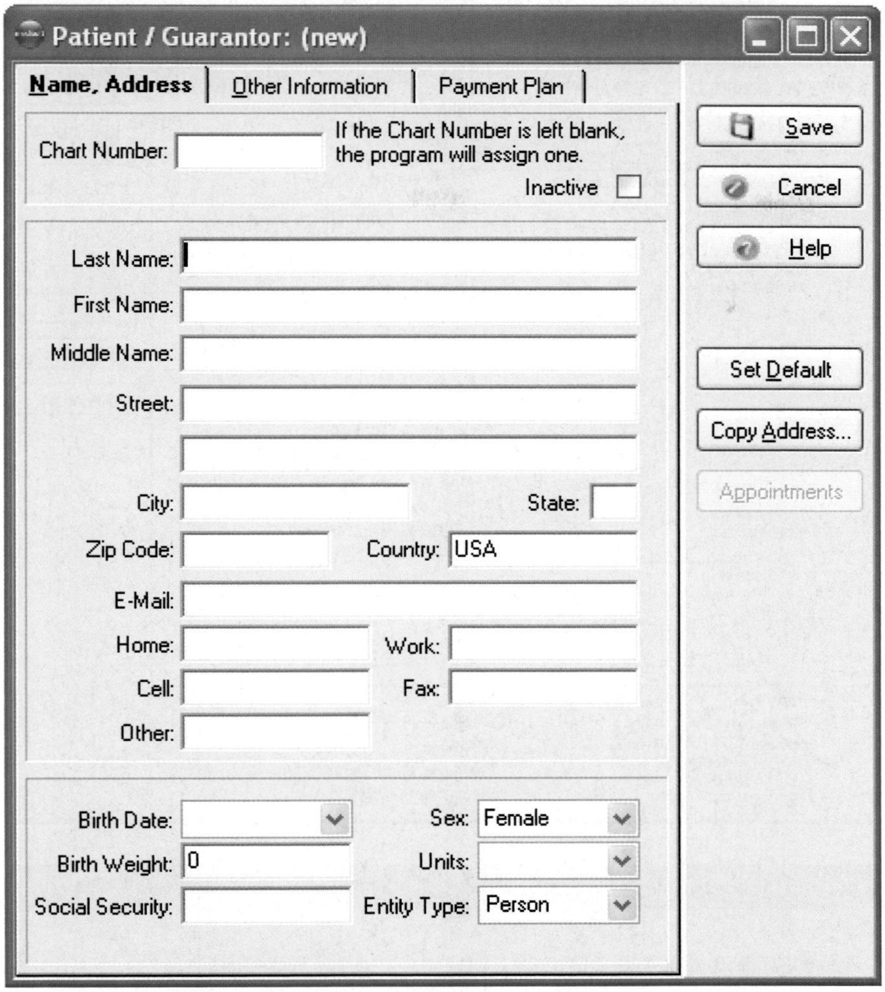

Patient / Guarantor: (new)

Name, Address | Other Information | Payment Plan

Chart Number: [ ] If the Chart Number is left blank, the program will assign one.

Inactive [ ]

Last Name:
First Name:
Middle Name:
Street:
City: State:
Zip Code: Country: USA
E-Mail:
Home: Work:
Cell: Fax:
Other:

Birth Date: Sex: Female
Birth Weight: 0 Units:
Social Security: Entity Type: Person

Save
Cancel
Help
Set Default
Copy Address...
Appointments

Figure 3.9 Patient/Guarantor Dialog Box

a new case is created, and the chief complaint is entered in the Description field of the Personal tab. Figure 3.10 displays the Case dialog box with the Personal tab selected.

Scheduling Appointments

The preferences of physician practices vary in regard to scheduling software. Some practices prefer to schedule appointments in a separate scheduling program, while others use a scheduling program that is built into a practice management or electronic health record program. In the exercises in this text/workbook, we will use Office Hours for patient appointments. Office Hours is a scheduling program included with Medisoft Network Professional. The main Office Hours screen is shown in Figure 3.11.

The following steps are used to enter an appointment in Office Hours:

1. Select a provider in the provider box in the upper-right corner of the Office Hours window.
2. Select a date in the calendar in the upper left corner of the window.

Figure 3.10 Case Dialog Box

Case: FITZWJ00 Fitzwilliams, John [Acute gastric ulcer]

Condition | Miscellaneous | Medicaid and Tricare | Multimedia | Comment | EDI
Personal | Account | Diagnosis | Policy 1 | Policy 2 | Policy 3

Save
Cancel
Help

Case Number: 7
Case Closed

Description: Acute gastric ulcer
Cash Case
Global Coverage Until:
Print Patient Statement
Guarantor: FITZWJ00 Fitzwilliams, John
Marital Status: Married
Student Status:

Eligibility...
Face Sheet
Set Default

Employment
Employer: ESE00 Self-employed
Status: Full time
Retirement Date:
Work Phone: (614)002-1112
Location:
Extension:

Patient Information
Name: Fitzwilliams, John
Address: 1627 Forest Avenue
Jefferson, OH
60093
Home Phone: (614)002-1111
Work Phone:
Cell Phone: (614)002-7947
Date of Birth: 11/15/1967

Case
7

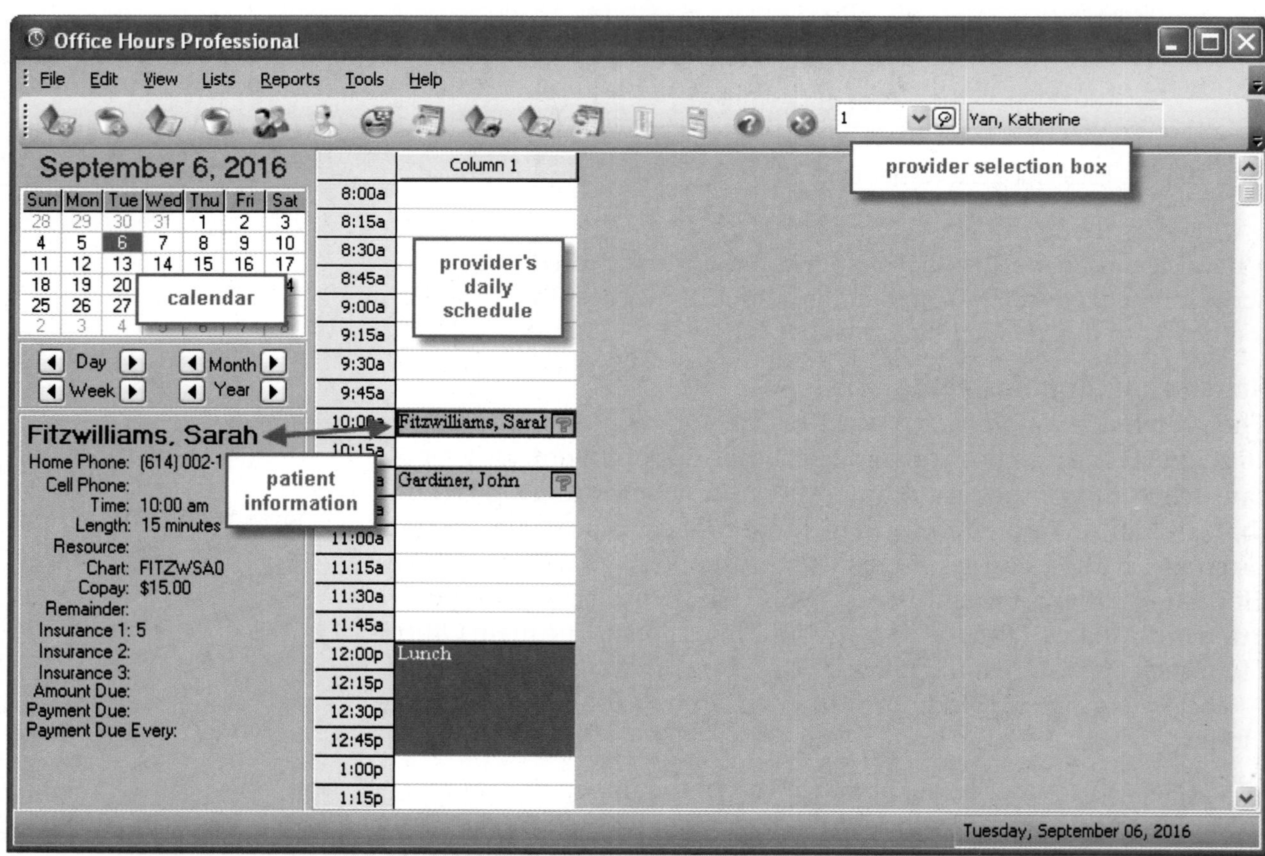

Figure 3.11 Main Areas of the Office Hours Window

THINKING IT THROUGH 3.2

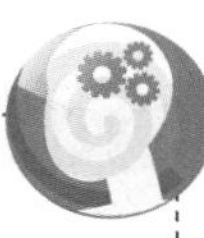

Most physician practices use computerized scheduling programs. Think about the steps required to find an open time slot and to enter a patient appointment. What do you think are the main advantages of a computerized scheduling program?

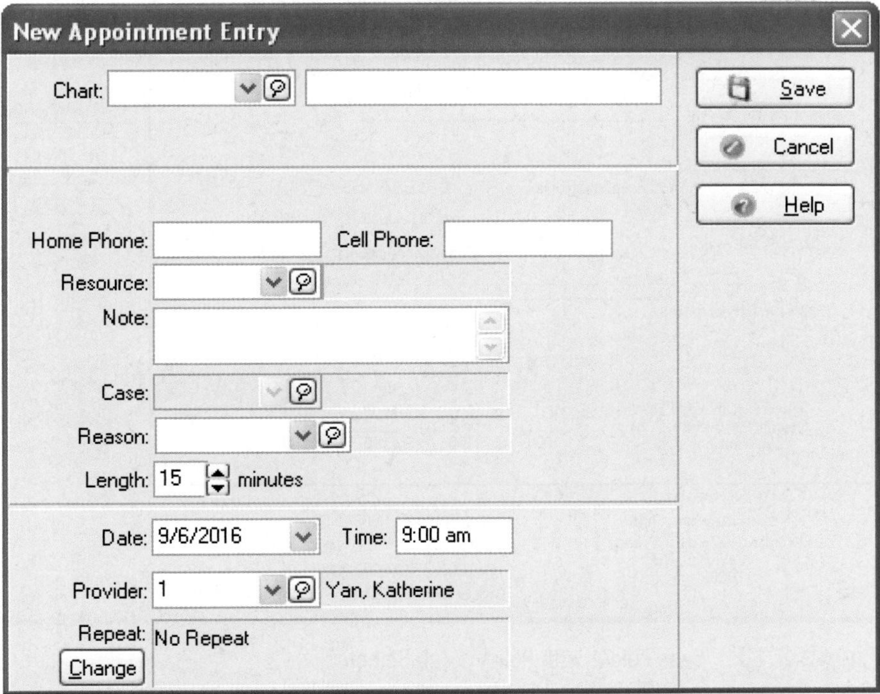

Figure 3.12 The New Appointment Entry Dialog Box

3. Click a time slot in the provider's daily schedule in Column 1. The New Appointment Entry dialog box is displayed (see Figure 3.12).
4. Complete the New Appointment Entry dialog box, and click Save.

Preregistration and scheduling are covered in detail in Chapter 4.

3.6 Using Medisoft Clinical to Complete Encounter Tasks

The encounter steps include all activities that take place from the time the patient arrives for an office visit until the patient leaves the office.

Establishing Financial Responsibility

In Medisoft Network Professional, the patient's insurance information is entered in one or more of the Policy tabs in the Case folder (see Figure 3.13). If the patient has just one policy, only the Policy 1 tab is completed. If the patient has additional plans, the Policy 2 tab and possibly the Policy 3 tab must also be completed. The Policy

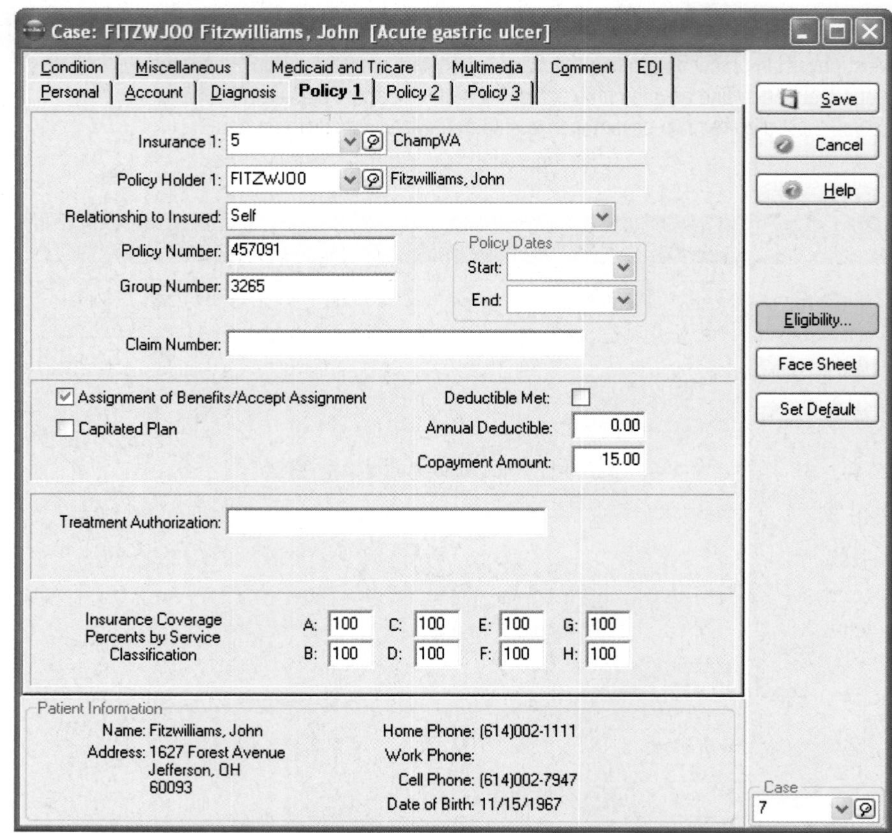

Figure 3.13 Case Folder with Policy 1 Tab Selected

tabs contain information about the patient's health plan coverage, including the name of the policyholder, the policy number, the co-payment or deductible amount, and more.

Checking Insurance Eligibility

The Policy tabs also contain a button that is used to make a real-time eligibility inquiry about a patient. In Figure 3.13, the button used to begin an eligibility check is highlighted in yellow. Using an Internet connection, the program sends an eligibility verification request to the patient's health plan and, in response, receives an eligibility response report that states whether the patient is eligible for benefits under the health plan.

The topic of eligibility verification is covered in detail Chapter 4.

Check-in

The check-in step includes a number of administrative and clinical activities, including:

- Checking in the patient and reviewing the patient's account balance
- Gathering and recording additional patient information
- Examining the patient and documenting the examination
- Coding the services performed and exporting the information to Medisoft Network Professional for claims and billing

Checking In and Reviewing Account Balance

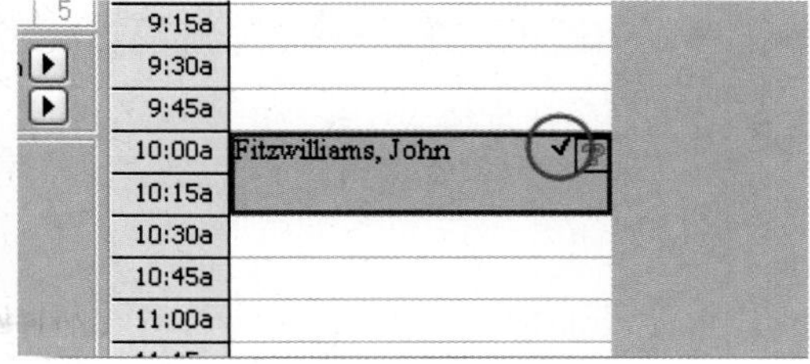

Figure 3.14 Patient Appointment with Checked-in Status

As patients assume more of the financial responsibility for health care, medical offices look for more efficient ways to check patients' balances and discuss any payments that are due while the patient is in the office. For this reason, the appointment schedulers inside Medisoft Clinical Patient Records and Medisoft Network Professional contain features to help facilitate the collection of time-of-service payments. Since this text/workbook uses Office Hours, a program within MNP, for scheduling, that is where check-in will take place. Figure 3.14 shows an appointment on the provider's schedule with a check mark to indicate that the patient has checked in. Figure 3.15 illustrates the Quick Balance dialog box, a feature within the scheduling program that enables front desk personnel to easily view a patient's balance during check-in.

Gathering and Recording Additional Patient Information

After patients check in at the front desk, they are given additional forms to complete, including a patient information form and a medical history form. Patients are also given several HIPAA documents, such as a Notice of Privacy Practices, an Acknowledgment of Receipt of Notice of Privacy Practices, and an Authorization to Use or Disclose Health Information. Most practices also provide patients with a copy of the practice's financial policy.

The information obtained during check-in is entered in several places in MNP. Most of the information on the patient information form is recorded in the Patient/Guarantor dialog box and in the Personal, Account, and Policy tabs of the Case folder. The data from the medical history form are reviewed by a medical assistant once the patient is taken to an exam room.

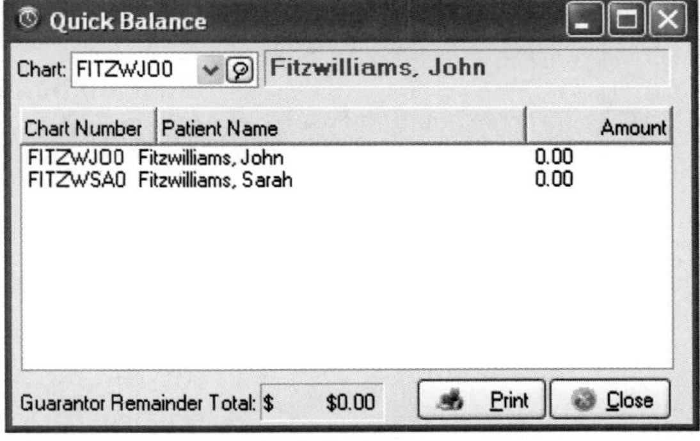

Figure 3.15 Quick Balance Dialog Box

The HIPAA forms that are signed by the patient and returned to the front desk may be scanned and included in the patient record.

Check-in, patient registration, and account balance review are covered in Chapter 5.

Documentation and Examination

After waiting to be called, the patient is escorted to the exam room, and a medical assistant or other clinical staff member interviews the patient and measures the patient's vital signs. The type and length of the interview depends on a number of factors, including whether the patient is new to the practice, the nature of the chief complaint, and the purpose of the visit (for example, new condition or routine follow-up). When a provider sees a patient for the first time, it is important to obtain the patient's medical history, allergies, and medications, as well as the chief complaint/reason for visit.

Medical History The medical history information is entered in the Past Medical History, Social History, and Family History tabs in Medisoft Clinical Patient Records (see Figure 3.16).

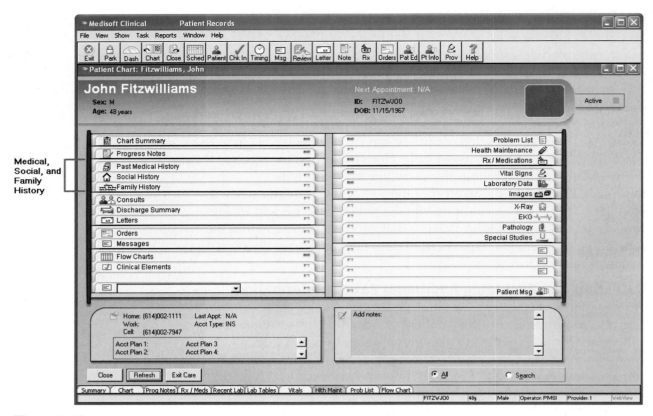

Figure 3.16 Patient Chart with Medical, Social, and Family History Folders Identified

Chief Complaint The chief complaint/reason for visit is recorded in the Problem List folder. The Problem List folder lists major problems, other problems, procedures, diagnoses, risks, and hospitalizations (see Figure 3.17).

Allergies and Medications A patient's allergies and medications are entered in the Rx/Medications folder. Allergies are listed at the top of the dialog box, and medications are grouped into current, ineffective, and historical categories. A date box indicates the last date on which the allergies were reviewed (see Figure 3.18).

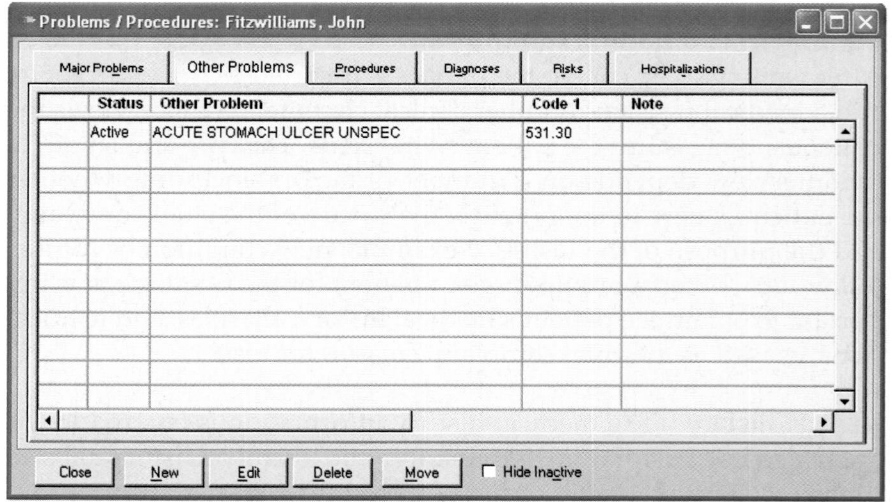

Figure 3.17 Problem List Folder with Other Problems Tab Selected

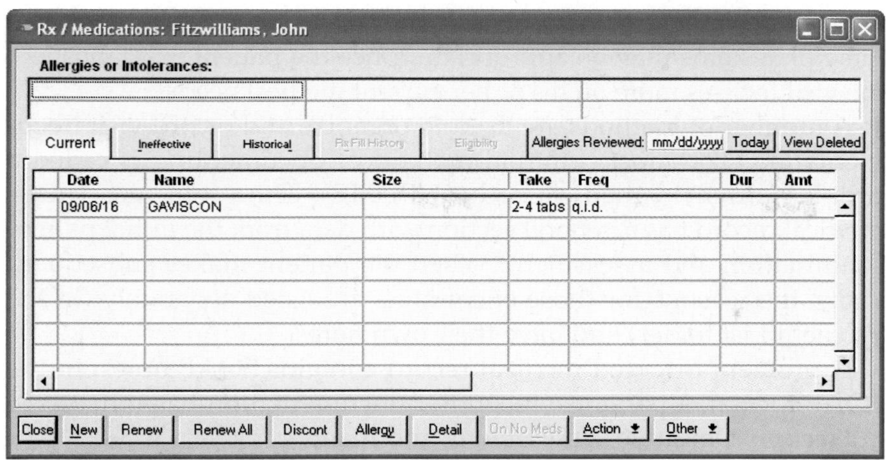

Figure 3.18 Rx/Medications Folder with Current Folder Selected

Measuring and Recording Vital Signs Vital signs are recorded and entered in the Vital Signs folder in MCPR. The Vital Signs dialog box contains fields for all commonly used vital signs and measurements (see Figure 3.19). As each measurement is taken, it is entered in the appropriate field.

The topics of medical history, chief complaint, allergies and medications, and entering vital signs are covered in Chapter 6.

Physician Examination During the office visit, a physician evaluates, treats, and documents a patient's condition. The visit documentation varies depending on a number of factors, including whether the patient

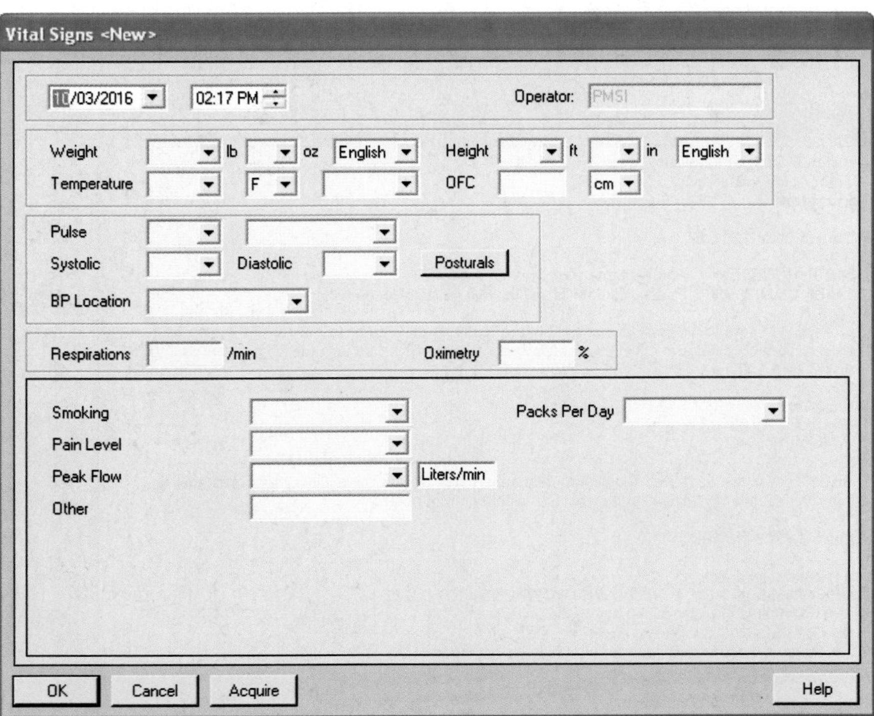

Figure 3.19 Vital Signs Dialog Box

is new or established. When examining a new patient, a complete review of systems may be appropriate. Once the patient is established, the visit focuses more on his or her current medical needs.

A number of methods are used to organize and record visit documentation. The most common method of documenting is called a problem-oriented medical record (POMR). The problem-oriented medical record has a general section with data from the initial patient examination and assessment. When the patient makes subsequent visits, the reasons for those encounters are listed separately (in the Problem List folder) and have their own notes.

A problem-oriented medical record contains SOAP notes. In the SOAP format, a patient's encounter documentation has four parts: Subjective, Objective, Assessment, and Plan:

S: The subjective information is what the patient names as the problems or complaints.

O: The objective information includes relevant positive and negative physical findings; it may include data from laboratory tests and other procedures.

A: The assessment, also called the impression or conclusion, is the physician's diagnosis.

P: The plan, also called advice or recommendations, is the course of treatment for the patient, such as surgery, medication, or other tests, including instructions to the patient and necessary patient monitoring and follow-up.

In Figure 3.20, a SOAP note entered in MCPR has been color-coded to show the S, O, A, and P sections. The SOAP format is used for the exercises in this text/workbook.

Figure 3.20 Progress Note in SOAP Format

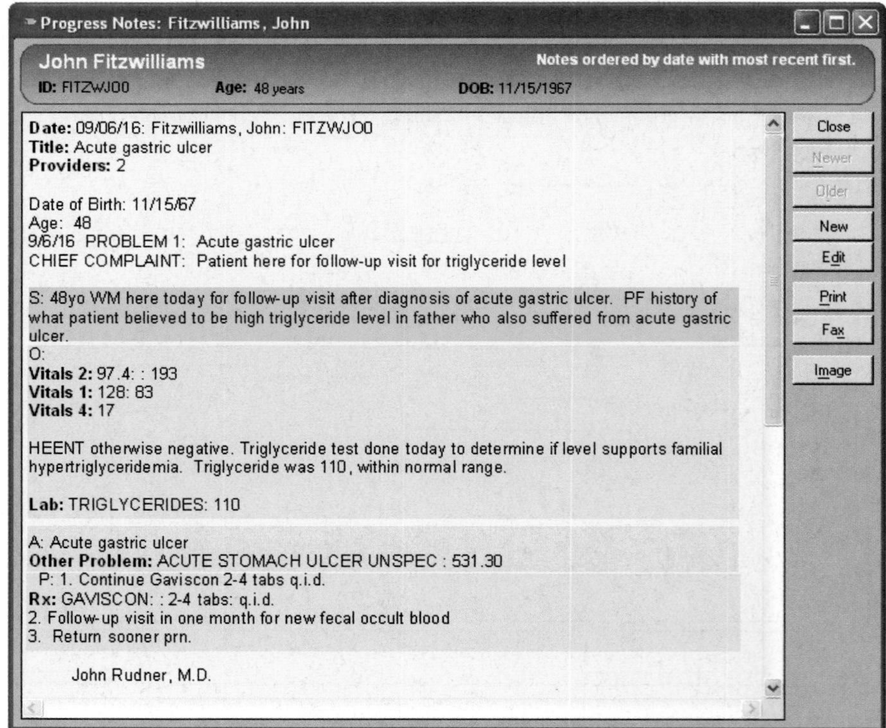

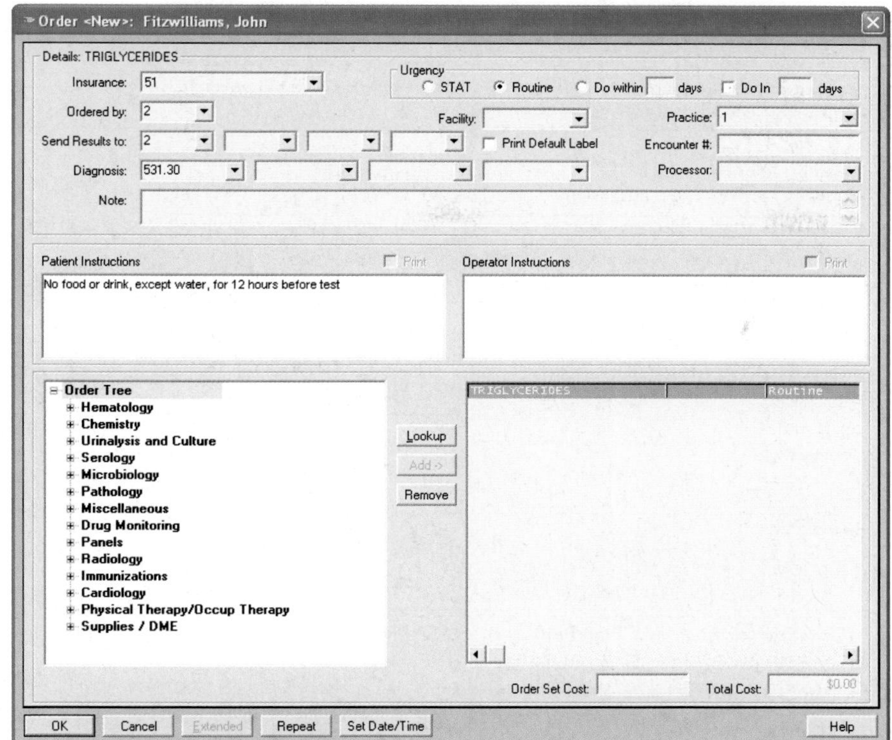

Figure 3.21 Order Dialog Box with Order for a Triglycerides Test

If the physician wants laboratory or radiological tests performed, orders are entered in the Orders folder of the patient chart. Figure 3.21 displays an order for a blood test for triglycerides.

Orders for new medications or renewals of existing prescriptions are entered in the Rx/Medications folder. An order for a new prescription is displayed in Figure 3.22. Prescriptions can be printed and given to the patient, or they can be electronically transmitted to the patient's pharmacy.

Coding

Once the examination is complete and the documentation has been entered in MCPR, the services provided and the provider's determination of the patient's diagnoses must be assigned numeric codes. In some cases, physicians assign these codes; in others, medical coders or medical billers perform this task. In either instance, the codes are determined by reviewing the documentation. Whether physicians receive payment from health plans depends in part on the diagnosis and procedure codes assigned to the visit. Both types of information are used to calculate the charges for the visit, and must be reported to insurance plans in order to receive payment for services.

In MCPR, codes are selected from lists provided on an electronic encounter form (see Figure 3.23). In this example, the procedures performed were coded as 99212 and 84478. The diagnosis code, 531.30, was assigned to both procedures.

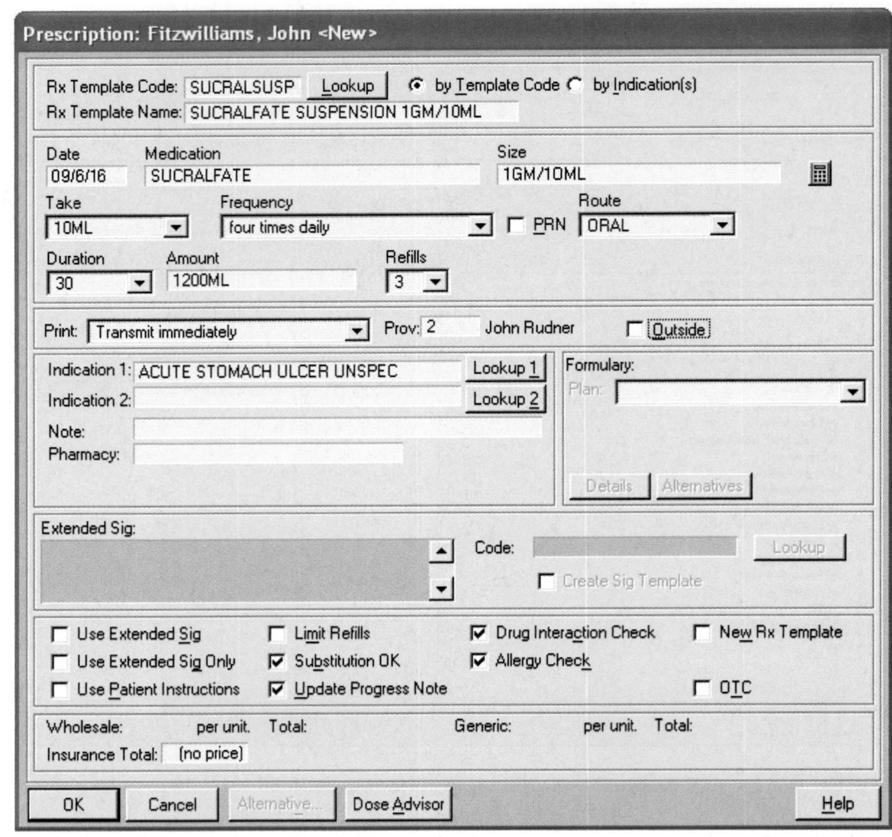

Figure 3.22 Prescription Dialog Box

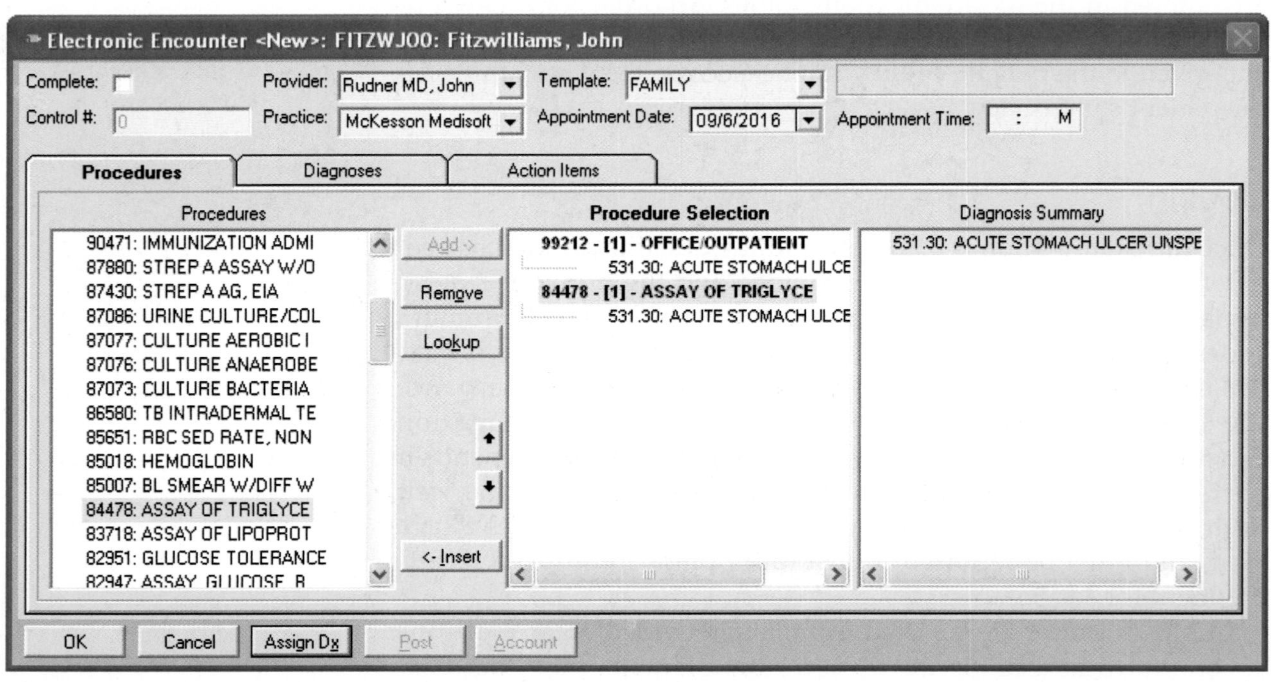

Figure 3.23 Electronic Encounter Dialog Box

Transmit Charges to Medisoft Network Professional for Billing

Once the coding is complete, the visit charges are transmitted electronically to Medisoft Network Professional. The charges are automatically transmitted every few minutes, with the exact amount of time specified by the user.

The charges appear in MNP in the Unprocessed Transactions dialog box, which is accessed by selecting Unprocessed Transactions > Unprocessed EMR Charges on the Activities menu (see Figure 3.24).

The topics of documenting a patient visit, coding a visit, and transferring charges to Medisoft Network Professional are described in Chapter 7.

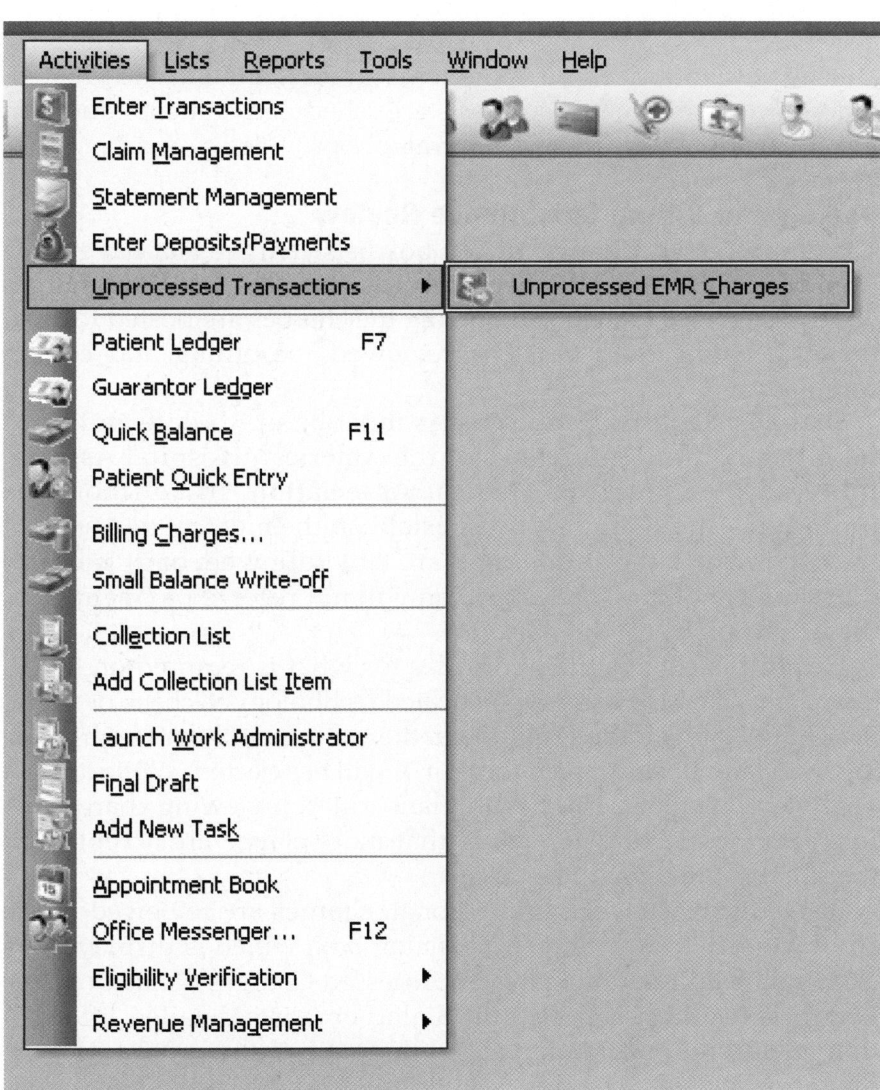

Figure 3.24 The Activities Menu with Unprocessed Transactions > Unprocessed EMR Charges Selected

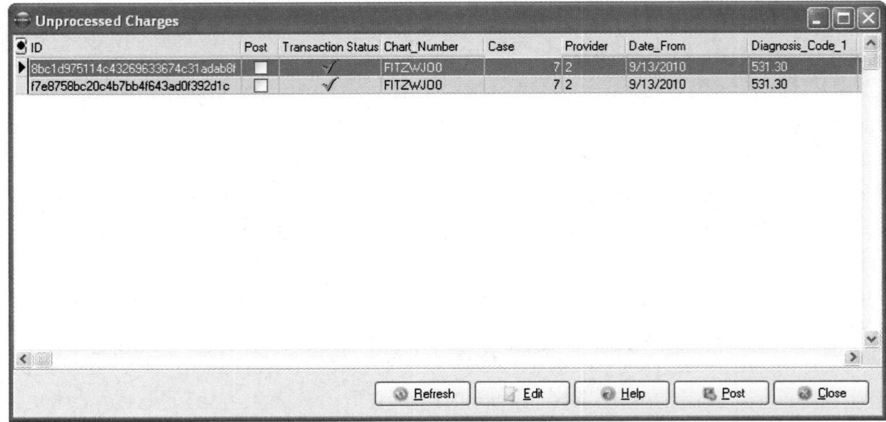

Figure 3.25 Unprocessed Charges Dialog Box

Checkout

During patient checkout, payments are calculated and posted, follow-up appointments and tests are scheduled, patient education materials are dispensed, and referrals are provided.

Coding and Billing Compliance Review

The Unprocessed Charges dialog box lists charges that have come from Medisoft Clinical Patient Records since the last time charges were posted (see Figure 3.25). Before the charges are posted to a patient's account, they must be reviewed for billing and coding compliance.

Diagnosis and procedure codes must be up-to-date and must follow the official guidelines of the American Hospital Association and the American Medical Association. In addition, the procedures and diagnosis must establish the medical necessity of the charges. If the guidelines are not followed or if medical necessity is not met, the physician will not receive payment from the health plan.

Health plans have different rules for what is required on health care claims, and they use sophisticated technology to check or "edit" incoming claims to determine whether to accept them for processing. If a claim does not pass the edit, it will be rejected. While it is not possible to memorize all health plans' rules, reviewing charges before sending claims will ensure that more claims are accepted on their first submission.

In Medisoft Network Professional, charges are reviewed in the Unprocessed Transactions Edit dialog box, which is displayed by clicking the Edit button in the Unprocessed Charges dialog box. The Unprocessed Transactions Edit dialog box lists detailed information, including information about the patient, the procedures, the diagnosis, and the charges (see Figure 3.26). If the billing compliance review finds a problem with the transaction, the charges can be held as unprocessed until the problem is corrected. If the review determines that the transaction is complete and accurate, the

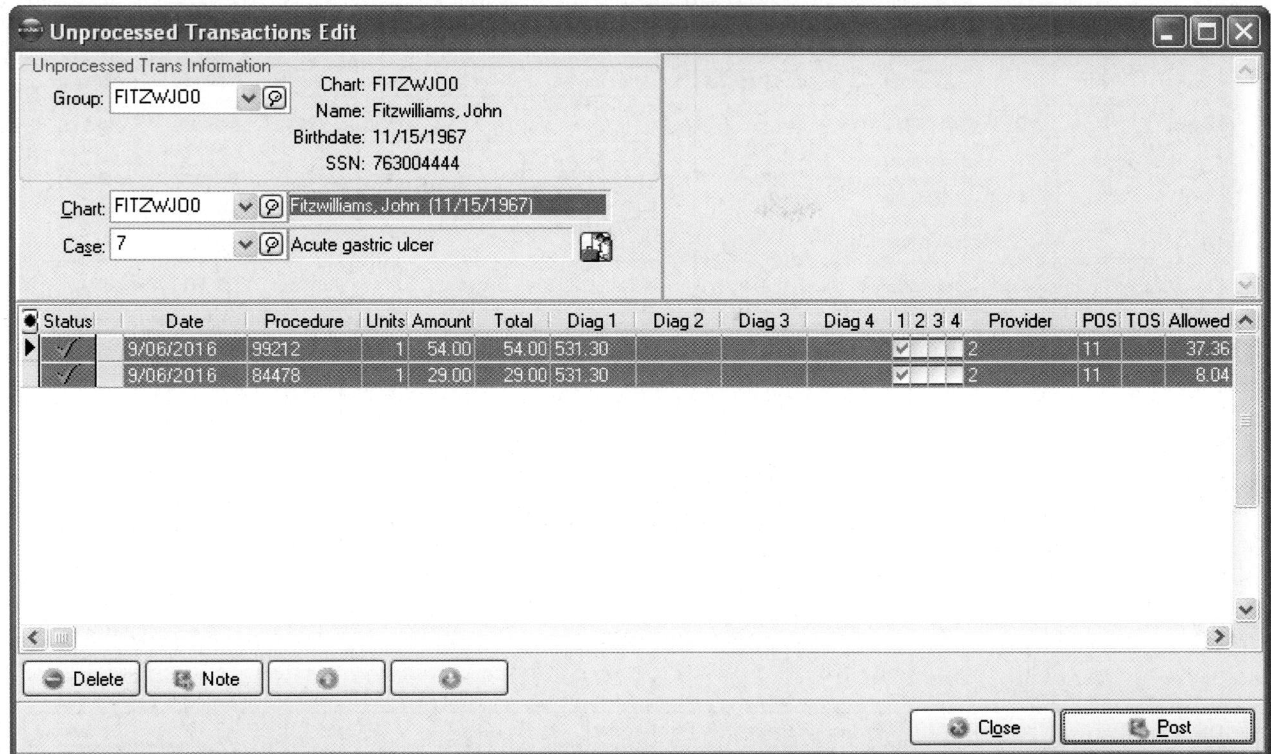

Figure 3.26 Unprocessed Transactions Edit Dialog Box

charges are posted to a patient's account. Clicking the Post button enters the charges into the Transaction Entry dialog box in MNP (see Figure 3.27). Transactions are not finalized until the Save button is clicked.

Billing and coding compliance is covered in Chapter 9.

Calculate and Post Time-of-Service (TOS) Payments

When a patient goes to the checkout desk, a staff member reviews the amount that the patient owes for the visit. In some cases, nothing is owed at the time of service. The claim will be submitted to the patient's health plan, and the patient will not be billed until the claim is processed. In other cases, patients pay for all or a portion of services at the time of the visit. A patient may be responsible for a small copayment or a percentage of estimated charges.

Patient payments are entered in the Transaction Entry dialog box. Figure 3.28 shows the Transaction Entry dialog box after a $15.00 patient copayment has been recorded. The payment line is highlighted in yellow.

If a patient makes a payment at the time of service, a receipt is typically printed. The Print Receipt button at the bottom of the Transaction Entry dialog box generates a receipt, which can be printed and given to the patient. Figure 3.29 displays a sample patient receipt.

Posting time-of-service payments is discussed in depth in Chapter 9.

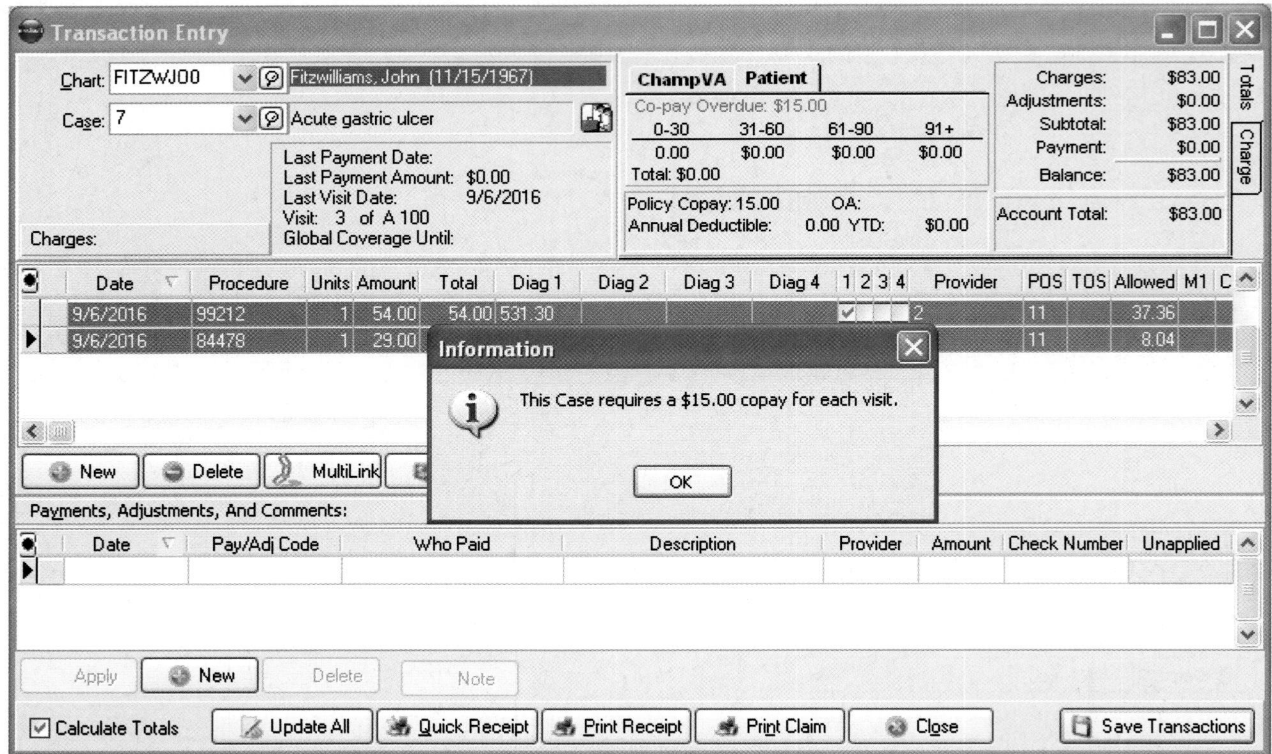

Figure 3.27 Transaction Entry Dialog Box with Transactions Posted

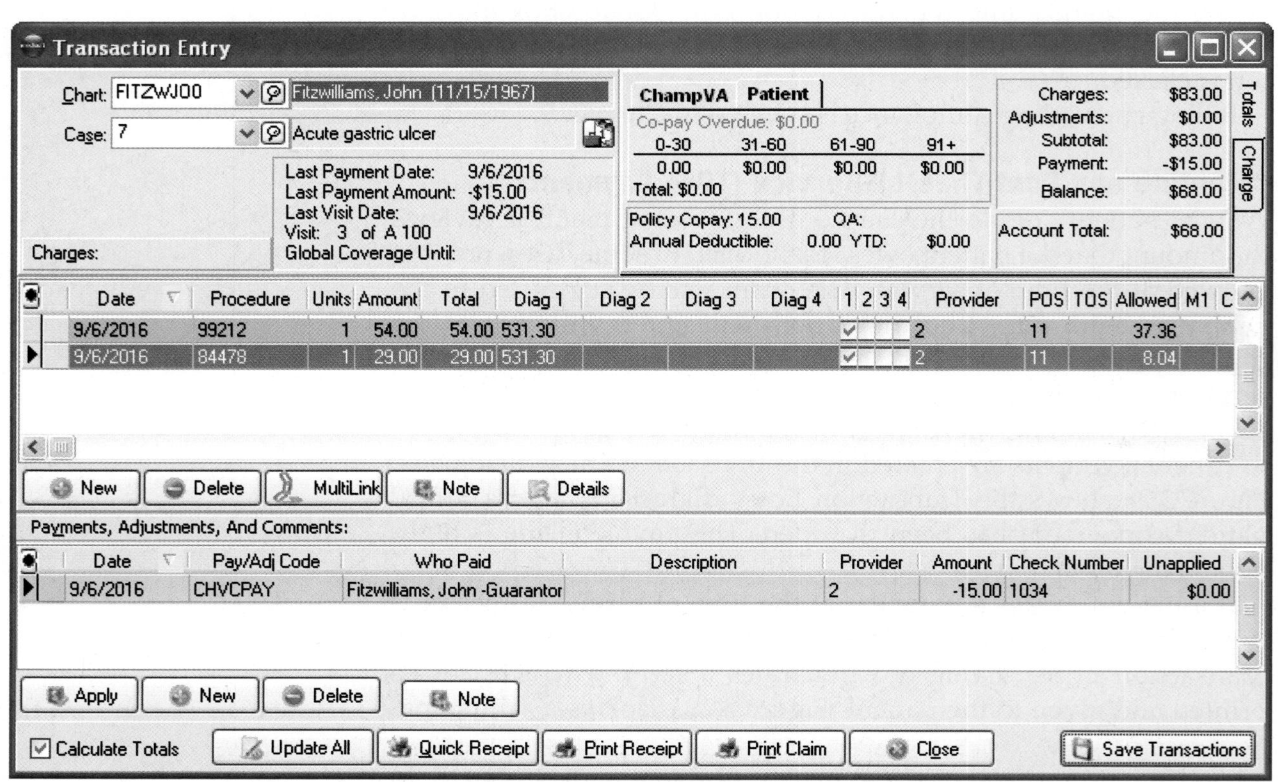

Figure 3.28 Transaction Entry Dialog Box with Patient Copayment Posted

Family Care Clinic
285 Stephenson Boulevard
Stephenson, OH 60089
(614)555-0000

Page: 1 9/6/2016

Patient: John Fitzwilliams
1627 Forest Avenue
Jefferson, OH 60093

Chart #: FITZWJO0
Case #: 7

Instructions:
Complete the patient information portion of your insurance claim form. Attach this bill, signed and dated, and all other bills pertaining to the claim. If you have a deductible policy, hold your claim forms until you have met your deductible. Mail directly to your insurance carrier.

Date	Description	Procedure	Modify	Dx 1	Dx 2	Dx 3	Dx 4	Units	Charge
9/6/2016	OF--established patient, low	99212		531.30				1	54.00
9/6/2016	Triglycerides test	84478		531.30				1	29.00
9/6/2016	ChampVA Copayment	CHVCPAY						1	-15.00

Provider Information
Provider Name: John Rudner MD
License: 84701
Champ VA PIN:
SSN or EIN: 339-67-5000

Total Charges:	$ 83.00
Total Payments:	-$ 15.00
Total Adjustments:	$ 0.00
Total Due This Visit:	**$ 68.00**
Total Account Balance:	$ 68.00

Assign and Release: I hereby authorize payment of medical benefits to this physician for the services described above. I also authorize the release of any information necessary to process this claim.

Patient Signature: ______________________ Date: ____________

Figure 3.29 Patient Receipt for Payment

Additional Checkout Activities

The final step of the checkout process includes scheduling any follow-up appointments ordered by the provider, such as return office visits, laboratory tests, or radiology services; providing referrals or prescriptions as required; and providing related patient education materials as ordered by the provider.

Scheduling is performed in Office Hours, the Medisoft Network Professional scheduling program. Referrals and prescriptions are created from within Medisoft Clinical Patient Records, as are patient education materials. Figure 3.30 shows a sample patient education handout selected in MCPR.

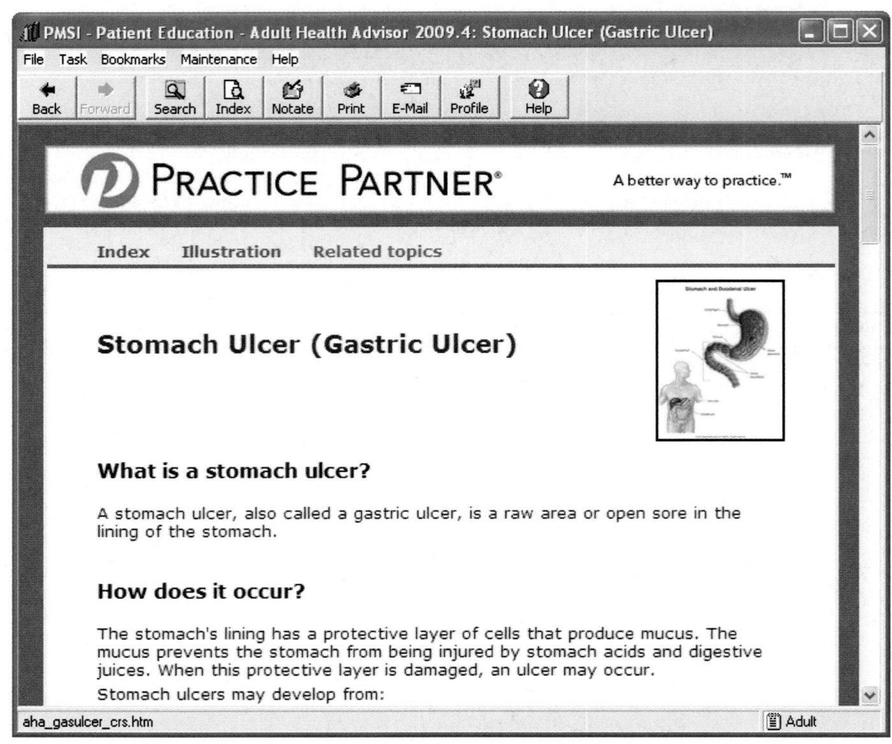

Figure 3.30 Patient Education Selection

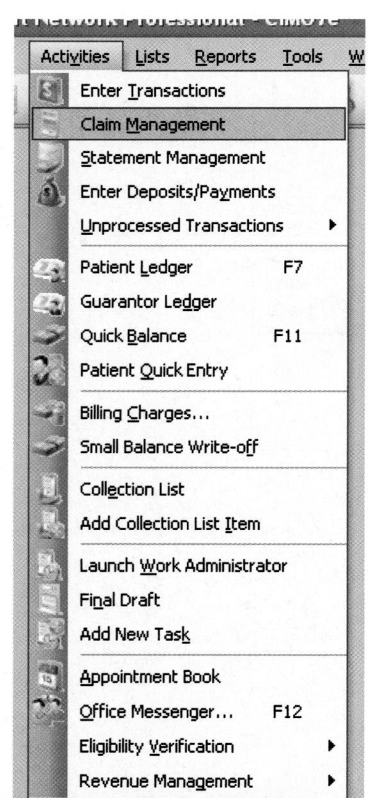

Figure 3.31 Activities Menu with Claim Management Selected

THINKING IT THROUGH 3.3

Electronic health record programs store patients' vital signs and laboratory results. Most programs provide an option to view patient results from a specified period of time in a graph. What is an advantage of viewing vital signs or test results in a graph?

3.7 Using Medisoft Clinical to Complete Post-Encounter Tasks

After the patient visit is complete, activities focus on payment for services, including preparing and transmitting claims, monitoring payer adjudication, generating patient statements, and following up on payments and collections.

Preparing and Transmitting Claims

To receive payment, a medical practice must create and submit claims to health plans. In Medisoft Network Professional, claim functions are located on the Activities menu (see Figure 3.31).

The Claim Management dialog box lists current claims. New claims are created in the Create Claims dialog box (see Figure 3.32).

Claims are transmitted to health plans through MNP's Revenue Management feature. In addition to transmitting electronic

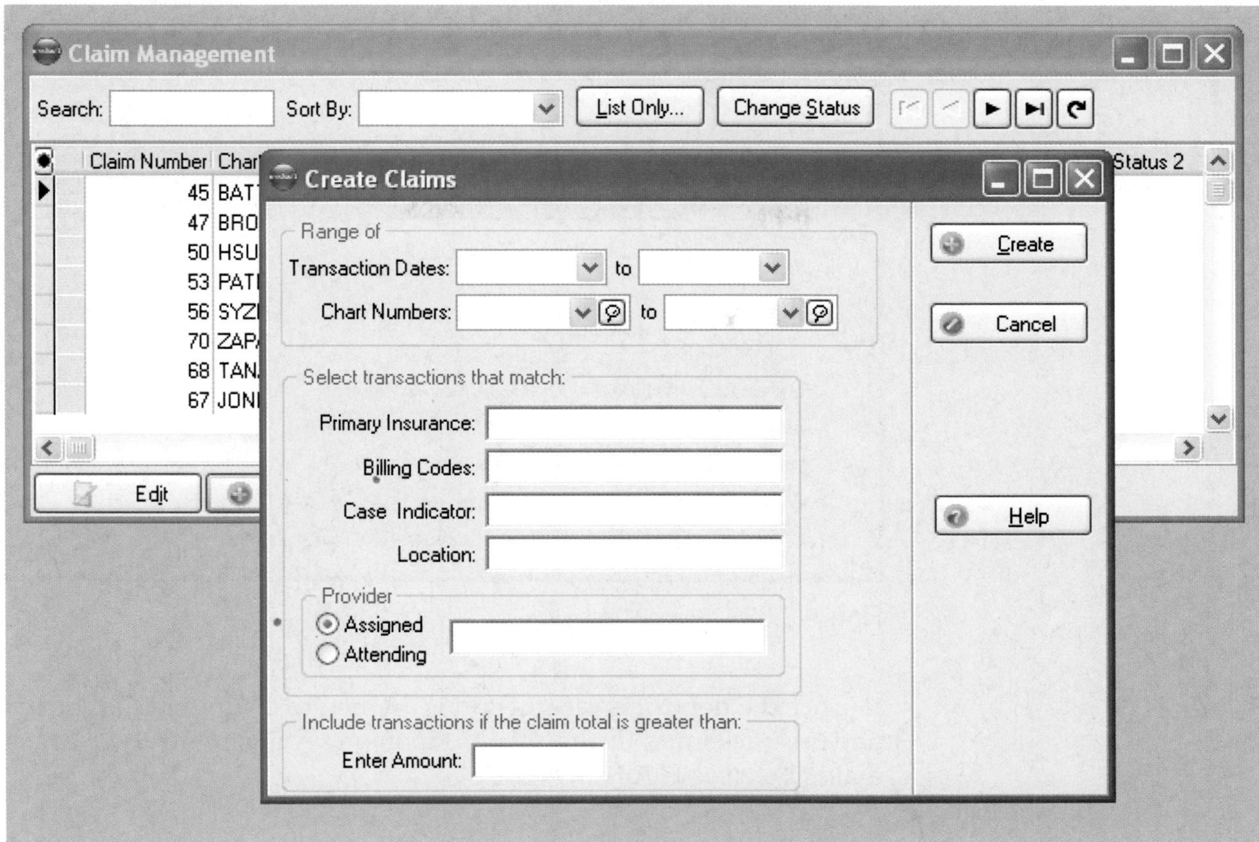

Figure 3.32 Create Claims Dialog Box

claims, Revenue Management checks outgoing claims for errors before sending them to the health plan. Claim management is covered in detail in Chapter 10.

Monitoring Payer Adjudication

The health plan reviews the claim and determines whether it will be paid in full, partially paid, or denied. The results of the claim review, including an explanation of why charges were not paid in full or were denied entirely, are sent to the provider along with the payment. This information is reviewed for accuracy by a member of the billing staff, such as a medical insurance specialist. If any discrepancies are found, a request for a review of the claim is filed with the payer. If no issues are discovered, the amount of the payment is recorded. The payment may be in the form of a paper check, or it may be sent electronically to the practice's bank.

In Medisoft Network Professional, the first step in entering health plan payments is to select Enter Deposits/Payments on the Activities menu. The Deposit List window is displayed. Clicking the New button brings up the dialog box used to enter payment information (see Figure 3.33).

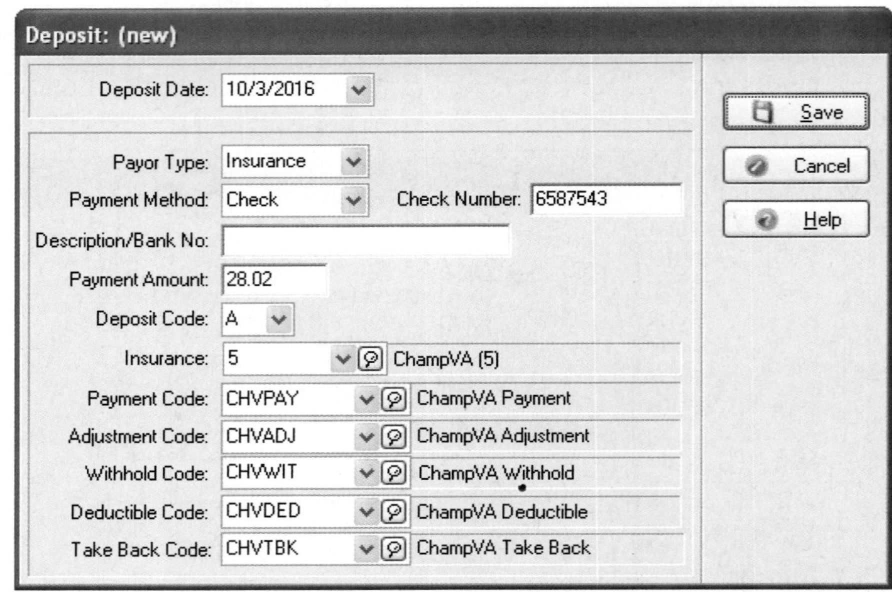

Figure 3.33 Deposit Dialog Box

Once the deposit is recorded, it is applied to charges in individual patients' accounts in the Apply Payment/Adjustment to Charges dialog box (see Figure 3.34).

Generating Patient Statements

After payments from health plans have been received, patients are billed for any remaining balances. Patient statements are created in Medisoft Network Professional and are sent to patients. A statement lists all services performed, along with the charges for each service.

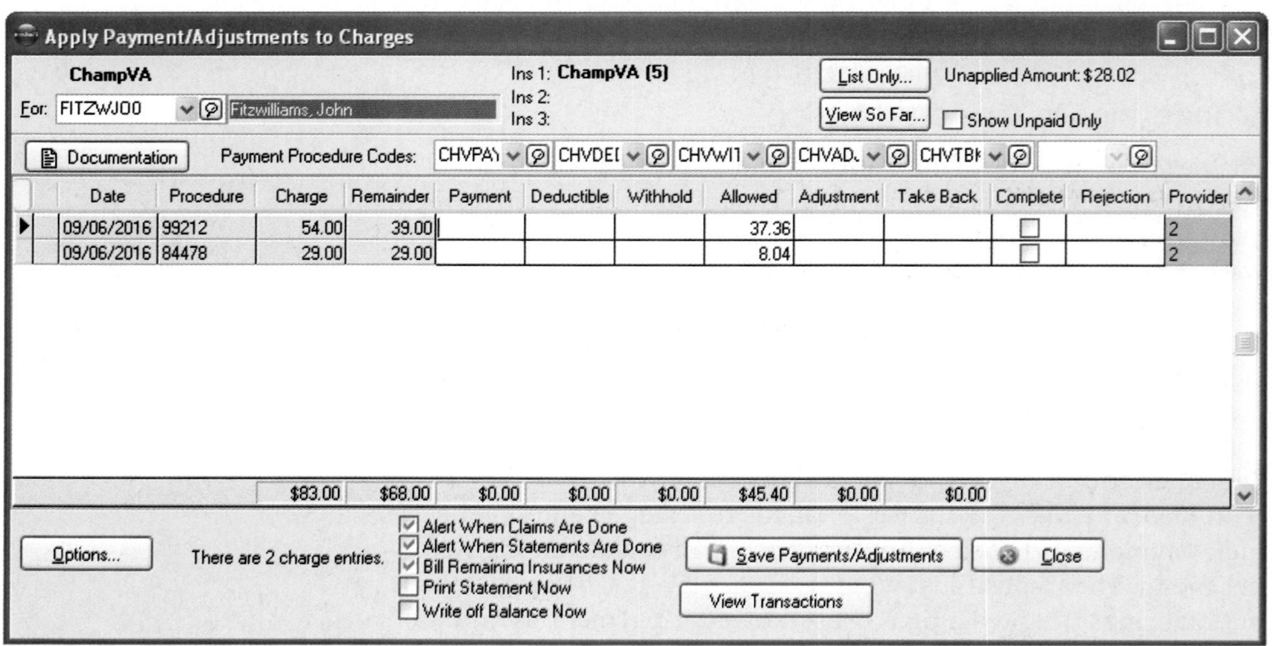

Figure 3.34 Apply Payment/Adjustments to Charges Dialog Box

It also lists the amount paid by the health plan and the remaining balance that is the responsibility of the patient. While some practices send statements electronically via e-mail, some practices still mail paper statements.

The Statement Management option on the Activities menu contains options for creating and printing patient statements (see Figure 3.35).

Selections in the Create Statements dialog box determine which statements will be created. The program allows filtering by patient, date, minimum amount owed, and other criteria (see Figure 3.36).

A sample patient statement is displayed in Figure 3.37.

The topics of posting insurance payments and creating patient statements are presented in Chapter 11.

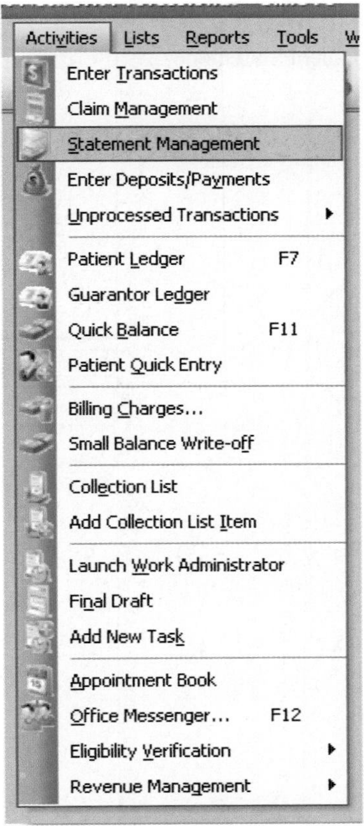

Figure 3.35 Activities Menu with Statement Management Selected

Following Up on Payments and Collections

Because a medical practice must be successful as a business as well as a provider of health care services, it must track the money that is coming in and going out. Medisoft Network Professional provides a large number of reports that enable office managers to closely monitor accounts.

For example, practices regularly print a report that lists outstanding patient balances (see Figure 3.38). The information in this report identifies accounts that require follow-up.

Most physician practices have financial policies that specify when an account should be placed in collections. In Medisoft

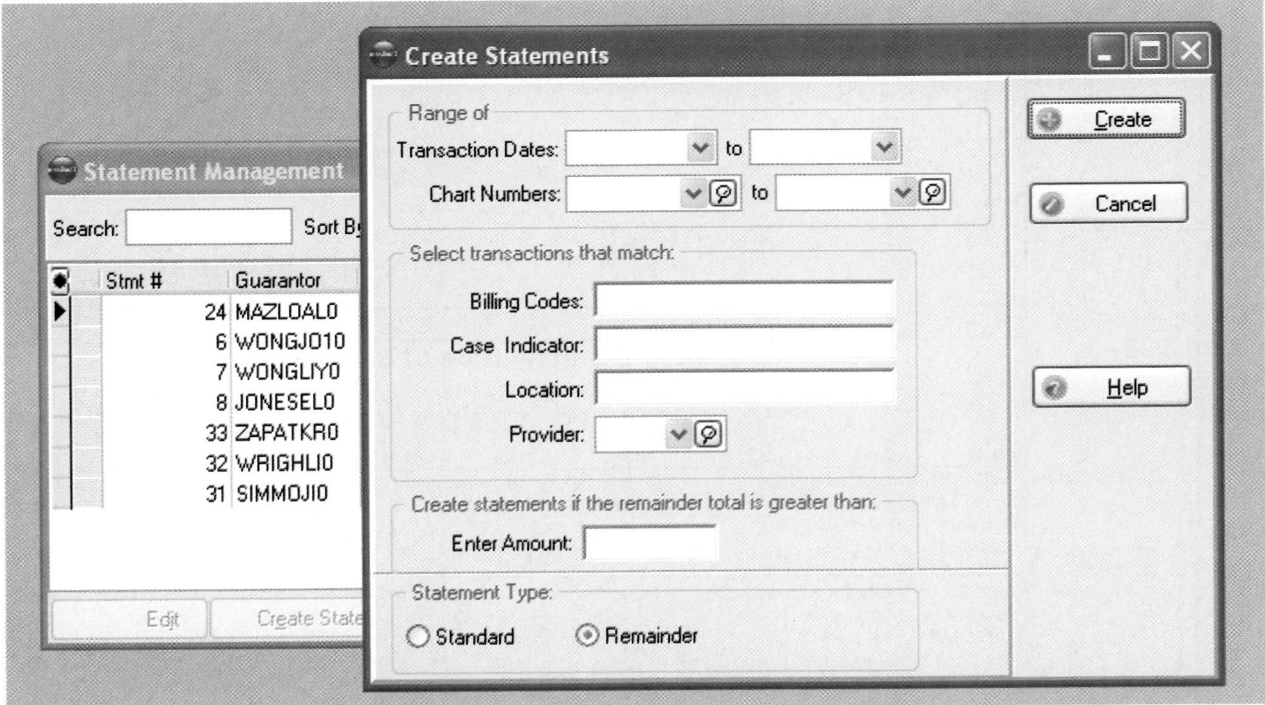

Figure 3.36 Create Statements Dialog Box

Figure 3.37
Patient Statement

Family Care Clinic
285 Stephenson Boulevard
Stephenson, OH 60089
(614)555-0000

Statement Date	Chart Number	Page
09/30/2016	**FITZWJO0**	**1**

Make Checks Payable To:
Family Care Clinic
285 Stephenson Boulevard
Stephenson, OH 60089
(614)555-0000

John Fitzwilliams
1627 Forest Avenue
Jefferson, OH 60093

Date of Last Payment: 9/6/2016 Amount: -15.00 Previous Balance: 0.00

Patient: John Fitzwilliams Chart Number: FITZWJO0 Case: Acute gastric ulcer

Dates	Procedure	Charge	Paid by Primary	Paid By Guarantor	Adjustments	Remainder
09/06/16	84478	29.00	0.00		-20.96	8.04

Amount Due
8.04

Figure 3.38
Patient Aging Report

Patient Aging by Date of Service

Family Care Clinic

Show all data where the Charges/Payments/Adj is on or before 11/30/2016

Chart	Name	0-30	31-60	61-90	91-120	121+	Total
BATTIAN0	Battistuta, Anthony		79.00				79.00
BROOKLA0	Brooks, Lawana		130.00				130.00
FITZWJO0	Fitzwilliams, John			8.04			8.04
GILESSH0	Giles, Sheila		61.60				61.60
HSUDIAN0	Hsu, Diane		102.00				102.00
JONESEL0	Jones, Elizabeth		72.00	21.17	7.47		100.64
MAZLOAL0	Mazloum, Ali					720.50	720.50
PATELRA0	Patel, Raji		34.00				34.00
SIMMOJI0	Simmons, Jill		21.00				21.00
SYZMAMI0	Syzmanski, Michael		34.00				34.00
WONGJO10	Wong, Jo			7.47		7.47	14.94
WONGLIY0	Wong, Li			4.14			4.14
WRIGHLI0	Wright, Lisa		46.40				46.40
ZAPATKR0	Zapata, Kristin		35.00		247.50		282.50
Report Totals:		0.00	615.00	40.82	254.97	727.97	1,638.76

THINKING IT THROUGH 3.4

In an office with an integrated PM/EHR, charges from an office visit are sent electronically to the practice management application. However, they are not immediately posted to patient accounts. A member of the billing staff must intervene and click a Post button to enter the charges. Since posting charges immediately seems more efficient, why do you think the program does not work that way? What is the reason for the delay?

Network Professional, collection functions are located on the Activities menu and on the Reports menu. Selecting Collection List on the Activities menu is the first step in placing an account in collections (see Figure 3.39).

When Collection List is selected, the Collection List dialog box appears. Clicking the New button displays the Tickler Item dialog box (see Figure 3.40). Once the Tickler Item dialog box has been completed, the account appears in the Collection List.

Medisoft Network Professional also facilitates the creation of collection letters. The option for creating collection letters is located on the Reports menu (see Figure 3.41).

Figure 3.42 shows a sample collection letter.

Follow-up on patient accounts and the collections process are discussed in Chapter 13.

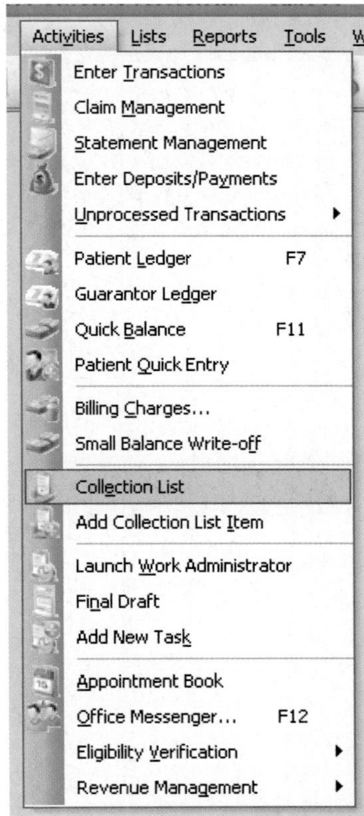

Figure 3.39 Activities Menu with Collection List Selected

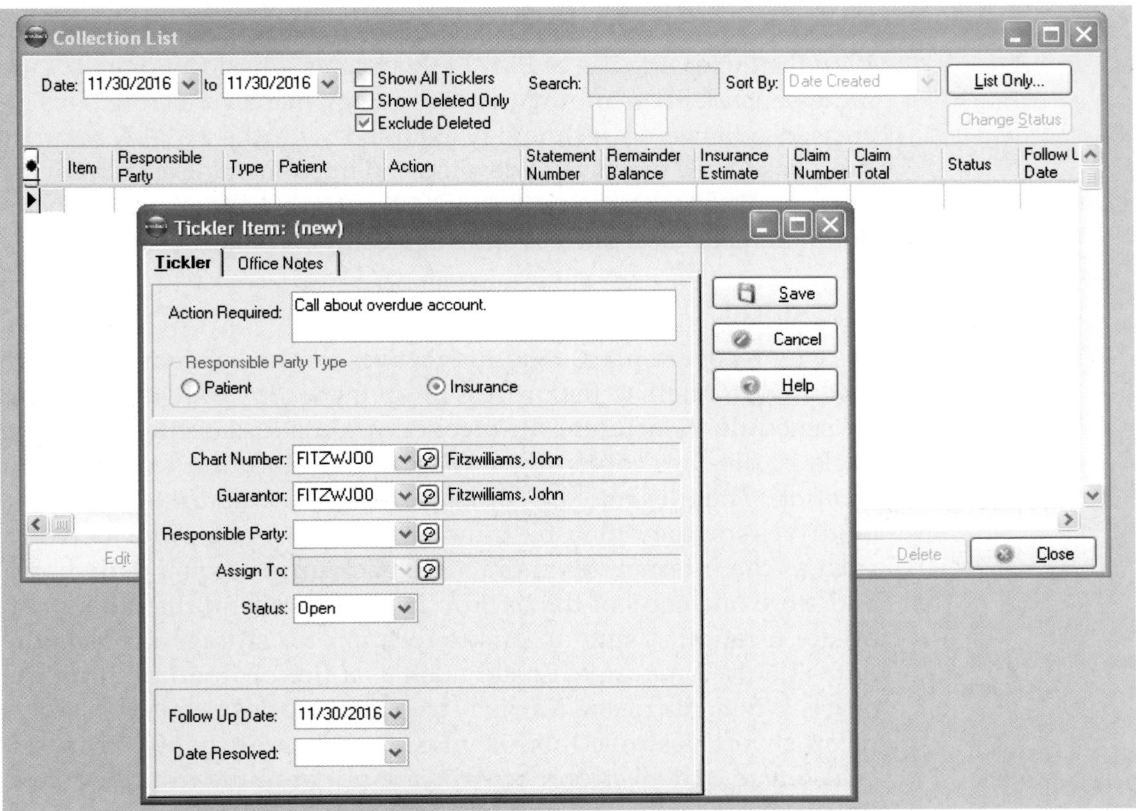

Figure 3.40 Tickler Item Dialog Box

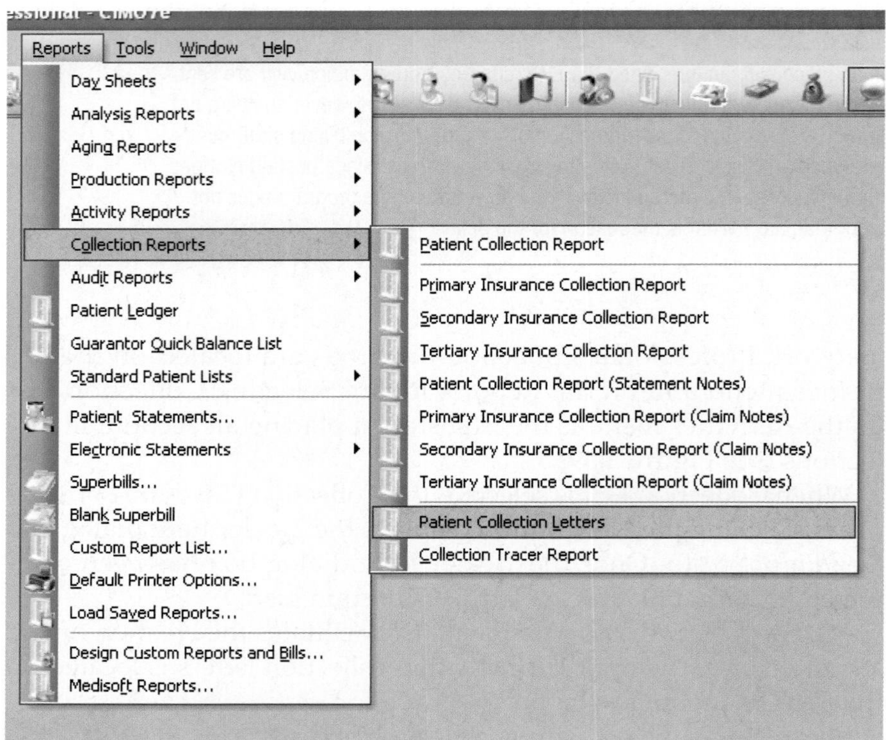

Figure 3.41 Reports Menu with Collection Reports >Patient Collection Letters Selected

3.8 Backing Up and Restoring Files

With the increasing use of PM/EHR systems, physician practices are more dependent on information technology than ever before. This increased reliance on technology, coupled with the HIPAA Security Rule, has forced practices to develop and implement disaster recovery plans. A **disaster recovery plan** is a plan for resuming normal operations after a disaster such as a fire or a computer malfunction.

disaster recovery plan plan for resuming normal operations after a disaster such as a fire or a computer malfunction

backing up making a copy of data files at a specific point in time that can be used to restore data

Backing Up Files

Disaster recovery plans require practices to back up computer data. **Backing up** refers to the process of saving a copy of files on a regular schedule to facilitate file recovery if data loss occurs. During a backup, files are copied from their normal location to a different location. The files may be copied to portable media, such as tapes or drives, or they may be transferred over a computer network such as the Internet. Most practices back up data on a daily basis, and store one copy of the backup in the office, and the other at an offsite location. Using an offsite location for storage protects the data should a natural disaster such as a fire or flood occur at the office. When Hurricane Katrina struck New Orleans, many medical records were destroyed. While most of these were paper records, it is also true that electronic records are not immune from disasters. In fact, computerized records are subject to additional threats, such as computer viruses and hardware malfunctions. As a result of the

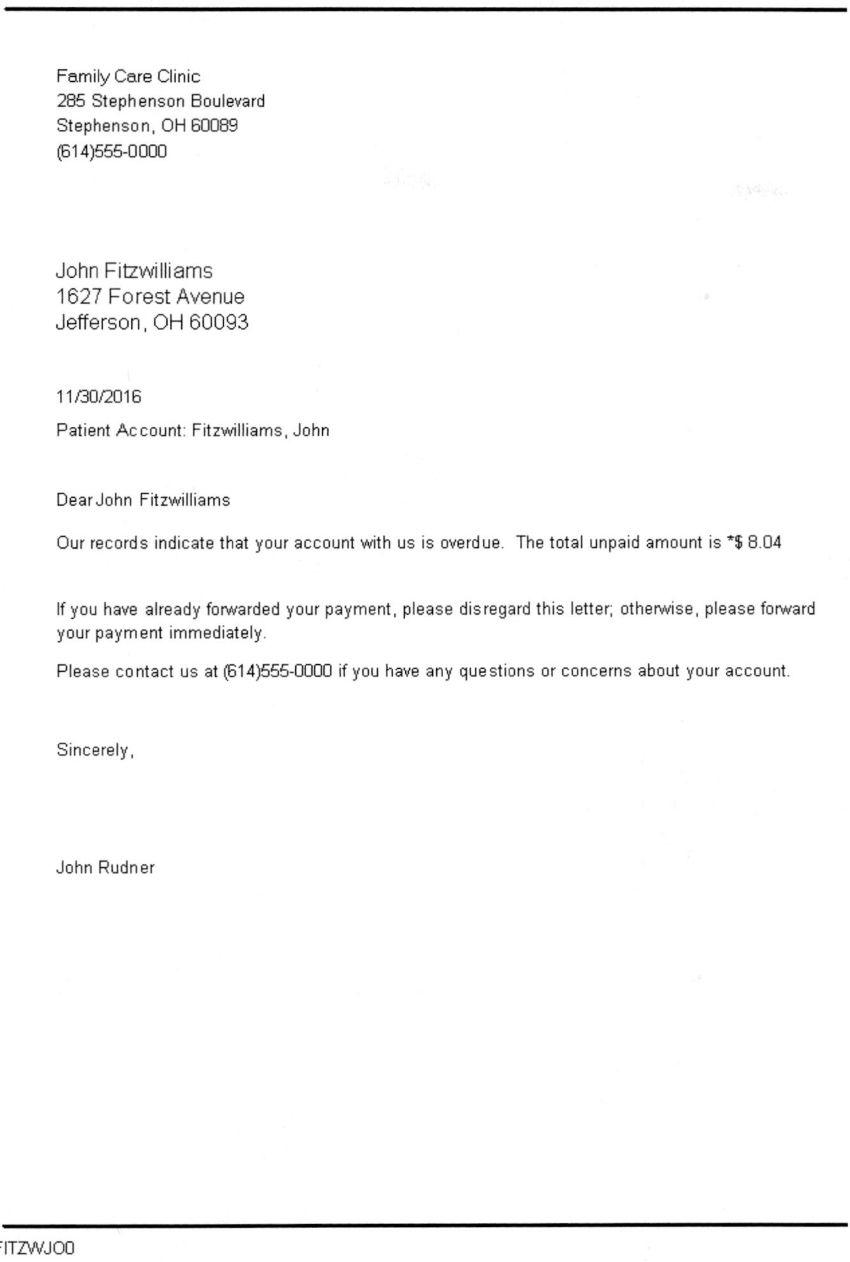

Family Care Clinic
285 Stephenson Boulevard
Stephenson, OH 60089
(614)555-0000

John Fitzwilliams
1627 Forest Avenue
Jefferson, OH 60093

11/30/2016

Patient Account: Fitzwilliams, John

Dear John Fitzwilliams

Our records indicate that your account with us is overdue. The total unpaid amount is *$ 8.04

If you have already forwarded your payment, please disregard this letter; otherwise, please forward your payment immediately.

Please contact us at (614)555-0000 if you have any questions or concerns about your account.

Sincerely,

John Rudner

FITZWJO0

*Balance does not reflect any outstanding insurance payments

Figure 3.42 Collection Letter

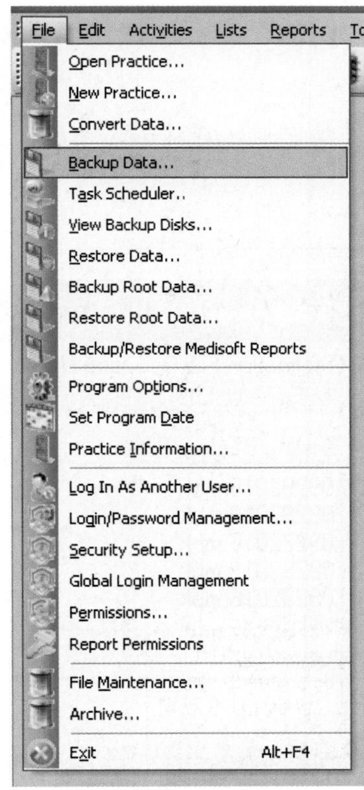

Figure 3.43 File Menu with Backup Data Selected

lessons learned from Hurricane Katrina, medical facilities are more aware of the importance of backing up data.

Files that are backed up can be restored. **Restoring** is the process of copying backup files onto the office's computer systems, facilitating a return to normal business activities.

restoring process of retrieving data from a backup storage device

In Medisoft Network Professional, the Backup Data option on the File menu can be used to make a backup copy of the database at any time (see Figure 3.43).

The Medisoft Backup dialog box pictured in Figure 3.44 lists the destination file path and name of the file being created, and also lists existing backup files.

EXERCISE 3.7

Mc Graw Hill connect plus+

BACKING UP

Practice creating a backup file in Medisoft Network Professional.

1. Select Backup Data on the File menu. The Medisoft Backup dialog box is displayed.
2. In the Destination File Path and Name box, enter ***C:\FCC\Backup_Files\2016\09\09302016.mbk.***
3. Medisoft automatically displays the location of the database files to be backed up in the Source Path box in the lower half of the dialog box.
4. Click the Start Backup button.
5. The program backs up the latest database files and displays an Information dialog box indicating that the backup is complete. Click OK.
6. Close the Medisoft Backup dialog box by clicking the Close button.

You have completed Exercise 3.7

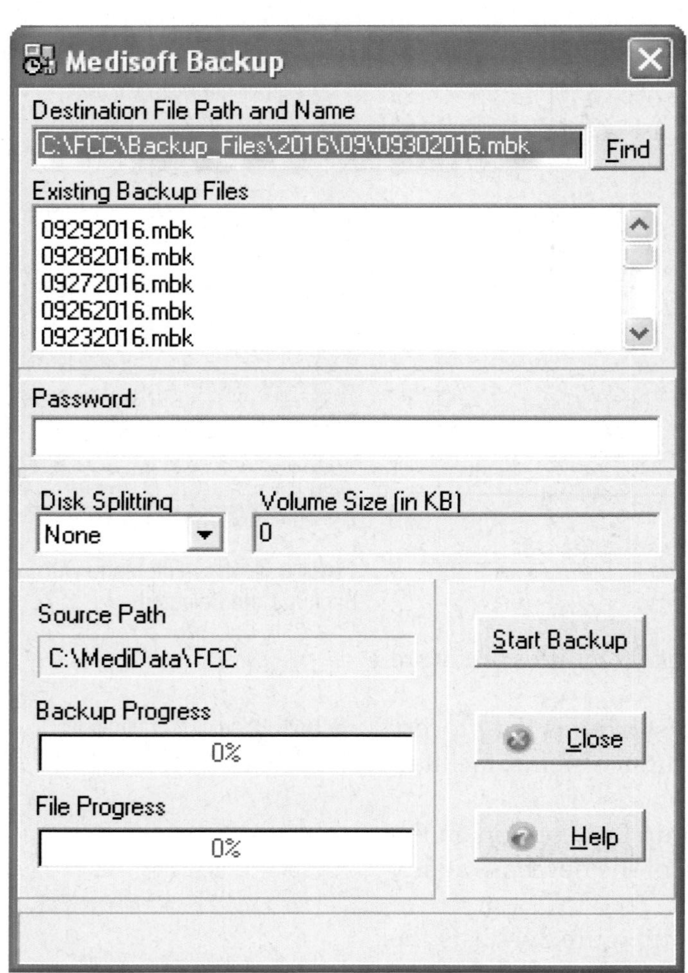

Figure 3.44 Medisoft Backup Dialog Box

Restoring Files

The steps required to restore a backup file are very similar to the steps used to back up a file. To restore 09302016.mbk to the Medisoft Network Professional directory on the C drive (C:\MediData\FCC):

1. Select Restore Data on the File menu.
2. When the Warning box appears, click OK. The Restore dialog box appears.
3. In the Backup File Path and Name box at the top of the dialog box, enter the location of the backup file, if this name is not already displayed.
4. The Destination Path at the bottom of the box should already show C:\MediData\FCC.
5. Click the Start Restore button.
6. When the Confirm box appears, click OK.
7. An Information dialog box appears indicating that the restore is complete. Click OK to continue.
8. Click the Close button to close the Restore dialog box.

3.9 The Medisoft Clinical Help Feature

Medisoft Network Professional and Medisoft Clinical Patient Records offer built-in and online help files. These resources provide detailed explanations of program features, list common errors, and offer tips designed to improve user productivity.

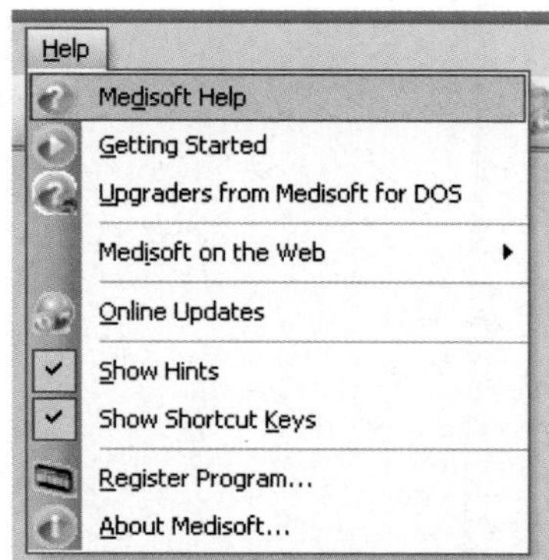

Figure 3.45 Medisoft Help Selection on Help Menu

Built-in Help

The built-in help feature is accessed by selecting an option on the Help menu. Figure 3.45 shows the Medisoft Help selection on the Help menu in MNP.

When this option is selected, the Help dialog box opens, and the contents of the Help feature are displayed (see Figure 3.46).

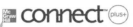

connect plus+ EXERCISE 3.8

USING MEDISOFT CLINICAL HELP

Practice using MNP's built-in help.

1. Click the Help menu.
2. Click Medisoft Help. Medisoft displays a list of topics for which help is available.
3. Click the plus sign to the left of the entry for Entering Payments. A list of subtopics is displayed.
4. Click Apply Payment to Charges. The article appears in the right column.
5. Use the scroll bar to view the rest of the article.
6. Click the Close box in the upper-right corner to close the Help window.

You have completed Exercise 3.8

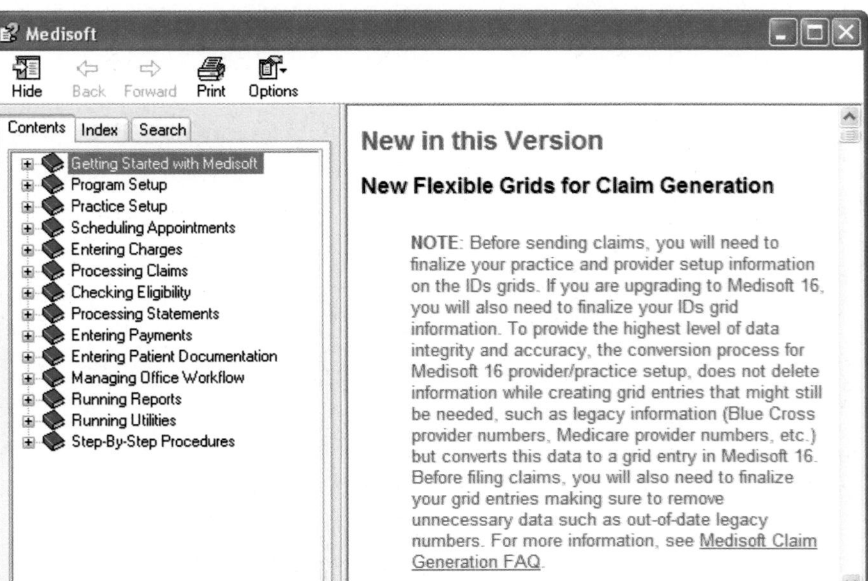

Figure 3.46 Contents of Medisoft Help Feature

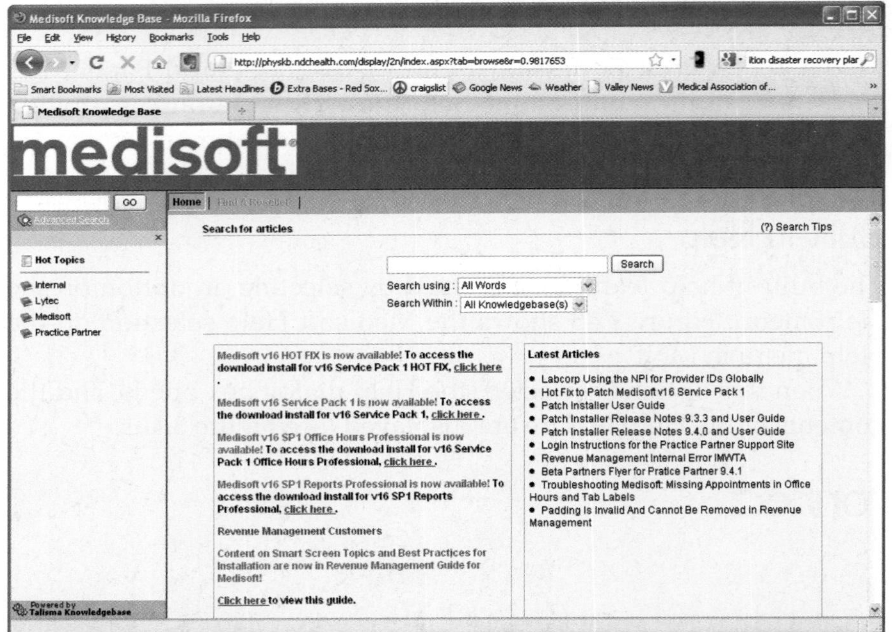

Figure 3.47 MNP Online Knowledge Base

Online Help

knowledge base a collection of up-to-date technical information

The Help menu also provides access to help available on the MNP website at www.medisoft.com. The website contains a searchable **knowledge base**, which is a collection of up-to-date technical information about Medisoft products (see Figure 3.47).

chapter 3 summary

LEARNING OUTCOME	KEY CONCEPTS/EXAMPLES
3.1 List the practice management and electronic health record applications in Medisoft Clinical. Page 106	The practice management application in Medisoft Clinical is called Medisoft Network Professional (MNP), and the electronic health record application is Medisoft Clinical Patient Records (MCPR).
3.2 Discuss three security features in Medisoft Clinical that protect patients' health information. Pages 106–108	- User names and passwords are assigned to individuals to protect unauthorized access, safeguard patient information, and protect patient confidentiality. - Access levels are assigned to job functions to specify who has access to information on a need-to-know basis; the user must enter a user name and password to see the information and to have editing and other privileges. - The park feature allows a user to walk away from the computer and still safeguard the information; it requires the next user to enter a user name and password to gain access. The Auto Log Off feature logs off a user after a specified period of inactivity. Both keep passers-by from viewing or accessing information.
3.3 List the menus in Medisoft Clinical Patient Records. Pages 109–113	The names of the standard menus in Medisoft Clinical Patient Records are File, View, Task, Maintenance, Reports, Window, and Help. The menus and commands available may change depending on the task being performed.
3.4 List the menus in Medisoft Network Professional. Pages 113–117	The menus in Medisoft Network Professional are File, Edit, Activities, Lists, Reports, Tools, Window, and Help.
3.5 Describe how pre-encounter tasks are completed in Medisoft Clinical. Pages 117–121	The pre-encounter steps include preregistration and appointment scheduling. Preregistration consists of entering basic information about the patient in Medisoft Network Professional. The demographic information is entered in the Patient/Guarantor dialog box, which is accessed via the Lists menu. A case is created, and the chief complaint is entered in the Personal tab. An appointment is scheduled in Office Hours.

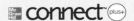

Enhance your learning at **mcgrawhillconnect.com**!

- *Practice Exercises*
- *Worksheets*
- *Activities*
- *Integrated eBook*

LEARNING OUTCOME	KEY CONCEPTS/EXAMPLES
3.6 Describe how encounter tasks are completed in Medisoft Clinical. Pages 121–134	The following tasks are handled in Medisoft Clinical during the encounter: - Insurance information is entered and eligibility is checked in the Policy tab. - At check-in, the account balance is reviewed, payment may be obtained, and additional patient information is gathered and recorded. - Documentation and examination take place, with the medical assistant or other clinical staff member doing part of it, and a physician doing and documenting the actual physical examination. - The diagnosis and procedures are coded, and charges are transmitted to MNP for billing. These are reviewed for coding and billing compliance.
3.7 Describe how post-encounter tasks are completed in Medisoft Clinical. Pages 134–139	- Claims are prepared and transmitted in the Claim Management dialog box of MNP. - The health plan's determination and payment are reviewed, starting with the Deposit dialog box. - Patient statements are generated in the Create Statements dialog box. - Follow-up takes place by creating a patient aging report.
3.8 Explain how to create and restore backup files in Medisoft Clinical. Pages 140–142	Files are backed up by choosing Backup Data on the File menu and entering the information in the Backup dialog box. They are restored by choosing Restore Data on the File menu and providing the required information in the dialog box.
3.9 Discuss the types of help available in Medisoft Clinical. Pages 143–144	Medisoft Clinical offers two types of help. Built-in help is available on the Help menu. Online help is obtained from the knowledge base on the MNP website.

chapter review

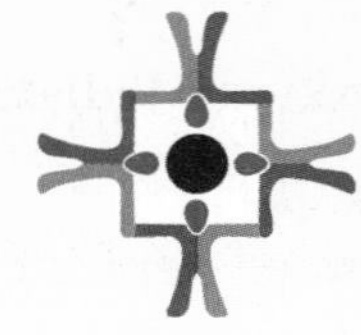

MATCHING QUESTIONS

Match the key terms with their definitions.

_____ 1. ***[LO 3.2]*** password

_____ 2. ***[LO 3.8]*** restoring

_____ 3. ***[LO 3.3]*** chart

_____ 4. ***[LO 3.3]*** dashboard

_____ 5. ***[LO 3.1]*** Medisoft Clinical Patient Records (MCPR)

_____ 6. ***[LO 3.5]*** chief complaint

_____ 7. ***[LO 3.2]*** user name

_____ 8. ***[LO 3.3]*** database

_____ 9. ***[LO 3.9]*** knowledge base

_____ 10. ***[LO 3.8]*** backing up

a. Panel in MCPR that offers providers a convenient view of important information.

b. Confidential authentication information.

c. Name that an individual uses for identification purposes when logging onto a computer or an application.

d. Making a copy of data files at a specific point in time that can be used to restore data.

e. Collection of up-to-date technical information.

f. Electronic health record application within Medisoft Clinical.

g. Folder that contains all records pertaining to a patient.

h. Patient's description of the symptoms or reasons for seeking medical care.

i. Process of retrieving data from a backup storage device.

j. Collection of related bits of information.

TRUE-FALSE QUESTIONS

Decide whether each statement is true or false.

_____ 1. ***[LO 3.2]*** Access levels define which areas of the program a user can view, and whether the user can only view the information or can also add, edit, or delete it.

_____ 2. ***[LO 3.6]*** The encounter steps include only activities that take place before the patient arrives for an office visit.

_____ 3. ***[LO 3.8]*** Disaster recovery plans require practices to back up computer data.

_____ 4. ***[LO 3.9]*** A user must be online to access any of the help features for Medisoft Network Professional and Medisoft Clinical Patient Records.

_____ 5. ***[LO 3.1]*** Medisoft Clinical is a practice management and electronic health record program for physician practices.

_____ 6. ***[LO 3.4]*** Medisoft Network Professional is the Medisoft application used for patient accounting.

_____ 7. ***[LO 3.2]*** In order to log in to Medisoft Clinical, an individual needs to have only a user name.

_____ 8. ***[LO 3.5]*** The pre-encounter steps include preregistration and appointment scheduling.

_____ 9. ***[LO 3.3]*** Medisoft Clinical Patient Records is the personal health record component of Medisoft Clinical.

_____ 10. ***[LO 3.7]*** The results of a claim review are sent to the provider along with the payment.

MULTIPLE-CHOICE QUESTIONS

Select the letter that best completes the statement or answers the question.

1. ***[LO 3.6]*** Once an examination is complete and the documentation has been entered in MCPR, the services provided and the provider's determination of the patient's diagnoses must be assigned __________.
   a. letters
   b. numeric codes
   c. names
   d. all of the above

2. ***[LO 3.8]*** A plan for resuming normal operations after a disaster such as a fire or a computer malfunction is a __________.
   a. back up plan
   b. restoring plan
   c. disaster recovery plan
   d. all of the above

3. ***[LO 3.2]*** Which of the following is a built-in security feature of Medisoft Clinical?
   a. user names
   b. passwords
   c. access levels
   d. all of the above

4. ***[LO 3.9]*** The website contains a searchable __________ which is a collection of up-to-date technical information about Medisoft products.
   a. database
   b. dashboard
   c. knowledge base
   d. user name

5. ***[LO 3.5]*** The pre-encounter steps include ____________.
   a. appointment scheduling
   b. preregistration
   c. claim preparation
   d. both a and b

6. ***[LO 3.3]*** The term ____________ refers to a patient's medical record.
   a. chart
   b. database
   c. dashboard
   d. consult

7. ***[LO 3.8]*** What is the process of copying backup files onto the office's computer systems, facilitating a return to normal business activities?
   a. restoring
   b. backing up
   c. parking
   d. both a and b

8. ***[LO 3.7]*** To receive payment, a medical practice must create and submit ____________ to health plans.
   a. diagnoses
   b. claims
   c. statements
   d. adjudication

9. ***[LO 3.7]*** A statement lists ____________.
   a. all service performed
   b. the amount paid by the health plan
   c. the charges for each service performed
   d. all of the above

10. ***[LO 3.4]*** Medisoft Network Professional includes ____________, a schedule program.
   a. Medisoft Clinical Patient Records
   b. Auto Log Off
   c. Office Hours
   d. none of the above

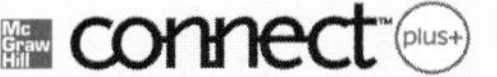

Enhance your learning at **mcgrawhillconnect.com**!
- *Practice Exercises*
- *Worksheets*
- *Activities*
- *Integrated eBook*

SHORT-ANSWER QUESTIONS

Define the following abbreviations.

1. ***[LO 3.1]*** MCPR ______________________

2. ***[LO 3.1]*** MNP ______________________

APPLYING YOUR KNOWLEDGE

Answer the questions below in the space provided.

3.1. ***[LO 3.2]*** How do access levels contribute to the security of patients' health information?

____

____

3.2. ***[LO 3.5]*** Some practices use built-in scheduling programs such as Office Hours, while others prefer to have scheduling programs separate from their PM programs. What advantages do you think using a built-in scheduling program offers?

____

____

3.3. ***[LO 3.6]*** What advantages are offered by the ability to make a real-time eligibility check on patients' insurance?

____

____

3.4. ***[LO 3.7]*** Why is it important for medical practices to monitor payer adjudication?

____

____

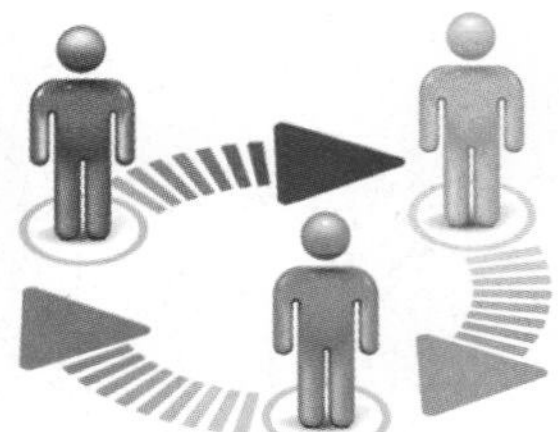

part two

Documenting Patient Encounters

chapter 4

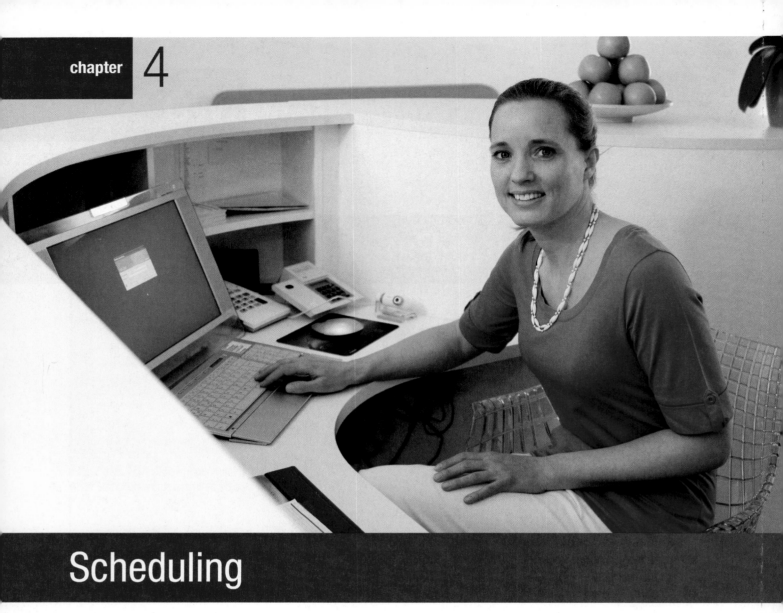

Scheduling

KEY TERMS

benefits
capitation
coinsurance
copayment (copay)
covered services
deductible
established patient (EP)
fee-for-service
health plan
indemnity plan
managed care
medical insurance
new patient (NP)
noncovered services
nonparticipating (nonPAR) provider
Office Hours break
Office Hours calendar
Office Hours patient information
out-of-network
out-of-pocket
participating (PAR) provider
patient portal
payer
policyholder
preauthorization
preexisting condition
premium
preregistration
preventive medical services
provider
provider's daily schedule
provider selection box
referral
referral number
schedule of benefits

LEARNING OUTCOMES

When you finish this chapter, you will be able to:

4.1 Describe the two methods used to schedule appointments.
4.2 Explain the method used to classify patients as new or established.
4.3 List the three categories of information new patients provide during telephone preregistration.
4.4 Identify the information that needs to be verified for established patients when making an appointment.
4.5 Describe covered and noncovered services under medical insurance policies.
4.6 List the three main points to verify with the payer regarding a patient's benefits prior to a visit.
4.7 Explain when a preauthorization number or referral document is required for a patient's encounter.
4.8 List the four main areas of Medisoft Network Professional's Office Hours window.
4.9 Demonstrate how to enter an appointment.
4.10 Demonstrate how to book follow-up and repeating appointments.
4.11 Demonstrate how to reschedule an appointment.
4.12 Demonstrate how to create a recall list.
4.13 Demonstrate how to enter provider breaks in the schedule.
4.14 Demonstrate how to print a provider's schedule.

Making Changes

As the receptionist, Laurie Harcourt does most of the scheduling for the Family Care Clinic. The first call to the office this morning is from Mrs. Jones, who is very upset because she needs to reschedule her appointment again. "You know, I had a little accident and my daughter made me stop driving. Honestly, I don't blame her, but I hate having to depend on her to get me where I need to go." Laurie reassures Mrs. Jones that it's easy to reschedule her appointment on the computer, "Making changes to the schedule is getting easier and easier. In fact, once we finish our new website, you'll be able to do it yourself online."

In this chapter, you will learn to navigate the scheduler with confidence. In the example given above: How does ease of scheduling serve the office staff? How does it serve the patient?

WHEN YOU FINISH THIS CHAPTER, YOU WILL ALSO BE ABLE TO USE MEDISOFT TO:

1. Enter appointments for patients, in Medisoft Network Professional's Office Hours program including follow-up, repeating, and rescheduled appointments.
2. Add patients to the recall list.
3. Create provider breaks in the Office Hours schedule.
4. Use Office Hours to print a provider's schedule.

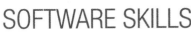

SOFTWARE SKILLS

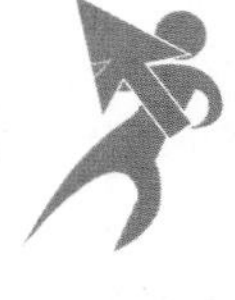

4.1 Scheduling Methods

The first step in a patient encounter occurs when the patient contacts the medical office to make an appointment. If the appointment will be for the patient's first visit to the practice, this initial contact is the patient's first impression of the medical office. Registration staff help make this a good impression by having a caring attitude and being attentive to the patient's needs.

Making Appointments via Telephone or Online

In most offices, patients use the traditional method of telephoning to contact the office. The medical office keeps the electronic scheduling program open so that it is easy to access when a patient calls to make an appointment. The scheduling program is usually a separate but integrated part of the practice management program. It houses a calendar that can be set to display a provider's schedule for the day, the week, or the month (see Figure 4.1).

When a patient calls to schedule a new appointment, the receptionist or other member of the front desk staff views the scheduling program, selects a provider, and has instant access to an electronic calendar displaying the provider's schedule. The staff member then selects the open time slot on the calendar that best suits the patient, and the program blocks off that slot with the patient's name. If a patient calls to cancel or reschedule an appointment, the scheduler's search feature can be used to locate the original appointment and reschedule or cancel it in a matter of seconds.

patient portal secure website that enables communication between patients and health care providers for tasks such as scheduling, completing registration forms, and making payments

More and more practices are using the Internet to communicate with their patients. **Patient portals** are websites that enable communication between patients and health care providers (see Figure 4.2). The portals are designed to benefit both patients and health care

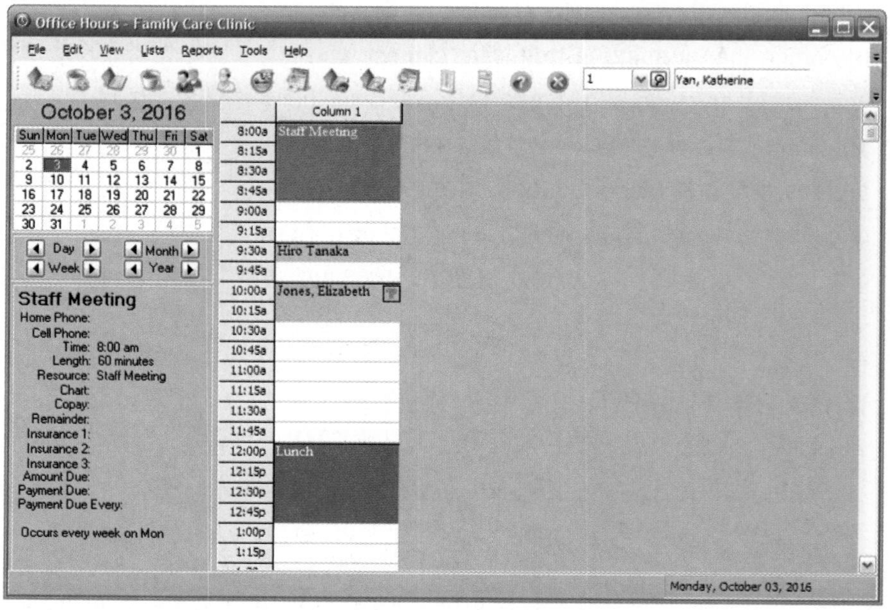

Figure 4.1 Sample Screen from Scheduling Program

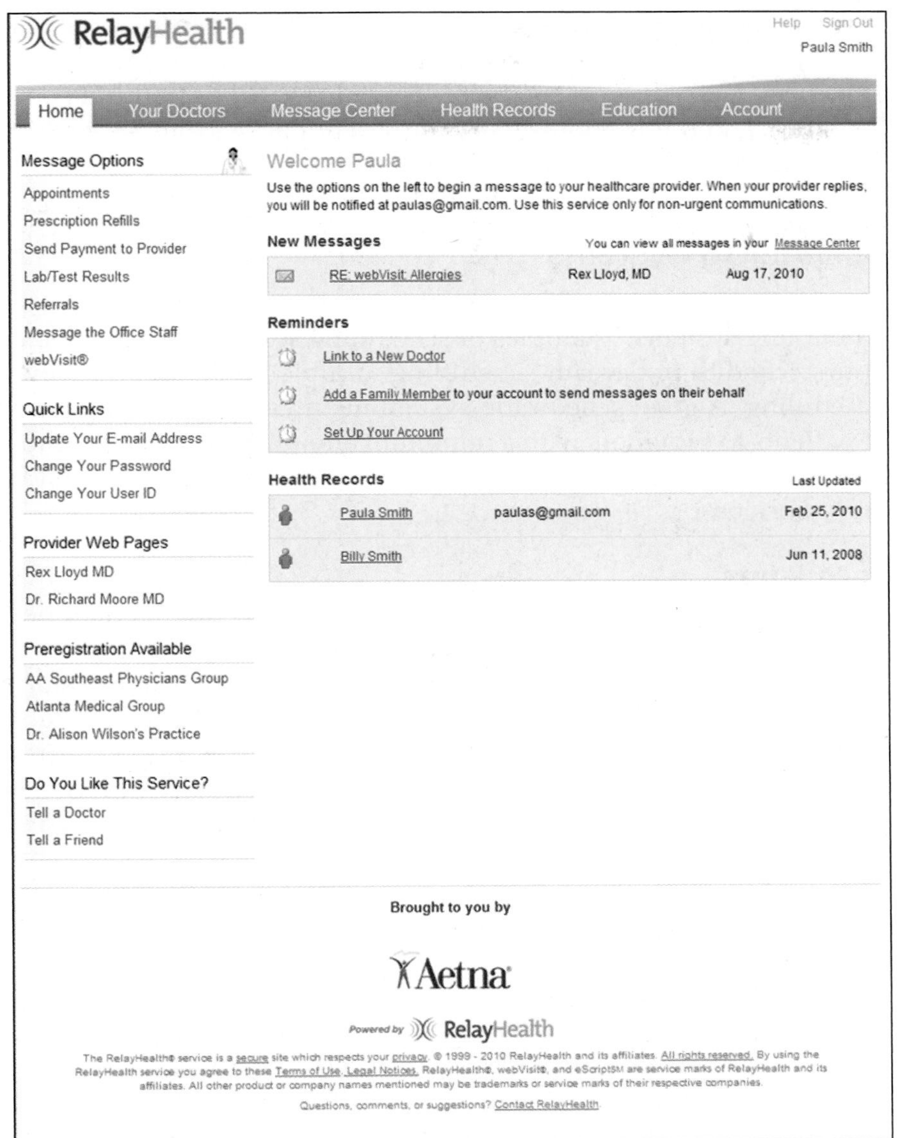

Figure 4.2 A Patient Portal Website

providers by increasing efficiency and productivity. Using a secure user name and password, a patient can perform a variety of tasks, such as:

- Request an appointment
- Review lab results
- Review an account and make payments
- Request a prescription refill
- Complete registration forms
- Send secure messages to the provider

The patient portal is also used by providers to send messages to patients, such as reminders for appointments. If a practice has a patient portal, patients may have the option of making appointments online. They can view an electronic calendar showing available openings and select a time slot. Making appointments online reduces the amount of time the front desk staff spend scheduling, since appointments are initially made without their assistance. This information is transmitted to the office, and if it is approved by the scheduling system, the patient receives an e-mail confirmation.

Scheduling Systems

Electronic schedulers can be set up to accommodate various types of scheduling systems. Examples of scheduling systems include open-hours scheduling, stream scheduling, double-booking, and wave scheduling. A good scheduling system maintains a consistent flow of patients to providers with a minimum amount of waiting time for patients. Depending on the type of facility, different scheduling systems work best.

Open Hours

In urgent care clinics and many walk-in clinics, patients may not have the option of making appointments. It is understood that they will be seen within a given window of time, say between the hours of 10:00 A.M. and 2:00 P.M., on a first-come, first-served basis—except in the case of an emergency. In this setting, the scheduler is set up using an open-hours scheduling system. The hours when a given provider is available to see patients is blocked off, and patients are added to the schedule as they arrive. Although the provider may have a steady stream of patients, the waiting time is often long because there are no prearranged appointments.

Stream Scheduling

Small medical practices commonly use a stream scheduling system, designed to give the provider a steady stream of patients throughout the day at regular, blocked-off intervals. The intervals are usually fifteen minutes long. If an appointment, such as a physical exam, requires more than fifteen minutes, additional fifteen-minute slots are blocked off. Stream scheduling is used in the Medisoft Clinical exercises in this text. Each patient is given a specific amount of time for an appointment based on the estimated length of time for the procedure. Time for lunch, weekly staff meetings, or monthly meetings with drug representatives from pharmaceutical companies, for example, can also be blocked off on a recurring basis.

Double-Booking

Another kind of scheduling system relies on double-booking appointments. In double-booking scheduling systems, two or more patients are scheduled in the same time slot. The provider speaks with one patient while the medical assistant records the vital signs of another patient or an X-ray technician sees the second patient for a specific procedure such as a chest X-ray. This system works well in larger offices where providers have enough examining rooms and medical staff to accommodate several patients at one time. Double-booking also works well in offices where patients come in

THINKING IT THROUGH 4.1

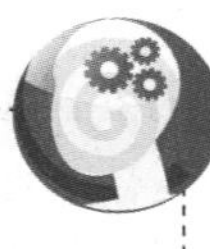

Why is it important to have both verbal and computer skills when scheduling patient appointments?

for routine checkups for conditions such as high blood pressure or diabetes and do not have to see the physician each time.

Wave Scheduling

In wave scheduling, patients are scheduled in waves at the beginning of each hour, with the rest of the hour left open. The patient who arrives first or has the most serious condition is usually seen first. Ideally, each member of the group for that hour is taken care of by the end of the hour, when the next wave arrives. Wave scheduling, like double-booking, is designed in part to accommodate patients who arrive late or do not show up (no-shows). Both types of scheduling also require a facility and staff that can accommodate several patients simultaneously. Otherwise, patients may become frustrated when they are not taken in the usual order and have to wait for stretches of time.

Regardless of the scheduling system used, every system should be evaluated regularly to make sure the average waiting time for patients is acceptable and to analyze whether medical staff and equipment are being used in the most efficient way. Electronic schedulers can be customized to accommodate any scheduling system a practice desires. In addition, electronic schedulers usually come with various reporting capabilities for analyzing the medical office's scheduling practices in order to help improve overall efficiency in scheduling.

4.2 New Versus Established Patients

When scheduling a patient appointment, it is important to determine whether the patient is new to the practice or is returning. Different information will be gathered in each case, and, for some procedures, different codes will be assigned. A **new patient (NP)** is someone who has not received any services from the provider (or another provider of the same specialty who is a member of the same practice) within the past three years. A returning patient is called an **established patient (EP).** This patient has seen the provider (or another provider in the practice who has the same specialty) within the past three years.

New patients complete many forms before their first appointment. Established patients review and update the information that is already on file about them. Figure 4.3 illustrates how to decide which category—new or established—fits the patient. Some of this information may be obtained over the phone while the patient is scheduling the appointment or online if the practice has a secure website. The process of gathering new patient information before an appointment is known as **preregistration.**

new patient (NP) a patient who has not received professional services from a provider (or another provider with the same specialty in the same practice) within the past three years

established patient (EP) patient who has received professional services from a provider (or another provider with the same specialty in the same practice) within the past three years

preregistration the process of gathering basic contact, insurance, and reason for visit information before a new patient comes into the office for an encounter

THINKING IT THROUGH 4.2

If a returning patient telephones to make an appointment for her young daughter who has not yet been seen by any of the practice's providers, is the daughter listed as a new or an established patient?

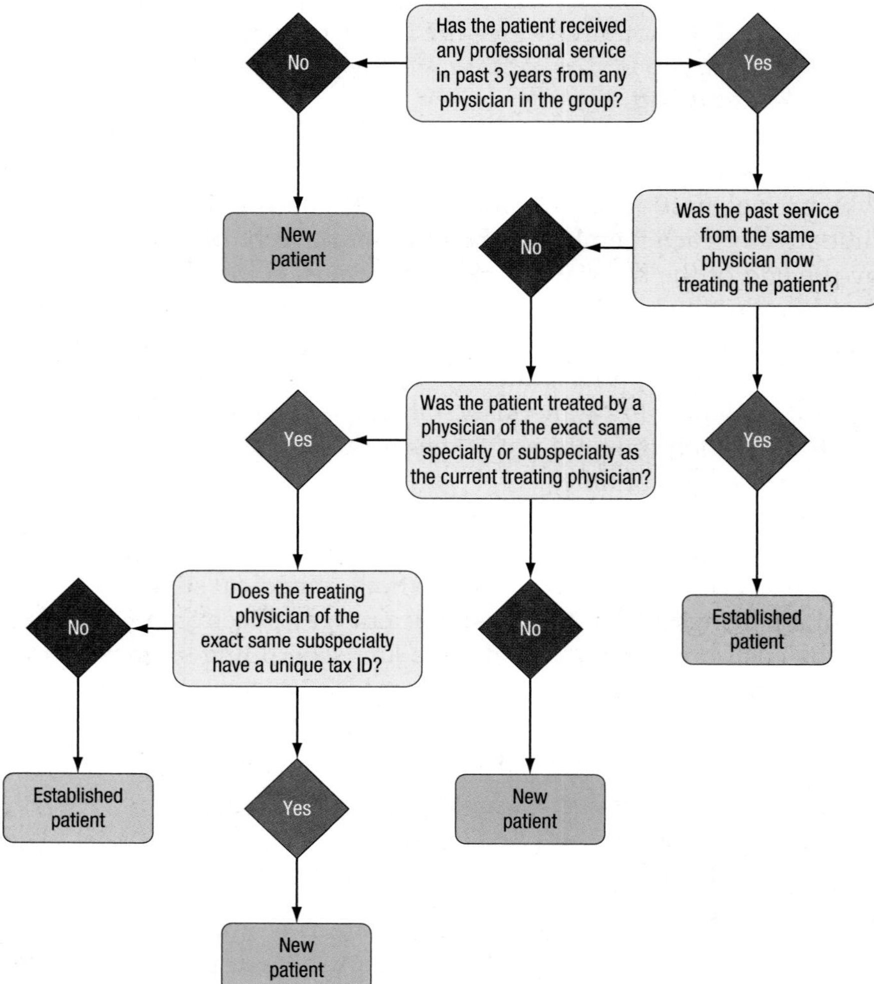

Figure 4.3 Decision Tree for New Versus Established Patients

4.3 Preregistration for New Patients

During preregistration, new patients usually provide three types of information: patient demographics, basic insurance information, and the reason for the visit, also known as the chief complaint.

Gathering Patient Demographics

Basic information about the patient, known as patient demographics, is obtained first. Patient demographics include the person's:

- Name
- Address

THINKING IT THROUGH 4.3

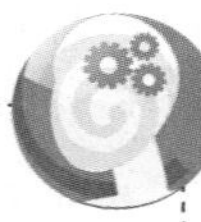

During preregistration, why is it important for the physician practice's health care team to be knowledgeable about the practice's participation with different insurance carriers?

- Gender
- Date of birth
- Home, work, and cell telephone numbers
- E-mail address (if preregistering online)

Additional details about the patient, such as marital status, Social Security number, and a contact person, are normally obtained during registration at the time of the appointment.

Gathering Insurance Information

If the patient has health insurance, basic information about the insurance is also gathered during preregistration, including the:

- Name of the patient's health plan
- Plan member's identification number
- Name of the policyholder, who may be the patient, a spouse, a divorced spouse, a guardian, or another relation
- Type of plan, and whether a copay is required
- Name of the referring physician, if the patient was referred by another physician

Before deciding to make an appointment, a new patient may need information about provider participation in a health insurance plan. Members of the medical administrative team need to know which plans their providers participate in. In most managed care insurance plans, patients are required to use network physicians to avoid paying higher charges. For this reason, patients check whether the provider is a **participating (PAR) provider** in their health plan. When patients see **nonparticipating (nonPAR) providers,** they must pay more—a higher copayment, greater coinsurance, or both—so a patient may choose not to make an appointment because of the additional expense.

participating (PAR) provider a provider who agrees to provide medical services to a payer's policyholders according to the terms of the plan's contract

nonparticipating (nonPAR) provider a provider who chooses not to join a particular government or other health plan

Recording the Reason for the Visit

When scheduling a patient's appointment, in addition to gathering personal and insurance information, it is important to establish the reason for the patient's visit. The reason for the visit will determine the length of time required for the appointment. A complete physical exam for a new patient may require forty-five minutes or an hour, whereas a follow-up visit for a bladder infection may require only fifteen minutes. Many providers require that new patients come in for a complete physical before they will provide other routine services. In most electronic schedulers, the length of time required for a procedure can be set up in the practice management program's database along with the procedure code and description.

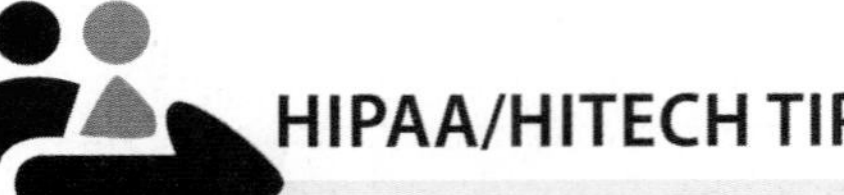

HIPAA/HITECH TIP

Documenting Appointments

As is true of other aspects of a patient visit, it is important to document appointments carefully and consistently. The practice should keep a permanent record of all appointments, including cancellations, walk-ins, emergencies, and no-shows. If a legal issue arises—for example, if a provider is accused of neglect—the record of appointments can be used to prove that a patient was or was not seen, how many times a patient canceled an appointment or did not show up, and whether the patient or the practice attempted to reschedule. Traditionally, a paper sign-in sheet was used for this purpose. Today, electronic schedulers are designed to keep track of all appointments and changes made to them.

4.4 Appointments for Established Patients

When an established patient contacts the office for an appointment, the members of the front desk staff verify that the information they have on file for the patient is still correct. If the electronic scheduling program is integrated with the practice management program, simple changes to a patient's address are usually made in the scheduler and are automatically carried over to the practice management program. More detailed changes, such as changes to a patient's health plan or employment, need to be made in the practice management program.

The front desk staff member also inquires about the reason for the visit so that the correct amount of time can be blocked off for the encounter. The office may want to know whether the patient is carrying a balance on his or her account. Most practice management programs contain reports that will identify patients with upcoming appointments who have overdue balances. Patients are increasingly paying for a greater percentage of their health care bills. Medical practices, in response, have had to assume a greater role in monitoring and collecting overdue amounts from patients. A patient who is late in paying can be reminded of the amount due while on the phone or via an e-mail message and can be asked to take care of it during the upcoming visit.

4.5 Insurance Basics

To be paid for services, medical practices need to establish financial responsibility for each visit. Although some patients pay the costs of medical care directly, the costs of most medical services are covered, in part or in full, by medical insurance. Nearly 250 million people in the United States have some form of insurance through either their employers or government programs.

The first step in establishing financial responsibility for insured patients is to verify the patient's eligibility. This is done by obtaining answers to questions such as:

- Has the policyholder paid the latest premium?
- What are the billing rules of the plan?

THINKING IT THROUGH 4.4

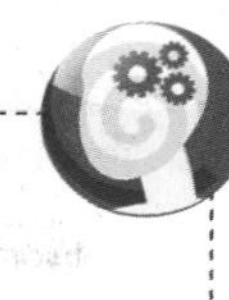

Imagine a telephone call with an established patient ten years ago. A traditional paper calendar is being used to set up an appointment. Now picture a contemporary office. How has using a computer changed the amount of information documented before a patient visit?

- What is the patient responsible for paying?
- What services are covered under the plan, and what medical conditions establish medical necessity for these services?
- What services are not covered?

Knowing the answers to these questions is essential in order to correctly bill payers for patients' covered services. This knowledge is also needed to determine what patients are responsible for so that they can be asked to pay their bills when benefits do not apply. To be able to answer questions about patients' benefits, the medical administrative team needs to be familiar with the basic terminology of medical insurance policies, what a standard set of health care benefits normally includes, and the types of insurance plans available.

Medical Insurance Policies

What is medical insurance? **Medical insurance** (health insurance) is a written policy between an individual or entity, called the **policyholder,** and a **health plan**—an insurance company or government program that is the **payer.** The policyholder pays a specified amount of money, usually monthly, called a **premium.** In exchange, the payer provides **benefits**—defined by America's Health Insurance Plans (AHIP) as payments for covered medical services—for a specific period of time.

There are actually three participants in the medical insurance relationship. The patient (policyholder) is the first party, and the physician is the second party. Legally, a patient–physician contract is created when a physician agrees to treat a patient who is seeking medical services. Through this unwritten contract, the patient is legally responsible for paying for services. The patient may have a policy with a health plan, the third party, that agrees to carry some of the risk of paying for those services and therefore is called a third-party payer.

The major types of third-party payers are:

- *Private payers:* Nationwide insurance companies that dominate the national market offer all types of health plans. They include such companies as WellPoint, UnitedHealth Group, Aetna, Kaiser Permanente, and the member companies of the Blue Cross and Blue Shield Association.
- *Self-funded health plans:* These are health plans set up by employers that assume the risk of paying directly for medical services.

medical insurance financial plan that covers the cost of hospital and medical care

policyholder person who buys an insurance plan; the insured, subscriber, or guarantor

health plan an individual or group plan that either provides or pays for the cost of medical care; includes group health plans, health insurance issuers, health maintenance organizations, Medicare Part A and B, Medicaid, TRICARE, and other government and nongovernment plans

payer health plan or program

premium money the insured pays to a health plan for a health care policy; usually paid monthly

benefits the amount of money a health plan pays for services covered in an insurance policy

- *Government-sponsored health care programs:* Four major government-sponsored health care programs offer benefits for which various groups in the population are eligible.
  - Medicare is a 100 percent federally funded health plan that covers people who are sixty-five and over and those who are disabled or have permanent kidney failure (end-stage renal disease, or ESRD).
  - Medicaid, a federal program that is jointly funded by the federal and state governments, covers low-income people who cannot afford medical care. Each state administers its own Medicaid program, determining the program's qualifications and benefits under broad federal guidelines.
  - TRICARE, a Department of Defense program, covers medical expenses for active-duty members of the uniformed services and their spouses, children, and other dependents; retired military personnel and their dependents; and family members of deceased active-duty personnel.
  - CHAMPVA, the Civilian Health and Medical Program of the Department of Veterans Affairs, covers veterans with permanent service-related disabilities and their dependents. It also covers surviving spouses and dependent children of veterans who died from service-related disabilities.

Health Care Benefits

Although most plans contain standard benefits for inpatient and outpatient care, the amount the patient owes for different services varies depending on the type of plan. The medical insurance policy for each health plan contains a **schedule of benefits** that summarizes the payments that may be made for medically necessary medical services. Figure 4.4 illustrates the range of benefits included in a popular managed care plan.

schedule of benefits list of the medical expenses that a health plan covers

provider person or entity that supplies medical or health services and bills for or is paid for the services in the normal course of business; may be a professional member of the health care team, such as a physician, or a facility, such as a hospital or skilled nursing home

covered services medical procedures and treatments that are included as benefits under an insured's health plan

The payer's definition of *medical necessity* is the key to coverage and payment. A medically necessary service is reasonable and is consistent with generally accepted professional medical standards for the diagnosis or treatment of illness or injury. Payers scrutinize the need for medical procedures, examining each bill to make sure it meets their medical necessity guidelines.

The **provider** of the service must also meet the payer's professional standards. Providers include physicians, nurse-practitioners, physician assistants, therapists, hospitals, laboratories, long-term care facilities, and suppliers such as pharmacies and medical supply companies.

Covered Services

Covered services are listed on the schedule of benefits. They may include primary care, emergency care, medical specialists' services, and surgery. Coverage of some services is mandated by state or federal law; coverage of others is optional. Some policies provide benefits only for loss resulting from illnesses or diseases, while others also cover accidents or injuries. The policies of many managed

Standard Benefits

This is a preferred provider organization (PPO) plan. That means members can receive the highest level of benefits when they use any of the more than 5,000 physicians and other health care professionals in this network. When members receive covered in-network services, they simply pay a copayment. Members can also receive care from providers that are not part of the network, however benefits are often lower and covered claims are subject to deductible, coinsurance and charges above the maximum allowable amount. Referrals are not needed from a Primary Care Physician to receive care from a specialist.

PREVENTIVE CARE	In-Network	Out-of-Network
Well child care		
Birth through 12 years	OV Copayment	Deductible & Coinsurance
All others	OV Copayment	Deductible & Coinsurance
Periodic, routine health examinations	OV Copayment	Deductible & Coinsurance
Routine eye exams	OV Copayment	Deductible & Coinsurance
Routine OB/GYN visits	OV Copayment	Deductible & Coinsurance
Mammography	No Charge	Deductible & Coinsurance
Hearing Screening	OV Copayment	Deductible & Coinsurance
MEDICAL CARE	**In-Network**	**Out-of-Network**
PCP office visits	OV Copayment	Deductible & Coinsurance
Specialist office visits	OV Copayment	Deductible & Coinsurance
Outpatient mental health & substance abuse – *prior authorization required*	OV Copayment	Deductible & Coinsurance
Maternity care – *initial visit subject to copayment, no charge thereafter*	OV Copayment	Deductible & Coinsurance
Diagnostic lab, x-ray and testing	No Charge	Deductible & Coinsurance
High-cost outpatient diagnostics – *prior authorization required. The following are subject to copayment: MRI, MRA, CAT, CTA, PET, SPECT scans*	No Charge OR $200 Copayment	Deductible & Coinsurance Deductible & Coinsurance
Allergy Services		
Office visits/testing	OV Copayment	Deductible & Coinsurance
Injections – *90 visits in 3 years*	$25 Copayment	Deductible & Coinsurance
HOSPITAL CARE – Prior authorization required	**In-Network**	**Out-of-Network**
Semi-private room *(General/Medical/Surgical/Maternity)*	HSP Copayment	Deductible & Coinsurance
Skilled nursing facility – *up to 120 days per calendar year*	HSP Copayment	Deductible & Coinsurance
Rehabilitative services – *up to 60 days per calendar year*	No Charge	Deductible & Coinsurance
Outpatient surgery – *in a hospital or surgi-center*	OS Copayment	Deductible & Coinsurance
EMERGENCY CARE	**In-Network**	**Out-of-Network**
Walk-in centers	OV Copayment	Deductible & Coinsurance
Urgent care centers – *at participating centers only*	UR Copayment	Not Covered
Emergency care – *copayment waived if admitted*	ER Copayment	ER Copayment
Ambulance	No Charge	No Charge
OTHER HEALTH CARE	**In-Network**	**Out-of-Network**
Outpatient rehabilitative services – *30 visits maximum for PT, OT, and ST per year, 20 visit maximum for Chiro, per year*	OV Copayment	Deductible & Coinsurance
Durable medical equipment/Prosthetic devices – *Unlimited maximum per calendar year*	No Charge OR 20%	Deductible & Coinsurance
Infertility Services (diagnosis and treatment)	Not Covered	Not Covered
Home Health Care	No Charge	$50 Deductible & 20% Coinsurance

KEY: Office Visit (OV) Copayment; Hospital (HSP) Copayment; Emergency Room (ER) Copayment; Outpatient Surgery (OS) Copayment; Urgent Care (UR) Copayment

PREVENTIVE CARE SCHEDULES

Well Child Care (including immunizations)
- 6 exams, birth to age 1
- 6 exams, ages 1–5
- 1 exam every 2 years, ages 6–10
- 1 exam every year, ages 11–21

Adult Exams
- 1 exam every 5 years, ages 22–29
- 1 exam every 3 years, ages 30–39
- 1 exam every 2 years, ages 40–49
- 1 exam every year, ages 50+

Mammography
- 1 baseline screening, ages 35–39
- 1 screening per year, ages 40+

Vision Exams
- 1 exam every 2 calendar years

Hearing Exams
- 1 exam per calendar year

OB/GYN Exams
- 1 exam per calendar year

Figure 4.4 Example of Range of Benefits for a Popular Plan

preventive medical services care that is provided to keep patients healthy or to prevent illness, such as routine checkups and screening tests

noncovered services medical procedures that are not included in a plan's benefits

preexisting condition illness or disorder of a beneficiary that existed before the effective date of insurance coverage

indemnity plan type of medical insurance that reimburses a policyholder for medical services under the terms of its schedule of benefits

care plans, such as the one illustrated in Figure 4.4 on page 163, also cover **preventive medical services,** such as annual physical examinations, pediatric and adolescent immunizations, prenatal care, and routine screening procedures. Not all services that are covered have the same benefits; for example, a policy may pay a smaller proportion of the charges for vision or hearing services. Many services are also limited in frequency. A payer may cover just three physical therapy treatments for a condition, or a certain screening test every five years, not every year. In the example shown in Figure 4.4, the outpatient rehabilitative services for physical, occupational, and speech therapy are limited to thirty visits per year.

Noncovered Services

The medical insurance policy also describes **noncovered services**—those for which it does not pay. Such excluded services may include all or some of the following:

- Most medical policies do not cover dental services, eye examinations or eyeglasses, employment-related injuries, cosmetic procedures, infertility services, or experimental procedures.
- Policies may exclude specific items such as vocational rehabilitation or surgical treatment of obesity.
- Many policies do not have prescription drug benefits.
- If a new policyholder has a medical condition that was diagnosed before the policy took effect—known as a **preexisting condition**—medical services to treat it are often not covered. Note that health care reform legislation that is being implemented will disallow payers from this exclusion in the future.

Types of Health Care Plans

All health plans are based on one of the two essential types of insurance, indemnity and managed care. Knowing which type of plan a patient has is an indicator of the type of benefits the patient has, as well as of how much the plan is likely to pay for covered services. Chapter 8 explains health care plans in detail and the different methods of reimbursement used by each. This section introduces the different types of plans as they relate to understanding a patient's basic set of benefits.

Indemnity

Indemnity is protection against loss. Under an **indemnity plan,** the payer indemnifies the policyholder against costs of medical services and procedures as listed on the benefits schedule. Patients choose the providers they wish to see. The physician usually sends the health care claim—the formal insurance claim that reports data about the patient and the services provided by the physician—to the payer on behalf of the patient. Figure 4.5 shows the enrollment trends for the different types of health plans.

BILLING TIP

Filing Claims for Patients

The provider usually bills the insurance company for patients. Patients are generally more satisfied with their medical encounters when billing is done for them, and the provider receives payment more quickly.

Conditions for Payment Four conditions must be met before the insurance company will make a payment on a claim processed by an indemnity plan:

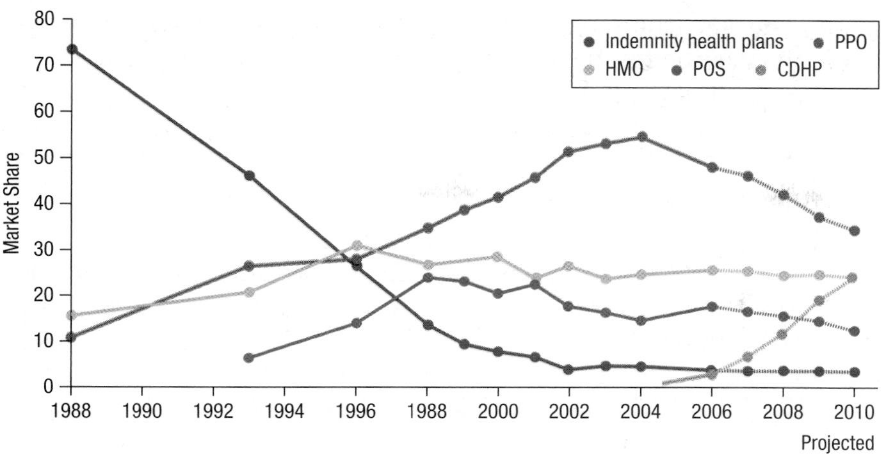

Figure 4.5 Trends in Health Plan Enrollment

1. The medical charge must be for medically necessary services that are covered by the insured's health plan.
2. The patient's payment of the premium—the periodic payment the patient is required to make to keep the policy in effect—must be up-to-date. Unless the premium is current, the patient is not eligible for benefits, and the insurance company will not make any payment.
3. If it is part of the policy, the **deductible**—the amount that the insured pays on covered services before benefits begin—must have been paid. Deductibles range widely, usually between two hundred dollars and thousands of dollars annually. Higher deductibles generally mean lower premiums.
4. Any **coinsurance**—the percentage of each claim that the insured pays—that is due must be taken into account. The coinsurance rate, such as 80-20, states the health plan's percentage of the charge, followed by the insured's percentage. This means that the plan pays 80 percent of the covered amount and the patient pays 20 percent after the premiums and deductibles are paid. The formula is as follows:

Charge − Deductible − Coinsurance = Health plan payment

deductible an amount that an insured person must pay, usually on an annual basis, for health care services before a health plan's payment begins

coinsurance the portion of charges that an insured person must pay for health care services after payment of the deductible amount; usually stated as a percentage

Example An indemnity policy states that the deductible is the first $200 in covered annual medical fees and that the coinsurance rate is 80-20. A patient whose first medical charge of the year was $2,000 would owe $560:

EXAMPLE

Charge	$2,000
Patient owes the deductible	$200
Balance	$1,800
Patient also owes coinsurance (20 percent of the balance)	$360
Total balance due from patient	$200 + $360 = $560

out-of-pocket expenses the insured must pay before benefits begin

fee-for-service health plan that repays the policyholder for covered medical expenses

In this case, the patient must pay an **out-of-pocket** expense of $560 this year before benefits begin. The health plan will pay $1,440, or 80 percent of the balance:

EXAMPLE

Charge	$2,000
Patient payment	− $560
Health plan payment	$1,440

If the patient has already met the annual deductible, the patient's benefits apply to the charge, as in this example:

EXAMPLE

Charge	$2,000
Patient coinsurance (20 percent)	$400
Health plan payment (80 percent)	$1,600

Fee-for-Service Payment Approach Indemnity plans usually reimburse medical costs on a fee-for-service basis. The **fee-for-service** payment method is retroactive; the fee is paid after the patient receives services from the physician (see Figure 4.6).

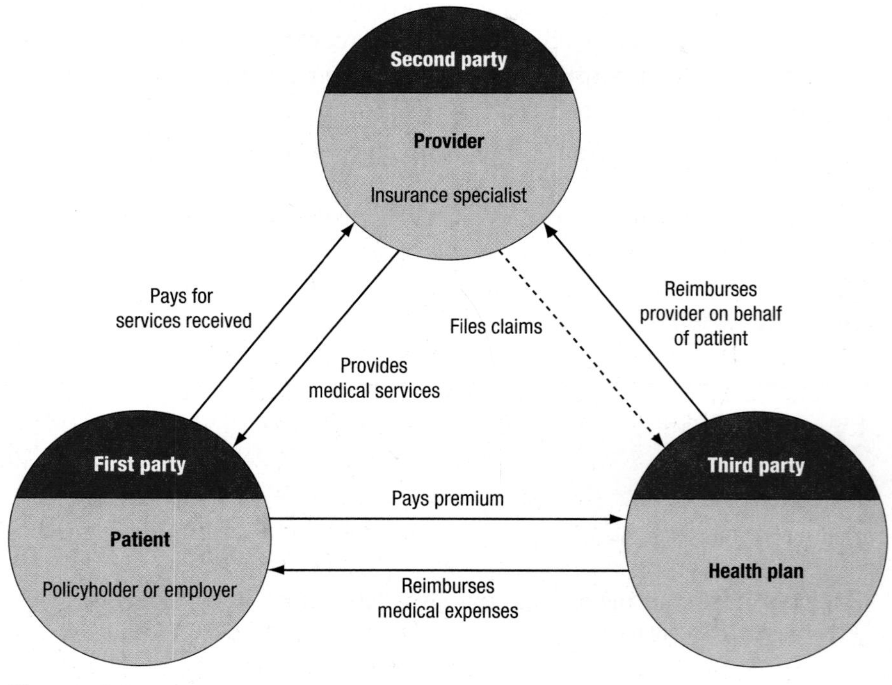

Figure 4.6 Payment Under Fee-for-Service

Managed Care

The other type of insurance plan available is a managed care plan. **Managed care** offers a more restricted choice of (and access to) providers and treatments in exchange for lower premiums, deductibles, and other charges than does traditional indemnity insurance. This approach to insurance combines the financing and management of health care with the delivery of services. A managed care organization (MCO) establishes links between provider, patient, and payer. Instead of only the patient having a policy with the health plan, the provider also has an agreement with the MCO. This arrangement gives the MCO more control over what services the provider performs and the fees for the services.

managed care system that combines the financing and delivery of appropriate, cost-effective health care services to its members

capitation a prepayment covering provider's services for a plan member for a specified period

Managed care plans, first introduced in California in 1929, are now the predominant type of insurance. Over 90 percent of all insured employees are enrolled in some type of managed care plan, and thousands of different plans are offered. The basic types are health maintenance organizations (HMOs), point-of-service (POS) plans, preferred provider organizations (PPOs), and consumer-driven health plans (CDHPs).

In addition to ensuring correct billing and reimbursement for the services provided, being familiar with the different types of managed care plans is the best way to help patients obtain the highest level of care they are entitled to under their current plan. Descriptions of the four different types of managed care follow.

Health Maintenance Organizations

A health maintenance organization (HMO) combines coverage of medical costs and delivery of health care for a prepaid premium. Approximately 20 percent of insured employees are enrolled in HMOs.

The HMO creates a network of physicians, hospitals, and other providers by employing them or negotiating contracts with them. The HMO then enrolls members in a health plan under which they use the services of those network providers. In most states, HMOs are licensed and are legally required to provide certain services to members and their dependents. Preventive care as appropriate for each age group is often required, such as immunizations and well-baby checkups for infants and screening mammograms for women.

BILLING TIP

Participation as a Provider

Participation means that a provider has contracted with a health plan to provide services to the plan's beneficiaries. Participation brings benefits, such as more patients, as well as contractual duties and, usually, reduced fees.

Capitation in HMOs **Capitation** (from *capit*, Latin for *head*) is a fixed prepayment to a medical provider for all necessary contracted services provided to each patient who is a plan member (see Figure 4.7). The capitated rate is a prospective payment—it is determined before the patient visit, and it covers a specific period of time. The health plan makes the payment whether the patient receives many or no medical services during the specified period.

In capitation, the physician agrees to share the risk that an insured person will use more services than the fee covers. The physician also shares in the prospect that an insured person will use fewer services. In fee-for-service, the more patients the provider sees, the more charges the health plan reimburses. In capitation, the payment remains the same, and the provider risks receiving lower per-visit revenue.

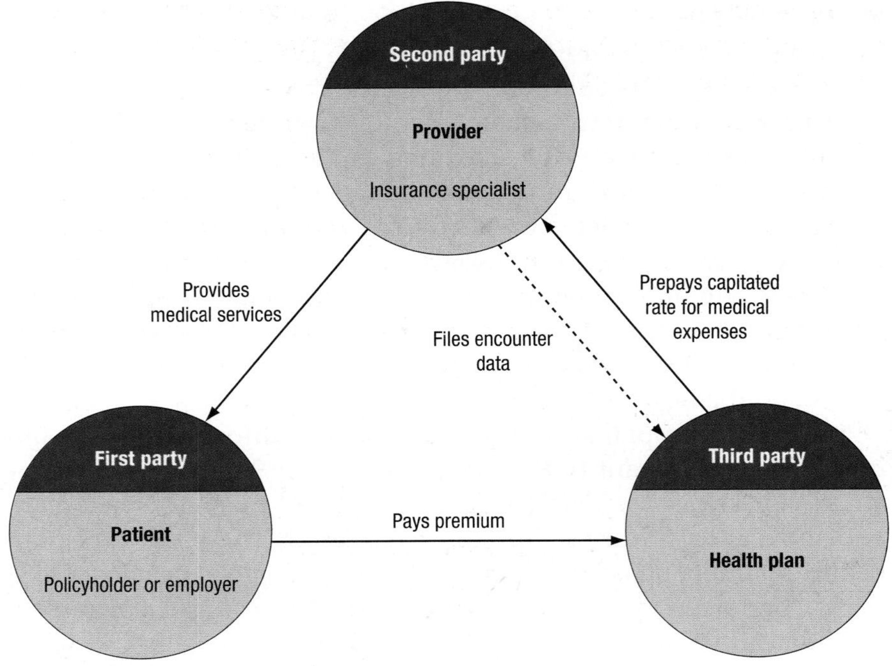

Figure 4.7 Payment Under Capitation

EXAMPLE

A family physician has a contract for a capitated payment of $30 a month for each of a hundred patients in a plan. This $3,000 monthly fee ($30 × 100 patients = $3,000) covers all office visits from all the patients. If half of the patients see the physician once during a given month, the provider in effect receives $60 for each visit ($3,000 divided by 50 visits). If, however, half of the patients see the physician four times in a month, the average fee is $3,000 divided by 200 visits, or $15 for each visit.

A patient is enrolled in a capitated health plan for a specific time period, such as a month, a quarter, or a year. The capitated rate, which is called *per member per month (PMPM),* is usually based on the health-related characteristics of the enrollees, such as age and gender. The health plan analyzes these factors and sets a rate based on its prediction of the amount of health care each person will need. The capitated rate of prepayment covers only services listed on the schedule of benefits for the plan. The provider may bill the patient for any other services.

Medical Management Practices in HMOs Health maintenance organizations seek to control rising medical costs and at the same time improve health care. An HMO uses the following cost-containment methods:

out-of-network a provider that does not have a participation agreement with a plan; using an out-of-network provider is more expensive for the plan's enrollees

- *Restricting patients' choice of providers:* After enrolling in an HMO, members must receive services from the network of physicians, hospitals, and other providers who are employed by or under contract to the HMO. Visits to **out-of-network** providers are not covered, except for emergency care or urgent health problems that arise when the member is temporarily away from the geographical service area.

- *Requiring preauthorization for services:* HMOs often require **preauthorization** (also called *precertification* or *prior authorization*) before the patient receives many types of services. Services that are not preauthorized are not covered. Preauthorization is almost always needed for nonemergency hospital admission, and it is usually required within a certain number of days after an emergency admission. It is also usually required for outpatient behavioral health care, including mental health care and substance abuse services.
- *Controlling the use of services:* HMOs develop medical necessity guidelines for the use of medical services. The HMO holds the provider accountable for a questionable service and may deny a patient's or provider's request for preauthorization. For example, a patient who has a rotator cuff shoulder injury repair can receive a specific number of physical therapy sessions. More sessions will not be covered unless additional approval is obtained. These guidelines are also applied to hospitals in the network, which, for instance, limit the number of days patients can remain in the hospital following particular surgeries.
- *Controlling drug costs:* Providers may prescribe only drugs that are listed on the HMO's list of selected pharmaceuticals and approved dosages, called a *formulary*. Drugs that are not on the list require preauthorization, which is often denied.
- *Requiring cost-sharing:* When HMO members see providers, they pay a specified charge called a **copayment (copay).** A lower copayment may be charged for an office visit to the primary care physician, and a higher copayment may be required for a visit to the office of a specialist or for the use of emergency department services.

preauthorization prior authorization from a payer for services to be provided; if preauthorization is not received, the charge is usually not covered

copayment (copay) an amount that a health plan requires a beneficiary to pay at the time of service for each health care encounter

referral transfer of patient care from one physician to another

One other cost-control method is now used less frequently but was a major feature of initial HMOs. This required a patient to select a primary care physician (PCP)—also called a *gatekeeper*—from the HMO's list of general or family practitioners, internists, and pediatricians. A PCP coordinates patients' overall care to ensure that all services are, in the PCP's judgment, necessary. In gatekeeper plans, an HMO member needs a medical **referral** from the PCP before seeing a specialist or a consultant and for hospital admission. Members who visit providers without referrals are directly responsible for the total cost of the services.

Historically, the first HMOs used all these cost-containment methods and reduced operating costs. However, both physicians and patients became dissatisfied with the policies. Physicians working under managed care contracts complained that they were not allowed to order needed treatments and tests. Patients often reported that needed referrals were denied. In response, the medical management practices of HMOs increasingly emphasize the quality of health care as well as the cost of its delivery.

BILLING TIP

Open-Access Plans

Many HMOs have switched from gatekeeper plans that require referrals to all specialists to plans that permit members to visit any specialists in the network without referrals. Even if referrals are required for specialists, patients can usually see OB-GYN specialists without referrals.

Point-of-Service Plans

Many patients dislike HMO rules that restrict their access to physicians. In order to better compete for membership, a point-of-service (POS) plan, also called an open HMO, reduces restrictions and allows members to choose providers who are not in the HMO's network. Over 20 percent of employees covered by employers' health care plans are enrolled in this type of plan.

Members must pay additional fees that are set by the plan when they use out-of-network providers. Typically, 20 to 30 percent of the charge for out-of-network service must be paid by the patient, and the deductible can be very high. The HMO pays out-of-network providers on a fee-for-service basis.

Preferred Provider Organizations

A preferred provider organization (PPO) is another health care delivery system that manages care. PPOs are the most popular type of insurance plan. They create a network of physicians, hospitals, and other providers with whom they have negotiated discounts from the usual fees. For example, a PPO might sign a contract with a practice stating that the fee for a brief appointment will be $60, although the practice's physicians usually charge $80. In exchange for accepting lower fees, providers—in theory, at least—see more patients, thus making up the revenue that is lost through the reduced fees. PPOs enroll almost 50 percent of the American workers who are insured through their employers.

In addition to requiring a payment of a premium, as seen in Figure 4.4 on page 163, a PPO often requires a copayment for visits. It does not require a primary care physician to oversee patients' care. Referrals to specialists are also not required. Premiums and copayments, however, are higher than in HMO or POS plans. Members choose from many in-network generalists and specialists. PPO members also can use out-of-network providers, usually for increased deductibles and coinsurance, higher copayments, or both.

EXAMPLE

A PPO member using an in-network provider pays a $20 copayment at the time of service, and the PPO pays the full balance of the charge for the visit. A member who sees an out-of-network provider pays a $40 copayment and is also responsible for coinsurance covering part of the visit charge.

As managed care organizations, PPOs also control the cost of health care by:

- *Directing patients' choices of providers:* PPO members have financial incentives to receive services from the PPO's network of providers.
- *Controlling use of services:* PPOs have guidelines for appropriate and necessary medical care.

- *Requiring preauthorization for services:* PPOs may require preauthorization for nonemergency hospital admission and for some outpatient procedures.
- *Requiring cost-sharing:* PPO members are also required to pay copayments for general or specialist services.

Consumer-Driven Health Plans

Consumer-driven health plans (CDHPs) combine two elements. The first element is a health plan, usually a PPO, that has a high deductible (such as $1,000) and low premiums. The second element is a special savings account that is used to pay medical bills before the deductible has been met. The savings account, which is similar to an individual retirement account (IRA), lets people put aside untaxed wages that they may use to cover their out-of-pocket medical expenses. Some employers contribute to employees' accounts as a benefit. Enrollment in CDHPs, as illustrated in Figure 4.5 on page 165, has increased steadily since 2005.

Cost containment in consumer-driven health plans begins with consumerism—the idea that patients who themselves pay for health care services become more careful consumers. Both insurance companies and employers believe that asking patients to pay a larger portion of medical expenses reduces costs. To this are added the other controls typical of a PPO, such as in-network savings and higher costs for out-of-network visits.

The most recent trend in health care plans is to replace copayments with coinsurance, thereby moving even more of the burden of health care onto the patient. The major types of plans are summarized in Table 4.1.

TABLE 4.1 Health Plan Options

Plan Type	Provider Options	Cost-Containment Methods	Features
Indemnity plan	Any provider	• Few or none • Preauthorization required for some procedures	• Higher costs • Deductibles • Coinsurance • Preventive care usually not covered
Health maintenance organization (HMO)	HMO network providers only	• Primary care physician manages care; referral required • No payment for out-of-network nonemergency services • Preauthorization required	• Low copayment • Limited provider network • Covers preventive care
Point-of-service (POS)	Network or out-of-network providers	• Within network, primary care physician manages care	• Lower copayments for network providers • Higher costs for out-of-network providers • Covers preventive care
Preferred provider organization (PPO)	Network or out-of-network providers	• Referral not required for specialists • Discounted fees • Preauthorization for some procedures	• Higher cost for out-of-network providers • Preventive care coverage varies
Consumer-driven health plan (CDHP)	Usually network or out-of-network providers	• Increases patient awareness of health care costs • Patient pays directly until high deductible is met	• High deductible, low premium • Savings account

THINKING IT THROUGH 4.5

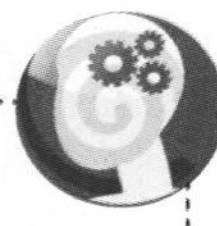

If a patient has met the annual deductible for her health plan and the coinsurance rate is 35 percent, how much does she owe for a charge of $310? How much will the health plan pay?

4.6 Eligibility and Benefits Verification

After scheduling an appointment, the front desk staff or the medical biller contacts the patient's health plan to verify the patient's eligibility for insurance benefits. What items need to be checked? Except in a medical emergency, where care is provided immediately and insurance is checked after the encounter, the following information should be obtained before a patient encounter:

- The patient's general eligibility for benefits
- The amount of the copayment for the visit, if one is required
- Whether the planned encounter is for a covered service that is medically necessary under the payer's rules

Factors Affecting General Eligibility

General eligibility for benefits depends on a number of factors. If premiums are required, patients must have paid them on time. For government-sponsored plans, like Medicaid, in which income is the criterion, eligibility can change monthly. For patients with employer-sponsored health plans, employment status can be the deciding factor:

- Coverage may end on the last day of the month in which the employee's active full-time service ends, such as for disability, layoff, or termination.
- The employee may no longer qualify as a member of the group. For example, some companies do not provide benefits for part-time employees. If a full-time employee changes to part-time employment, the coverage ends.
- An eligible dependent's coverage may end on the last day of the month in which the dependent status ends, such as for reaching the age limit stated in the policy.

If the patient's plan is an HMO that requires a primary care provider (PCP), the practice must verify that (1) the provider is a plan participant, (2) the patient is listed on the plan's enrollment master list, and (3) the patient is assigned to the PCP as of the date of service.

The office also checks with the payer to confirm whether the patient is currently covered. If online access is used, the office and the payer's provider representative exchange information over the Internet and via e-mail messages. If the payer requires verification to be checked on the telephone, the provider representative is called. Based on the patient's plan, eligibility for these specific benefits may also need to be checked:

- Office visits
- Laboratory work
- Diagnostic X-rays
- Maternity services
- Pap smears
- Psychiatric visits
- Physical or occupational therapy
- Durable medical equipment (DME)
- Foot care

Checking Out-of-Network Benefits

If a patient has insurance coverage but the practice does not participate in the plan, the office staff checks whether the patient has out-of-network benefits. When the patient has out-of-network benefits, the payer's rules concerning copayments and coverage are followed. If a patient does not have out-of-network benefits, as is common when the health plan is an HMO, the patient is responsible for the entire bill, rather than simply a copayment. This must be communicated to the patient before the appointment.

Verifying the Amount of the Copayment and Coinsurance

The amount of the copayment, if required, must be checked. Sometimes the copay information on the insurance card is out-of-date, and the correct copay is different. If the plan requires coinsurance, the percentage of coinsurance the patient must pay also should be verified.

Determining Whether the Planned Encounter Is for a Covered Service

The office staff must also attempt to determine whether the planned encounter is for a covered service. If the service will not be covered, the patient can be made aware of the financial responsibility in advance.

The resources for determining what services are covered under a given plan include knowledge of the major plans held by the practice's patients, information from payer websites, and the electronic benefit inquiries described below. Most members of the medical administrative team are familiar with the services covered under typical plans. For example, most plans cover regular office visits, but they may not cover preventive services or some therapeutic services. For unusual or unfamiliar services, the office needs to query the payer.

Electronic Benefit Inquiries and Responses

Previously, to query a payer—to find out about coverage, about whether a patient was up-to-date on insurance premiums, or about what percentage the plan would pay for a given procedure—the staff member in charge of patient eligibility had to refer to the latest

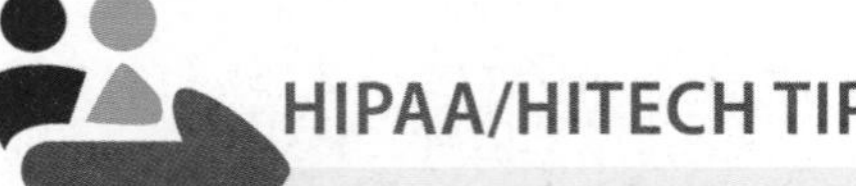

HIPAA/HITECH TIP

X12 270/271 Eligibility for a Health Plan Inquiry and Response

The HIPAA Eligibility for a Health Plan transaction is also called the X12 270/271. The number 270 refers to the inquiry that is sent, and 271 to the answer returned by the payer.

paperwork from the insurance company or phone a representative. This process has changed because of easy access to the Internet.

Instead of making telephone calls or sending faxes medical practices most often use electronic transactions to communicate with payers. Electronic transactions are the most efficient because they take only seconds. Most practice management programs have a feature that enables online inquiries to a payer to be sent from within the program. When an eligibility benefits transaction is sent, the computer program assigns a unique trace number to the inquiry. Often, eligibility transactions are sent the day before patients arrive for appointments.

The health plan responds to an inquiry with this information:

- Trace number, as a double-check on the inquiry
- Benefit information, such as whether the insurance coverage is active
- Covered period—the period of dates that the coverage is active
- Benefit units, such as the number of physical therapy visits
- Coverage level—who is covered, such as spouse and family or individual

The following information may also be transmitted:

- The copay amount
- The yearly deductible amount
- The coinsurance amount
- The out-of-pocket expenses
- The health plan's information on the insured's/patient's first and last names, dates of birth, and identification numbers
- The primary care provider

Online Eligibility Services

Some practice management programs also offer electronic eligibility checking through an online service. Rather than having the medical practice contact the payer directly, the online service acts as the relay, or go-between, for a practice and all the major payers. The online service provides a computer network for instant communication of clinical, financial, and administrative data with the major insurance payers. The responses retrieved via the service come directly from payers. Figure 4.8 illustrates an eligibility verification response received from a payer that was requested through RelayHealth, an online connectivity service that can be accessed from within the Medisoft Professional Network software.

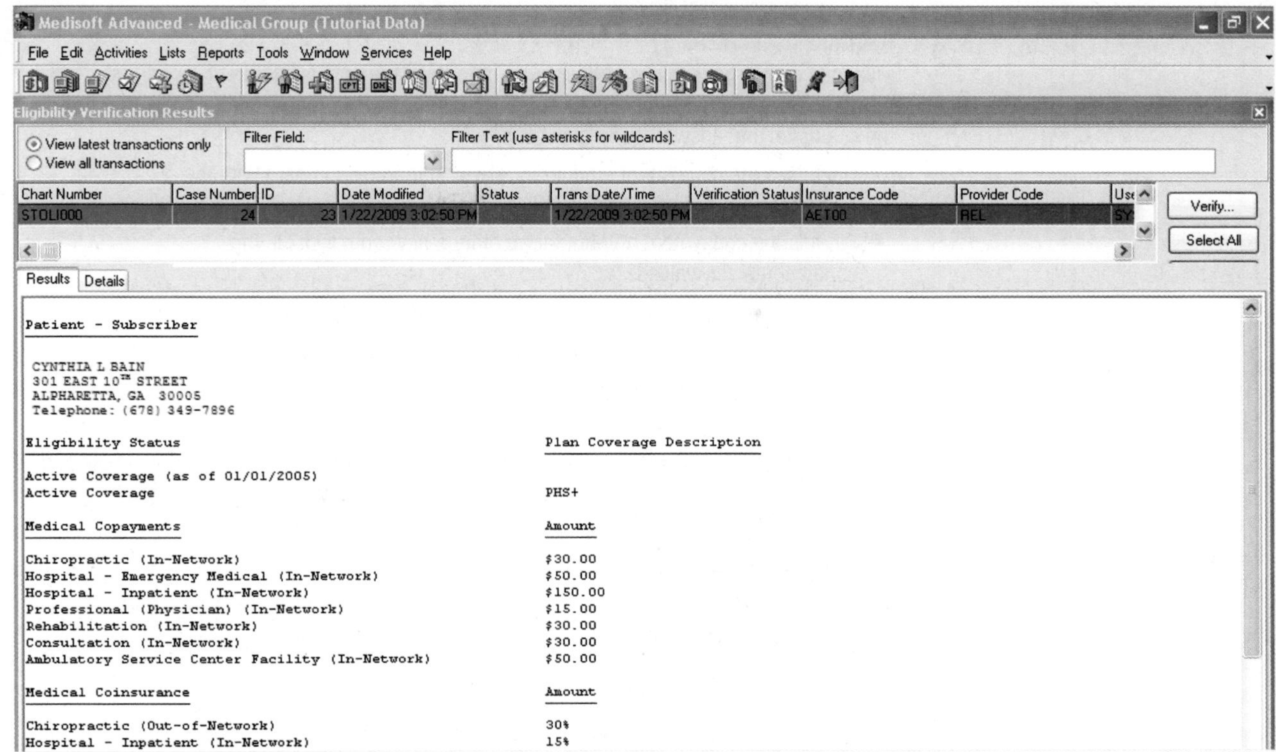

Figure 4.8 A Medisoft Screen Showing Eligibility Verification Results

Procedures When the Patient Is Not Covered

If an insured patient's policy does not cover a planned service, the patient should be informed that the payer does not pay for the service and that he or she is responsible for the charges. For example, some plans do not pay for preventive services such as annual physical examinations. Many patients, however, consider preventive services a good idea and are willing to pay for them.

Some payers require the physician to use specific forms to tell the patient about noncovered services. These financial agreement forms, which patients must sign, prove that patients were told—before the services were given—about their obligation to pay the bill. Figure 4.9 is an example of a form used to tell patients in advance of the probable cost of procedures that are not going to be covered by their plan and to secure their agreement to pay.

Service to be performed: ______________________
Estimated charge: ______________________
Date of planned service: ______________________
Reason for exclusion: ______________________

I, ______________, a patient of ______________, understand the service described above is excluded from my health insurance. I am responsible for payment in full of the charges for this service.

Figure 4.9 Sample Financial Agreement for Patient Payment of Noncovered Services

THINKING IT THROUGH 4.6

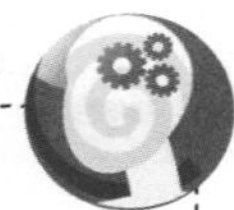

Managed care organizations often require different payments for different services. The table below shows the copayments for an HMO health plan. Study the schedule, and answer these questions:

- How does the copayment amount for physical therapy compare with the copayment for seeing a specialist?
- What is the copayment amount for an emergency room visit? Is the copayment ever waived?
- Does this health plan cover chiropractic care? Contraceptives? Eye exams?
- How much does an insured have to pay on prescriptions each year before prescription benefits begin?

Example of Benefits Under an HMO

Service	Copayment
Primary Care Physician Visits	
During office hours	$20 copay
After hours/home visits	$20 copay
Specialty Care	
During office hours	$30 copay
For diagnostic outpatient testing	$20 copay
Physical, occupational, speech therapy	$20 copay
Surgery in Special Purpose Unit	$250 copay
Hospitalization	$250 copay
Emergency Room (copay waived if admitted)	$35 copay
Maternity	
First OB visit	$30 copay
Hospital	$250 copay
Mental Health	
Inpatient	$250 copay, 60 days
Outpatient	30% copay
Substance Abuse	
Detoxification	$250 copay
Inpatient rehab (combined w/mental health amount)	$250 copay
Outpatient rehabilitation	30% copay
Preventive Care	
Routine eye exam	Not covered
Routine gynecological exam	$30 copay
Pediatric preventive dental exam	Not covered
Chiropractic Care (20 visits/condition)	$20 copay
Prescriptions	$15/$20/$20 copay; $150 deductible/calendar year
Contraceptives	Covered
Diabetic supplies	Covered
31–90 day supply	$30/$40/$60 copay
Durable Medical Equipment	No copay

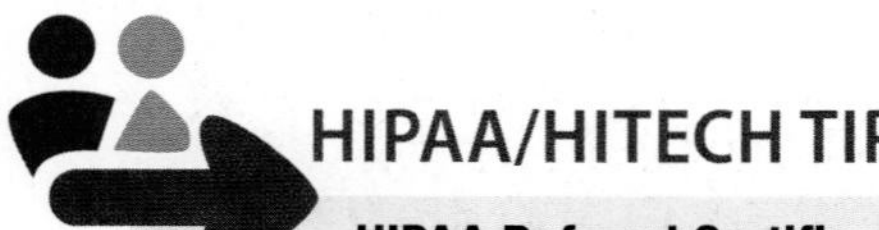

HIPAA/HITECH TIP

HIPAA Referral Certification and Authorization

The electronic transaction that must be used for preauthorization or referral is the HIPAA Referral Certification and Authorization transaction, also called the X12 278.

4.7 Preauthorization, Referrals, and Outside Procedures

In addition to verifying a patient's eligibility for benefits, the medical administrative team needs to check for preauthorization or referral requirements that may be part of the patient's plan prior to the office visit. Preauthorization and referrals are required for many services in managed care plans, such as HMOs.

Preauthorization

A managed care payer often requires preauthorization before the patient sees a specialist, is admitted to the hospital, or has a particular procedure. The office's medical insurance specialist may request preauthorization over the phone, by e-mail or fax, or in an electronic transaction. If the payer approves the service, it issues a preauthorization number that must be entered in the practice management program so it will be stored and appear later on the health care claim for the encounter. (This number may also be called a certification number.)

To help secure preauthorization, best practice is to:

- Be as specific as possible about the planned procedure when exchanging information with the payer
- Collect and have available all diagnosis information related to the procedure, including any pertinent history
- Query the provider about all procedures that may potentially be used to treat the patient, and then request preauthorization for all of them

Referrals

Often, a physician needs to send a patient to another physician for evaluation and/or treatment. For example, an internist might send a patient to a gastroenterologist for a colonoscopy. If a patient's plan requires it, the patient must obtain a **referral number** and a referral document for the specialist before the visit. Usually the office of the primary care physician contacts the payer to obtain the referral number and then prepares the referral document.

referral number authorization number given by a referring physician to the referred physician

The referral document is either given to the patient to take to the visit or sent directly to the specialist on the patient's behalf. A paper referral document (see Figure 4.10) describes the services the patient is certified to receive. It is a specific set of instructions from the primary care physician that directs the patient to a specialist or facility for medically necessary care. This approval may instead be communicated electronically using the HIPAA referral transaction.

Referral Form

Label with Patient's Demographic & Insurance Information

Physician referred to: __________

Referred for:

- ❑ Consult only
- ❑ Follow-up
- ❑ Lab
- ❑ X-ray
- ❑ Procedure
- ❑ Other

Reason for visit: __________

Number of visits: __________

Appointment requested: Please contact patient; phone: __________

Primary care physician

Name: __________

Signature: __________

Phone: __________

Figure 4.10 Referral Document

The specialist's office handling a referred patient must:

- Check that the patient has a referral number
- Verify patient enrollment in the plan
- Understand restrictions to services, such as regulations that require the patient to visit a specialist in a specific amount of time after receiving the referral or that limit the number of times the patient can receive services from the specialist

Sometimes a managed care patient may "self-refer"—come for specialty care without a referral number when one is required. In such a case, the medical insurance specialist asks the patient to sign a form acknowledging responsibility for the services. A sample form is shown in Figure 4.11a.

In other cases, a patient who is required to have a referral document may not bring one. When this occurs, the medical insurance specialist asks the patient to sign a referral waiver document, such as that shown in Figure 4.11b, to ensure that the patient will pay for services if a referral is not documented in the time specified.

Outside Procedures

The medical administrative team is also responsible for scheduling patients for inpatient (defined as requiring an overnight stay) or outpatient admissions procedures. Most plans require preauthorization for such procedures if they are not emergencies.

After obtaining the preauthorization, the staff member in charge of scheduling outside appointments asks the doctor for an order that

Member Self-Referral Acknowledgment

I, ____________________, understand that I am seeking the care of this specialty physician or health care provider, ____________________, without a referral from my primary care physician. I understand that the terms of my plan coverage required that I obtain that referral, and that if I fail to do so, my plan will not cover any part of the charges, costs, or expenses related to this specialist's services to me.

Signed,

____________________ ____________________
(member's name) (date)

****

Specialty physician or other health care provider:

Please keep a copy of this form in your patient's file

(a)

Referral Waiver

I did not bring a referral for the medical services I will receive today. If my primary care physician does not provide a referral within two days, I understand that I am responsible for paying for the services I am requesting.

Signature: ____________________

Date: ____________________

(b)

Figure 4.11 (a) Self-Referral Document, (b) Referral Waiver

specifies all the details related to the procedure, including when the results are required. The provider of the outside procedures requires such an order to do the medical work. The staff member then contacts the outside lab or hospital where the procedure will be performed to verify that the facility or referring physician accepts the patient's insurance. In preparation for the appointment, the staff member also:

- Finds out what days and times are available for scheduling the procedure
- Provides the facility with detailed information about the test or procedure
- Obtains instructions the patient needs in order to prepare for the procedure
- Contacts the operating room secretary about reserving a room and time, if required
- Provides the facility with the patient's demographics and insurance information for admission and billing purposes
- Obtains a telephone number and contact person for the patient to use when calling back to set up the appointment

After this information is obtained, the staff member can contact the patient with an idea of what times are available and provide the

THINKING IT THROUGH 4.7

What is the difference between a preauthorization and a referral?

patient with the phone number to use for making the appointment. The patient is also given instructions on how to prepare for the procedure. Patients generally feel less stressed about making an appointment for an inpatient or outpatient admissions procedure when given this information ahead of time.

4.8 Using Office Hours—Medisoft Network Professional's Appointment Scheduler

Chapter 3 introduced a special program called Office Hours that is used to handle appointment scheduling in Medisoft Network Professional. This section provides practice in using Office Hours. Exercises are provided for entering appointments, changing and deleting appointments, creating provider breaks in the schedule, and printing provider schedules.

The Office Hours Window

The Office Hours program has its own window (see Figure 4.12), including its own menu bar and toolbar. The Office Hours menu

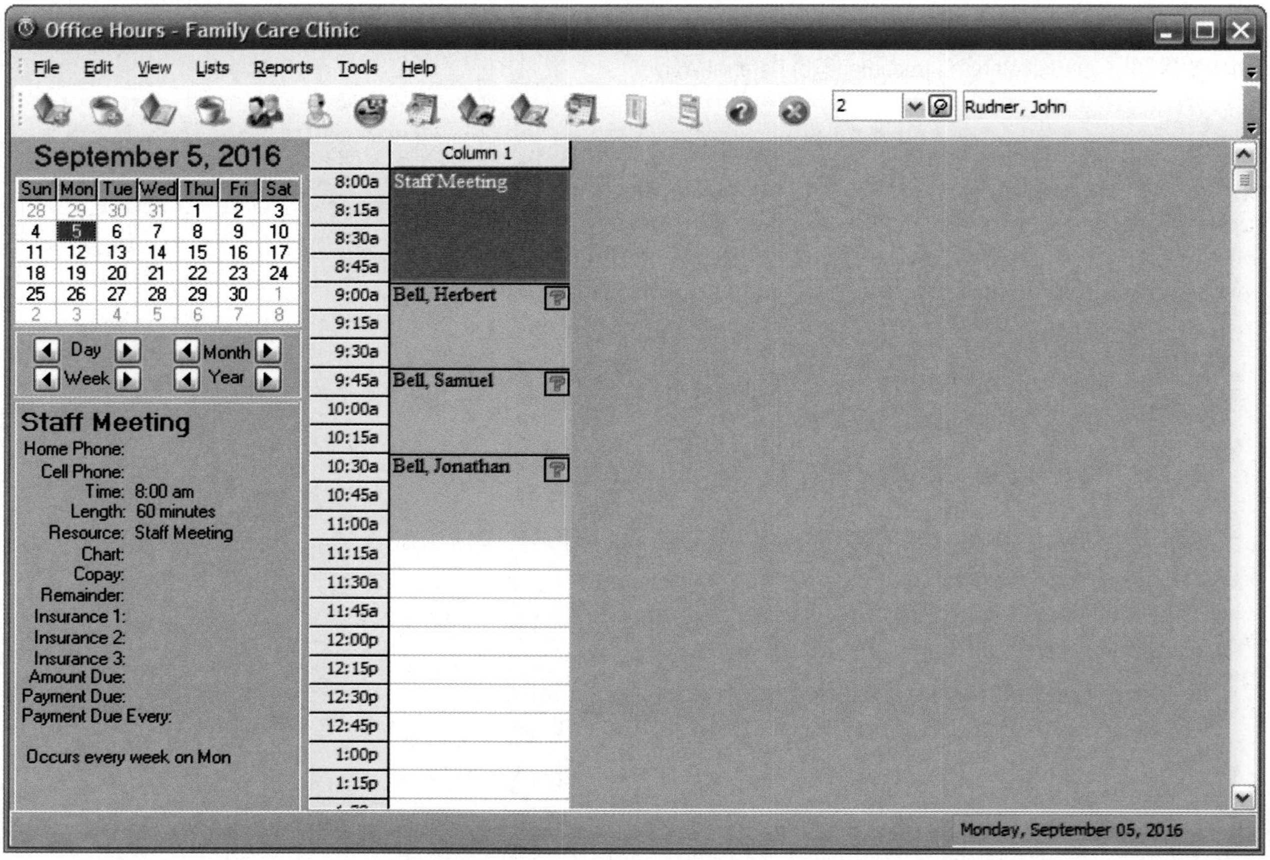

Figure 4.12 The Office Hours Window

bar lists the menus available: File, Edit, View, Lists, Reports, Tools, and Help (see Figure 4.13). Under the menu bar is a toolbar with shortcut buttons. The functions of Office Hours are accessed by selecting a choice from one of the menus or by clicking a button on the toolbar.

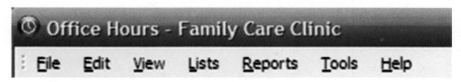

Figure 4.13 The Office Hours Menu Bar

Located just below the menu bar, the toolbar contains a series of buttons that represent the most common activities performed in Office Hours. These buttons are shortcuts for frequently used menu commands. The toolbar displays fifteen buttons (see Figure 4.14 and Table 4.2).

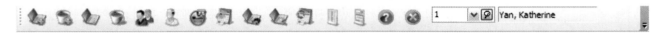

Figure 4.14 The Office Hours Toolbar

In addition to the menu bar and toolbar, the Office Hours window contains four main areas (see Figure 4.15).

Provider Selection Box The **provider selection box,** located at the far-right end of the toolbar, is where you select a provider. This selection determines which provider's schedule is displayed in the provider's daily schedule.

provider selection box a selection box that determines which provider's schedule is displayed in the provider's daily schedule

provider's daily schedule a listing of time slots for a particular day for a specific provider that corresponds to the date selected in the calendar

Office Hours calendar an interactive calendar that is used to select or change dates in Office Hours

Office Hours patient information the area of the Office Hours window that displays information about the patient who is selected in the provider's daily schedule

Provider's Daily Schedule The **provider's daily schedule,** shown in Column 1, is a listing of time slots for a particular day for a specific provider. The schedule displayed corresponds to the date selected in the calendar, which is located on the left side of the window.

Calendar The **Office Hours calendar** is used to select or change dates. The right and left arrows that surround Day, Week, Month, and Year are used to move back or ahead on the calendar. When a different date on the calendar is clicked, the calendar switches to the new date.

Patient Information The area just below the calendar contains **Office Hours patient information** about the patient who is selected in the provider's daily schedule.

Program Options

When Office Hours is installed in a medical practice, it is set up to reflect the needs of that particular practice. Most offices that use Medisoft Network Professional already have Office Hours set up and

TABLE 4.2	Office Hours Toolbar Buttons		
Button	**Button Name**	**Associated Function**	**Activity**
	Appointment Entry	New Appointment Entry dialog box	Enter appointments
	Break Entry	New Break Entry dialog box	Enter breaks
	Appointment List	Appointment List dialog box	Display list of appointments
	Break List	Break List dialog box	Display list of breaks
	Patient List	Patient List dialog box	Display list of patients
	Provider List	Provider List dialog box	Display list of providers
	Resource List	Resource List dialog box	Display list of resources
	Go to a Date	Go to Date dialog box	Change calendar to a different date
	Search for Open Time Slot	Find Open Time dialog box	Locate first available time slot
	Search Again	Find Open Time dialog box	Locate next available time slot
	Go to Today		Return calendar to current date
	Print Appointment List		Print appointment list
	Edit Patient Notes in Final Draft	Final Draft word processor	Use Final Draft word processor
	Help	Office Hours Help	Display Office Hours Help contents
	Exit	Exit	Exit the Office Hours program

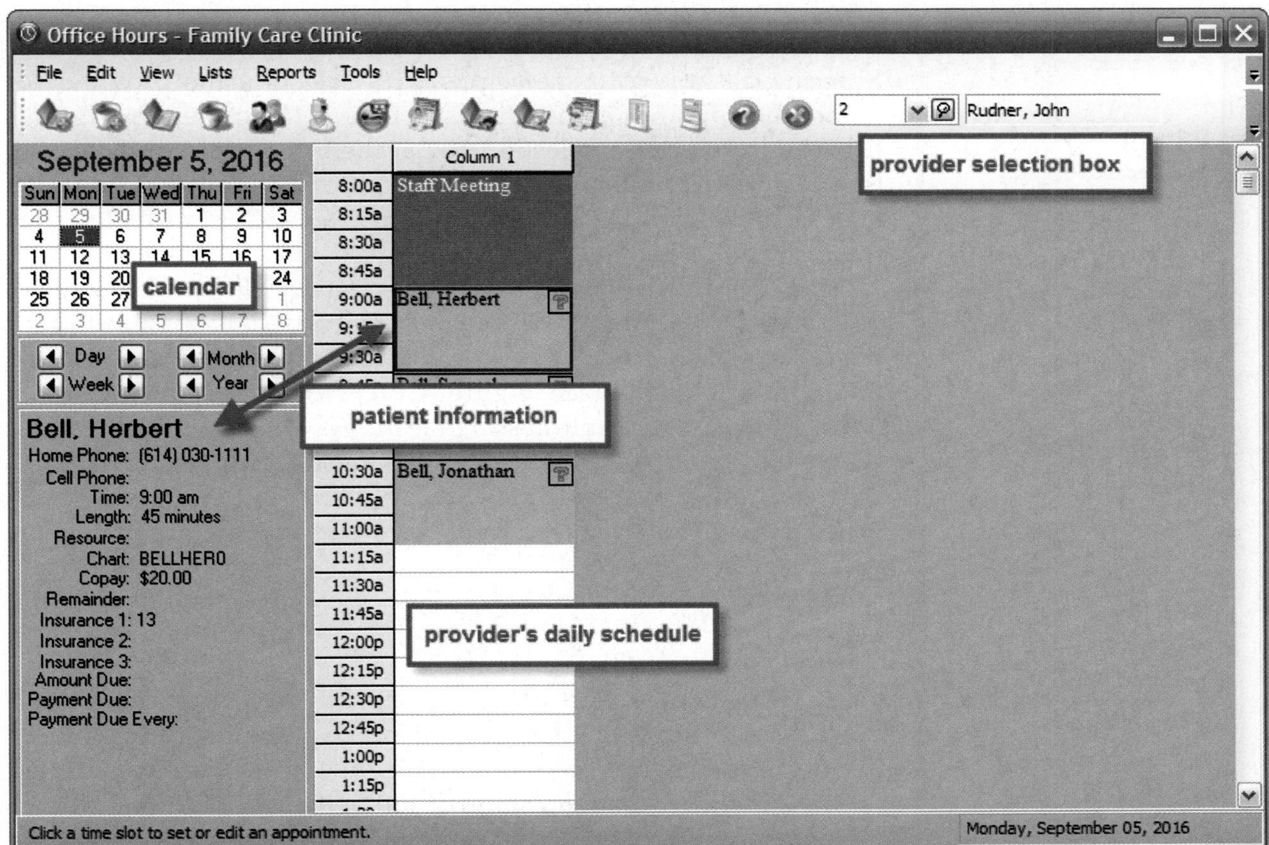

Figure 4.15 The Main Areas of the Office Hours Window

running. However, if Medisoft Network Professional is just being installed, the options to set up the Office Hours program can be found in the Program Options dialog box, which is accessed by clicking Program Options on the Office Hours File menu.

Entering and Exiting Office Hours

Office Hours can be started from within Medisoft Network Professional or directly from Windows. To access Office Hours from within Medisoft Network Professional, Appointment Book is clicked on the Activities menu (see Figure 4.16). Office Hours can also be started by clicking the corresponding shortcut button on the toolbar (see Figure 4.17).

To start Office Hours without entering Medisoft Network Professional:

1. Click Start > All Programs.
2. Click Medisoft on the Programs submenu.
3. Click Office Hours on the Medisoft submenu.

The Office Hours program is closed by clicking Exit on the Office Hours File menu or by clicking the Exit button on its toolbar. If Office Hours was started from within Medisoft Network Professional, exiting will return you to Medisoft Network Professional. If Office Hours was started directly from Windows, clicking Exit will return you to the Windows desktop.

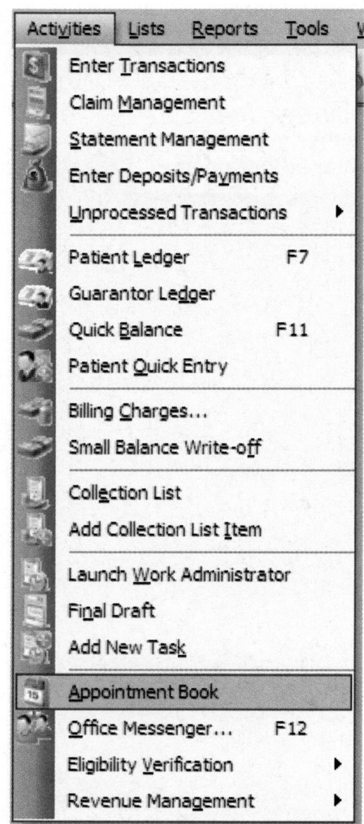

Figure 4.16 The Appointment Book Selection on the Activities Menu

Figure 4.17 The Office Hours Shortcut Button

4.9 Entering Appointments

Entering an appointment begins with selecting the provider for whom the appointment is being scheduled. The current provider is listed in the provider selection box at the upper right of the screen (see Figure 4.18). Clicking the arrow button displays a drop-down list of providers in the system. To choose a different provider, click the name of the provider on the drop-down list.

After the provider is selected, an appointment slot must be located. To change the date on the Office Hours calendar, it is possible to click the Day, Week, Month, and Year right and left arrow buttons located under the calendar (see Figure 4.19). However, many times it is quicker to use the built-in search features.

Appointments are entered by clicking the Appointment Entry shortcut button or by double clicking a time slot on the schedule. When either action is taken, the New Appointment Entry dialog box is displayed (see Figure 4.20).

The New Appointment Entry dialog box contains the following fields:

Chart A patient's chart number is chosen from the Chart drop-down list. To select the desired patient, click the patient's name in the drop-down list and press Tab. If an appointment is being created for an established patient, some of the fields will automatically be filled in once the patient's chart number is selected. If you are setting up an appointment for a new patient who has not been assigned a chart number, skip the Chart box, and key the patient's name in the blank box to the right of the Chart box.

Home Phone After a patient's chart is selected, that patient's home phone number is automatically entered in the Home Phone box.

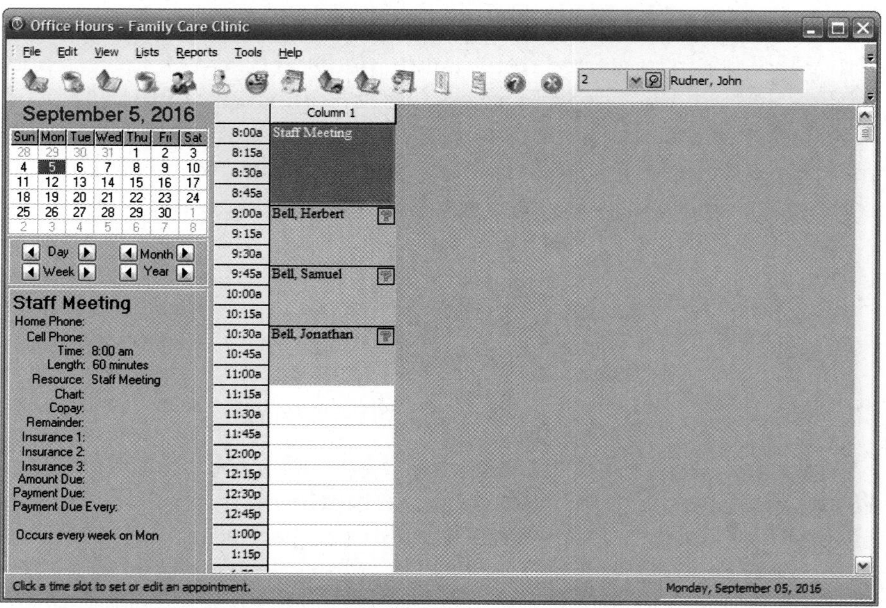

Figure 4.18 Office Hours Window with Provider Box Highlighted

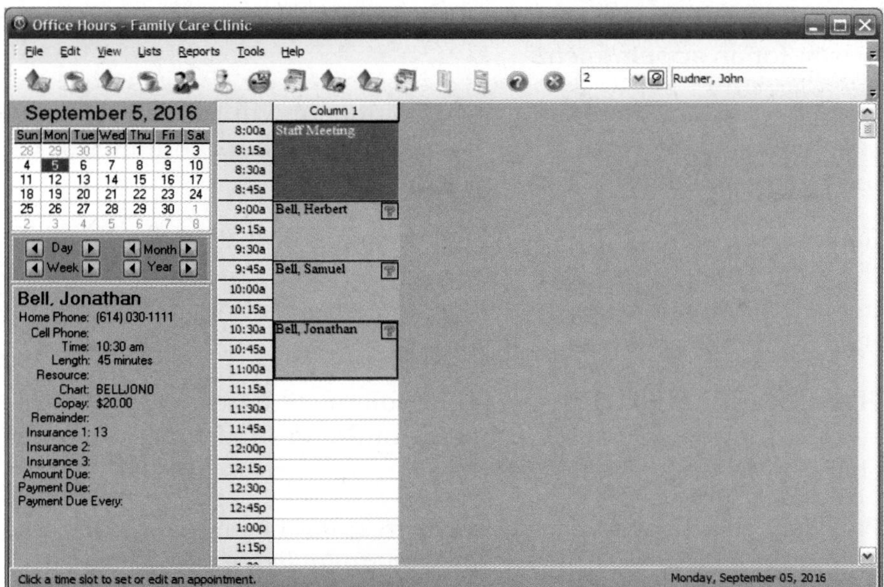

Figure 4.19 Office Hours Window with Day, Week, Month, and Year Arrow Buttons Highlighted

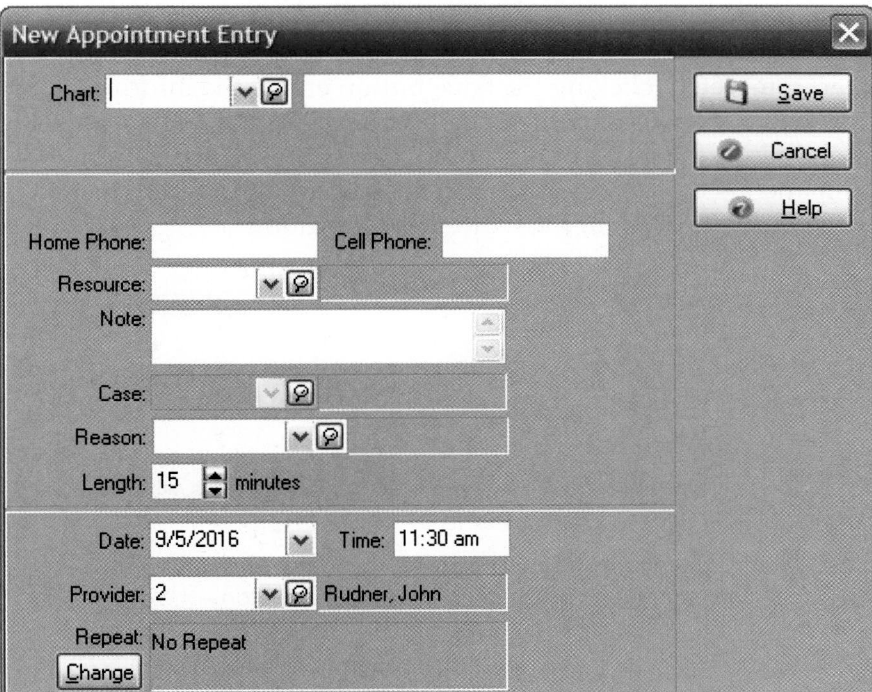

Figure 4.20 New Appointment Entry Dialog Box

Cell Phone After a patient's chart is selected, that patient's cell phone number is automatically entered in the Cell Phone box.

Resource This box is used if the practice assigns codes to resources, such as exam rooms and equipment.

Note Any special information about an appointment is entered in the Note box.

Case The case that pertains to the appointment is selected from the drop-down list of cases.

Reason Reason codes can be set up in the program to reflect the reason for an appointment.

Length The amount of time an appointment will take (in minutes) is entered in the Length box by keying the number of minutes or using the up and down arrows.

Date The Date box displays the date that is currently displayed on the calendar. If this is not the desired date, it may be changed by keying in a different date or by clicking the arrow button and selecting a date from the pop-up calendar that appears.

Time The Time box displays the appointment time that is currently selected on the schedule. If this is not the desired time, it may be changed by keying in a different time.

Provider The provider who will be treating the patient during this appointment is selected from the drop-down list of providers.

Repeat The Repeat box is used to enter appointments that recur on a regular basis.

After the boxes in the New Appointment Entry dialog box have been completed, clicking the Save button enters the information on the schedule. The patient's name appears in the time slot corresponding to the appointment time. In addition, information about the patient's insurance appears in the patient information section in the lower-left corner of the Office Hours window.

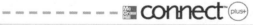

EXERCISE 4.1

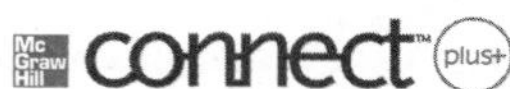

ENTERING AN APPOINTMENT FOR AN ESTABLISHED PATIENT (HERBERT BELL)

Enter an appointment for Herbert Bell at 3:00 P.M. on Monday, November 14, 2016. The appointment is sixty minutes in length and is with Dr. John Rudner.

1. Start Office Hours from within Medisoft Network Professional by clicking the Appointment Book shortcut button—the sixth icon from the left—on the toolbar.
2. The provider selection box in the upper-right corner currently displays "1–Yan, Katherine." To change the selection to Dr. John Rudner, open the drop-down list and select "2–Rudner, John."
3. The Office Hours calendar in the upper-left corner displays today's Windows System Date (Monday, October 3, 2016) by default. To change the calendar to the date for the new appointment (Monday, November 14, 2016), first click the Month right arrow button.
4. The calendar moves to November.
5. Then click 14 on the calendar so that the date is now Monday, November 14, 2016.
6. Click the down arrow button on the scroll bar to the far right to scroll down the provider's daily schedule until the 3:00 P.M. time slot is visible.

7. To enter an appointment for Herbert Bell at this time, double click the time slot.
8. The New Appointment Entry dialog box is displayed.
9. Click the down arrow to the right of the Chart box to open the drop-down list of names.
10. Click Herbert Bell on the list displayed, and then press Tab.
11. The system automatically fills in several boxes in the dialog box, including the patient's name and home and cell phone numbers.
12. Notice that the Length box already contains an entry of fifteen minutes. This is the default appointment length. Since Herbert Bell's appointment is for an annual exam, this entry must be changed to sixty minutes. Click the up arrow next to the Length box three times to change the appointment length to sixty minutes.
13. To save the appointment, click the Save button. The program saves the appointment and closes the dialog box.
14. Notice that Herbert Bell's name is displayed in the 3:00 P.M. time slot on the schedule as well as in the patient information section on the left.

 **You have completed Exercise 4.1**

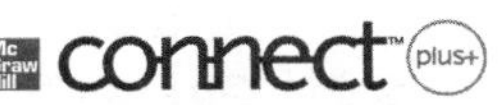

EXERCISE 4.2

LOOKING UP A PROVIDER AND ENTERING AN APPOINTMENT (JOHN GARDINER)

Enter a thirty-minute appointment on Thursday, November 10, 2016, at 9:00 A.M. for John Gardiner. You do not know his provider, so this information must be looked up before you enter the appointment.

1. Open the Lists menu in Office Hours, and select Patient List. The Patient List dialog box is displayed.
2. Enter ***G*** in the Search For box at the top of the dialog box to select John Gardiner.
3. Double click the line that contains John Gardiner's chart number and name in the left pane, or click the Edit Patient button. The Patient/Guarantor dialog box appears.
4. Click the Other Information tab. Look in the Assigned Provider field to determine that John Gardiner's provider is Dr. Katherine Yan.
5. With this information, you can return to the Office Hours window and enter the appointment. Click the Cancel button to close the Patient/Guarantor dialog box.
6. Click the Close button to close the Patient List dialog box. You are back to the main Office Hours window.
7. To enter the appointment, select John Gardiner's provider in the provider selection box.

(continued)

(Continued)

8. Change the Office Hours calendar in the upper-left corner to November 10, 2016, by clicking 10 on the calendar.
9. Scroll up to the correct appointment time in the daily schedule (9:00 A.M.), and double click the "9:00a" appointment slot.
10. The New Appointment Entry dialog box appears.
11. Key ***G*** in the Chart box to display the list of names that begin with the letter *G*.
12. Click John Gardiner's name to select it, and then press Tab.
13. Change the entry in the Length box from 15 to 30 by clicking the up arrow.
14. Verify that the date and time boxes are correct.
15. Click the Save button.
16. Notice that the new appointment—9:00 A.M on Thursday, November 10, for John Gardiner—is listed in the provider's daily schedule.

 **You have completed Exercise 4.2**

Searching for Available Time Slots

Often it is necessary to search for available appointment space on a particular day of the week and at a specific time. For example, a patient needs a thirty-minute appointment and would like it to be during his lunch hour, which is from 12:00 P.M. to 1:00 P.M. He can get away from the office only on Mondays and Fridays. Office Hours makes it easy to locate an appointment slot that meets these requirements with the Search for Open Time Slot shortcut button.

EXERCISE 4.3

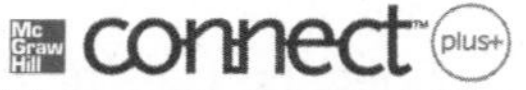

SEARCHING FOR OPEN TIME (MARITZA RAMOS)

Maritza Ramos needs an appointment, but she has very limited times she can come to the office. Search for the next available appointment slot with Dr. Yan on a Tuesday, thirty minutes in length, between 11:00 A.M. and 2:00 P.M., beginning November 10, 2016.

1. Verify that Dr. Katherine Yan is selected in the provider selection box.
2. Verify that the date on the calendar is November 10, 2016.
3. On the Edit menu, click Find Open Time, or click the Search for Open Time Slot shortcut button.
4. The Find Open Time dialog box is displayed.
5. Double click inside the Length box to highlight the current entry. Key ***30*** over the current entry. Press the Tab key.
6. Key ***11*** in the Start Time box. Press the Tab key.
7. Key ***2*** in the End Time box. Press the Tab key.

8. To search for an appointment on Tuesday, click the Tuesday box in the Day of Week area of the dialog box. If necessary, deselect any other days that are selected.
9. Click the Search button to begin looking for an appointment slot. The Find Open Time dialog box closes and the program locates the first available time slot that meets these specifications (Tuesday, November 15, 2016, at 11:00 A.M.). The time slot is outlined on the schedule.
10. Double click the selected time slot. The New Appointment Entry dialog box appears.
11. Key ***R*** in the Chart box to select Maritza Ramos's name. Click Tab.
12. Press the Tab key to move through each field until the cursor is in the Length box.
13. Key ***30*** in the Length box, and press the Tab key.
14. Click the Save button to save the appointment.
15. Verify that a thirty-minute appointment for Maritza Ramos has been entered on the schedule for November 15, 2016, at 11:00 A.M.

 **You have completed Exercise 4.3**

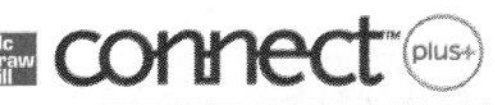

EXERCISE 4.4

SEARCHING FOR OPEN TIME (RANDALL KLEIN)

Schedule Randall Klein for a thirty-minute appointment with Dr. John Rudner sometime after November 14, 2016. Mr. Klein is available only on Mondays between 3:00 P.M. and 5:00 P.M.

1. Click the desired provider, John Rudner, in the Provider box.
2. Verify that the date on the calendar is November 15, 2016.
3. Click Find Open Time on the Edit menu to display the Find Open Time dialog box.
4. Double click in the Length box, and then key ***30***. Press the Tab key to move the cursor to the Start Time box.
5. Key ***3*** in the Start Time box. Click on "am" to highlight it, and then key ***p*** to change "am" to "pm." Press Tab to move to the End Time box.
6. Key ***5*** in the End Time box. Press Tab.
7. In the Day of Week boxes, select Monday. If necessary, deselect any other days that are selected.
8. Click the Search button. The first available slot that meets the requirements is outlined on the schedule (Monday, November 21, 3:00 P.M.).
9. Double click the time slot to open the New Appointment Entry dialog box.
10. Key ***K*** to select Randall Klein in the drop-down list in the Chart box, and then press Tab.

(continued)

(Continued)

11. Click the up arrow in the Length box once to change the length of the appointment from 15 to 30 minutes.
12. Click the Save button to save the new appointment. The dialog box closes. Verify that a thirty-minute appointment for Randall Klein appears on the schedule for Monday, November 21, 2016, at 3:00 P.M.

 **You have completed Exercise 4.4**

Entering Appointments for New Patients

When a new patient phones the office for an appointment, the appointment can be scheduled in Office Hours before the patient information is entered in Medisoft Network Professional. It is possible to enter an appointment before a chart number has been assigned to the patient. However, while the prospective patient is still on the phone, most offices obtain basic data and enter them in the appropriate Medisoft Network Professional dialog boxes. You will learn how to enter this information in Chapter 5.

EXERCISE 4.5

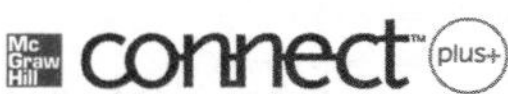

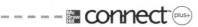

ENTERING AN APPOINTMENT FOR A NEW PATIENT (JORGE BARRETT)

Schedule Jorge Barrett, a new patient, for a forty-five-minute appointment with Dr. Patricia McGrath on October 21, 2016, at 1:15 P.M.

1. Select Dr. Patricia McGrath in the provider selection box.
2. Change the month on the Office Hours calendar to October.
3. Change the date on the Office Hours calendar to October 21.
4. Double click the 1:15 P.M. time slot.
5. Click in the blank box to the right of the Chart box, and key ***Barrett, Jorge.*** Press the Tab key to move the cursor to the Home Phone box.
6. Key ***6145093637*** in the Home Phone box, and press Tab to go to the Cell Phone box.
7. Enter ***6149637682*** in the Cell Phone box. Press Tab four times to go to the Length box.
8. Key ***45*** in the Length box.
9. Click the Save button. Verify that a forty-five-minute appointment is scheduled for Jorge Barrett on October 21, 2016, starting at 1:15 P.M.

 **You have completed Exercise 4.5**

4.10 Booking Follow-up and Repeating Appointments

Some patients need either follow-up or repeating appointments. Follow-up appointments are scheduled at a certain time in the future. For example, suppose a physician would like a patient to return for a checkup in three weeks. Repeating appointments occur at the same time for a limited period of time. For example, a patient may need an appointment once a month for three months to monitor the effectiveness of a new medication.

Booking Follow-up Appointments

The most efficient way to create a follow-up appointment in Office Hours is to use the Go to a Date shortcut button on the toolbar. (This feature can also be accessed on the Edit menu.)

Clicking the Go to a Date shortcut button displays the Go To Date dialog box (see Figure 4.21). Within the dialog box, five boxes offer options for choosing a future date.

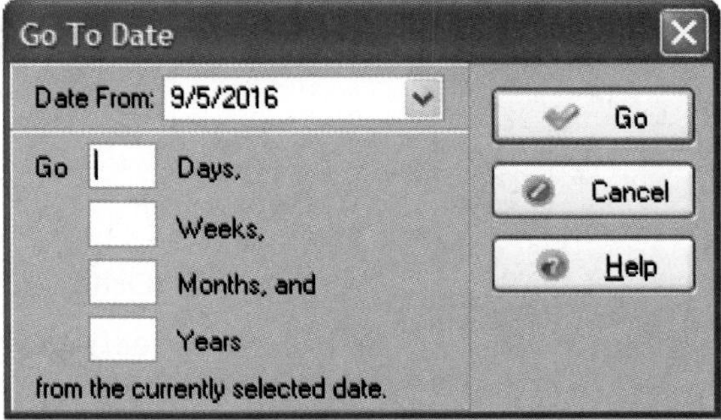

Figure 4.21 Go To Date Dialog Box

Date From This box indicates the current date in the appointment search.

Go __ Days This box is used to locate a date that is a specific number of days in the future. For example, if a patient needs an appointment ten days from the current day, ***10*** is entered in this box.

Go __ Weeks This box is used when a patient needs an appointment a specific number of weeks in the future, such as six weeks from the current day.

Go __ Months This box is used when a patient needs an appointment a specific number of months in the future, such as three months from the current day.

Go __ Years Similar to the weeks and months options, this box is used when an appointment is needed in one year or several years in the future.

After a future date option has been selected, clicking the Go button closes the dialog box and begins the search. The system locates the future date and displays the calendar schedule for that date.

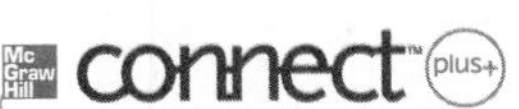

EXERCISE 4.6

BOOKING A FOLLOW-UP APPOINTMENT (JOHN GARDINER)

Enter the following follow-up appointment with Dr. Katherine Yan, using the Go to a Date shortcut button.

1. Click Dr. Katherine Yan from the list of providers in the Provider drop-down list.
2. Change the month on the Office Hours calendar to November.

(continued)

(Continued)

3. Change the date to November 10.
4. Click on John Gardiner's 9:00 A.M. appointment.
5. To schedule a follow-up appointment at the same time in two weeks, fifteen minutes in length, click the Go to a Date shortcut button (the eighth icon from the left) on the toolbar.
6. Click inside the Go ____ Weeks box, and key ***2.***
7. Click the Go button.
8. The program closes the Go To Date box and displays the appointment schedule for November 24, 2016, at 9:00 A.M.. Double click the time slot to make the appointment.
9. The New Appointment Entry dialog box appears. Key **G** in the Chart box, and then press Tab to select John Gardiner.
10. Note that the Length box is already set to 15 minutes, the default setting. Click the Save button to save the appointment.
11. Verify that a fifteen-minute appointment for John Gardiner appears on the schedule for November 24 (two weeks after November 10) at 9:00 A.M.

 **You have completed Exercise 4.6**

Booking Repeating Appointments

Repeating appointments are set up in the New Appointment Entry dialog box. The Repeat feature is located at the bottom of the dialog box (see Figure 4.22). When the Change button is clicked, the Repeat

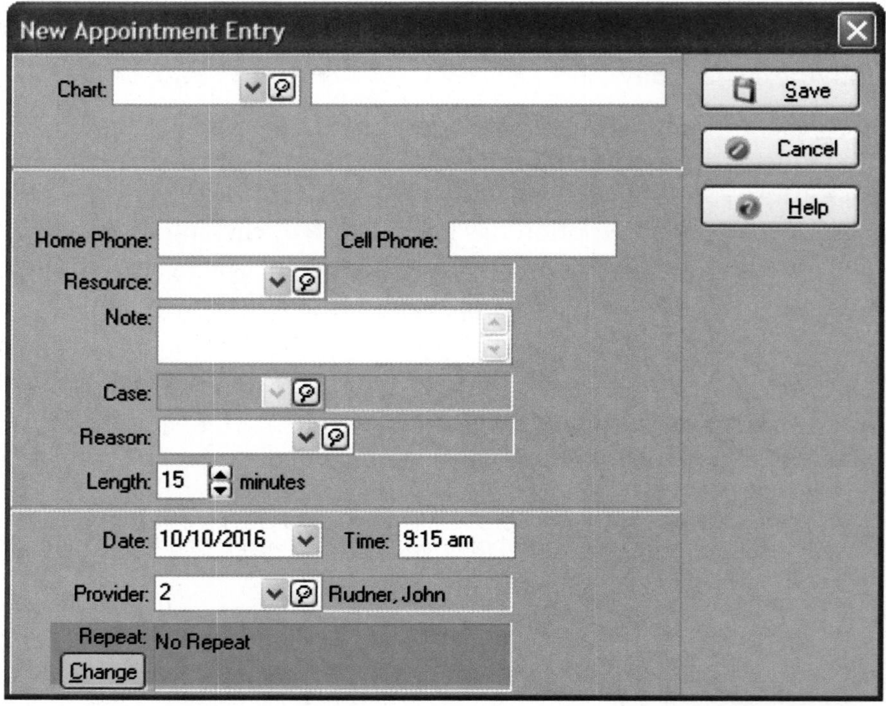

Figure 4.22 New Appointment Entry Dialog Box with Repeat Change Area Highlighted

Change dialog box is displayed. The Repeat Change dialog box provides a number of choices for setting up repeating appointments (see Figure 4.23).

The left side of the dialog box contains information about the frequency of the appointments. The default is set to None. Other options include Daily, Weekly, Monthly, and Yearly. When an option other than None is selected, the center section of the dialog box changes and displays additional options for setting up the appointments (see Figure 4.24).

In the center section, an option is provided to indicate how often the appointments should be scheduled, such as once every week. Below that there is an option to indicate the day of the week on which the appointments should be scheduled. Finally, there is a box to indicate when the repeating appointments should stop. When all the information has been entered, clicking the OK button closes the Repeat Change dialog box, and the New Appointment Entry dialog box is once again visible. Clicking the Save button enters the repeating appointments on the schedule.

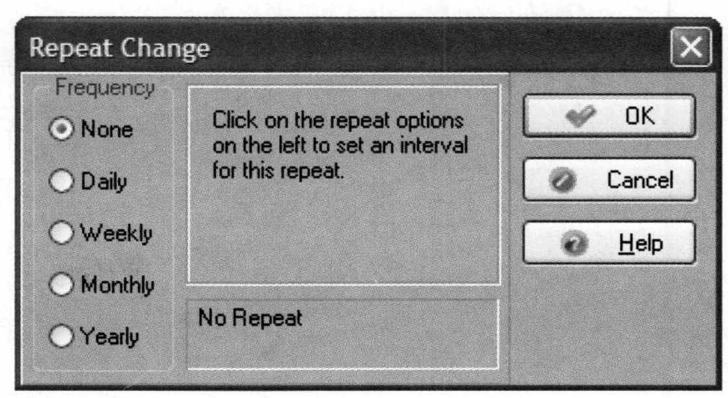

Figure 4.23 Repeat Change Dialog Box with the Default Settings (None Button Selected)

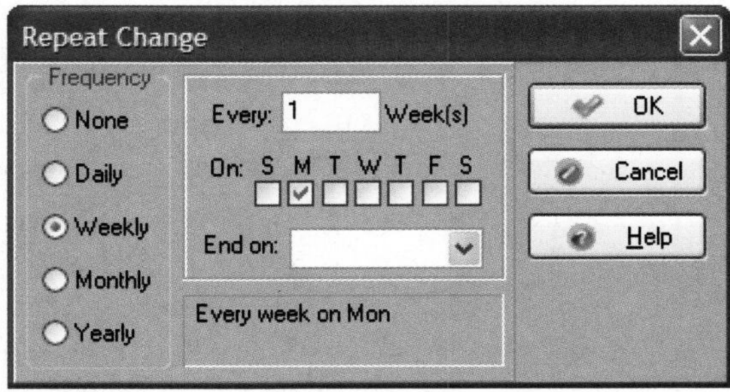

Figure 4.24 Repeat Change Dialog Box When an Option Other than None Is Selected

connect plus+

EXERCISE 4.7

BOOKING REPEATING APPOINTMENTS (JO WONG)

Schedule Jo Wong for a fifteen-minute appointment once a week for six weeks with Dr. Katherine Yan. Mr. Wong has requested that the appointments be at the same time every week, preferably in the early morning, beginning on Wednesday, November 16, 2016.

1. Verify that Dr. Katherine Yan is selected as the provider.
2. Change the Office Hours schedule to November 16, 2016.
3. Double click the 8:00 A.M. time slot. The New Appointment Entry dialog box is displayed.
4. Key ***W*** to select Jo Wong from the Chart drop-down list, and then press the Tab key.
5. Confirm that the entry in the Length box is fifteen minutes.
6. Click the Change button to schedule the repeating appointments.
7. The Repeat Change dialog box appears. In the Frequency column, select Weekly.
8. Accept the default entry of 1 in the Every __ Week(s) box.
9. Accept the default entry of W to accept Wednesday as the day of the week.
10. Click the arrow for the drop-down list in the End on box.
11. A calendar box pops up, displaying today's date, October 3, 2016. To determine the End on date for the repeating appointments, locate the date for the first repeating

(continued)

(Continued)

appointment—Wednesday, November 16. Change the month in the calendar box to November by clicking the right arrow button at the top of the pop-up calendar box. Then click 16 inside the calendar box.

12. Click the down arrow in the End on box again to display the pop-up calendar with the November 16, 2016, date.
13. If Wednesday, November 16, is counted as the first Wednesday, then six appointments later is Wednesday, December 21. Click the right arrow button at the top of the pop-up calendar to move the calendar to December.
14. Click 21 in the pop-up calendar.
15. The pop-up calendar closes, and the date 12/21/2016 appears in the End on box in the Repeat Change dialog box. Click the OK button.
16. Notice that "Every week on Wed" is displayed in the Repeat area at the bottom of the New Appointment Entry dialog box.
17. Click the Save button to enter the appointments.
18. Notice that "Occurs every week on Wed" appears in the lower-left corner of the Office Hours window, below the patient information.
19. Go to December 21, 2016, in the Office Hours schedule: Click the Month right arrow button below the Office Hours calendar to go to December, and then click 21 on the calendar.
20. Verify that Mr. Wong is scheduled for a fifteen-minute appointment at 8:00 A.M.
21. Go to December 28 by clicking 28 on the calendar.
22. Confirm that Mr. Wong is not scheduled. This is the seventh week, and his repeating appointments were scheduled for six weeks, so no appointment appears on December 28, 2016.

You have completed Exercise 4.7

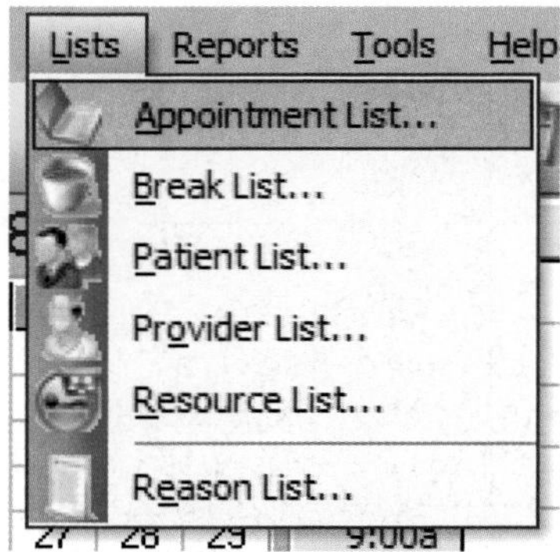

Figure 4.25 Appointment List Option on the Office Hours Lists Menu

4.11 Rescheduling and Canceling Appointments

It is often necessary to reschedule a patient's appointment. The Appointment List option on the Office Hours Lists menu can be used to locate an appointment that needs to be rescheduled (see Figure 4.25).

When the Appointment List option is selected, the Appointment List dialog box appears (see Figure 4.26).

The Appointment List dialog box lists appointments currently in the database. Appointments can be listed from today forward

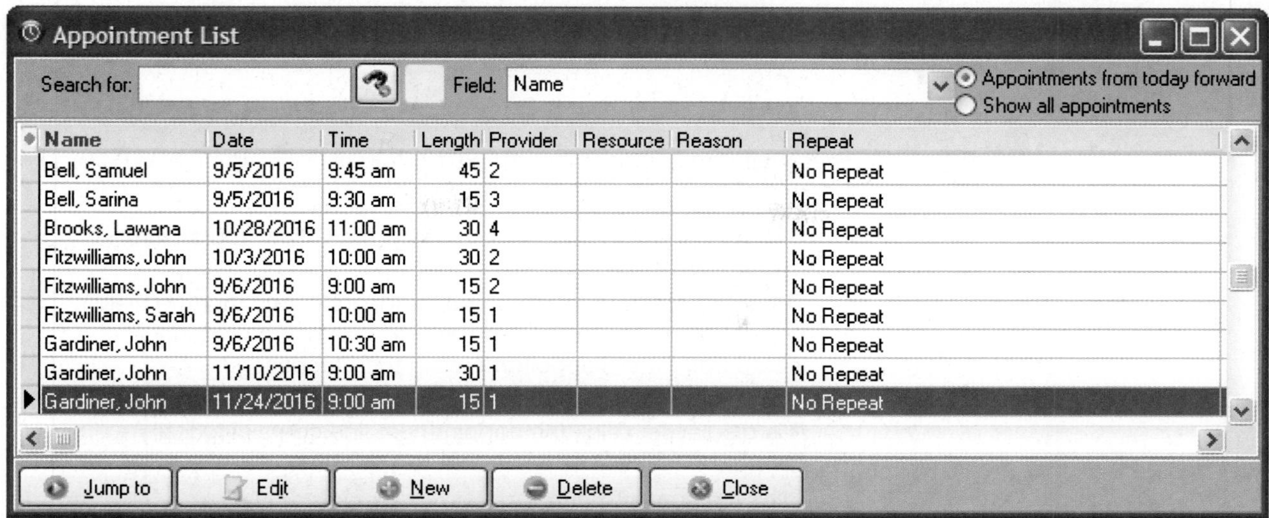

Name	Date	Time	Length	Provider	Resource	Reason	Repeat
Bell, Samuel	9/5/2016	9:45 am	45	2			No Repeat
Bell, Sarina	9/5/2016	9:30 am	15	3			No Repeat
Brooks, Lawana	10/28/2016	11:00 am	30	4			No Repeat
Fitzwilliams, John	10/3/2016	10:00 am	30	2			No Repeat
Fitzwilliams, John	9/6/2016	9:00 am	15	2			No Repeat
Fitzwilliams, Sarah	9/6/2016	10:00 am	15	1			No Repeat
Gardiner, John	9/6/2016	10:30 am	15	1			No Repeat
Gardiner, John	11/10/2016	9:00 am	30	1			No Repeat
Gardiner, John	11/24/2016	9:00 am	15	1			No Repeat

Figure 4.26 Appointment List Dialog Box

or all appointments can be listed. Using the Search For and Field boxes, appointments can be filtered by Name, Date, or Provider. After an appointment is located, the Jump To button is used to jump to that appointment in the Office Hours schedule.

Changing an appointment in Office Hours is accomplished with the Cut and Paste commands on the Office Hours Edit menu. Similarly, an appointment can be canceled and not rescheduled simply by using the Cut command.

The following steps are used to reschedule an appointment:

1. Locate the appointment that needs to be changed. Make sure the appointment slot is visible on the schedule.
2. Click the existing time-slot box. A black border surrounds the slot to indicate that it is selected.
3. Click Cut on the Edit menu. The appointment disappears from the schedule.
4. Click the date on the calendar when the appointment is to be rescheduled.
5. Click the desired time-slot box on the schedule. The slot becomes active.
6. Click Paste on the Edit menu. The patient's name appears in the new time-slot box.

The following steps are used to cancel an appointment without rescheduling:

1. Locate the appointment on the schedule.
2. Click the time-slot box to select the appointment.
3. Click Cut on the Edit menu. The appointment disappears from the schedule.

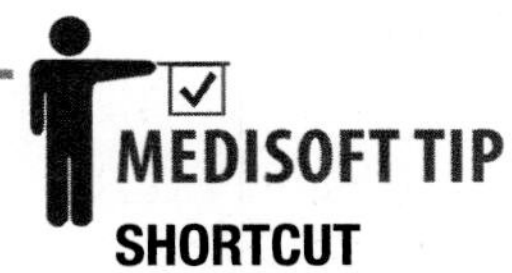

MEDISOFT TIP

SHORTCUT

Instead of using the Cut and Paste commands to change or delete an appointment, select the appointment, and press the right mouse button. A shortcut menu appears with several options, including Cut, Copy, and Delete.

EXERCISE 4.8 connect plus+

RESCHEDULING AN APPOINTMENT (RAJI PATEL)

Change Raji Patel's December 10, 2016, appointment from 10:30 A.M. to 1:00 P.M.

1. Click the Appointment List option on the Office Hours Lists menu.
2. The Appointment List dialog box appears. Verify that the Field box at the top is set to Name. In the Search For box, key ***P*** to locate Raji Patel's appointments in the database.
3. A list of appointments for patients whose last names begin with *P* is displayed. Click the appointment line containing Raji Patel's 12/10/2016 appointment to select it.
4. Click the Jump To button.
5. The Office Hours program jumps to December 10, 2016, with Raji Patel's 10:30 A.M. appointment selected on the schedule. Notice that Raji Patel's provider, Dr. Dana Banu, is listed in the provider selection box.
6. Click the right mouse button to display a shortcut menu.
7. Click the Cut option on the shortcut menu.
8. Raji Patel's appointment is removed from the 10:30 A.M. time-slot box.
9. Click the 1:00 P.M. time-slot box.
10. Click the right mouse button again to display the shortcut menu, and then select Paste to paste the appointment to the new time.
11. Raji Patel's name is displayed in the 1:00 P.M. time-slot box.
12. Click the X in the upper-right corner of the Office Hours window to close the Office Hours program for the time being.

 **You have completed Exercise 4.8**

4.12 Creating a Patient Recall List

Medical offices frequently must keep track of patients who need to return for future appointments. Some offices schedule future appointments when the patient is leaving the office. For example, if a patient has just seen a physician and needs to return for a follow-up appointment in six weeks, the appointment is usually made before the patient leaves the office. However, when the appointment is needed further in the future, such as one year later, it is not always practical to set up the appointment. It is difficult for the patient and the physician to know their schedules a year in advance. For this reason, many offices keep lists of patients who need to be contacted for future appointments.

In Medisoft Network Professional, a recall list can be created and maintained by clicking Patient Recall on the Lists menu. *Note:* The

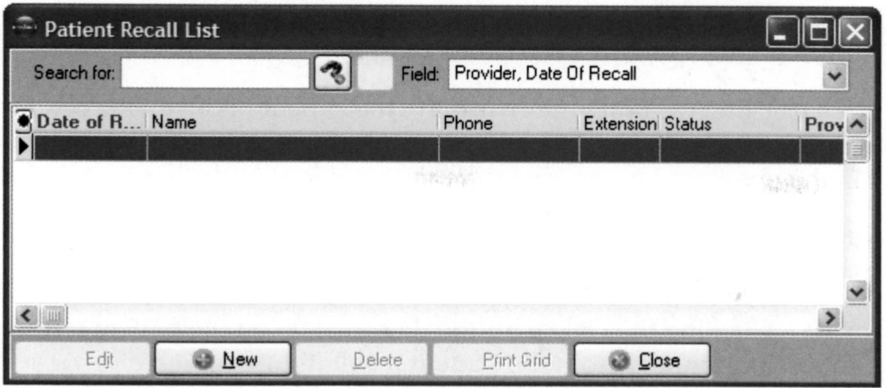

Figure 4.27 Patient Recall List Dialog Box

Patient Recall feature is located in Medisoft Network Professional, not in Office Hours. When Patient Recall is selected from the Lists menu, the Patient Recall List dialog box is displayed (see Figure 4.27). This dialog box organizes the recall information in a column format. The scroll bar is used to display the last three columns on the right.

Date of Recall Lists the date on which the recall is scheduled.

Name Displays the patient's name.

Phone Lists the patient's phone number, making it easy to call patients for appointments without having to look up phone numbers in another dialog box.

Extension Lists the patient's phone extension.

Status Indicates the patient's recall status: Call, Call Again, Appointment Set, or No Appointment.

Provider Displays the provider code for the patient's provider.

Message Displays the entry made in the Message box of the Patient Recall dialog box.

Chart Number Displays the patient's chart number.

Procedure Code Lists the procedure code for the procedure for which the patient is being recalled.

The Patient Recall List dialog box contains the following boxes:

Search For The Search For box is used to locate a specific patient on the recall list. Entering the first few letters or numbers in the Search For box displays the selection that is the closest match to the search criteria.

Field The choices in the Field box determine the order in which patients are listed in the dialog box. There are three sorting options:

1. Provider, Date of Recall
2. Chart Number, Date of Recall
3. Date of Recall, Provider, Chart Number

The Patient Recall List dialog box also contains these buttons: Edit, New, Delete, Print Grid, and Close.

Edit Clicking the Edit button displays the Patient Recall dialog box for the patient whose entry is highlighted. The information on the patient can then be edited by making different selections in the boxes.

New Clicking the New button displays an empty Patient Recall dialog box in which data on a new recall patient can be entered.

Delete Clicking the Delete button deletes data on the patient whose entry is highlighted from the patient recall list.

Print Grid Clicking the Print Grid button displays options to print the grid that is used in the Patient Recall dialog box.

Close The Close button is used to exit the Patient Recall List dialog box.

Adding a Patient to the Recall List

Patients are added to the recall list by clicking the New button in the Patient Recall List dialog box or by clicking the Patient Recall Entry shortcut button. When either of these actions is performed, the Patient Recall dialog box is displayed (see Figure 4.28).

The Patient Recall dialog box contains the following boxes:

Recall Date The date a patient needs to return to see a physician is entered in the Recall Date box.

Provider A patient's provider is selected from the drop-down list.

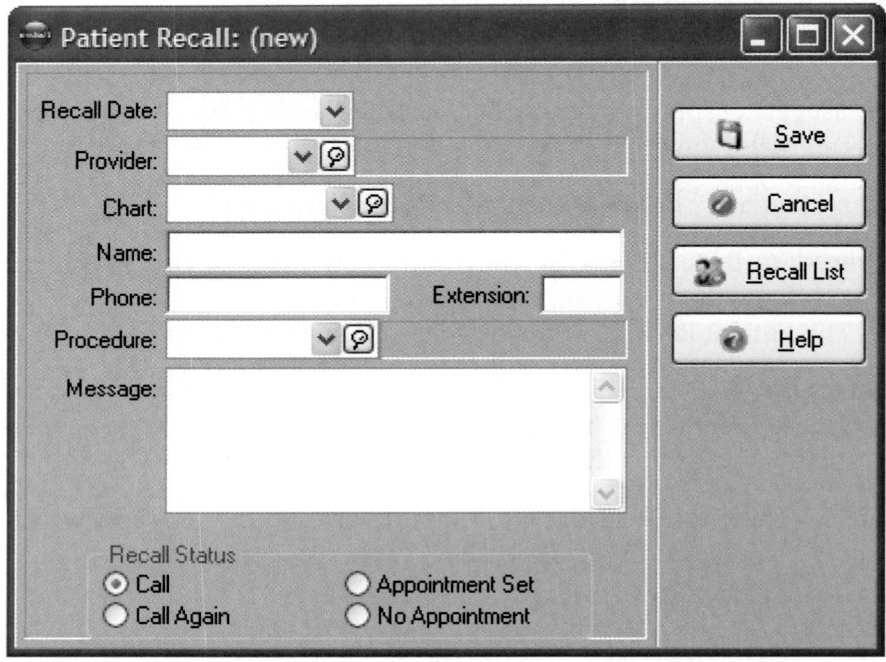

Figure 4.28 Patient Recall (new) Dialog Box

Chart A patient's chart number is selected from the drop-down list, or the first few letters of a patient's chart number are entered in the Chart box.

Name, Phone, Extension After a chart number is entered, the system automatically completes the Name, Phone, and Extension boxes.

Procedure If the procedure for which a patient is returning is known, it is entered in the Procedure box in one of two ways. The procedure code can be selected from the drop-down list, or the first few numbers can be entered so that the drop-down list will display the entry that most closely matches the entered numbers. This is especially valuable in practices that use hundreds of procedure codes because it eliminates the need to scroll through the codes to locate the desired one.

Message The Message box is used to record any special notes, reminders, or instructions about a patient and his or her appointment.

Recall Status The choices in the Recall Status box are used to indicate the action that needs to be taken. They include:

- *Call* The Call button is used when a patient needs to be telephoned about a future appointment.
- *Call Again* The Call Again button is used when a patient has been called once, but contact was not made and an additional call is necessary.
- *Appointment Set* The Appointment Set button is used when a patient has an appointment already scheduled.
- *No Appointment* The No Appointment button is used when a patient has been contacted for an appointment but has declined for some reason.

After the information has been entered in the dialog box, clicking the Save button saves the data and adds the patient to the recall list. In addition to the Save button, the Patient Recall dialog box contains Cancel, Recall List, and Help buttons. The Cancel button exits the dialog box without saving the data entered. The Recall List button in the Patient Recall dialog box is used to display the Patient Recall List dialog box. The Help button displays Medisoft Network Professional's online help for the Patient Recall dialog box.

connect plus+ EXERCISE 4.9

ADDING A PATIENT TO THE RECALL LIST (JOHN FITZWILLIAMS)

John Fitzwilliams needs to receive a phone call one year from November 14, 2016, to set up an appointment for an annual physical. Add John Fitzwilliams to the recall list.

1. In Medisoft Network Professional, click the Patient Recall Entry shortcut button (the eleventh icon from the right). The Patient Recall dialog box is displayed.

(continued)

(Continued)

2. Click inside the Recall Date box, and key ***11/14/2017.*** Press Tab.
3. Click John Fitzwilliams's provider, Dr. John Rudner, on the drop-down list in the Provider box. Press Tab.
4. Enter John Fitzwilliams's chart number in the Chart box by keying ***F*** and pressing Tab. Notice that the system automatically completes the Name and Phone boxes. (The Extension box would also be completed if there were an extension.)
5. Click inside the Procedure box and select the procedure code by keying ***99396*** (Preventive est., 40–64 years) and pressing Tab.
6. Verify that the Call radio button in the Recall Status box is selected.
7. Click the Save button to save the entry.
8. The Patient Recall dialog box closes. Click Patient Recall on the Lists menu.
9. Verify that the 11/14/2017 entry for John Fitzwilliams has been added to the recall list.
10. Click the Close button at the bottom of the dialog box to close the Patient Recall List dialog box.

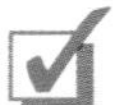
You have completed Exercise 4.9

4.13 Creating Provider Breaks

Office Hours break a block of time when a physician is unavailable for appointments with patients

Office Hours provides features for inserting standard breaks in providers' schedules. The **Office Hours break** is a block of time when a physician is unavailable for appointments with patients. Some examples of breaks include Lunch, Meeting, Personal, Emergency, Break, Vacation, Seminar, Holiday, Trip, and Surgery. In Office Hours, breaks can be created one at a time or on a recurring basis for all providers. One-time breaks, such as those for vacations, are set up for individual providers. Other breaks, such as staff meetings, can be entered once for multiple providers.

Often breaks need to be inserted into a provider's schedule when he or she is not available for appointments with patients. For example, if a physician will be in surgery on Thursday from 9 A.M. until 12:00 P.M., that time period must be marked as unavailable on his or her schedule.

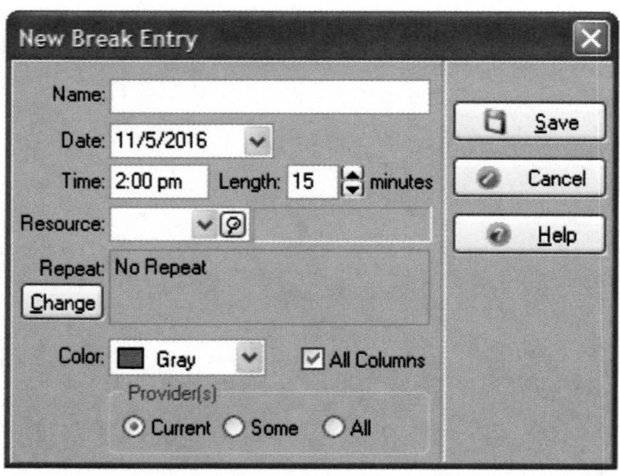

Figure 4.29 New Break Entry Dialog Box

To set up a break for a current provider (that is, the provider listed in the Office Hours Provider box), click the Break Entry shortcut button. This action causes the New Break Entry dialog box to appear (see Figure 4.29).

The dialog box contains the following options:

Name The Name field is used to store a name or description of the break.

Date The Date field displays the current date on the Office Hours calendar. If this is not the correct date for the break entry, a different date can be entered.

Time The starting time of the break is entered in this box.

Length This box indicates the length of the break in minutes (from 0 to 720).

Resource The drop-down list entries in the Resource box display the different types of breaks already set up in Office Hours.

Change The Change button next to the Repeat box is used to enter breaks that recur at a regular interval.

Color By selecting a different color from the drop-down list, the color of the break time slot in the schedule can be changed.

All Columns If the All Columns box is checked, the break will appear across all columns of the schedule (if a practice uses multiple columns in Office Hours).

Provider(s) The Provider(s) buttons are used to indicate whether a break is to be set for the current provider (the provider selected in the Provider box in Office Hours), some providers, or all providers. If Some is selected, a Provider Selection dialog box will be displayed when the Save button is clicked. The appropriate providers can then be selected.

When all the information has been entered, clicking the Save button closes the dialog box and enters the break(s).

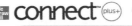

EXERCISE 4.10

ENTERING A PROVIDER BREAK (DR. JESSICA RUDNER)

Dr. Jessica Rudner will be attending a seminar from 10:00 A.M. to 12:00 P.M. on Monday, Tuesday, and Wednesday, December 12–14, 2016. Enter this as a break on her schedule.

1. Click the Appointment Book shortcut option on the Medisoft Network Professional toolbar to open Office Hours.
2. Select Jessica Rudner from the Provider drop-down list.
3. The calendar displays today's date—Monday, October 3, 2016. Change the month on the calendar to December, and then change the date to December 12.
4. Click once in the 10:00 A.M. time slot to select it (do not double click).
5. Click the Break Entry shortcut button (the second icon from the left on the Office Hours toolbar) to display the New Break Entry dialog box.
6. Enter ***HITECH Update Seminar*** in the Name box.

(continued)

(Continued)

7. Confirm that the date and time are correct.
8. Press Tab three times to move the cursor to the Length box. Enter ***120*** in the Length box to change the length of time to 120 minutes.
9. Click the down arrow next to the Resource box to display the list of resource options.
10. Select Seminar Break from the list.
11. Click the Change button (to repeat the break for two additional days). The Repeat Change dialog box is displayed.
12. If it is not already selected, click the Daily button in the Frequency column.
13. Accept the default entry of 1 in the Every __ Day(s) box, since the break occurs every day for a period of three days.
14. Click in the End on box, and key ***12/14/2016.***
15. Click the OK button. You are returned to the New Break Entry dialog box.
16. Click the Save button to enter the break in Office Hours. Notice that the time slot from 10:00 A.M. to 12:00 P.M. on December 12, 2016, has been filled in on the calendar.
17. Change the calendar to December 13 and 14, 2016, to verify that the break has been entered correctly.

 **You have completed Exercise 4.10**

4.14 Printing Schedules

While provider schedules can be viewed from within Office Hours, most medical offices still print schedules on a daily basis. To view a list of all appointments for a provider for a given day, the Appointment List option on the Office Hours Reports menu is used. A single provider and date are specified in the Data Selection dialog box for the report. (If the Provider boxes are left blank, schedules are created for all providers.) The schedule created is based on the provider and date specified in the Data Selection dialog box rather than the provider and date selected in the Office Hours window.

The report can be previewed on the screen or sent directly to the printer. If the preview option is selected, the appointment list is displayed in a preview window (see Figure 4.30). Various buttons are used to view the schedule at different sizes, to move from page to page, to print the schedule, and to save the schedule as a file. Clicking the Close button closes the preview window.

The schedule can also be printed without using the Appointment List option on the Office Hours Reports menu by clicking the Print Appointment List shortcut button. If this option is chosen, Office Hours prints the schedule for the date selected in the calendar and for the provider listed in the Provider box. To print the schedule for a different date or provider, change the date on the calendar and the entry in the Provider box before printing the schedule.

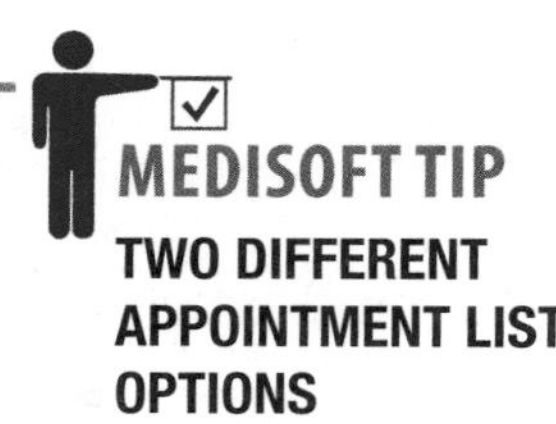

MEDISOFT TIP

TWO DIFFERENT APPOINTMENT LIST OPTIONS

In Office Hours, there are two different Appointment List options. The Appointment List option on the Lists menu displays a list of all appointments in the database and is used to search for a particular patient's appointment. The Appointment List option on the Reports menu is used to view and print a list of the provider's appointments for a given day.

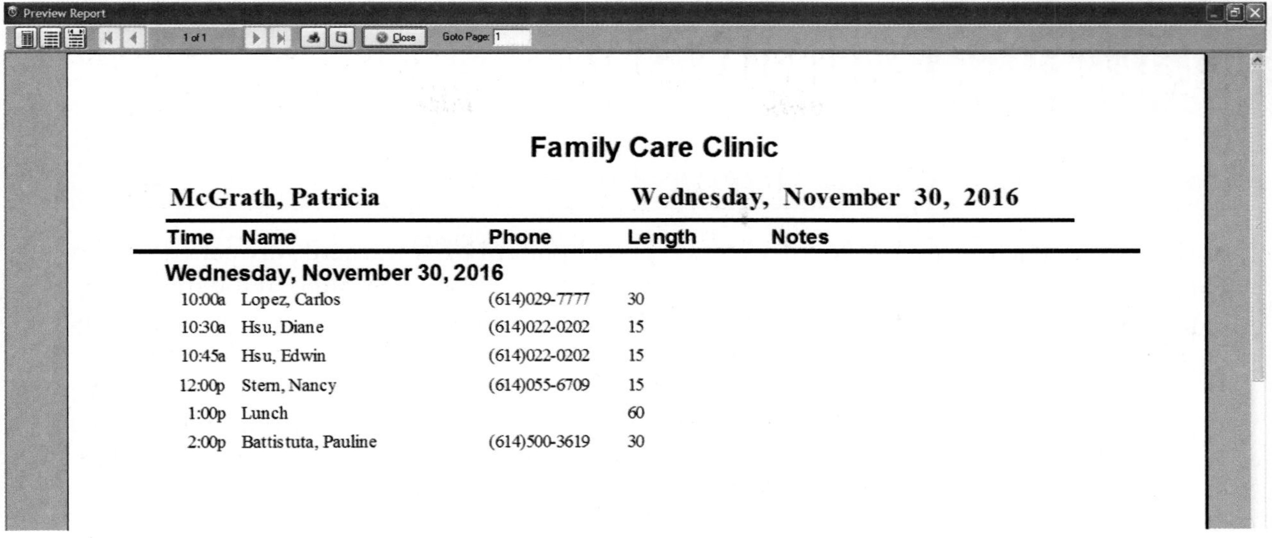
Preview Report

1 of 1 | Close | Goto Page: 1

Family Care Clinic

McGrath, Patricia | **Wednesday, November 30, 2016**

Time	Name	Phone	Length	Notes
Wednesday, November 30, 2016				
10:00a	Lopez, Carlos	(614)029-7777	30	
10:30a	Hsu, Diane	(614)022-0202	15	
10:45a	Hsu, Edwin	(614)022-0202	15	
12:00p	Stern, Nancy	(614)055-6709	15	
1:00p	Lunch		60	
2:00p	Battistuta, Pauline	(614)500-3619	30	

Figure 4.30 Preview Report Window with Appointment List Displayed

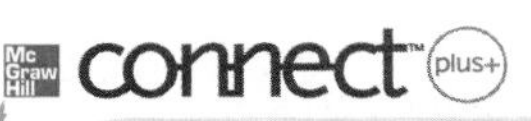

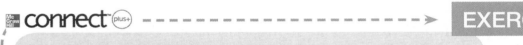

EXERCISE 4.11

VIEWING A PROVIDER SCHEDULE (DR. KATHERINE YAN)

View Dr. Katherine Yan's schedule for October 3, 2016, using the Appointment List option on the Office Hours Reports menu.

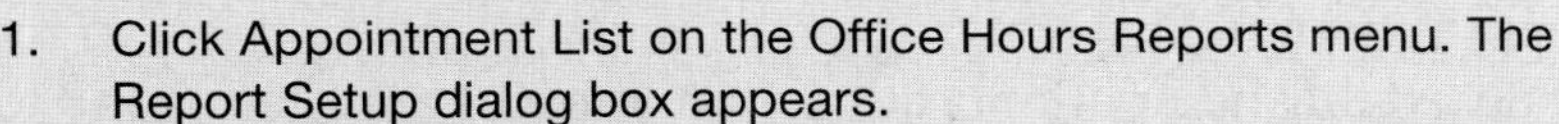

1. Click Appointment List on the Office Hours Reports menu. The Report Setup dialog box appears.
2. Under Print Selection, click the button that previews the report on the screen.
3. Click the Start button. The Data Selection dialog box is displayed.
4. Verify that the Date boxes display the computer's current system date—10/3/2016.
5. In both Provider boxes, click the down arrow and select Katherine Yan from the drop-down list.
6. Click the OK button. The Preview Report window appears with Dr. Yan's schedule for the day.
7. Note that the printer icon at the top of the window can be used to print the report. You do not need to print the report at this time.
8. Click the Close button at the top of the window to close the Preview Report window.
9. Click Exit on the Office Hours File menu to close the Office Hours program.

You have completed Exercise 4.11

chapter 4 summary

LEARNING OUTCOME	KEY CONCEPTS/EXAMPLES
4.1 Describe the two methods used to schedule appointments. Pages 154–157	In medical offices, most patient appointments are scheduled over the telephone, and some are scheduled online. If a patient requests an appointment via telephone (or in person after a visit), the offices' electronic scheduling program can be easily accessed to set up the appointment. If the medical office has a website, patients may have the option of scheduling appointments online through a patient portal. Patients can view an online calendar with available openings, select a time, and receive an e-mail confirmation.
4.2 Explain the method used to classify patients as new or established. Pages 157–158	A patient is classified as a new patient (NP) if he or she has not received any services from the provider (or another provider of the same specialty who is a member of the same practice) within the past three years. The patient is classified as an established patient (EP) if he or she has seen the provider (or another provider in the practice who has the same specialty) within the past three years.
4.3 List the three categories of information new patients provide during telephone preregistration. Pages 158–160	1. Patient demographics such as name, address, gender, date of birth, and telephone number 2. Basic information about insurance coverage 3. The reason for the visit
4.4 Identify the information that needs to be verified for established patients when making an appointment. Page 160	When an established patient calls for an appointment, the front desk verifies that the demographic and insurance information on file for the patient is still up-to-date. The reason for the visit is determined so that the correct length of time can be scheduled. In addition, the patient's account is reviewed to check for any overdue amounts so that the patient can be asked to take care of them during the upcoming visit.
4.5 Describe covered and noncovered services under medical insurance policies. Pages 160–172	Covered services are listed on each plan's schedule of benefits and usually include primary care, emergency care, medical specialists' services, and surgery. Managed care plans generally cover preventive medical services as well, including annual physical examinations, prenatal care, and screening procedures such as mammograms. The services for which the payer does not pay, called noncovered services, are listed separately in the medical insurance policy, and may include dental services, eye examinations or eyeglasses, employment-related injuries, cosmetic procedures, infertility services, or experimental procedures. Many policies also do not offer prescription drug benefits.

LEARNING OUTCOME	KEY CONCEPTS/EXAMPLES
4.6 List the three main points to verify with the payer regarding a patient's benefits prior to a visit. Pages 172–177	The medical insurance specialist verifies: 1. The patient's general eligibility for benefits 2. The amount of the copayment for the visit (if one is required) 3. Whether the planned encounter is for a covered service that is medically necessary under the payer's rules
4.7 Explain when a preauthorization number or referral document is required for a patient's encounter. Pages 177–180	Preauthorization from a payer is required to certify that the services the patient is scheduled to receive will be covered under the policy. A referral to another provider requires a similar certification, along with a referral letter from the referring physician with specific instructions regarding the medically necessary services that are being requested.
4.8 List the four main areas of the Office Hours window. Pages 180–183	The four main areas of the Office Hours window are: 1. Provider selection box 2. Provider's daily schedule 3. Office Hours calendar 4. Office Hours patient information
4.9 Demonstrate how to enter an appointment. Pages 184–190	To enter an appointment for an established patient: 1. Start Office Hours. 2. Select the appropriate provider in the Provider box. 3. Change the date on the calendar to the desired date. 4. Locate the desired time slot in the schedule. 5. Double click the time slot. 6. Select the patient in the Chart box. 7. Complete the other fields as required, being sure to enter the appointment length in the Length box. 8. When you are finished entering information, click the Save button.

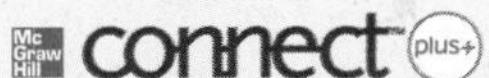

Enhance your learning at **mcgrawhillconnect.com**!

- *Practice Exercises*
- *Worksheets*
- *Activities*
- *Integrated eBook*

LEARNING OUTCOME	KEY CONCEPTS/EXAMPLES
	To search for an available time slot: 1. Verify that the correct provider is selected in the Provider box. 2. Click the Search Open Time Slot button. 3. Make appropriate entries in the Length, Start Time, End Time, and Day of Week boxes. 4. Click the Search button. 5. The calendar displays the first available time slot that matches the specifications. 6. Double click the time slot. 7. Select the patient in the Chart box. 8. Complete the other fields as required, being sure to enter the appointment length in the Length box. 9. When you are finished entering information, click the Save button.
	To book an appointment for a new patient: 1. Verify that the correct provider is selected in the Provider box. 2. Locate the desired date and time for the appointment. 3. Double click the desired time slot. 4. Click in the blank box to the right of the Chart box, and enter the patient's name (last name, first name). Press the Tab key to move the cursor to the Home Phone box. 5. Enter the patient's home phone. Press Tab to go to the Cell Phone box. 6. Finish entering information in the boxes, as appropriate. 7. Click the Save button.
4.10 Demonstrate how to book follow-up and repeating appointments. Pages 191–194	To book a follow-up appointment: 1. Verify that the correct provider is selected in the Provider box. 2. Click the Go to a Date shortcut button. 3. Confirm the entry in the Date From box. 4. Make an entry in the Go ___ Days, Weeks, Months, or Years boxes. 5. Click the Go button. 6. The calendar changes to the specified date. 7. Double click the time slot. 8. Select the patient in the Chart box. 9. Complete the other fields as required, being sure to enter the appointment length in the Length box. 10. When you are finished entering information, click the Save button.

LEARNING OUTCOME	KEY CONCEPTS/EXAMPLES
	To book repeating appointments: 1. Click the desired provider on the Provider drop-down list. 2. Change the calendar to the appropriate date. 3. Double click the desired time slot. The New Appointment Entry dialog box is displayed. 4. Select the patient in the Chart box. 5. Finish completing the boxes in the dialog box. 6. Click the Change button to schedule the repeating appointments. The Repeat Change dialog box appears. 7. Make a selection in the Frequency column. 8. Make entries in the additional boxes that appear. (These will vary depending on whether you selected Daily, Weekly, Monthly, or Yearly in the Frequency column.) 9. Click the arrow for the drop-down list in the End on box. A calendar pops up. Set the calendar to the date when the repeating appointment should stop. 10. Click the OK button. 11. Check the calendar to be sure the repeating appointments are correct.
4.11 Demonstrate how to reschedule an appointment. Pages 194–196	To reschedule an appointment: 1. Locate the appointment that needs to be changed. Make sure the appointment slot is visible on the provider's daily schedule. 2. Click the existing time-slot box. A black border surrounds the slot to indicate that it is selected. 3. Click Cut on the Edit menu. The appointment disappears from the schedule. 4. Click the date on the calendar when the appointment is to be rescheduled. 5. Click the desired time-slot box on the schedule. The slot becomes active. 6. Click Paste on the Edit menu. The patient's name appears in the new time-slot box.

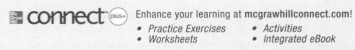

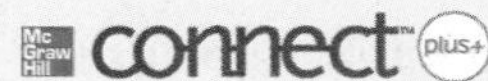

LEARNING OUTCOME	KEY CONCEPTS/EXAMPLES
4.12 Demonstrate how to create a recall list. Pages 196–200	To create a recall list: 1. In Medisoft, click the Patient Recall Entry shortcut button. The Patient Recall dialog box is displayed. 2. In the Recall Date box, enter the date the patient needs to have a follow-up appointment. Press Tab. 3. Select the patient's provider from the drop-down list in the Provider box. Press Tab. 4. Select the patient in the Chart box. 5. Enter the procedure code that corresponds to the appointment, if known. 6. Verify that the appropriate radio button is selected in the Recall Status box. 7. Click the Save button to save the entry.
4.13 Demonstrate how to enter provider breaks in the schedule. Pages 200–202	To enter provider breaks: 1. Select the provider from the Provider drop-down list. 2. Change the date on the calendar to the date of the break. 3. Click once in the appropriate time slot (do not double click). 4. Click the Break Entry shortcut button. The New Break Entry dialog box appears. 5. Enter a description of the break in the Name box. 6. Confirm that the date and time are correct. 7. Make the appropriate selection in the Length box. 8. Make a selection in the Resource box. 9. If the break is for more than one day, press the Change button. The Repeat Change dialog box is displayed. 10. Complete the Repeat Change box if necessary, and click OK. 11. Click the Save button to enter the break in Office Hours. 12. Verify that the break has been entered correctly.
4.14 Demonstrate how to print a provider's schedule. Pages 202–203	To print a provider's schedule: 1. Click Appointment List on the Office Hours Reports menu. The Report Setup dialog box appears. 2. Under Print Selection, click the button that sends the report directly to the printer. 3. Click the Start button. The Data Selection box is displayed. 4. Enter the desired date in both Date boxes. 5. Select the appropriate provider in both Provider boxes. 6. Click the OK button. The Print dialog box appears. 7. Click OK to print the report.

chapter review

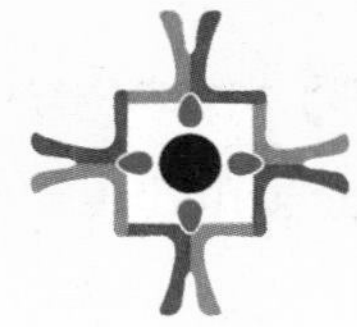

MATCHING QUESTIONS

Match the key terms with their definitions.

_____ 1. ***[LO 4.5]*** preexisting condition

_____ 2. ***[LO 4.5]*** indemnity plan

_____ 3. ***[LO 4.5]*** deductible

_____ 4. ***[LO 4.5]*** coinsurance

_____ 5. ***[LO 4.5]*** payer

_____ 6. ***[LO 4.5]*** benefits

_____ 7. ***[LO 4.5]*** provider

_____ 8. ***[LO 4.5]*** referral

_____ 9. ***[LO 4.5]*** premium

_____ 10. ***[LO 4.5]*** medical insurance

a. An amount that an insured person must pay, usually on an annual basis, for health care services before a health plan's payment begins.

b. Illness or disorder of a beneficiary that existed before the effective date of insurance coverage.

c. Health plan or program.

d. Person or entity that supplies medical or health services and bills for the services in the normal course of business.

e. The portion of charges that an insured person must pay for health care services after payment of the deductible amount.

f. Type of medical insurance that reimburses a policyholder for medical services under the terms of its schedule of benefits.

g. Money the insured pays to a health plan for a health care policy; usually paid monthly.

h. Financial plan that covers the cost of hospital and medical care.

i. Transfer of patient care from one physician to another.

j. The amount of money a health plan pays for services covered in an insurance policy.

TRUE/FALSE QUESTIONS

Decide whether each statement is true or false.

_____ 1. ***[LO 4.5]*** Preferred provider organizations are the most popular type of managed care plans.

_____ 2. ***[LO 4.5]*** A consumer-driven health plan involves a high-deductible health plan coupled with a tax-preferred savings account.

_____ 3. ***[LO 4.5]*** The third party to a medical insurance contract is the policyholder.

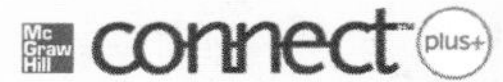

Enhance your learning at **mcgrawhillconnect.com**!

- *Practice Exercises*
- *Worksheets*
- *Activities*
- *Integrated eBook*

_____ 4. ***[LO 4.5]*** Health plans pay for covered and noncovered services.

_____ 5. ***[LO 4.1]*** On an electronic scheduler, each provider's schedule must be viewed separately.

_____ 6. ***[LO 4.5]*** Many managed care plans also cover preventive medical services.

_____ 7. ***[LO 4.2]*** A new patient is someone who has not received any services from the provider (or another provider of the same specialty who is a member of the same practice) within the past two years.

_____ 8. ***[LO 4.3]*** It is best to wait to obtain the patient's reason for the visit at the time of the encounter.

_____ 9. ***[LO 4.7]*** A paper referral document is a specific set of instructions from the primary care physician that directs the patient to a specialist or facility for medically necessary care.

_____ 10. ***[LO 4.3]*** The three categories of information new patients provide during telephone preregistration are patient demographics, basic insurance information, and the reason for the visit.

MULTIPLE-CHOICE QUESTIONS

Select the letter that best completes the statement or answers the question.

1. ***[LO 4.7]*** The preauthorization number may also be called the _________ number.
   a. eligibility
   b. verification
   c. certification
   d. demographic

2. ***[LO 4.1]*** Websites that can be used by patients to make appointments or receive messages from their health care providers are known as _________.
   a. patient portals
   b. health care networks
   c. electronic health records
   d. medical alerts

3. ***[LO 4.1]*** Examples of different scheduling systems include open-hours scheduling, _________ scheduling, double-booking, and wave scheduling.
   a. rotating
   b. ripple
   c. stream
   d. flow

4. ***[LO 4.3]*** The process of gathering information about a new patient before an appointment is known as _________.
   a. prerecording
   b. preregistration
   c. preauthorization
   d. predetermination

5. ***[LO 4.5]*** In most managed care insurance plans, patients must use network physicians to avoid paying higher charges. For this reason, patients check whether the provider is ________ in their plan.
   a. a practicing physician
   b. a participating provider
   c. an authorized provider
   d. a preferred provider
6. ***[LO 4.5]*** At the time an HMO member sees a provider, he or she pays a specified charge called the ________.
   a. copayment
   b. coinsurance
   c. premium
   d. indemnity
7. ***[LO 4.5]*** The medical insurance policy for each health plan contains the ________ that summarizes the payments that may be made for medically necessary services received by policyholders.
   a. schedule of referrals
   b. diagnostic code list
   c. formulary of benefits
   d. schedule of benefits
8. ***[LO 4.5]*** Although there are many variations in the way health plans are structured, indemnity and ________ plans are the basis of all of them.
   a. workers' compensation
   b. individual
   c. managed care
   d. group
9. ***[LO 4.11]*** To display a shortcut menu with cut and paste commands for cutting and pasting appointments in Office Hours, press the ________.
   a. Enter key
   b. Delete key
   c. left mouse button
   d. right mouse button
10. ***[LO 4.7]*** A certification number for a procedure is the result of the ________ transaction and process.
    a. coordination of benefits
    b. referral and authorization
    c. claims status
    d. eligibility for a health plan

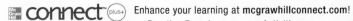

CHAPTER 4 REVIEW CHAPTER REVIEW

SHORT-ANSWER QUESTIONS

Define the following abbreviations.

1. ***[LO 4.2]*** EP ____________________________

2. ***[LO 4.5]*** MCO __________________________

3. ***[LO 4.3]*** nonPAR _______________________

4. ***[LO 4.2]*** NP____________________________

5. ***[LO 4.3]*** PAR __________________________

APPLYING YOUR KNOWLEDGE

Sequencing Tasks

4.1 ***[LO 4.1]*** Assume that you are scheduling a follow-up appointment over the phone for a patient who was in the office several months ago for a heart condition. Number the steps below in the order that best accommodates the patient's needs while on the phone.

_____ Review the patient's account to see if there is an outstanding balance.

_____ Book the appointment.

_____ Ask the patient to verify the reason for the visit.

_____ Ask the patient to verify his or her name and date of birth.

_____ Ask the patient if he or she would like to set up a payment plan for an overdue balance of $250 from several earlier visits.

_____ Greet the patient while opening the scheduling program.

_____ Look for the first suitable day and time in the schedule.

Using Insurance Terms

4.2 ***[LO 4.5]*** The following passage describes a patient's insurance plan. Using the insurance terms provided after the passage, fill in the missing words.

If you have paid your _________ and your _________ policy is up-to-date, the _________ services, listed on your _________, will be paid by your insurance. However, you will still be responsible for the _________ for each visit.

medical insurance

copay

premium

covered

schedule of benefits

4.3 ***[LO 4.5]*** The following passage describes an insurance contract. Using the insurance terms provided after the passage, fill in the missing words.

_________ is a written policy between an individual, called the _________, and a _________, an insurance company or government program that is the _________. The policyholder pays a specified amount of money called a _________. In exchange, the policyholder receives _________, defined by America's Health Insurance Plans (AHIP) as payments for covered medical services for a specific period of time.

policyholder

health plan

benefits

medical insurance

premium

payer

Calculating Amounts Due

Calculate the amounts billed in each of the following situations.

4.4 ***[LO 4.5]*** The patient is enrolled in a capitated HMO. Previously, the patient paid a $25 copay for mental health care services. Due to a change in policy, the patient is now required to pay 10 percent coinsurance. The provider charges $450 for a visit. What amount is the patient responsible for? How much will the health insurance plan pay for the visit? Which costs the patient more, the copay or the coinsurance?

4.5 ***[LO 4.5]*** A patient's total surgery charges are $4,300. The patient's health plan has a $100 annual deductible. The coinsurance percentage listed in the policy is 80-20. What does the patient owe? The plan?

4.6 ***[LO 4.5]*** A patient has a high-deductible consumer-driven health plan. The annual deductible is $3,000. Of that deductible, the patient has paid $400 this year. The patient now faces minor surgery, and the procedure will cost $2,200. What percentage of this cost will the insurance plan pay?

chapter 5

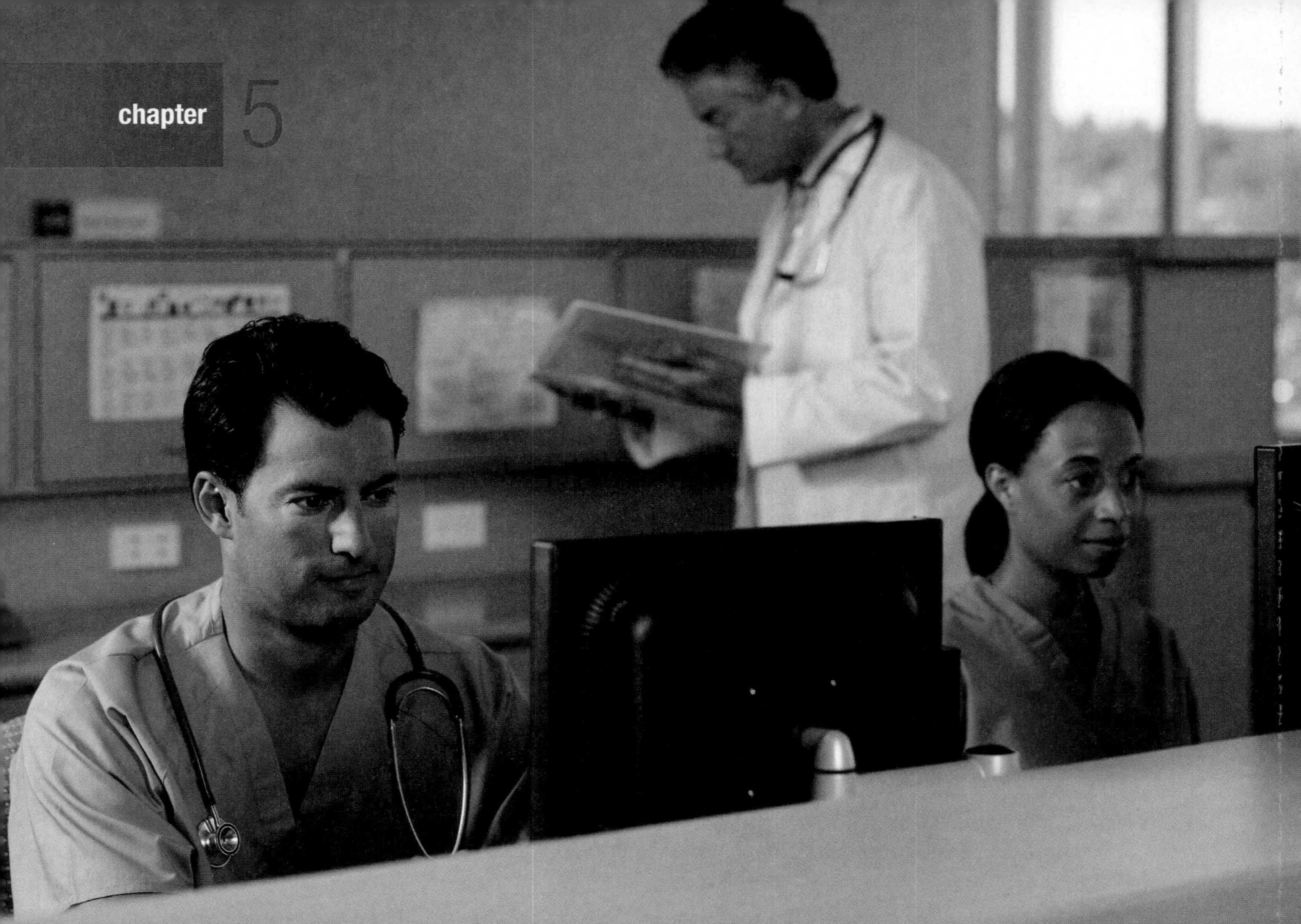

Check-in Procedures

KEY TERMS

accept assignment
advance beneficiary notice of noncoverage (ABN)
assignment of benefits
birthday rule
capitated plan
case
chart
chart number
coordination of benefits (COB)
financial policy
guarantor
patient information form
patient tracking features
primary insurance plan
record of treatment and progress
referring provider
registration
secondary insurance plan
sponsor

LEARNING OUTCOMES

When you finish this chapter, you will be able to:

5.1 List the six types of information that are gathered as part of the registration process for new patients.
5.2 Determine which health plan is primary when there is more than one.
5.3 Describe the purpose of a practice's financial policy.
5.4 List the types of payments that may be collected from patients at check-in.
5.5 Discuss the advantages of tracking patients electronically during a visit.
5.6 In Medisoft Network Professional, describe the organization of patient data.
5.7 Discuss how a new patient is added to the database.
5.8 Name the two options used to conduct searches.
5.9 Describe when it is necessary to create a new case or to utilize an existing case.
5.10 Analyze the information contained in the Personal and Account tabs.
5.11 Discuss the information recorded in the Policy 1, 2, 3, and Medicaid and Tricare tabs.
5.12 Describe the information contained in the Diagnosis and Condition tabs.
5.13 Discuss the purpose of the Miscellaneous, Multimedia, Comment, and EDI tabs.

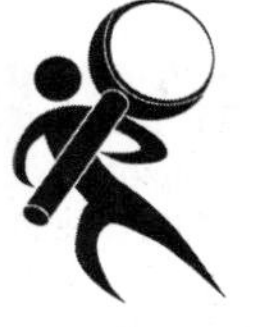

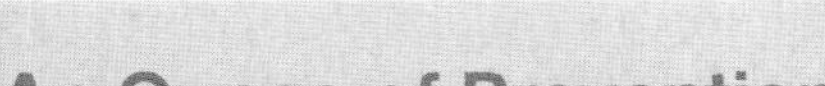

An Ounce of Prevention

As a receptionist for a busy practice like the Family Care Clinic, Laurie Harcourt is at her desk most of the day. Usually, she tries to go out for a short walk during her lunch break, but today she's decided to stay at her desk. Laurie came in this morning feeling a bit out of sorts—too bad, because the busy morning included two new patients, plus an emergency case she had to squeeze in! "I think I should double-check the two new patient records that I put into the system this morning." She remembers the mistake she made when she chose the wrong insurance company from the pull-down menu. A simple slip of her curser had caused a lot of trouble! Now Laurie makes a point of looking over her work.

The receptionist in the example has developed a number of habits that help her maintain her balance in the office. What self-awareness skills has she developed? Why are they important?

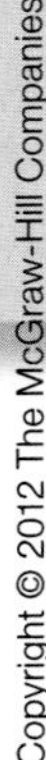

WHEN YOU FINISH THIS CHAPTER, YOU WILL ALSO BE ABLE TO USE MEDISOFT CLINICAL TO:

1. Check the balance of a patient account during check-in using Office Hours.
2. Use Medisoft Network Professional to create a chart number and enter a new patient.
3. Search for and update patient information.
4. Create a new case.

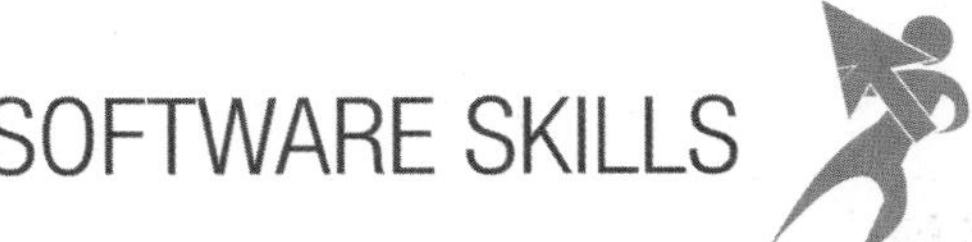

5.1 Patient Registration

Preregistration, as explained in Chapter 4, is the process of obtaining basic patient information and setting up an appointment time that suits the patient's needs. When patients arrive at the front desk for their appointments, registration staff follow the process of **registration** to obtain more detailed information about patients and their particular health plans before their encounters with providers.

registration process of gathering personal and insurance information about a patient before an encounter with a provider

patient information form form that includes a patient's personal, employment, and insurance data needed to complete a health care claim; also known as a registration form

Information for New Patients

If the patient is new to the practice, these six types of information are gathered:

1. Medical history
2. Detailed patient and insurance information
3. Identification verification
4. Financial agreement and authorization for treatment
5. Assignment of benefits statement
6. Acknowledgment of Receipt of Notice of Privacy Practices

To communicate this information, a new patient fills out several forms and signs others.

Medical History Form

Each new patient is asked to complete a medical history form. This form asks for information about the patient's pertinent personal medical history, the family's medical history, and the patient's social history. Social history covers lifestyle factors such as smoking, exercise, and alcohol use. Some practices give printed forms to patients when they come in. Others make the form available for completion ahead of time by posting it online or mailing it to the patient. For patients with long medical histories, particularly elderly patients, the option to complete a medical history form ahead of time can be useful, as it can be difficult to recall this information in five minutes in a waiting room.

During the encounter, the physician reviews the information on the medical history form with the patient and documents the patient's answers and the physician's observations. If the practice uses EHRs, the physician can enter this information into the record during the visit. EHRs offer physicians a number of methods for documenting patients' histories and other clinical information during or after a visit. The methods range from traditional dictation to the use of medical history templates to voice-activated software. Chapters 6 and 7 discuss some of these methods.

Patient Information Form

New patients also complete a **patient information form.** Also referred to as a *patient registration form*, it is used to collect information about the patient, including employment and insurance data needed to complete an insurance claim. As with the medical history form, some practices provide patients with printed patient information forms to fill in when they arrive. Others make the form available for completion ahead of time by posting it online or mailing it to patients.

A patient information form, as illustrated in Figure 5.1, contains the following information:

- First name, middle initial, and last name.
- Gender (*F* for female or *M* for male).
- Birth date, using four digits for the year.
- Home address and telephone number (area code with seven-digit number).
- Marital status (*S* for single, *M* for married, *D* for divorced, *W* for widowed).
- Student status.
- Social Security number.
- E-mail address.
- Allergies.
- Employer's name, address, and telephone number.
- For a patient who is a minor (under the age of majority according to state law) or has a medical power of attorney in place, meaning that another person is handling the patient's medical decisions, the responsible person's name, gender, birth date, address, Social Security number, telephone number, and employer information. In most cases, the responsible person is a parent, guardian, adult child, or other person acting with legal authority to make health care decisions on behalf of the patient. A minor's status as a full-time or part-time student is also recorded.
- The name of the patient's primary insurance carrier.
- The insured's (policyholder's) name, the patient's relationship to the insured, and the insured's identification number and other details of the plan (group number, insurance address, telephone number, copay and deductible amounts).
- If the patient is covered by another insurance carrier, the name and policyholder information for that plan.

It is important to understand the difference between the insured and the patient. The insured is the holder of the insurance policy that covers the patient. If a patient has his or her own insurance policy, the patient and the insured are the same person. However, if a patient is covered by someone else's policy, such as a spouse's, that person is the insured. As mentioned in Chapter 4, when the patient is not the insured, the insured is usually a spouse, divorced spouse, guardian, or other relation. Other terms for insured are **guarantor,** *policyholder,* and *subscriber.*

guarantor person who is the insurance policyholder for a patient of the practice

Identification Verification

For an insured new patient, the front and the back of the insurance card are scanned or photocopied and added to the patient's chart

FAMILY CARE CLINIC
285 Stephenson Boulevard
Stephenson, OH 60089–4000
614-555-0000

PATIENT INFORMATION FORM

Patient

Last Name First Name MI	Sex __ M __ F	Date of Birth / /
Address City	State	Zip
Home Ph # ( ) Cell Ph # ( )	Marital Status	Student Status
SS# Email	Allergies	

Employment Status	Employer Name	Work Ph # ( )	Primary Insurance ID #
Employer Address	City	State	Zip
Referred By		Ph # of Referral ( )	

Responsible Party (Complete this section if the person responsible for the bill is not the patient)

Last Name First Name MI	Sex __ M __ F	Date of Birth / /
Address City State	Zip	SS#

Relation to Patient __ Spouse __ Parent __ Other	Employer Name	Work Phone # ( )
Spouse, or Parent (if minor):		Home Phone # ( )

Insurance (If you have multiple coverage, supply information from both carriers)

Primary Carrier Name		Secondary Carrier Name	
Name of the Insured (Name on ID Card)		Name of the Insured (Name on ID Card)	
Patient's relationship to the insured __ Self __ Spouse __ Child		Patient's relationship to the insured __ Self __ Spouse __ Child	
Insured ID #		Insured ID #	
Group # or Company Name		Group # or Company Name	
Insurance Address		Insurance Address	
Phone #	Copay $ Deductible $	Phone #	Copay $ Deductible $

Other Information

Is patient's condition related to: | Reason for visit:
__ Employment __ Auto Accident (if yes, state in which accident occurred: __) __Other Accident
Date of Accident: / / Date of First Symptom of Illness: / /

Financial Agreement and Authorization for Treatment

I authorize treatment and agree to pay all fees and charges for the person named above. I agree to pay all charges shown by statements, promptly upon their presentation, unless credit arrangements are agreed upon in writing.

I authorize payment directly to FAMILY CARE CLINIC of insurance benefits otherwise payable to me. I hereby authorize the release of any medical information necessary in order to process a claim for payment in my behalf.

Signed: ____________________ Date: ____________________

Figure 5.1 Patient Information (Registration) Form

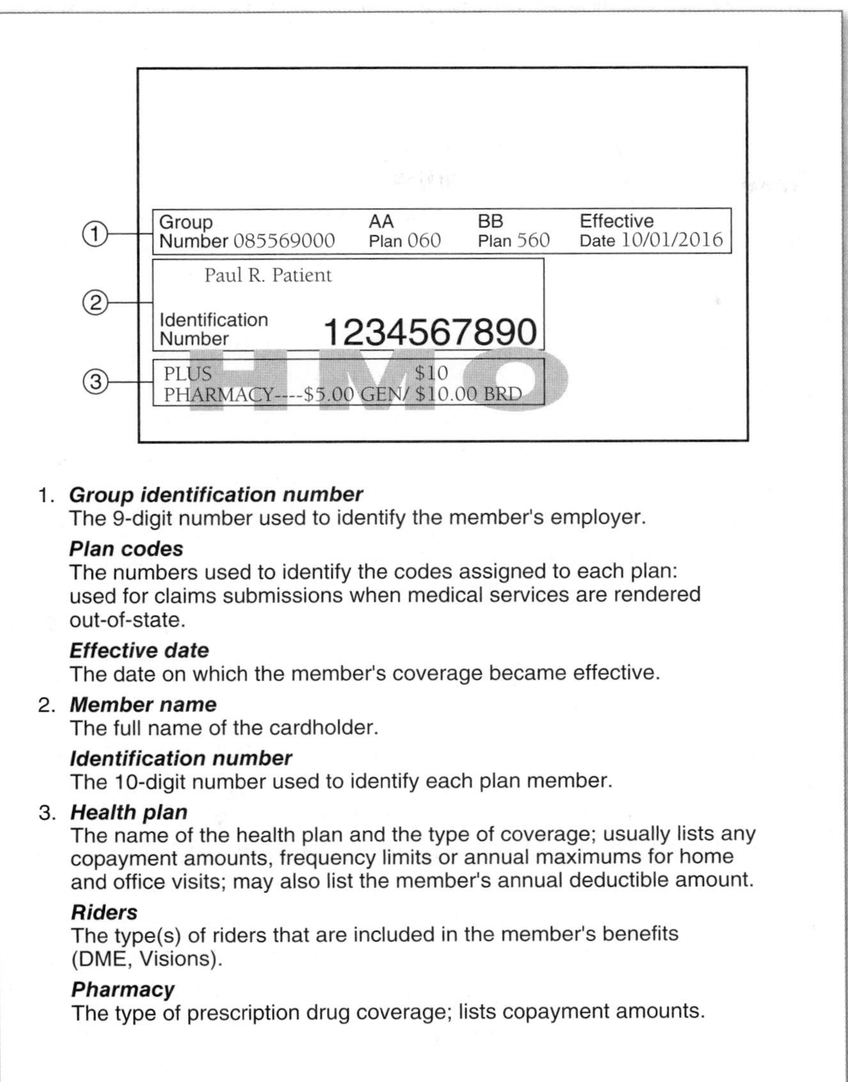

Group Number 085569000
AA Plan 060
BB Plan 560
Effective Date 10/01/2016
Paul R. Patient
Identification Number
1234567890
HMO
PLUS $10
PHARMACY----$5.00 GEN/ $10.00 BRD
1. Group identification number
The 9-digit number used to identify the member's employer.
Plan codes
The numbers used to identify the codes assigned to each plan: used for claims submissions when medical services are rendered out-of-state.
Effective date
The date on which the member's coverage became effective.
2. Member name
The full name of the cardholder.
Identification number
The 10-digit number used to identify each plan member.
3. Health plan
The name of the health plan and the type of coverage; usually lists any copayment amounts, frequency limits or annual maximums for home and office visits; may also list the member's annual deductible amount.
Riders
The type(s) of riders that are included in the member's benefits (DME, Visions).
Pharmacy
The type of prescription drug coverage; lists copayment amounts.

Figure 5.2 An Example of an Insurance Card

at registration. All data from the card that the patient has written on the patient information form are double-checked against the insurance card for accuracy before being entered into the practice's patient database.

Most insurance cards have the following information (see Figure 5.2):

- Group identification number
- Date on which the member's coverage became effective
- Member name
- Member identification number
- The health plan's name, type of coverage, copayment requirements, and frequency limits or annual maximums for services; sometimes the annual deductible
- Claim submission procedure and contact information

- Preauthorization/preadmission requirements
- Optional items, such as prescription drugs that are covered, with the copayment requirements

A common error message on returned or rejected insurance claims relates to the misspelling of the patient's name. Payers want the name of the patient on a claim to be exactly as it is shown on the insurance card. It is important, therefore, to check the patient information form to make sure the patient has not used a nickname, skipped a middle initial, or otherwise changed the name from the way it appears on the insurance card and thus in the health plan's records.

Patient Identification Many practices also require the patient to present a photo ID card, such as a driver's license. The practice scans the photo ID and stores it in the EHR, where it can be called up for billing purposes or to verify the patient's identity when the patient arrives for a visit. Family Care Clinic uses the new technology of a hand scanner for patient identification. The patient places his or her hand in the holder each time he or she checks in for an appointment.

Assignment of Benefits

Physicians usually submit claims for patients and receive payments directly from the payers. This saves patients paperwork and expedites payments to providers. The policyholder must authorize this procedure by signing and dating an **assignment of benefits** statement. This statement authorizes the provider to **accept assignment** for the patient—that is, to submit claims for the patient and receive payments directly from the payer. The assignment of benefits may be a separate form, as in Figure 5.3, or an entry on the patient information form. In Figure 5.1, an assignment of benefits statement is displayed at the bottom of the form: "I authorize payment directly to Family Care Clinic of insurance benefits otherwise payable to me."

assignment of benefits authorization by a policyholder that allows a health plan to pay benefits directly to a provider

accept assignment A participating physician's agreement to accept the allowed charge as payment in full

Financial Agreement and Authorization for Treatment

"I authorize treatment and agree to pay all fees and charges for the person named above. I agree to pay all charges shown by statements, promptly upon their presentation, unless credit arrangements are agreed upon in writing." This is a typical financial agreement and authorization for treatment statement. Like the

Figure 5.3 Assignment of Benefits Form

Assignment of Benefits

I hereby assign to Family Care Clinic, any insurance or other third-party benefits available for health care services provided to me. I understand that Family Care Clinic has the right to refuse or accept assignment of such benefits. If these benefits are not assigned to Family Care Clinic, I agree to forward to Family Care Clinic all health insurance and other third-party payments that I receive for services rendered to me immediately upon receipt.

Signature of Patient/Legal Guardian: ____________________

Date: ____________

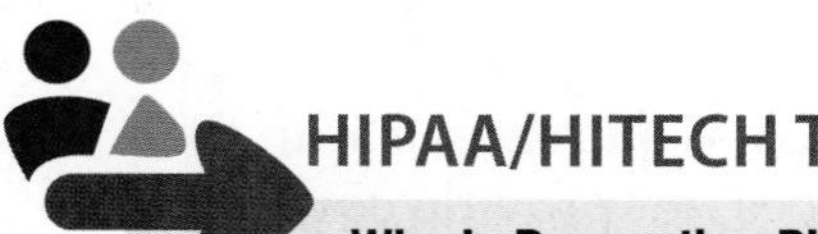

HIPAA/HITECH TIP

Who Is Requesting PHI?

Although the HIPAA Privacy Rule permits sharing PHI for treatment, payment, and operations (TPO) purposes without authorization, it also requires verification of the identity of the person who is asking for the information. The person's authority to access PHI must also be verified. If the requestor's right to the information is not certain, the best practice is to have the patient authorize the release of PHI.

assignment of benefits, this information may be provided on a separate form or as an entry on the patient information form, as in the example in Figure 5.1.

Acknowledgment of Receipt of Notice of Privacy Practices

HIPAA (see Chapter 2) requires medical practices to give each patient a copy of their Notice of Privacy Practices document at the time of the patient's first encounter and at least once every three years thereafter, and then to have the patient sign a separate form called an Acknowledgment of Receipt of Notice of Privacy Practices (see Figure 2.2 on page 61). This form indicates that the patient has received the document that states how the provider intends to protect the patient's rights to privacy under HIPAA.

The patient's acknowledgment is scanned and stored along with the patient's chart in the EHR. If the EHR program uses an electronic format for the Notice of Privacy Practices and acknowledgment, the documents may be read and signed online.

Other Forms and Documents

In addition to the six types of information just discussed, depending on the office's policies, several other forms and documents may be exchanged as part of the registration process.

Release Authorization

While the HIPAA Privacy Rule does not require an authorization to release patients' PHI for treatment, payment, and operations (TPO) purposes, state law may be more stringent and demand a release authorization. For this reason many practices routinely have patients sign release of information statements at the time of registration. Release statements are either separate documents or part of the patient information form. On the patient information form in Figure 5.1, the release of information statement—"I hereby authorize the release of any medical information necessary in order to process a claim for payment in my behalf"—is included with the other authorizations at the bottom of the form. Family Care Clinic patients also sign a form that includes the names of other individuals who are authorized to receive information about the patient, such as a sister, parents, or a spouse.

Forms Required by Particular Health Plans

At times, patients' health plans require the practice to inform beneficiaries in writing about the patients' likely financial responsibility.

One of the most typical examples of such plan requirements is in the Medicare program. By statute, Medicare does not provide coverage for all services and procedures. Claims are denied for services that are excluded by Medicare and for services not considered reasonable and necessary for the patient.

Physicians who participate in the Medicare program agree to not bill patients for services that Medicare declares are not reasonable and necessary unless the patients were informed ahead of time in writing and agreed to pay for the services. Local coverage determinations (LCDs) and national coverage determinations (NCDs) issued by Medicare help sort out medical necessity issues. LCDs and NCDs contain detailed and updated information about the coding and medical necessity of specific services.

advance beneficiary notice of noncoverage (ABN) Medicare form used to inform a patient that a service to be provided is not likely to be reimbursed by Medicare

If a provider thinks that a procedure will not be covered by Medicare because it is not reasonable and necessary, the patient is notified of this before the treatment by means of a standard **advance beneficiary notice of noncoverage (ABN)** from CMS (see Figure 5.4). A filled-in form is given to the patient for signature. The ABN form is designed to:

- Identify the service or item that Medicare is unlikely to pay for
- State the reason Medicare is unlikely to pay
- Estimate how much the service or item will cost the beneficiary if Medicare does not pay

The purpose of the ABN is to help the beneficiary make an informed decision about services that might have to be paid out-of-pocket. Medicare expects providers to know that certain services will not be covered. If a provider performs such a service without informing the patient in advance, the provider would not be allowed to bill the patient and thus would not be paid for the service.

When provided, the ABN must be verbally reviewed with the beneficiary or with his or her representative, and questions posed during that discussion must be answered before the form is signed. The form must be provided in advance to allow the beneficiary or representative time to consider options and make an informed choice. Either the physician or another member of the practice's health care team presents the ABN. After the form has been completely filled in and signed, a copy is given to the beneficiary or his or her representative. In all cases, the provider must retain the original notice on file.

Information for Established Patients

When established patients appear for appointments, their patient and insurance information is already stored in the practice management program. Registration staff, though, must ask returning patients whether any pertinent personal or insurance information has changed. This update process is important because different employment, marital status, dependent status, or plans may affect patients' coverage. Patients sometimes alert the practice about changes, such as new addresses or employers, in advance of an appointment.

(A) **Notifier(s):**
(B) **Patient Name:** ***(C)*** **Identification Number:**

ADVANCE BENEFICIARY NOTICE OF NONCOVERAGE (ABN)

NOTE: If Medicare doesn't pay for ***(D)***______________ below, you may have to pay.

Medicare does not pay for everything, even some care that you or your health care provider have good reason to think you need. We expect Medicare may not pay for the ***(D)***_____________ below.

(D)________________	***(E)*** **Reason Medicare May Not Pay:**	***(F)*** **Estimated Cost:**

WHAT YOU NEED TO DO NOW:

- Read this notice, so you can make an informed decision about your care.
- Ask us any questions that you may have after you finish reading.
- Choose an option below about whether to receive the ***(D)***______________listed above.

  Note: If you choose Option 1 or 2, we may help you to use any other insurance that you might have, but Medicare cannot require us to do this.

(G) **OPTIONS:** **Check only one box. We cannot choose a box for you.**

☐ **OPTION 1.** I want the ***(D)***___________ listed above. You may ask to be paid now, but I also want Medicare billed for an official decision on payment, which is sent to me on a Medicare Summary Notice (MSN). I understand that if Medicare doesn't pay, I am responsible for payment, but **I can appeal to Medicare** by following the directions on the MSN. If Medicare does pay, you will refund any payments I made to you, less co-pays or deductibles.

☐ **OPTION 2.** I want the ***(D)***___________ listed above, but do not bill Medicare. You may ask to be paid now as I am responsible for payment. **I cannot appeal if Medicare is not billed.**

☐ **OPTION 3.** I don't want the ***(D)***___________listed above. I understand with this choice I am **not** responsible for payment, and **I cannot appeal to see if Medicare would pay.**

(H) **Additional Information:**

This notice gives our opinion, not an official Medicare decision. If you have other questions on this notice or Medicare billing, call **1-800-MEDICARE** (1-800-633-4227/**TTY**: 1-877-486-2048).

Signing below means that you have received and understand this notice. You also receive a copy.

(I) **Signature:**	***(J)*** **Date:**

According to the Paperwork Reduction Act of 1995, no persons are required to respond to a collection of information unless it displays a valid OMB control number. The valid OMB control number for this information collection is 0938-0566. The time required to complete this information collection is estimated to average 7 minutes per response, including the time to review instructions, search existing data resources, gather the data needed, and complete and review the information collection. If you have comments concerning the accuracy of the time estimate or suggestions for improving this form, please write to: CMS, 7500 Security Boulevard, Attn: PRA Reports Clearance Officer, Baltimore, Maryland 21244-1850.

Form CMS-R-131 (03/08) Form Approved OMB No. 0938-0566

Figure 5.4 Advance Beneficiary Notice of Noncoverage (ABN)

To make sure information is current, most practices periodically ask established patients to review and sign off on their patient information forms when they come in. This review should be done at least once a year. A good time is an established patient's first appointment in a new year. The file is also checked to be sure that the patient has been given a current Notice of Privacy Practices.

THINKING IT THROUGH 5.1

The process of registration requires the patient to fill out numerous forms and to sign papers that may be difficult to understand. In addition, the patient may be under time constraints or may not be feeling well. In what ways can the medical administrative team show empathy to the patient? What advantages can be gained by establishing a clear line of communication with the patient during the registration process?

If the insurance of an established patient has changed, both sides of the new card are copied, and all data are checked. Many practices routinely scan or copy the card at each visit as a safeguard.

5.2 Other Insurance Plans: Coordination of Benefits

primary insurance plan health plan that pays benefits first when a patient is covered by more than one plan

secondary insurance plan health plan that pays benefits after the primary plan pays when a patient is covered by more than one plan

coordination of benefits (COB) clause in an insurance policy that explains how the policy will pay if more than one insurance policy applies to the claim

The registration staff also examines the patient information form and insurance card to see if other coverage is in effect. A patient may have more than one insurance carrier. The staff member, using the coordination of benefits guidelines described below, must then determine which carrier is the **primary insurance plan**—the plan that pays first when more than one plan is in effect—and which is the **secondary insurance plan**—an additional policy that provides benefits. Tertiary insurance, a third payer, is possible. Some patients have supplemental insurance, a "fill-the-gap" insurance plan that covers parts of expenses, such as coinsurance, that they must otherwise pay out-of-pocket under the primary plan.

Determining the primary insurance is important because this payer is sent the first claim for the encounter. A second claim is sent to the secondary payer after the payment is received for the primary claim. After both plans have made payments, any unpaid bills are submitted to the patient.

The HIPAA Coordination of Benefits transaction is used to send the necessary data to payers. This transaction is also called the HIPAA 837 or the X12 837—the same transaction used to send electronic claims—because it goes along with the claim.

Coordination of Benefits

Deciding which payer is primary is also important because insurance policies contain a provision called **coordination of benefits (COB).** The coordination of benefits guidelines ensure that when a patient has more than one policy, maximum appropriate benefits are paid, but without duplication. Under the law, to protect the insurance companies, if the patient has signed an assignment of benefits statement, the provider is responsible for reporting any additional insurance coverage to the primary payer.

Coordination of benefits in government-sponsored programs such as Medicare and Medicaid follow specific guidelines. Medicaid, for example, always pays last. If the patient has coverage through any other insurance plan or if the claim is covered by another program, such as

Medicare or workers' compensation, the other plan is billed first, and information from that payer is forwarded to Medicaid. For this reason, Medicaid is known as the payer of last resort, since it is always billed after another plan has been billed when other coverage exists.

Guidelines for Determining the Primary Plan

How do patients come to have more than one plan in effect? Possible answers are that a patient may have coverage under more than one group plan, such as a person who has both employer-sponsored insurance and a policy from union membership. A person may have primary insurance coverage from an employer but also be covered as a dependent under a spouse's insurance, making the spouse's plan the person's additional insurance. General guidelines for determining the primary insurance are shown in Table 5.1.

A common issue involves determining which of two parents' plans is primary for a child. If both parents cover dependents on their plans, the child's primary insurance is usually determined by the **birthday rule.** This rule states that the parent whose day of birth is earlier in the calendar year is primary. For example, Rachel Foster's mother and father both work and have employer-sponsored insurance policies. Her father, George Foster, was born on October 7, 1971, and her mother, Myrna, was born on May 15, 1972. Since the mother's date of birth is earlier in the calendar year (although the father is older), her plan is Rachel's primary insurance. The father's plan is secondary for Rachel.

birthday rule guideline that determines which of two parents with medical coverage has the primary insurance for a child; the parent whose day of birth is earlier in the calendar year is considered primary

TABLE 5.1 Determining Primary Coverage
• If the patient has only one policy, it is primary.
• If the patient has coverage under two plans, the plan that has been in effect for the patient for the longest period of time is primary. (However, if an active employee has a plan with the present employer and is still covered by a former employer's plan as a retiree or a laid-off employee, the current employer's plan is primary.)
• If the patient is also covered as a dependent under another insurance policy, the patient's plan is primary.
• If an employed patient has coverage under the employer's plan and additional coverage under a government-sponsored plan, the employer's plan is primary. For example, if a patient is enrolled in a PPO through employment and is also on Medicare, the PPO is primary.
• If a retired patient is covered by a spouse's employer's plan and the spouse is still employed, the spouse's plan is primary, even if the retired person has Medicare.
• If the patient is a dependent child covered by both parents' plans and the parents are not separated or divorced (or if the parents have joint custody of the child), the primary plan is determined by the birthday rule.
• If two or more plans cover a dependent child of separated or divorced parents who do not have joint custody of their child, the child's primary plan is determined in this order (or by court order): • The plan of the custodial parent • The plan of the spouse of the custodial parent if remarried • The plan of the parent without custody

THINKING IT THROUGH 5.2

When a patient has secondary insurance, the claim for the secondary payer is sent after the claim to the primary payer is paid. Why is that the case? What information do you think the medical biller provides to the secondary payer?

Note that if a dependent child's primary insurance does not provide for the complete reimbursement of a bill, the balance may usually be submitted to the other parent's plan for consideration.

5.3 Financial Policy of the Practice

financial policy practice's rules governing payment for medical services from patients

As part of the check-in procedures, patients should always be reminded of their financial obligations according to practice procedures. New patients are given information about the practice's financial policy so they understand that they are responsible for payment of charges that are not paid by their health plans. The practice's **financial policy** on payment for services is usually either displayed at the reception desk or included in a new patient information packet. An example of a financial policy is shown in Figure 5.5.

We sincerely wish to provide the best possible medical care. This involves mutual understanding between the patients, doctors, and staff. We encourage you, our patient, to discuss any questions you may have regarding this payment policy.

Payment is expected at the time of your visit for services not covered by your insurance plan. We accept cash, check, MasterCard, and Visa.

Credit will be extended as necessary.

Credit Policy

Requirements for maintaining your account in good standing are as follows:

1. All charges are due and payable within 30 days of the first billing.
2. For services not covered by your health plan, payment at the time of service is necessary.
3. If other circumstances warrant an extended payment plan, our credit counselor will assist you in these special circumstances at your request.

We welcome early discussion of financial problems. A credit counselor will assist you.

An itemized statement of all medical services will be mailed to you every 30 days. We will prepare and file your claim forms to the health plan. If further information is needed, we will provide an additional report.

Insurance

Unless we have a contract directly with your health plan, we cannot accept the responsibility of negotiating claims. You, the patient, are responsible for payment of medical care regardless of the status of the medical claim. In situations where a claim is pending or when treatment will be over an extended period of time, we will recommend that a payment plan be initiated. Your health plan is a contract between you and your insurance company. We cannot guarantee the payment of your claim. If your insurance company pays only a portion of the bill or denies the claim, any contact or explanation should be made to you, the policyholder. Reduction or rejection of your claim by your insurance company does not relieve the financial obligation you have incurred.

Figure 5.5 Example of a Financial Policy

THINKING IT THROUGH 5.3

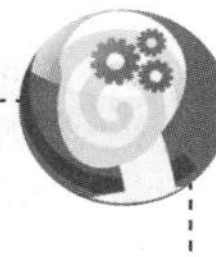

Who is ultimately responsible for payment of charges incurred for medical services?

The policy should explain what is required of the patient and when payment is due. For example, the policy may state the following:

Assigned claims	After your insurance claim is processed by your insurance company, you will be billed for any amount you owe. You are responsible for any charges that are denied or are not paid by the carrier. All patient accounts are due within thirty days of the date of the invoice.
Unassigned claims	Payment for the physician's services is expected at the end of your appointment unless you have made other arrangements with our practice manager.
Copayments	Copayments must be paid before patients leave the office.

If patients have large bills that they are unable to pay immediately, financial arrangements for series of payments may be made (see Figure 5.6). The patient may begin with a prepayment followed by monthly amounts. Such arrangements are governed by federal and state laws.

Patient Name and Account Number

Total of All Payments Due

FEE	$________	
PARTIAL PAYMENT	$________	
UNPAID BALANCE	$________	
AMOUNT FINANCED	$________	(amount of credit we have provided to you)
FINANCE CHARGE	$________	(dollar amount the interest on credit will cost)
ANNUAL PERCENTAGE RATE	$________	(cost of your credit as a yearly rate)
TOTAL OF PAYMENTS DUE	$________	(amount paid after all payments are made)

Rights and Duties

I (we) have reviewed the above fees. I agree to make ________ payments in monthly installments of $________, due on the ________ day of each month payable to ________, until the total amount is paid in full. The first payment is due on ________. I may request an itemization of the amount financed.

Delinquent Accounts

I (we) understand that I am financially responsible for all fees as stated. My account will be overdue if my scheduled payment is more than 7 days late. There will be a late payment charge of $________ or ________% of the payment, whichever is less. I understand that I will be legally responsible for all costs involved with the collection of this account including all court costs, reasonable attorney fees, and all other expenses incurred with collection if I default on this agreement.

Prepayment Penalty

There is no penalty if the total amount due is paid before the last scheduled payment.

I (we) agree to the terms of the above financial contract.

________________________ ________
Signature of Patient, Parent, or Legal Representative Date

________________________ ________
Witness Date

________________________ ________
Authorizing Signature Date

Figure 5.6 Financial Arrangement for Services Form

5.4 Estimating and Collecting Payment

Another aspect of check-in procedures is estimating and collecting payments from patients. Chapter 9 explains how most time-of-service payments are collected at checkout after the encounter. However, depending on office policy, some payments, including copayments, outstanding balances, and partial payments, may be collected from patients at check-in.

Copayments

Copayments are routinely collected during check-in. Payments may be made by cash, check, or credit or debit card. When a payment is made, a receipt is given to the patient. The copayment amount depends on the type of service and on whether the provider is in the patient's network. Copays for out-of-network providers are usually higher than for in-network providers. Different copay amounts may be required for office visits to primary care physicians (PCPs), for visits to specialists, and for lab work, radiology services such as X-rays, and surgery.

Established patients' copayment requirements are stored in the practice management program along with their insurance data. When the patient's appointment is selected in the practice management program at check-in, the scheduling screen displays the copayment amount due for the visit. If the plan's copayment requirements change, the patient informs the practice, and the amounts are easily updated in the program.

Outstanding Balances

In many practices, if a patient owes a balance to the practice, this amount is also collected at check-in, or arrangements for payment are made. Practice management programs usually have shortcut keys or quick check buttons for determining whether the patient has an overdue amount. Usually, the appointment scheduler that comes with the practice management program will also display this information. If the patient's account is overdue, the receptionist can talk with the patient about the possibility of making a payment while the patient is at the desk. The Office Hours appointment scheduler in Medisoft Network Professional displays the balance due for each patient's account in the patient information area when an appointment is selected.

EXERCISE 5.1

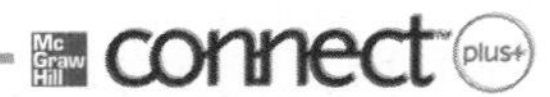

VIEWING A PATIENT'S BALANCE AT CHECK-IN

Elizabeth Jones has arrived for her 10:00 A.M. appointment with Dr. Yan. Use Office Hours to check the balance due on her account.

Date: October 3, 2016

1. Verify that Medisoft Network Professional is open and that the practice name in the title bar at the top of the screen is Family Care Clinic.

2. On the Activities menu, click the Appointment Book option to open the Office Hours program.
3. Select Elizabeth Jones's provider, Dr. Katherine Yan, from the Provider drop-down list at the top of the Office Hours window.
4. Verify that the date on the calendar is October 3, 2016.
5. Click once on Elizabeth Jones's 10:00 A.M. appointment on the schedule to select it.
6. Elizabeth Jones's appointment is outlined on the schedule, and her patient information is displayed under the calendar in the left side of the window. Notice that the Remainder field lists the amount $49.22, indicating the amount due on her account.
7. Click the X in the upper-right corner of the Office Hours window to close the program.

 **You have completed Exercise 5.1**

Partial Payment

While insurance companies require physician practices to collect co-payments from patients when they come in for care, some medical offices are now asking patients for partial payment of the office visit charges during check-in to increase cash flow. The amount of the partial payment is usually a percentage of the estimated patient responsibility for the procedure. For example, if the patient is expected to owe $200 for a procedure and practice policy is to collect 50 percent, the patient is asked to pay $100 on the day of the encounter and to expect to be billed $100 after the claim is processed. Since it is not always possible to estimate a patient's financial obligation accurately at check-in, offices usually base the patient's share on the average charge for the scheduled service. The prepayments are low enough that few patients overpay.

5.5 Patient Tracking

Patient tracking features are used during patient encounters to track the status of each appointment (this includes whether the appointment was kept, canceled, or rescheduled) as well as to track where patients are during the different steps of the encounter (this includes whether a patient has checked in, is in the exam room, is with a provider, or has checked out). In most PM and EHR programs, the patient tracking features are attached to the electronic scheduler. Tracking where patients are during a visit is especially helpful in large practices that see many patients at a time and may be double-booking them. Any member of the medical administrative team can see a patient's whereabouts at a glance.

patient tracking features function attached to the electronic scheduler that is used during a patient encounter to track where the patient is during the different steps of the encounter

Depending on the reporting capacity of the program, various reports can be created using the patient tracking information. For example, a report can be created that lists canceled appointments for all providers during the last week. If the scheduling program has a timing feature that keeps track of the amount of time patients spend for each part of a visit, more-detailed reports can be generated that list the average amount of time patients are being seen by physicians or the average time patients spend in the waiting room. The office manager can study the results of the tracking reports to help improve the day-to-day functions of the office.

Tracking Patients in Office Hours for Network Professional

The current version of Office Hours that comes with Medisoft Network Professional, does not include a patient tracking feature. Future versions of the software, however, will be packaged with a professional network version, called Office Hours for Network Professional. The professional network version contains the following appointment status options for tracking patients' visits:

- Unconfirmed
- Confirmed
- Checked In
- Missed
- Cancelled
- Being Seen
- Checked Out
- Rescheduled

The appointment status options are located in the Edit Appointment dialog box (see Figure 5.7), which is opened by double clicking on a patient's appointment slot in the Office Hours schedule.

To keep track of the patient's whereabouts during the course of the visit, the Checked In, Being Seen, and Checked Out status buttons are selected. If no option is selected, an Unconfirmed status is assumed. Other status options, such as Cancelled and Rescheduled, are selected to cancel or reschedule an appointment as necessary. Only one of the eight status buttons can be selected at a time.

Tracking Patients in the Medisoft Clinical Appointment Scheduler

Medisoft Clinical Patient Records, the EHR program used with the exercises in this text, has its own appointment scheduler and tracking features. Figure 5.8 shows the Medisoft Clinical Patient Check-in window with two tracking features highlighted: the appointment status feature and the appointment timing feature.

In the example shown in Figure 5.8, the appointment status feature displays "IN" to indicate the patient has checked in, and the appointment timing feature in the upper right shows the time the patient has entered each step of the patient encounter. With the timing feature, times are recorded in five fields: Check-in, In Exam Room,

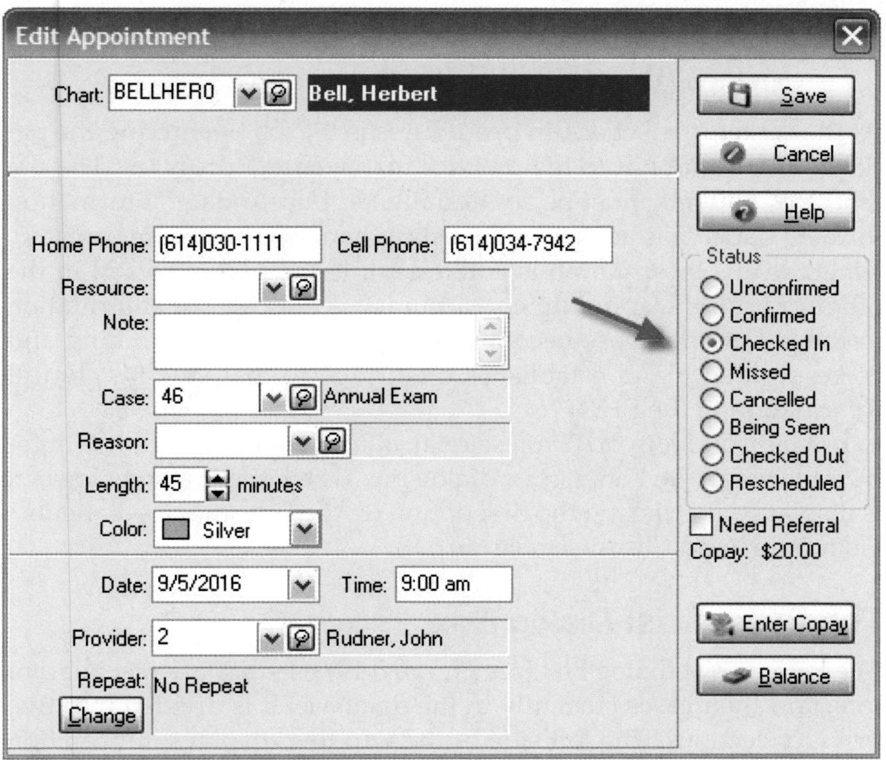

Figure 5.7 Status Options in the Edit Appointment Dialog Box

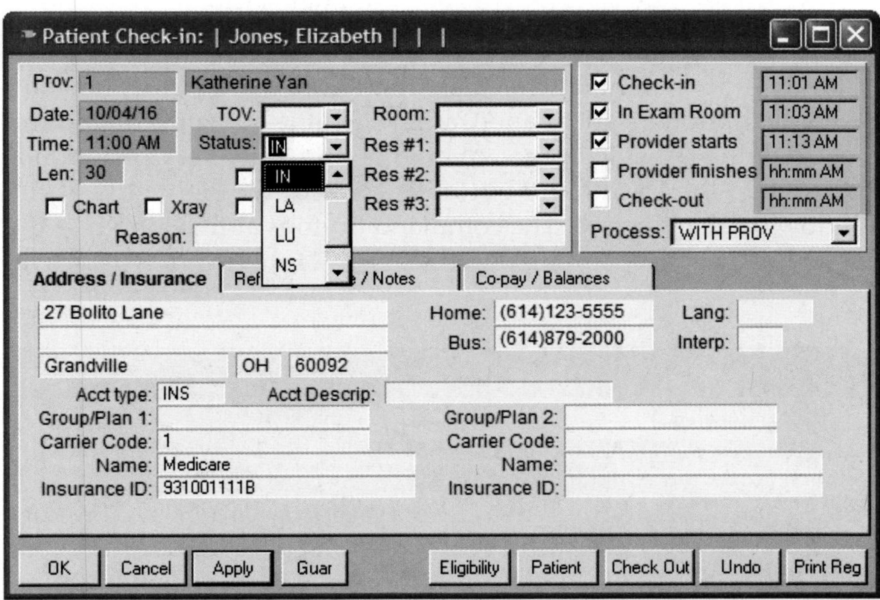

Figure 5.8 Medisoft Clinical Patient Check-in Window with Tracking Features Highlighted

Provider starts, Provider finishes, and Check-out. The use of the timing feature adds another step to the check-in procedure for staff members; however, the information collected can be useful in monitoring office workflow.

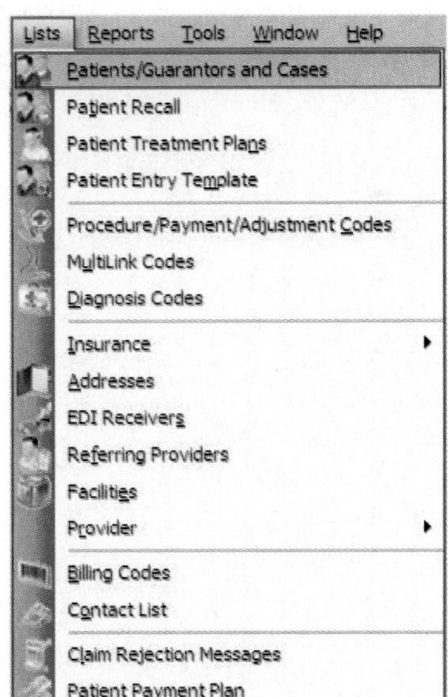

Figure 5.9 Lists Menu with Patients/Guarantors and Cases Option Highlighted

case grouping of transactions for visits to a physician office organized around a specific medical condition

5.6 Patient Information in Medisoft Network Professional

At the center of all check-in procedures is the job of entering the patient's information into the practice management program. The database of patients must be continually kept up-to-date: information for new patients is added, and existing patient records are updated. Whether this information is entered while the patient is still in the office or after the appointment, accuracy is critical. The information in the patient database becomes the basis for all future billing and correspondence and establishes the bridge to the patient's clinical information in the EHR.

In Medisoft Network Professional, all patient information is organized through the Patient List dialog box. The Patient List dialog box is displayed by clicking the first option on the Lists menu—Patients/Guarantors and Cases (see Figure 5.9).

The Patient List Dialog Box

The Patient List dialog box (see Figure 5.10) lists all patients, guarantors, and their cases currently in the database. It is divided into two primary sections. The left side of the window displays information about patients, and the right side of the window contains information about cases. A **case** is a grouping of transactions for visits to a physician office organized around a specific medical condition, such as hypertension, bronchitis, or an annual exam. Cases are covered later in the chapter.

On the upper-right side of the Patient List dialog box, there are two radio buttons: Patient and Case. When the Patient radio button is clicked, the left side of the window becomes active. Correspondingly, when the Case radio button is clicked, the right side of the window becomes active. The command buttons at the bottom of the dialog box vary, depending on which side of the window is active.

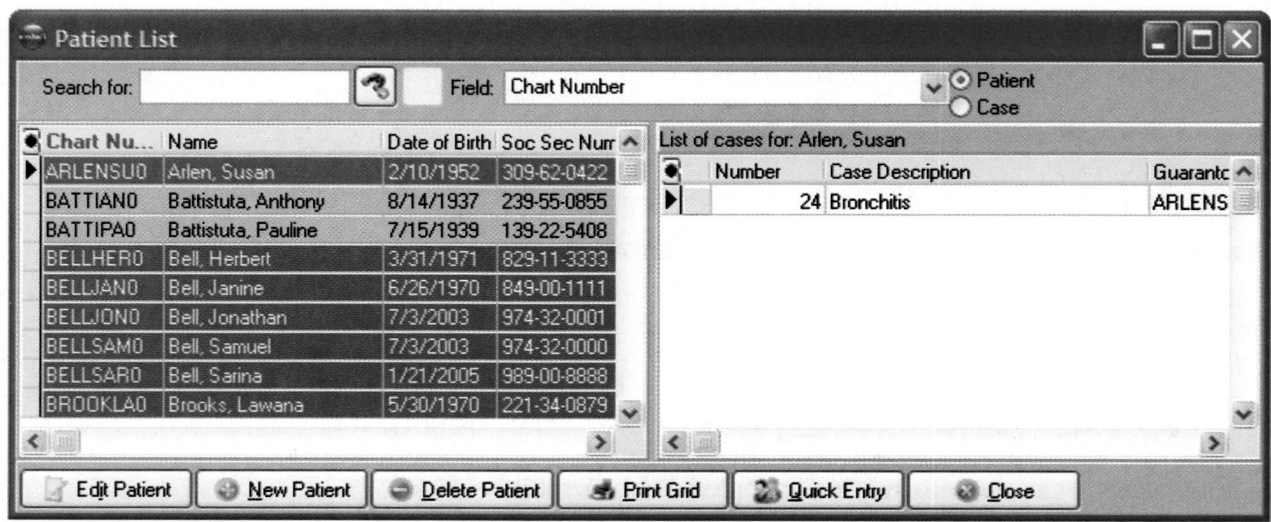

Figure 5.10 Patient List Dialog Box

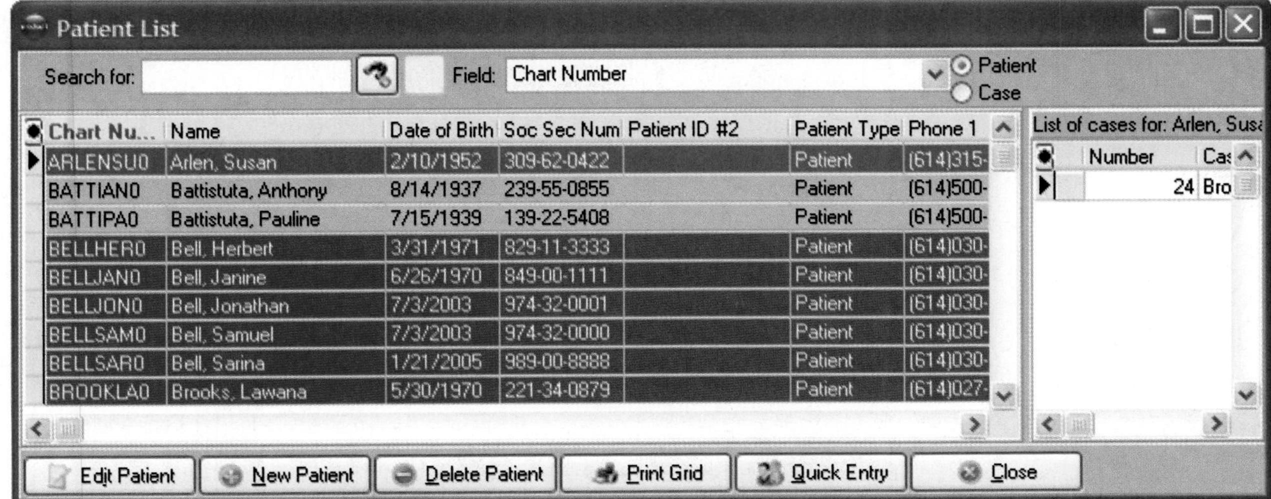

Figure 5.11 Patient Window Expanded to Show Additional Columns

When the Patient window is active, the command buttons at the bottom of the screen include Edit Patient, New Patient, Delete Patient, Print Grid, Quick Entry, and Close.

The Patient window contains the following data: Chart Number, Name, Date of Birth, Social Security Number, Patient ID #2, Patient Type, Phone 1, Provider, Last Name, Billing Code, and Patient Indicator. There is not enough room in the Patient window to display all this information, so only a portion is visible at one time. The additional patient information can be viewed by using the scroll bar, maximizing the dialog box, or resizing the Patient area of the dialog box (see Figure 5.11).

Information in the Patient window is color-coded. In the exercises in this text, the patient identification color codes represent the patient's insurance carrier (see Figure 5.12).

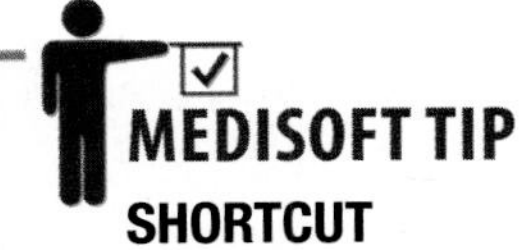

SHORTCUT

The quickest way to open a patient or case record is to double click the line associated with a patient or case.

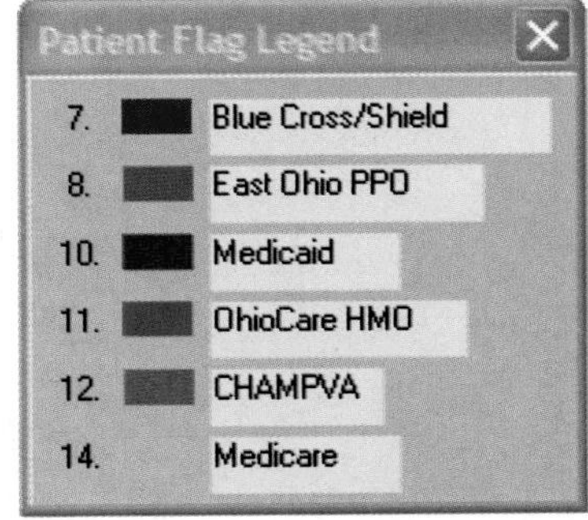

Figure 5.12 Color Legend for Patient List Window

5.7 Entering New Patient Information

After a new patient fills in a patient information form at registration, the information must be entered in Medisoft Network Professional. Information on a new patient is entered by clicking the New Patient button at the bottom of the Patient List dialog box (see Figure 5.13). This action opens the Patient/Guarantor dialog box (see Figure 5.14). The Patient/Guarantor dialog box contains three tabs: the Name, Address tab; the Other Information tab; and the Payment Plan tab. The information entered in the first two tabs is obtained from the patient information form. The third tab is used if the practice sets up a payment plan for the patient.

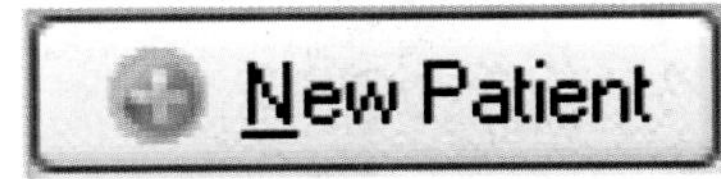

Figure 5.13 New Patient Button

Several buttons are located on the right side of the Patient/Guarantor dialog box. These buttons include the following:

Save Saves the information entered in the dialog box.

Cancel Closes the dialog box and discards any information entered.

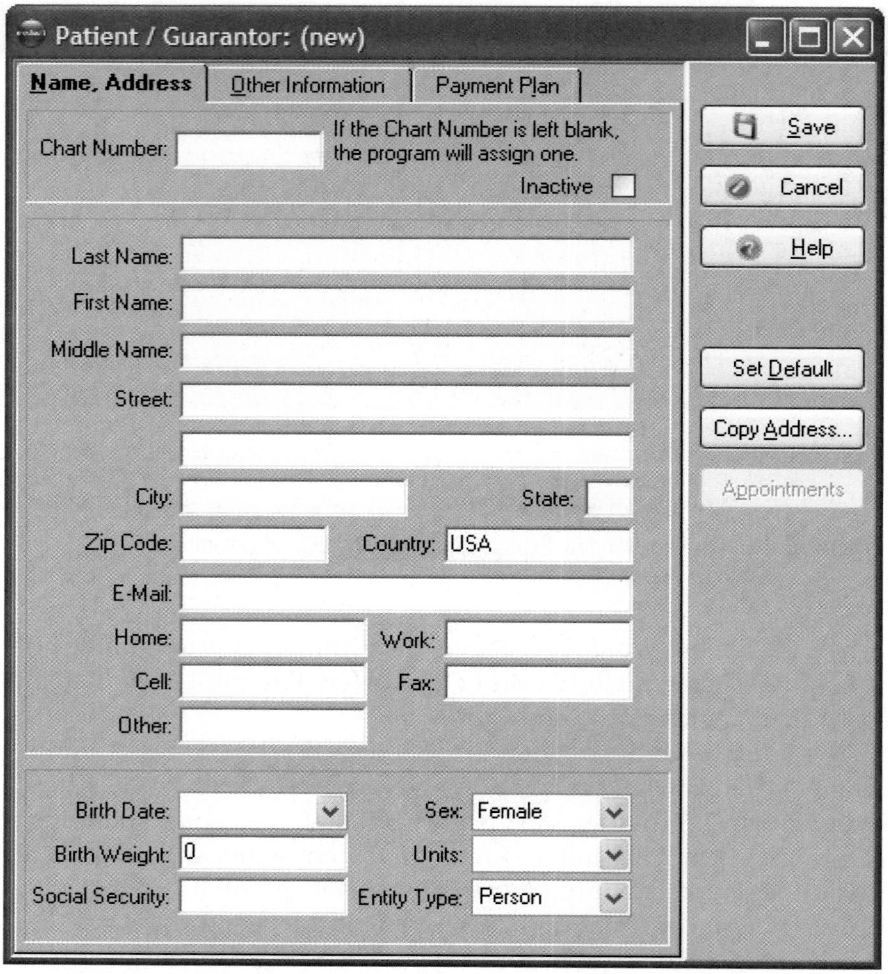

Figure 5.14 Patient/Guarantor Dialog Box with Name, Address Tab Active

Help Displays the Medisoft Network Professional help window for Patient/Guarantor Entry.

Set Default Sets the information in this window as the default for all new patients. (To undo, hold down the CTRL key, and this button will change to Remove Default.)

Copy Address Copies demographic information from another patient or guarantor entry.

Appointments Opens a window with a list of scheduled appointments for the patient. (The Appointments button is grayed and cannot be selected if a patient has no appointments scheduled.)

Name, Address Tab

The Name, Address tab is where basic patient information is entered (see Figure 5.14).

chart number unique alphanumeric code that identifies a patient

Chart Number

The **chart number** is a unique number that identifies a patient. In Medisoft Network Professional, a chart number links all the information about a patient that is stored in the different databases, such as name, address, charges, and insurance claims. Each patient is assigned an eight-character chart number. If the chart number box for a patient is left blank, the system will assign a number.

Medical practices may use different methods for assigning chart numbers, although two general guidelines must be followed: (1) no special characters, such as hyphens, periods, or spaces, are allowed; and (2) no two chart numbers can be the same.

For the purposes of this book, the following method will be used for assigning chart numbers:

- The first five characters of the chart number are the first five letters of a patient's last name. If the patient's last name has fewer than five characters, add the beginning letters of the patient's first name.
- The next two characters are the first two letters of a patient's first name. (If the first two letters of the first name were used to complete the first five letters, the next two letters of the patient's first name are used.)
- The last character is always a zero, displayed in this book with the symbol "Ø."

For example, the chart number for John Fitzwilliams begins with the first five letters of his last name (FITZW), followed by the first two characters of his first name (JO), followed by a zero (Ø). John's complete chart number is FITZWJOØ. Following the same rules, John's daughter Sarah has a chart number of FITZWSAØ.

connect plus+ EXERCISE 5.2

CREATING CHART NUMBERS

Create a chart number for each of these patients, and write it in the space provided.

Beth House ______________________

Robert Park ______________________

Rebecca Turner ______________________

You have completed Exercise 5.2

Personal Data

In addition to the chart number, personal information about a patient is entered in the Name, Address tab.

Name, Address, Phone Numbers, E-Mail Medisoft Network Professional provides fields for name and address as well as a number of fields for contact methods. There are boxes for e-mail address, home phone,

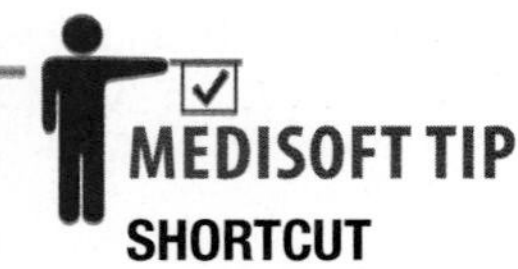

SHORTCUT

The Copy Address button saves time when entering patients with the same address, such as family members. Clicking on the Copy Address button provides an option to copy demographic information from a patient already in the database.

work phone, cell phone, fax, and other. To make data entry faster, phone and fax numbers are entered without parentheses or hyphens. The program adds the parentheses and hyphens automatically.

Birth Date The patient's birth date is entered in the Birth Date box using the pop-up calendar or by keying in the date using the MMDDCCYY format. In the MMDDCCYY format, *MM* stands for the month, *DD* stands for the day, *CC* represents the century, and *YY* stands for the year. Each month, day, century, and year entry must contain two digits, and no punctuation can be used. For example, March 5, 1958, would be keyed ***03051958***. Alternatively, the date can be entered using one or two digits for the day and month, four digits for the year, and separating each entry with a slash. Using this method, March 5, 1958, would be keyed ***3/5/1958***. Medisoft Network Professional accepts either format.

Sex This drop-down list contains choices for the patient's gender: male or female.

Birth Weight If the patient is a newborn, the birth weight is entered in this field.

Units This field indicates whether the birth weight is listed in pounds or grams.

Social Security The nine-digit Social Security number is entered without hyphens; the program adds the hyphens automatically.

Entity Type This field is used for the direct transmission of electronic claims to an insurance carrier. The options in this field are person or non-person.

Other Information Tab

The Other Information tab within the Patient/Guarantor dialog box contains facts about a patient's employment and other miscellaneous information (see Figure 5.15).

Type The Type drop-down list is used for billing purposes to designate whether an individual is a patient or guarantor.

In the Patient/Guarantor dialog box, individuals are classified into two categories: patient and guarantor. A patient is an individual who is a patient of the practice, whether or not he or she is also the insurance policyholder. The guarantor may or may not be a patient of the practice but is the insurance policyholder for a patient of the practice. For example, if the insurance policy of a parent who is not a patient provides coverage for a child who is a patient, the parent is listed in the database as the guarantor.

Information about the patient is always entered in the Name/Address tab. When the patient is not the policyholder, information about the guarantor must also be entered in the Medisoft Network Professional database for insurance claims to be processed. This information is collected from the patient information or patient update form.

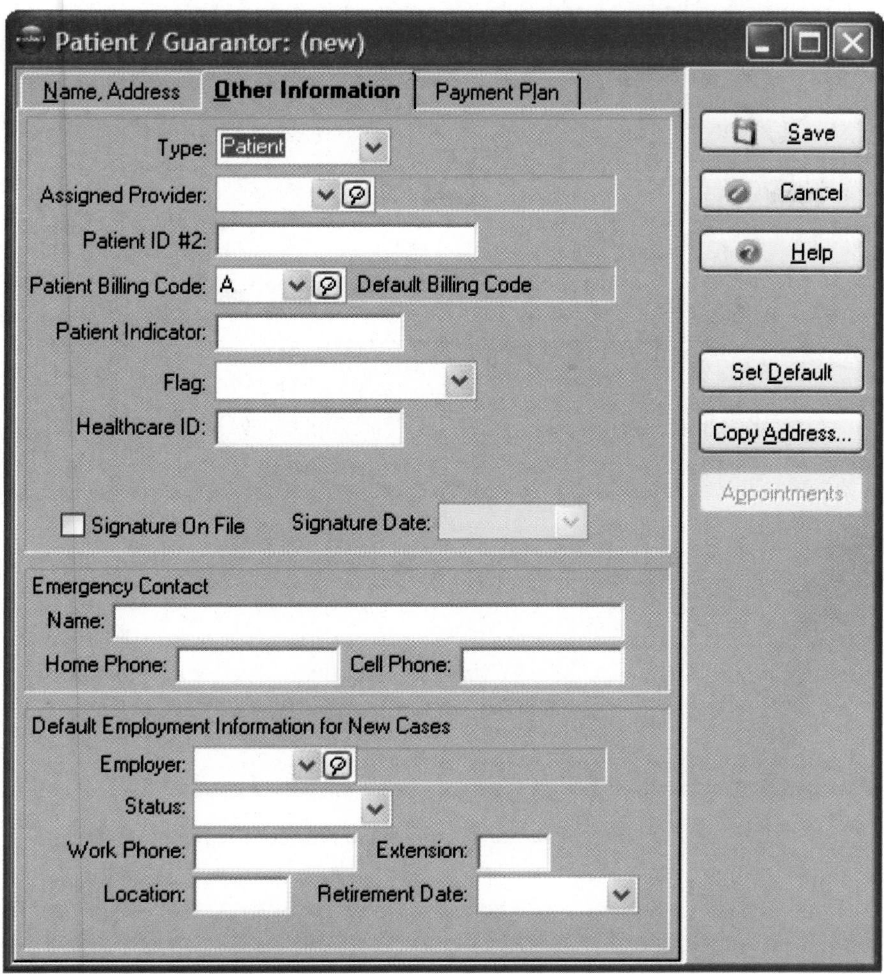

Figure 5.15 Other Information Tab

Assigned Provider The Assigned Provider drop-down list contains codes assigned to the doctors in the practice (see Figure 5.16). The code for the doctor who provides care to this patient is selected.

Patient ID #2 The Patient ID #2 box is used by some medical practices as a second identification system in addition to chart numbers.

Patient Billing Code The Patient Billing Code is an optional field used to categorize patients according to the billing codes that the practice has set up. For example, Billing Code A might be for patients with insurance coverage, B for cash patients, and so on. Some practices use billing codes to classify patients according to a billing cycle—patients with Billing Code A are billed on the first of the month, and those with Billing Code B on the fifteenth of the month. The Billing Code field is not used in the exercises in this book.

Patient Indicator The Patient Indicator is an optional field that practices can use to classify types of patients, such as workers' compensation patients, cash patients, and diabetic patients.

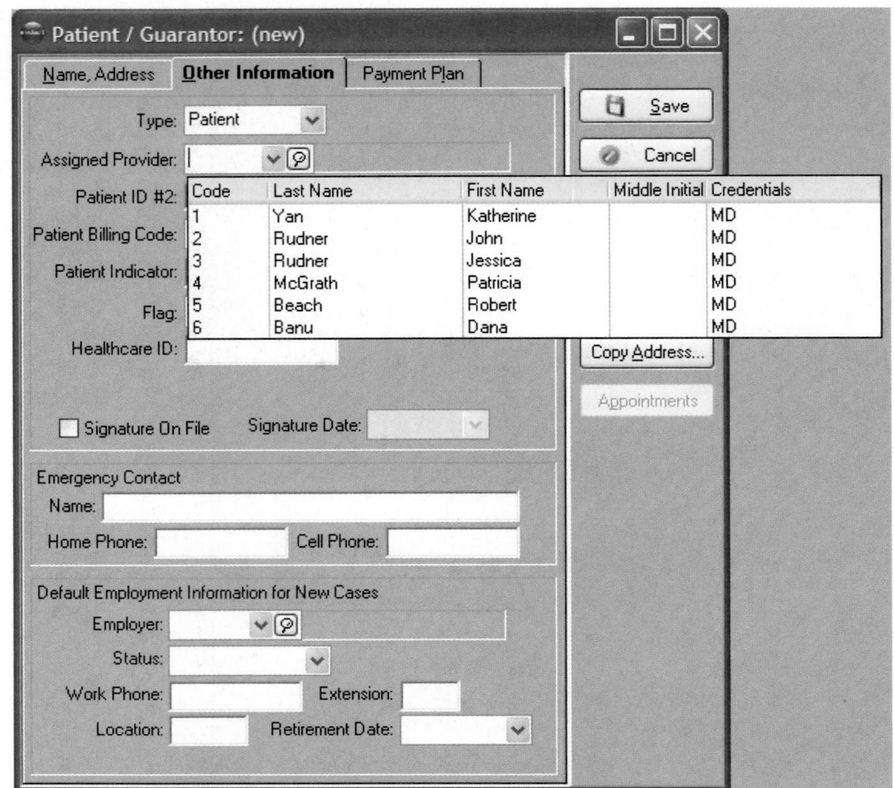

Figure 5.16 Other Information Tab with Assigned Provider Drop-down List Displayed

Flag This field can be used to organize patients into groups and assign a color code to each group. In this text, the flag is assigned to patients' insurance plans.

Healthcare ID The Healthcare ID is not used at present; it is included for future implementation of HIPAA legislation.

Signature on File A check mark in the Signature on File check box means that the patient's signature is on file for the purpose of submitting insurance claims. This box must be completed. If it is not, the insurance carrier will not accept and process insurance claims.

Signature Date The date keyed in the Signature Date box is the date the patient signed the insurance release form.

Emergency Contact The name and phone number of a person to contact in case of a patient emergency are entered in these fields.

Employer The code for the patient's employer is selected from the drop-down list of employers in the database (see Figure 5.17). If the patient's employer is not in the database, this information must be entered before the code can be selected.

Status The Status drop-down list displays the following choices for the patient's employment status: Not employed, Full time, Part time, Retired, and Unknown.

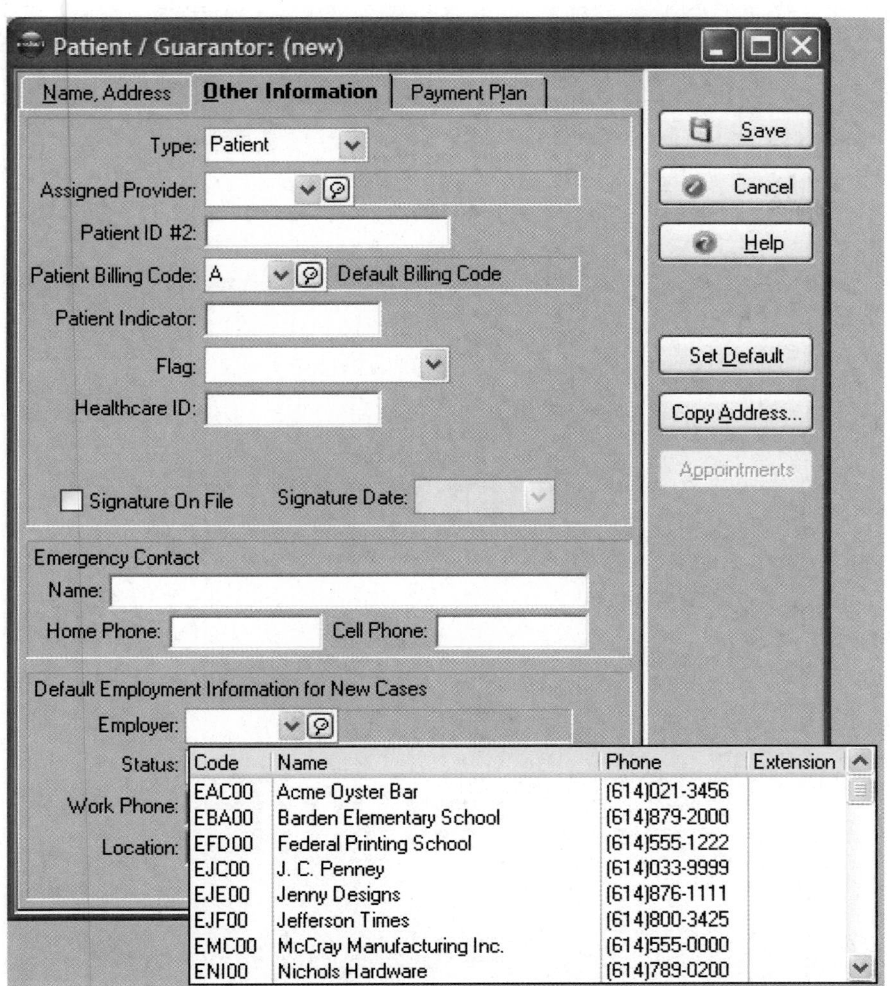

Figure 5.17 Other Information Tab with Employer Drop-down List Displayed

Work Phone and Extension Work phone numbers are entered without parentheses or hyphens.

Location Some companies have multiple locations. If the patient supplies information on the specific company location, it is entered in this box.

Retirement Date The Retirement Date box is filled in only if the patient is already retired. The date can be keyed directly in the box or it can be selected from the pop-up calendar that appears when the triangle button to the right of the box is clicked.

When all the fields in the Name, Address tab and the Other Information tab have been filled in, entries should be checked for accuracy. If any information needs to be corrected, it can easily be changed. Once the information has been checked and necessary corrections made, data are saved by clicking the Save button.

Payment Plan Tab

The Payment Plan tab is used when a patient's account is overdue and a payment plan has been created to pay down the remaining balance (see Figure 5.18).

Figure 5.18 Payment Plan Tab

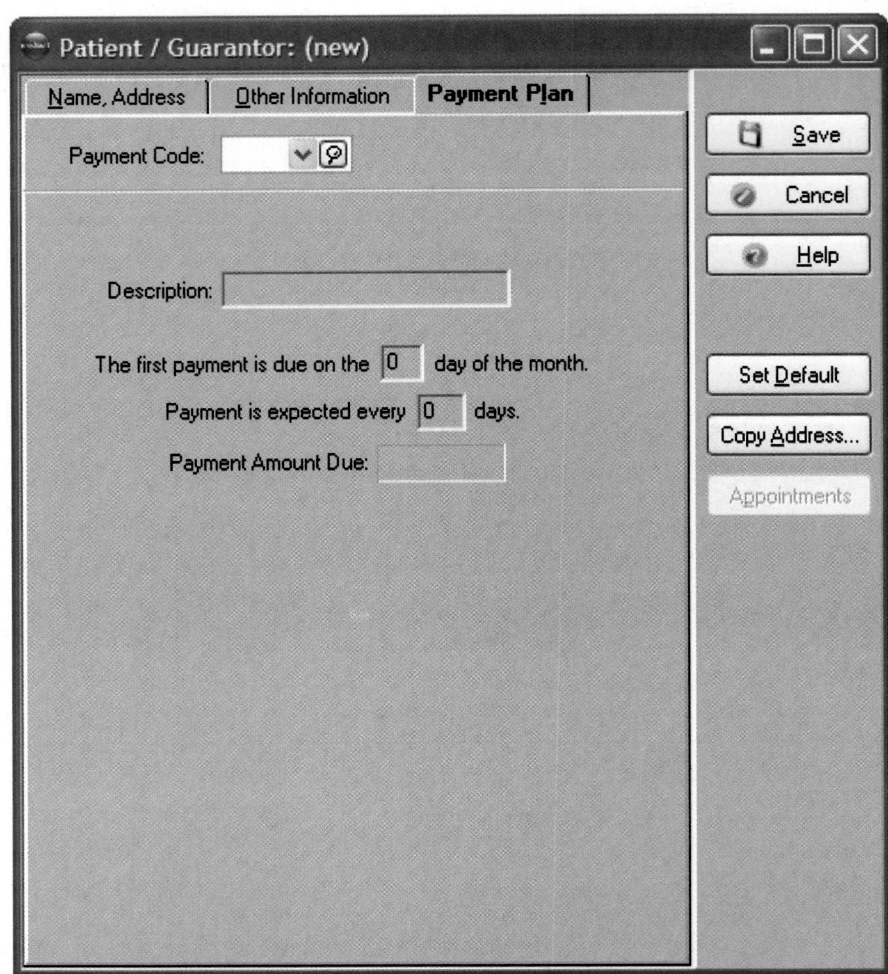

EXERCISE 5.3

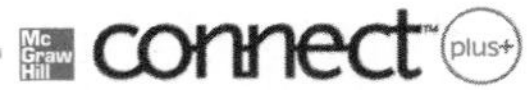

ENTERING PATIENT INFORMATION FOR A NEW PATIENT

Using Source Document 1 (located in Part 5 of this book), complete the Patient/Guarantor dialog box for Hiro Tanaka, a new patient of Dr. Yan.

Date: October 3, 2016

1. Verify that Medisoft Network Professional is open.
2. On the Lists menu, click Patients/Guarantors and Cases, or click the corresponding shortcut button on the toolbar.
3. Scroll down the list of patients to make sure Hiro Tanaka is not already in the patient database.
4. Click the New Patient button.
5. Create a chart number for this patient. Remember, in this text/workbook the chart number should be the first five letters of the patient's last name, followed by the first two letters of the patient's first name, followed by Ø. Click the Chart Number box, and enter the chart number.
6. Click the Last Name box, fill in the patient's last name, and then press Tab.

7. Using Source Document 1, fill in the rest of the boxes for which you have data, pressing the Tab key to move from box to box. This includes the following boxes:
   First Name
   Street, City, State, Zip Code
   E-mail
   Home, Work, and Cell phone numbers
   Birth Date
   Sex
   Social Security
8. Click the Other Information tab. Notice that the default setting for the Type box is Patient. Since Hiro Tanaka is being added to the database as a patient, keep this setting as it is, and press Tab.
9. In the Assigned Provider box, select Dr. Katherine Yan as Tanaka's provider.
10. Press Tab four times to move to the Flag box.
11. Select Tanaka's insurance carrier in the Flag box.
12. Press Tab twice to move to the Signature On File box.
13. Click inside the Signature On File box to insert a check mark, and press Tab.
14. Key Tanaka's signature date in the Signature Date box, and press Tab.
15. Click inside the Employer box to display a drop-down list of employers currently in the database.
16. Select Tanaka's employer from the drop-down list, and press Tab.
17. Select her employment status (Full time) in the Status drop-down box.
18. Click the Save button. The program saves the data that you entered in both the Name, Address and Other Information tabs.
19. Verify that Tanaka has been added to the list in the Patient List dialog box.
20. Close the Patient List dialog box.

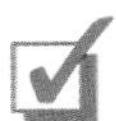 **You have completed Exercise 5.3**

5.8 Searching for and Updating Patient Information

From time to time, patients notify the practice that they have moved, changed jobs or insurance carriers, or made other changes. When this happens, information needs to be updated in Medisoft Network Professional's patient/guarantor database.

The process of updating patient information is similar to that of entering information for a new patient. The Patients/Guarantors and Cases option is selected from the Lists menu. A search is usually performed to locate the chart number of the patient whose record needs to be updated. The program provides two options for conducting searches: Search for and Field boxes and Locate buttons.

Search for and Field Options

The Search for and Field boxes at the top of many dialog boxes provide a quick way to search for information in the program (see Figure 5.19).

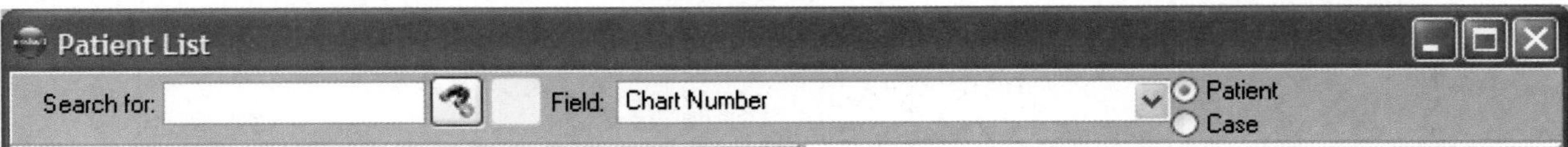

Figure 5.19 Search for and Field Boxes

The Search for box contains the text that is to be searched on. The entry in the Field box controls how the list is sorted. Figure 5.20 displays the Field options in the Patient List dialog box.

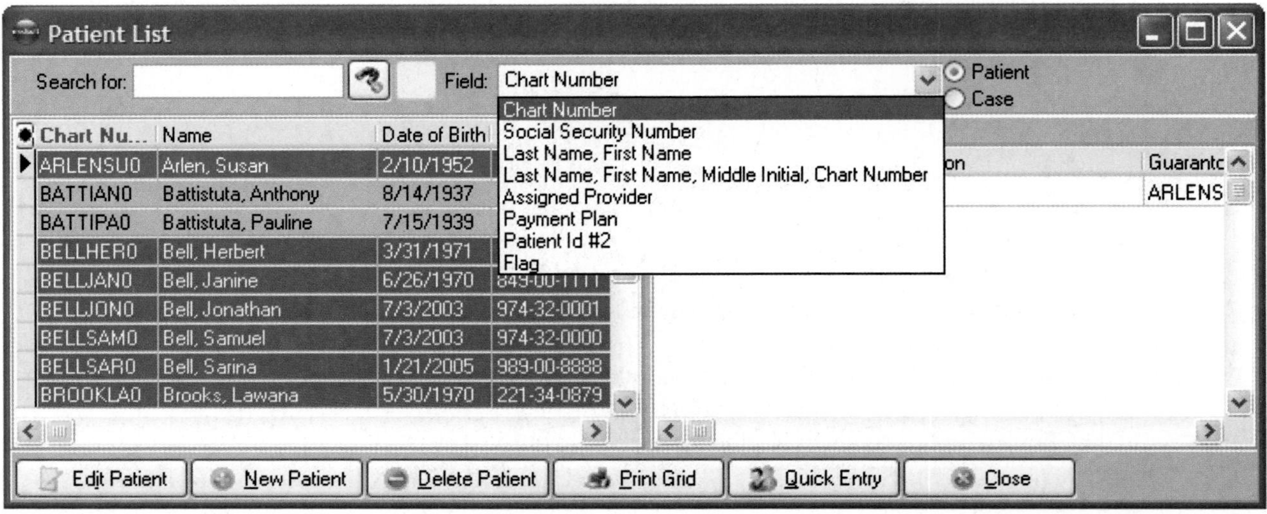

Figure 5.20 Field Options in the Patient List Dialog Box

When a selection is made in the Field box, the information is resorted by the selected criteria. For example, in the Patient List dialog box, if Social Security Number is selected in the Field box, the entries in the List window are listed in numerical order by Social Security number. The Search for and Field feature is available in many of the Medisoft Network Professional dialog boxes that list information, including the Insurance Carrier List, Diagnosis Code List, and Provider List dialog boxes.

After an entry is made in the Field box, the search criteria are entered in the Search field. As each letter or number is entered, the list automatically filters out records that do not match. For example, if the Field box is set to Last Name, First Name in the Patient List dialog box and *S* is entered in the Search field, the program eliminates all data from the list except patients whose last names begin with *S* (see Figure 5.21). To restore the Patient list to its default setting (all patients listed), the entry in the Search for box is deleted.

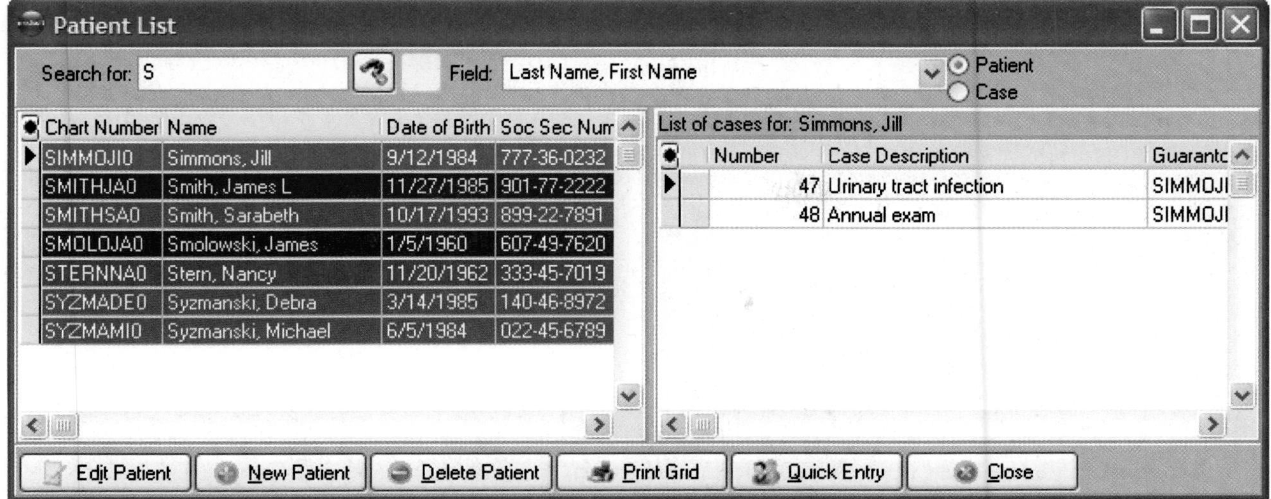

Figure 5.21 Patient List Dialog Box with Search for Patients Whose Last Names Begin with *S*

connect plus+ EXERCISE 5.4

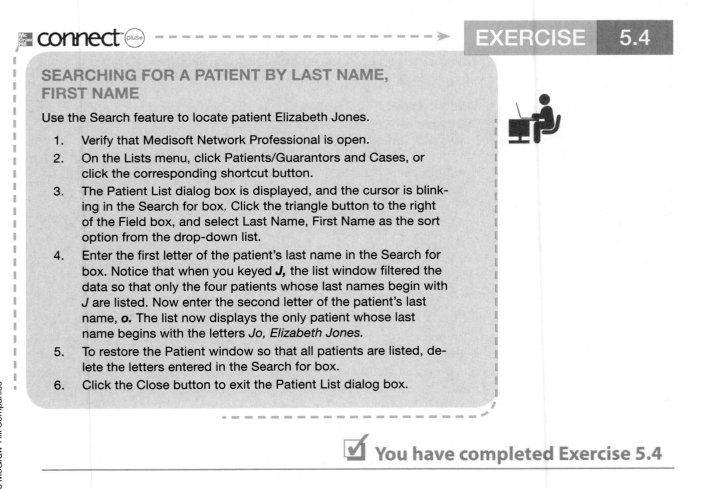

SEARCHING FOR A PATIENT BY LAST NAME, FIRST NAME

Use the Search feature to locate patient Elizabeth Jones.

1. Verify that Medisoft Network Professional is open.
2. On the Lists menu, click Patients/Guarantors and Cases, or click the corresponding shortcut button.
3. The Patient List dialog box is displayed, and the cursor is blinking in the Search for box. Click the triangle button to the right of the Field box, and select Last Name, First Name as the sort option from the drop-down list.
4. Enter the first letter of the patient's last name in the Search for box. Notice that when you keyed ***J,*** the list window filtered the data so that only the four patients whose last names begin with *J* are listed. Now enter the second letter of the patient's last name, ***o.*** The list now displays the only patient whose last name begins with the letters *Jo, Elizabeth Jones.*
5. To restore the Patient window so that all patients are listed, delete the letters entered in the Search for box.
6. Click the Close button to exit the Patient List dialog box.

You have completed Exercise 5.4

Locate Buttons Option

Another option for finding information in Medisoft Network Professional is to use the Locate buttons (see Figure 5.22).

When a Locate button is clicked, a Locate dialog box is displayed. Figure 5.23 shows the Locate Patient dialog box.

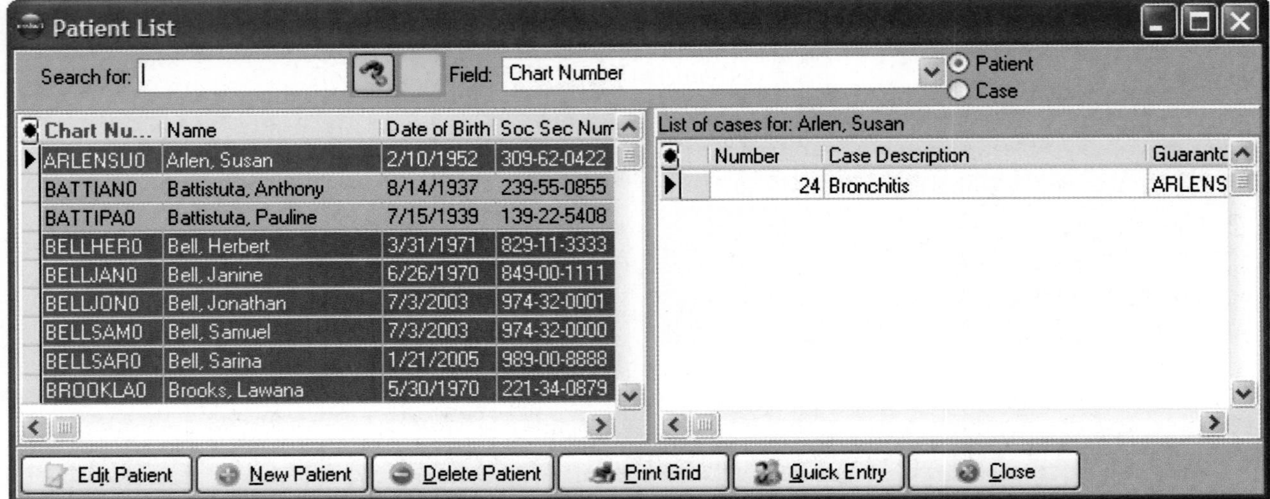

Figure 5.22 Locate Buttons Highlighted in Yellow

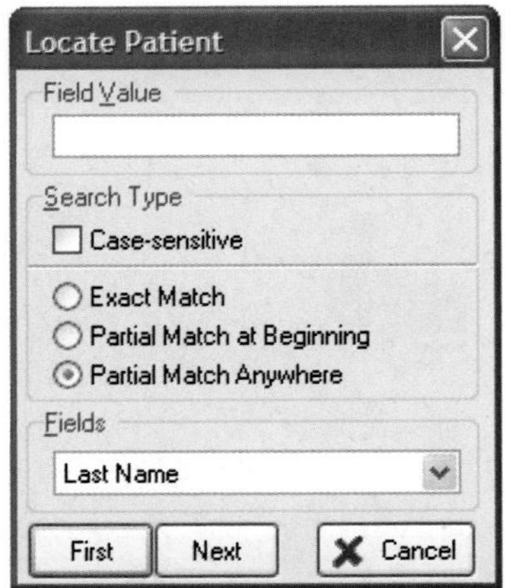

Figure 5.23 Locate Patient Dialog Box

Field Value

The information entered in the Field Value box at the top of the window can be part of a name, birth date, payment date or amount, or assigned provider. Any combination of numbers and letters can be used.

Search Type

Case-Sensitive Use to make the search sensitive to uppercase or lowercase letters.

Exact Match Use when an entry in the Field Value box is exactly as entered in the program.

Partial Match at Beginning Use when unsure of the correct spelling or entry at the end of the word.

Partial Match Anywhere Use when unsure of the correct spelling or entry.

Fields

The Fields box provides a drop-down list from which to choose the field that contains the information that is being matched. For example, if searching for a patient by last name, select the Last Name field. The available fields are determined by the type of information you are working with. For example, if you are looking for a particular chart number, you have nineteen fields from which to choose as the basis of your search. Searching for cases gives access to up to ninety-one fields.

Once the criteria are selected, clicking the First button starts a search for the first match to the criteria. If a match is found, the Locate window is closed, and the search result is highlighted in the Search window. If a match is not found, a message is displayed. Clicking the Next button begins a search for the next criteria match, and so on. When the program reaches the end of the list, a message is displayed indicating that the search is complete.

MEDISOFT TIP

SHORTCUT

To make searching easier, right click a column heading in a window that contains several columns. From the shortcut menu that appears, select Locate, or press ALT + L. This opens a Locate window that defaults the Fields selection to the column you selected.

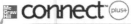

connect plus+

EXERCISE 5.5

SEARCHING FOR AND UPDATING PATIENT INFORMATION

Search for John Gardiner's name in the patient list, and then edit his patient information.

1. Verify that Medisoft Network Professional is open.
2. Open the Patient List dialog box. Confirm that the Field box entry is Last Name, First Name.
3. Search for John Gardiner by keying the first two letters of his last name in the Search for box. Notice that as soon as the *Ga* is entered, all patients except Gardiner disappear from the Patient List window, because Gardiner is the only patient whose last name begins with *Ga.*
4. Double click his name, or click the Edit Patient button to display his information in the Patient/Guarantor dialog box.
5. In the Name, Address tab, change his home phone number from 614-726-9898 to 614-726-5003 as follows: click inside the box, press Backspace four times, and key ***5003.*** The program inserts the hyphen for you.
6. Click the Save button to store the information you have entered.
7. A Confirm Phone Change dialog box appears, asking if you wish to update the home phone number for all future appointments. Click the Yes button.
8. Close the Patient List dialog box.

 **You have completed Exercise 5.5**

5.9 Navigating Cases in Medisoft Network Professional

The data stored in the Patient/Guarantor dialog box is primarily demographic, including a patient's name, address, date of birth, Social Security number, employer, and so on. There is no detailed information about the patient's condition, insurance coverage, allergies, and the like. This information is entered in a case. In Medisoft Network Professional, a case is a grouping of transactions that share a common element. These transactions represent the services and treatments that the physician provided to the patient during the visit. To receive payment, the office must transmit these transactions to the patient's insurance carrier in the form of an insurance claim.

When to Set Up a New Case

Most often, transactions are grouped into cases based on the medical condition for which the patient seeks treatment. For example, if a patient has a chronic condition such as diabetes, charges for all visits related to diabetes are stored in one case. If the same patient also has hypertension, all visits for treatment of hypertension are stored in another case. Patients with chronic conditions often have many transactions in a single case.

On the other hand, a patient may require more than one case per office visit if treatment is provided for two or more unrelated conditions. For example, a patient who visits the physician complaining of migraine headaches may also ask for an influenza vaccination. Since the two conditions are unrelated, two cases would need to be created: one for the migraine headaches, and the other for the vaccination. In contrast, a patient who is treated for shortness of breath and chest pain during exertion would require one case if the physician determines that the two complaints are related to the same diagnosis.

In the examples just described, the patient's medical condition determines whether more than one case is needed, since each different medical condition requires its own case. There are other instances when a separate case must be created, such as a change in insurance. When a patient changes insurance plans, a new case is set up, even if the same condition is being treated. This makes it easier to submit insurance claims to the appropriate carrier. Transactions that took place while the previous policy was in effect must be submitted under that policy. Transactions that occur after the change in policies must be submitted to the new carrier. By opening a new case, transactions for the two insurance carriers can be kept separate. The information needed to submit claims to the previous carrier is still intact, while information for claims under the new policy is current.

Similarly, when a patient is injured at work and is treated under workers' compensation insurance, a new case must be created so that the claims are billed to the workers' compensation plan, not to the patient's personal policy.

Case Examples

The following scenarios provide examples of when new cases are—and are not—required.

Example 1

Among Dr. Yan's patients today is Josephine Tremblay, a Medicare patient. Josephine has a number of chronic health conditions, including diabetes, arthritis, hypertension, and asthma. She has four cases already set up in the program, one for each of her chronic conditions. Today she is seeing Dr. Yan because she is experiencing lower back pain. From this information alone, we cannot determine whether to create a new case, since the back pain may be due to one of her existing conditions. When the billing assistant reviews the electronic encounter form, she sees that Dr. Yan has diagnosed Mrs. Tremblay with lower back pain due to arthritis. Since arthritis is one of Mrs. Tremblay's existing cases, no new case is needed.

Example 2

Dr. Jessica Rudner has just finished examining Kimberly DeJong. Ms. DeJong is a twenty-five-year-old woman who has an existing case for rosacea, a chronic skin condition. Today, Ms. DeJong received an antimalarial prescription in preparation for a trip to India. Since this visit is not related to her existing case for rosacea, a new case is created.

Example 3

Jose Gonzales has been a patient of Dr. John Rudner for three months. During that time, he was diagnosed with hypertension and started on medication. He has come in today for a follow-up visit to see how well the medication is working. The front desk staff asks him if any information has changed since his last visit, and he indicates that he changed jobs and has a new health plan. Even though he is being treated for the same condition (hypertension), claims for today's visit must be sent to the new insurance carrier. To ensure that today's charges are submitted to the new carrier, a new case must be created.

Example 4

David Weber is the seven-year-old son of Marcia and Ronald Weber, who are divorced. David has not been seen by Dr. Yan except for routine immunizations each year before school starts. David has been covered by his father's insurance plan since the divorce. David's father recently lost his job, and David is now covered by his mother's health plan. Today, David's father has brought him in for his annual immunizations. A new case must be created even though David has an existing case for annual immunizations because he is covered by a different insurance plan. If a new case were not created, the charges would be submitted to the insurance plan listed in the existing case, and the claim would be rejected.

Case Command Buttons

When the Case radio button in the Patient List dialog box is clicked, the following command buttons appear at the bottom of the Patient List dialog box: Edit Case, New Case, Delete Case, Copy Case, Print Grid, Quick Entry, and Close (see Figure 5.24).

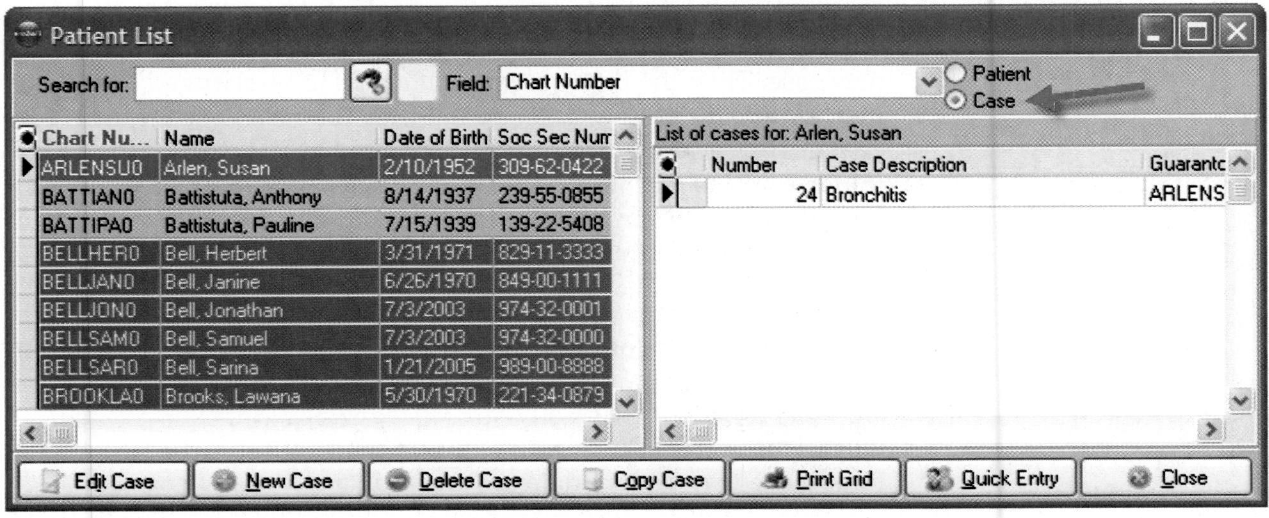

Figure 5.24 Patient List Dialog Box with Case Radio Button Selected

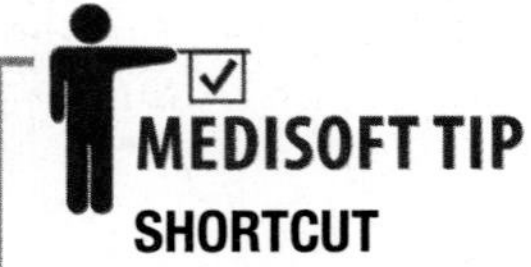

Cases can also be opened for editing by double clicking the case number or description in the Case window within the Patient List dialog box.

Edit Case The Edit Case button is used to add, delete, or change information in an existing case. When the Edit Case button is clicked, the Case dialog box is displayed. Case information to be updated is contained in twelve different tabs. For example, if a patient gets married, information needs to be updated in the Personal tab. The only item in the Case dialog box that cannot be changed is the case number. All other boxes are edited by moving the cursor to the box and making the change, whether this involves rekeying, selecting and deselecting check boxes, or clicking a different option on a drop-down list.

New Case The New Case button creates a new case.

Delete Case The Delete Case button deletes a case from the system if the case has no open transactions. Open transactions are charges that have not been fully paid by the insurance carrier or the policyholder. The Delete Case button should be used with caution; once deleted, information cannot be retrieved. Cases should be deleted only when it is definite that the patient's records will never be needed again. Medical offices usually have policies about when a patient's records are deleted, such as five years after the patient's last visit to the practice. In most instances, it is more appropriate to close a case than to delete it. Cases are closed by clicking the Case Closed box in the Personal tab of the Case dialog box.

Cases are deleted in the Patient List dialog box. With the Case radio button clicked, the specific case to be deleted is selected by clicking the line that displays the case number and description. The case is then deleted by clicking the Delete Case button at the bottom of the dialog box. The system will ask, "Are you sure you want to delete this case?" Clicking the Yes button deletes the case from the system.

Copy Case The Copy Case button copies all the information from an existing case into a new case. This feature is useful when creating a new case for a patient who already has a case in the system. Copy Case makes it unnecessary to reenter the information in all twelve tabs; instead, the information in the existing case is copied into a new case. Then the information that needs to be changed can be edited to reflect the new case. Sometimes the new case requires few changes; other times data must be changed in all the tabs of the Case folder. For this reason, when copying a case it is important to check each tab to make sure the copied information is accurate for the new case. The information that remains the same from the previous case can be left as is.

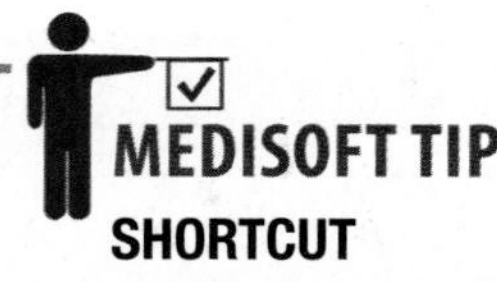

When creating a new case for an established patient, it is faster to use the Copy Case button than to create a new case using the New Case button.

Print Grid The Print Grid button is used to select or deselect columns of information for printing purposes.

Quick Entry The Quick Entry button is used in practices that customize the way patient data are entered.

Close The Close button closes the Patient List dialog box.

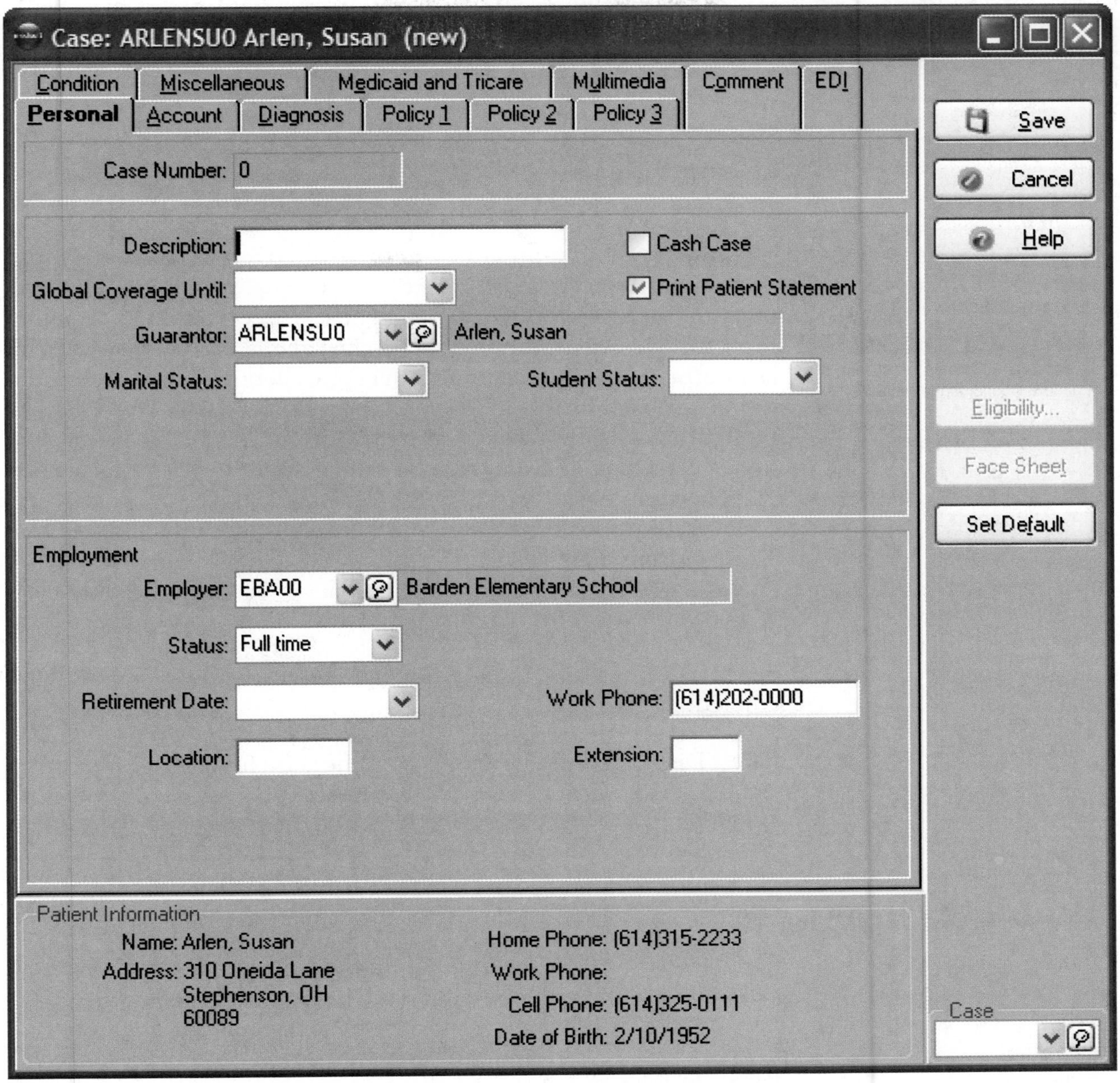

Figure 5.25 Case Dialog Box

The Case Dialog Box

Clicking the New Case button brings up the Case dialog box (see Figure 5.25). Information about a patient is entered in twelve different tabs in the Case dialog box:

1. Personal
2. Account
3. Diagnosis
4. Policy 1
5. Policy 2
6. Policy 3

7. Condition
8. Miscellaneous
9. Medicaid and Tricare
10. Multimedia
11. Comment
12. EDI

chart folder that contains all records pertaining to a patient

record of treatment and progress physician's notes about a patient's condition and diagnosis

The information required to complete the twelve tabs comes from documents found in a patient's chart. The **chart** is a folder that contains all records pertaining to a patient. The new patient information form supplies basic information, such as name and address, as well as information about insurance coverage, allergies, whether the condition is related to an accident, and the referral source. The **record of treatment and progress** contains the physician's notes about a patient's condition and diagnosis. The encounter form is a list of services performed and the charges for them.

Several buttons are located on the right side of the Case folder. These buttons are:

Save Saves the information entered in the dialog box.

Cancel Closes the dialog box and discards any information entered.

Help Displays the help window for the Case folder.

Eligibility Displays an option to verify eligibility for the patient and case.

Face Sheet Prints a sheet of information about the patient and case.

Set Default Sets the information in the case as the default for new cases for this patient. To remove the default, hold down the CTRL key, and this button changes to a Remove Default button.

Case Displays a list of the patient's cases.

5.10 Entering Patient and Account Information

The Personal tab and the Account tab contain basic information about the patient, such as name, address, date of birth, marital status, and employment status. Much of the information is filled in by the program, using the information already entered in the Patient/Guarantor dialog box. The Account tab lists the patient's assigned provider, referral source, authorized number of visits, and more.

Personal Tab

The Personal tab contains basic information about a patient and his or her employment (see Figure 5.26).

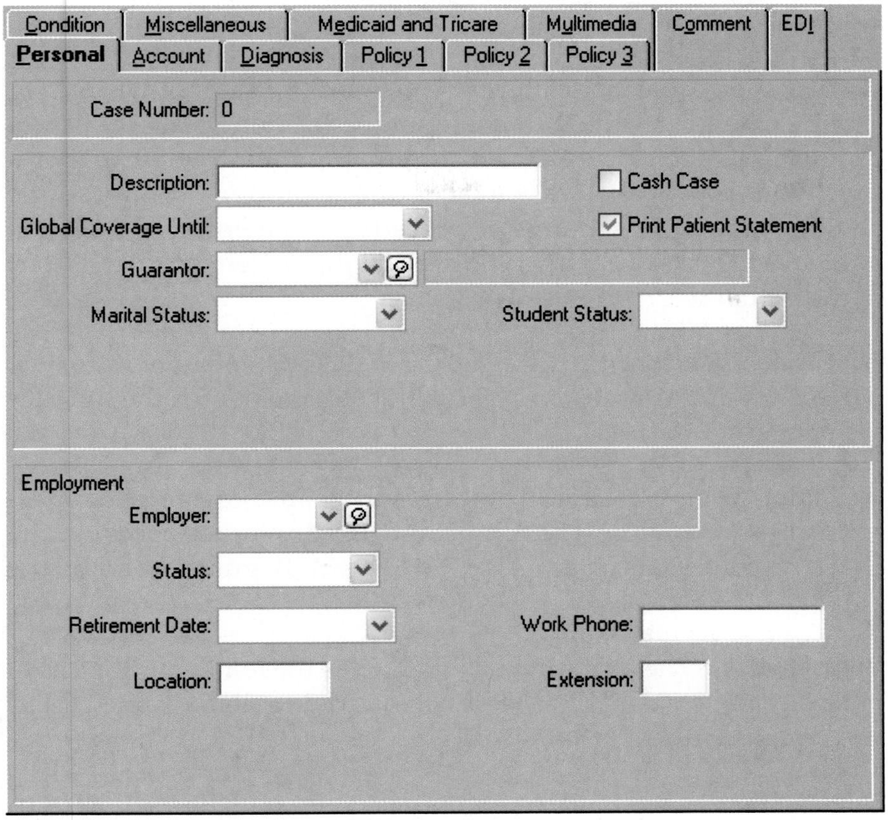

Figure 5.26 Personal Tab

Case Number The case number is a sequential number assigned by the program. To avoid confusion, case numbers are unique; no two patients ever have the same case number.

Case Closed A case is marked as closed by placing a check mark in the Case Closed box. At times it is appropriate to close a case. Closing a case indicates that no more data will be entered into the case. When is it appropriate to close a case? Policies vary from practice to practice, but generally cases are closed when a patient changes insurance carriers, has recovered completely from a condition (such as the flu), or is no longer a patient at the practice. *Note:* The Case Closed box does not appear until a case is created and saved.

Description Information entered in the Description box indicates a patient's complaint, or reason for seeing a physician. For example, if a patient comes to see a physician for an annual physical examination, the Description box would read "annual physical." Other examples of entries are sore throat, stomach pains, dog bite, and accident at work. A patient's complaint can be found in his or her chart.

Cash Case If the Cash Case box is checked, the patient is paying cash and has no insurance coverage.

Global Coverage Until Certain services are paid for under what are known as "global fees." These fees include reimbursement for services performed at different times by the same provider (or group) when performed in conjunction with one medical procedure or episode of care. For example, preoperative, intraoperative, and postoperative services are included in the single payment for a global surgical procedure. The entry in this field indicates the date on which charges are no longer considered part of the global fee.

Print Patient Statement If this box is checked, a statement for the patient is automatically printed when statements for the practice are printed.

Guarantor The Guarantor box lists the name of the person responsible for paying the bill. The drop-down list contains the chart numbers and names of all potential guarantors in the database.

Marital Status The drop-down list provides the following choices to indicate a patient's marital status: Divorced, Legally separated, Married, Single, Unknown, or Widowed.

Student Status The Student Status drop-down list is used to indicate whether a patient is a full-time student, a part-time student, or a non-student. If a patient's status is not known, the box should be left blank.

Employer The Employer box contains the default employer information that has been entered in the Patient/Guarantor dialog box. If it is necessary to change the employer, the default can be overridden by clicking another employer code on the drop-down list.

Status The Status box lists a patient's employment status as recorded in the Patient/Guarantor dialog box. To change the selection that appears in the Status box, another selection is clicked on the drop-down list. The options are Full-time, Not employed, Part-time, Retired, and Unknown.

Retirement Date The Retirement Date box should be filled in only when a patient is already retired. The date can be keyed directly in the box or it can be selected from the pop-up calendar that appears when the triangle button to the right of the box is clicked.

Work Phone The Work Phone box contains a patient's work phone number.

Location If a patient has supplied a specific work location, such as "Fifth Avenue Branch," it is entered in the Location box.

Extension The Extension box lists a patient's work phone extension.

connect plus+ EXERCISE 5.6

ENTERING DATA IN THE PERSONAL TAB

Create a new case for patient Hiro Tanaka, and enter information in the Personal tab. The information needed to complete this exercise is found on Source Document 1.

Date: October 3, 2016

1. Verify that Medisoft Network Professional is open.
2. On the Lists menu, click Patients/Guarantors and Cases to display the Patient List dialog box.
3. Search for Hiro Tanaka by keying ***T*** in the Search for box. The arrow should point to the entry line for Hiro Tanaka.
4. Click the Case radio button to activate the case portion of the Patient List dialog box.
5. Click the New Case button. The dialog box labeled Case: TANAKHIØ Tanaka, Hiro (new) is displayed. The Personal tab is the current active tab. Notice that some information is already filled in.
6. Enter Tanaka's reason for seeing the doctor in the Description box. This information is located in Source Document 1, under the Other Information section.
7. Choose the correct entry for Tanaka's marital status from the drop-down list in the Marital Status box. The Student Status box can be left blank.
8. Notice that the information on Tanaka's employment is already filled in. The system copies the information entered in the Patient/Guarantor dialog box to the case file.
9. Click the Save button to save the case information you just entered.
10. The Patient List dialog box redisplays. Notice that the case you just created is listed in the right side of the dialog box in the area labeled List of cases for: Tanaka, Hiro.
11. Leave the Patient List dialog box open.

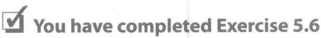

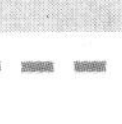 **You have completed Exercise 5.6**

Account Tab

The Account tab includes information on a patient's assigned provider, referring provider, and referral source, as well as other information that may be used in some medical practices but not others (see Figure 5.27).

Assigned Provider The Assigned Provider box is automatically filled in with the code number and name of the assigned provider listed in the Patient/Guarantor dialog box. The drop-down list includes a complete list of providers in the practice. If necessary, the Assigned Provider selection can be changed by clicking another provider on the list.

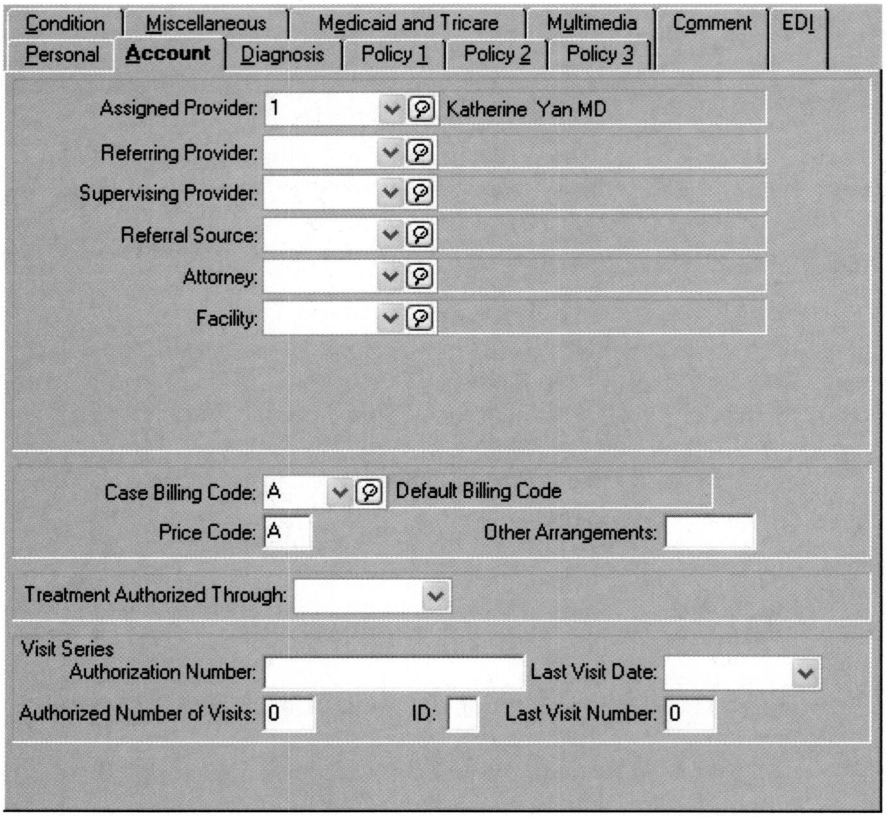

Figure 5.27 Account Tab

referring provider physician who refers the patient to another physician for treatment

Referring Provider A **referring provider** is a physician who recommends that a patient see a specific other physician. The Referring Provider box contains the name of the physician who referred the patient to the practice. The referring provider's name and code are selected from the drop-down list. If the referring provider is not listed on the drop-down list, he or she will need to be added to the Referring Provider list, which is found on the Lists menu. It is not necessary to close the Case dialog box to add a referring provider to the database. To add a new referring provider, click the Referring Provider box and press the F8 key, or click Referring Providers on the Lists menu. The Referring Provider List dialog box opens in front of the other dialog boxes displayed on the screen, and a new provider can be entered.

Supervising Provider When the provider rendering services is being supervised by a physician, the supervising physician's information is included on the claim.

Referral Source If known, the source of a patient's referral is selected from the drop-down list of choices.

Attorney When an attorney is involved in a patient's case, such as in an accident or disability case, the name of the patient's attorney should be selected from the drop-down list. If the attorney is not listed, he or she will need to be added to the system by clicking Addresses on the Lists menu and entering information about the attorney.

Facility The Facility box lists the place where a patient is receiving treatment. A facility is selected from the drop-down list. When necessary, facilities can be added to the database by clicking Facilities on the Lists menu and entering the necessary information.

Case Billing Code The Case Billing Code box is a one- or two-character box used by some practices to classify and sort patients by insurance carrier, diagnosis, billing cycle, or other kinds of information.

Price Code The Price Code box determines which set of fees is used when entering transactions for this case. The Price Code fees are entered and stored in the Amounts tab of the Procedure/Payment/Adjustment List dialog box, accessed through the Lists menu.

Other Arrangements If a special arrangement is made for billing, it is indicated in the Other Arrangements box.

Treatment Authorized Through A date can be entered in this box if the insurance carrier has authorized treatment only through a certain date.

Visit Series Information in the Visit Series section of the Account tab is reported whenever a patient seeks treatment that requires a preauthorized series of visits, such as visits to chiropractors, physical therapists, or for psychotherapy visits.

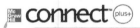

EXERCISE 5.7

ENTERING DATA IN THE ACCOUNT TAB

Complete the Account tab for Hiro Tanaka. The information needed to complete this exercise is found on Source Document 1.

Date: October 3, 2016

1. Verify that you are in Medisoft Network Professional, that Hiro Tanaka is still listed in the Patient List dialog box, and that the Case radio button is selected.
2. Click the Edit Case button to add information to Tanaka's case file. The Case dialog box is displayed, with the Personal tab active.
3. Make the Account tab active. The word *Account* should now be displayed in boldface type, and the boxes on the Account tab should be visible.
4. Notice that the Assigned Provider box is already filled in with the name of Tanaka's assigned provider, Katherine Yan. The system copies this information from data stored in the Patient/Guarantor dialog box.
5. Click the name of Tanaka's referring provider on the Referring Provider drop-down list, and press Tab.

(continued)

(Continued)

6. Accept the default entries in both the Case Billing Code and Price Code boxes.
7. Click the Save button to save the changes.
8. The Patient List dialog box is redisplayed.

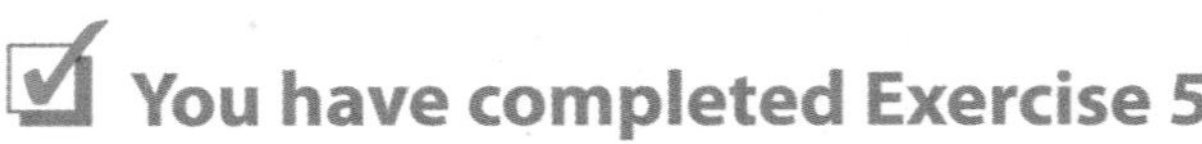

5.11 Entering Insurance Information

The primary insurance carrier is the first carrier to whom claims are submitted. There may also be a secondary carrier (Policy 2 tab) or a tertiary carrier (Policy 3 tab). The Medicaid and Tricare tab is used to enter specific information for Medicaid and TRICARE claims.

Policy 1 Tab

The Policy 1 tab is where information about a patient's primary insurance carrier and coverage is recorded (see Figure 5.28).

Insurance 1 The Insurance 1 box lists the code number and name of the insurance carrier. The drop-down list shows the carriers already in the system. If the carrier is not listed, it must be added to the database.

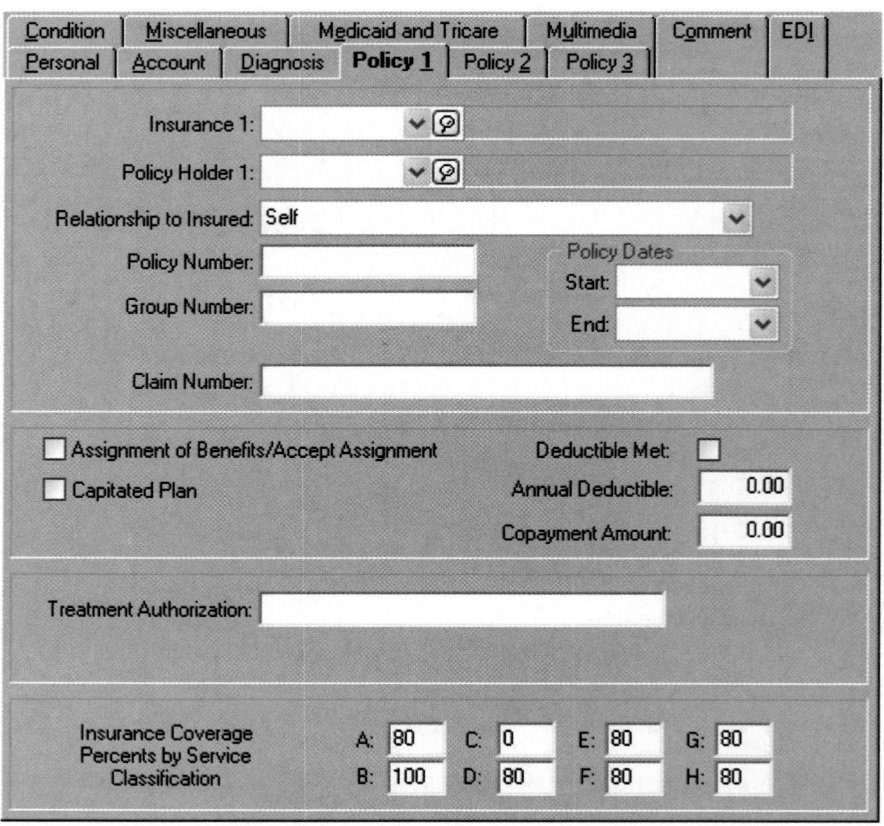

Figure 5.28 Policy 1 Tab

It is not necessary to close the Case dialog box to add an insurance carrier to the database. When Insurance is clicked on the Lists menu, and Carriers is clicked on the submenu, the Insurance Carrier List dialog box is displayed in front of the other dialog boxes on the screen.

Policy Holder 1 The Policy Holder box lists the person who is the insured under a particular policy. For example, if the patient is a child covered under his or her parent's insurance plan, the parent's chart number would be entered in this box. The insured's chart number is selected from the choices on the drop-down list. (If the insured is not a patient of the practice, he or she must be entered as a guarantor in the program, and a chart number must be established.)

Relationship to Insured This box describes a patient's relationship to the individual listed in the Policy Holder 1 box.

Policy Number A patient's policy number is entered in the Policy Number box.

Group Number The group number for a patient's policy is entered in the Group Number box.

Policy Dates—Start/End The date a patient's insurance policy went into effect is entered in the Policy Dates—Start box. If the date is not known, the date the patient first came to the practice for treatment can be entered. If the policy has ended, for example, because the carrier changed or the coverage expired, the date on which coverage terminated is entered in the Policy Dates—End box.

Claim Number This field is used on property, casualty, and auto claims. The number is assigned by the property and casualty payer, usually during eligibility determinations.

Assignment of Benefits/Accept Assignment For physicians who are participating in an insurance plan, a check mark in the Accept Assignment box indicates that the provider accepts payment directly from the insurance carrier. For the exercises in this book, this information is located on the bottom of the patient information form.

Capitated Plan In a **capitated plan,** prepayments are made to the physician from a managed care company to cover the physician's services to a plan member for a specified period of time, whether the member seeks medical care or not. A check mark in this box indicates that the insurance plan is capitated.

capitated plan insurance plan in which prepayments made to a physician cover the physician's services to a plan member for a specified period of time

Deductible Met This box is checked if the patient has met the deductible for the current year.

Annual Deductible The dollar amount of the insured's insurance plan deductible is entered in this box.

Copayment Amount The dollar amount of a patient's copayment per visit is entered in the Copayment Amount box.

Treatment Authorization This field is used to record the treatment authorization code from an insurance company for UB-04 claims. The UB-04 is the standard uniform bill (UB) that is used for institutional health care providers such as hospitals. The UB-04 replaced the UB-92 in 2007.

Insurance Coverage Percents by Service Classification The percentage of fees that an insurance carrier covers is entered in the Insurance Coverage Percents by Service Classification box. Some insurance plans pay different percentages of charges based on the type of service provided. For example, a plan may pay 80 percent of necessary medical procedures, 100 percent of lab work, and 50 percent of outpatient mental health charges.

EXERCISE 5.8

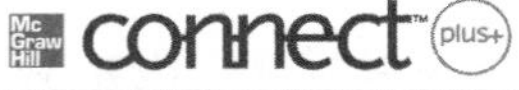

ENTERING DATA IN THE POLICY 1 TAB

Complete the Policy 1 tab for Hiro Tanaka. The information needed to complete this exercise is found on Source Document 1.

Date: October 3, 2016

1. Verify that Medisoft Network Professional is open, that Hiro Tanaka is still listed in the Patient List dialog box, and that the Case radio button is selected.
2. Double click the line with Hiro Tanaka's case in the Case window to edit it.
3. Make the Policy 1 tab active.
4. Select Tanaka's primary insurance carrier from the drop-down list in the Insurance 1 box. Press Tab.
5. The program completes the Policy Holder 1 field with the name of the patient. Since Tanaka is the policyholder, accept this entry.
6. Notice that the Relationship to Insured box already has "Self" entered. Since this is correct, do not make any changes.
7. Enter Tanaka's insurance policy number in the Policy Number box. Press Tab.
8. Enter Tanaka's group number in the Group Number box. Press Tab.
9. In the Policy Dates—Start box, key ***01012016*** or ***1/1/2016*** (January 1, 2016) as the start date of the policy. Press Tab.
10. Dr. Yan accepts assignment for this carrier, so click the Assignment of Benefits/Accept Assignment box.
11. The insurance plan is capitated, so check the Capitated Plan box.
12. Key ***20*** in the Copayment Amount box. Press Tab.
13. Key ***100*** in each of the Insurance Coverage Percents by Service Classification boxes, using the Tab key to move from box to box.
14. Save the changes. The Patient List dialog box is redisplayed.

 **You have completed Exercise 5.8**

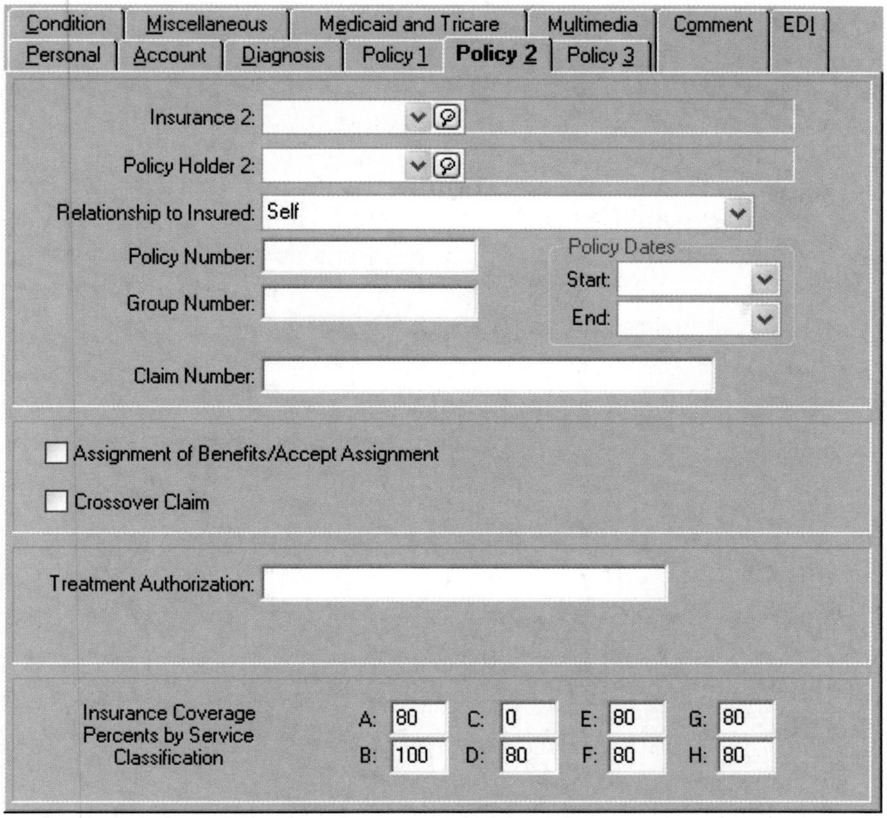

Condition | Miscellaneous | Medicaid and Tricare | Multimedia | Comment | EDI
Personal | Account | Diagnosis | Policy 1 | Policy 2 | Policy 3

Insurance 2:
Policy Holder 2:
Relationship to Insured: Self
Policy Number:
Group Number:
Policy Dates
Start:
End:
Claim Number:

Assignment of Benefits/Accept Assignment
Crossover Claim

Treatment Authorization:

Insurance Coverage Percents by Service Classification
A: 80 C: 0 E: 80 G: 80
B: 100 D: 80 F: 80 H: 80

Figure 5.29 Policy 2 Tab

Policy 2 Tab

Claims are usually not submitted to a secondary carrier until the primary carrier has paid. The secondary carrier must have access to the remittance advice of the primary carrier to see what has already been paid on the claim. Delayed secondary billing may be set up so a claim is not created for the secondary carrier until a response has been received from the primary carrier.

The boxes in the Policy 2 tab are the same as those in the Policy 1 tab, with a few exceptions. The Capitated Plan, Deductible Met, Annual Deductible, and Copayment Amount are in the Policy 1 tab only. The Policy 2 tab has only a Crossover Claim box (see Figure 5.29).

Crossover Claim The Crossover Claim box is used when a patient has Medicare as the primary carrier and Medicaid as the secondary carrier. Because Medicare is the primary carrier, it pays first on a claim and then submits the claim directly to the Medicaid carrier.

Policy 3 Tab

The Policy 3 tab does not contain the Capitated Plan, Deductible Met, Annual Deductible, Copayment Amount, or Crossover Claim boxes. Otherwise, the boxes are the same as those in the Policy 1 and Policy 2 tabs (see Figure 5.30).

Condition | Miscellaneous | Medicaid and Tricare | Multimedia | Comment | EDI
Personal | Account | Diagnosis | Policy 1 | Policy 2 | **Policy 3**

Insurance 3:

Policy Holder 3:

Relationship to Insured: Self

Policy Number:

Group Number:

Policy Dates
Start:
End:

Claim Number:

Assignment of Benefits/Accept Assignment

Treatment Authorization:

Insurance Coverage Percents by Service Classification

A: 80	C: 0	E: 80	G: 80
B: 100	D: 80	F: 80	H: 80

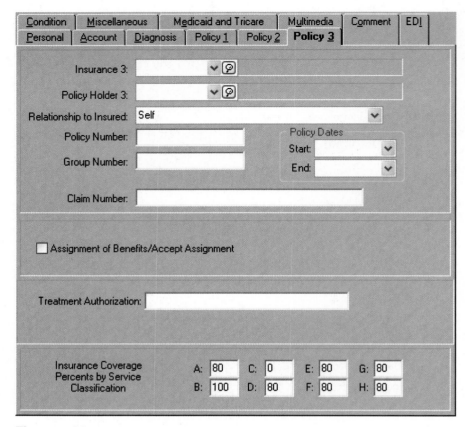

Figure 5.30 Policy 3 Tab

Medicaid and Tricare Tab

The Medicaid and Tricare tab is used to enter additional information about Medicaid or TRICARE for patients covered by the government programs (see Figure 5.31).

Medicaid

EPSDT *EPSDT* stands for Early and Periodic Screening, Diagnosis, and Treatment. This is a Medicaid program for patients under the age of twenty-one who need screening and diagnostic services to determine physical or mental problems as well as treatment for conditions discovered. It also includes well-baby checkup examinations. A check mark in the EPSDT box indicates that a patient's visit is part of the EPSDT program.

Family Planning A check mark in the Family Planning box specifies that a patient's condition is related to Medicaid family planning services.

Resubmission Number For claims being resubmitted to Medicaid, the resubmission number is entered in this box.

Original Reference For claims being resubmitted to Medicaid, the original reference number is recorded in the Original Reference box.

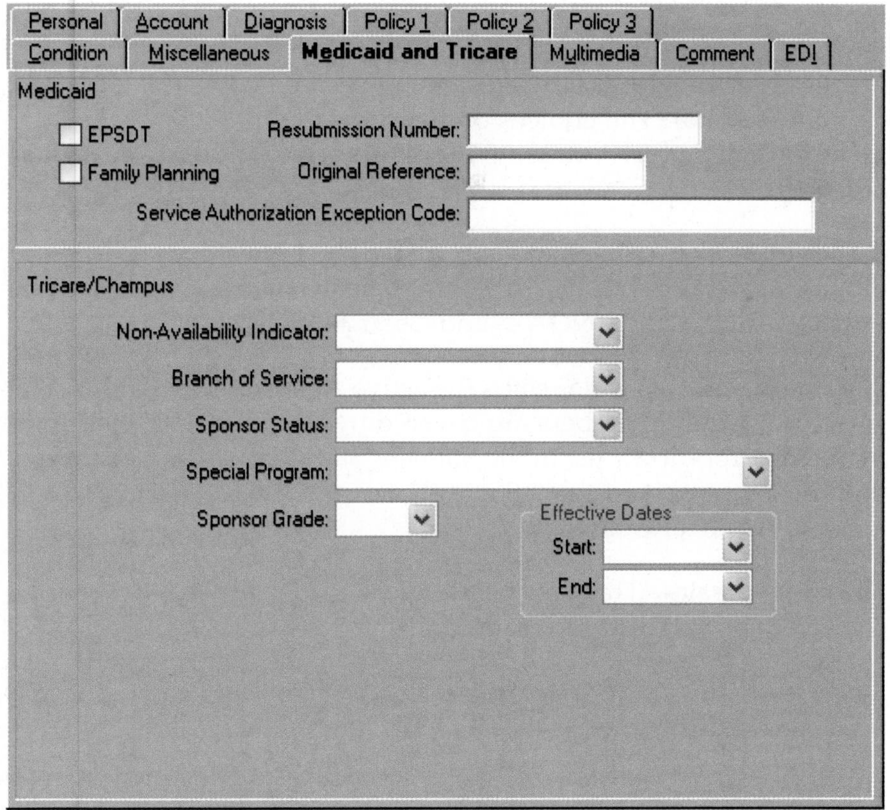

Figure 5.31 Medicaid and Tricare Tab

Service Authorization Exception Code This code is required on some Medicaid claims. If a service authorization code was not obtained before seeing the patient, enter one of the following codes:

1 Immediate/Urgent Care
2 Services Rendered in a Retroactive Period
3 Emergency Care
4 Client as Temporary Medicaid
5 Request from County for Second Opinion to Recipient Can Work
6 Request for Override Pending
7 Special Handling

TRICARE/CHAMPUS

TRICARE is the government insurance program that serves spouses and children of active-duty service members, military retirees and their families, some former spouses, and survivors of deceased military members (Army, Navy, Air Force, Marine Corps, Coast Guard, Public Health Service, and NOAA, the National Oceanic and Atmospheric Administration). TRICARE was previously known as CHAMPUS.

Non-Availability Indicator The Non-Availability Indicator box specifies whether a nonavailability (NA) statement is required. A *nonavailability statement* is an electronic document stating that the required service is not available at the nearby military facility. It is required for preauthorization for certain inpatient nonemergency procedures when a TRICARE member seeks medical services at a civilian hospital. The choices on the drop-down list are NA statement not needed, NA statement obtained, and Other carrier paid at least 75%.

Branch of Service The Branch of Service box indicates the particular branch of service: Army, Air Force, Marines, Navy, Coast Guard, Public Health Service, NOAA, and ChampVA.

sponsor in TRICARE, the active-duty service member

Sponsor Status The **sponsor** is the active-duty service member. The sponsor's family members are covered by the TRICARE insurance plan. The drop-down list in the Sponsor Status box provides choices to indicate the sponsor's status in the service, such as Active, Civilian, and National Guard.

Special Program The Special Program drop-down list contains codes for special TRICARE programs.

Sponsor Grade The two-character sponsor grade is entered in the Sponsor Grade box.

Effective Dates The start date of the TRICARE policy is entered in the Effective Dates—Start box. If there is an end date, it is entered in the Effective Dates—End box. Specific dates can be entered, or a selection can be made from the pop-up calendar.

5.12 Entering Health Information

Information about a patient's health is recorded in the Diagnosis and Condition tabs in Medisoft Network Professional.

Diagnosis Tab

The Diagnosis tab contains a patient's diagnosis, information about allergies, and electronic media claim (EDI) notes (see Figure 5.32).

Principal Diagnosis and Default Diagnosis 2, 3, and 4 A patient's diagnosis is selected from the drop-down list of diagnoses. If a patient has more than one diagnosis for the same condition, the primary diagnosis is entered in the Principal Diagnosis field. Additional diagnoses are entered in the Default Diagnosis 2, 3, and 4 fields. The program options can be changed to display up to eight diagnoses if required.

Allergies and Notes If a patient has allergies or other special conditions that need to be recorded, they are entered in the Allergies and Notes box.

EDI Notes If a patient's claims require special handling when submitted electronically, notes about the procedure, such as an explanation about the charges for supplies, are listed in this box.

Condition | Miscellaneous | Medicaid and Tricare | Multimedia | Comment | EDI
Personal | Account | **Diagnosis** | Policy 1 | Policy 2 | Policy 3

Principal Diagnosis:
Default Diagnosis 2:
Default Diagnosis 3:
Default Diagnosis 4:

Allergies and Notes
EDI Notes

EDI Report
Report Type Code: Report Transmission Code:
Attachment Control Number:

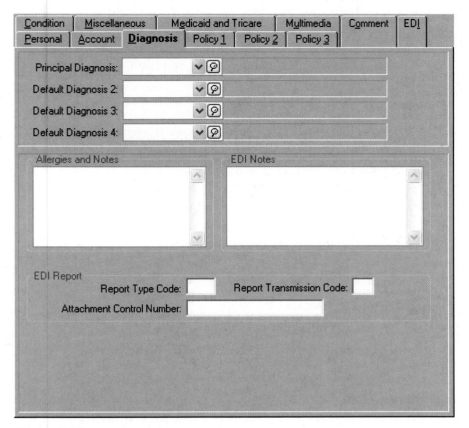

Figure 5.32 Diagnosis Tab

EDI Report The Report Type Code is a two-character code that indicates the title or contents of a document, report, or supporting item sent with electronic claims. The Report Transmission Code is a two-character code that defines the timing, transmission method, or format by which reports are sent with electronic claims. The value entered in the Attachment Control Number field is a unique reference number up to seven digits long.

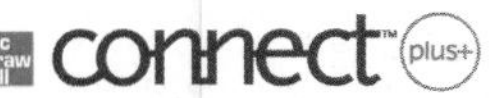

EXERCISE 5.9

ENTERING DATA IN THE DIAGNOSIS TAB

Complete the Diagnosis tab for Hiro Tanaka. The information needed to complete this exercise is found on Source Documents 1 and 6.

Date: October 3, 2016

1. Verify that Medisoft Network Professional is open, that Hiro Tanaka is still listed in the Patient List dialog box, and that the Case radio button is selected.
2. Double click the name of Hiro Tanaka's case in the Case window to edit it.
3. Make the Diagnosis tab active.
4. To enter Tanaka's diagnosis, click the triangle button in the Principal Diagnosis box. A drop-down list of codes and descriptions is displayed.

(continued)

(Continued)

5. Refer to Tanaka's electronic encounter form for the visit (Source Document 6) to locate the diagnosis code for the visit (724.2: Lumbago). Key the first number of the code in the Principal Diagnosis box to narrow the search.
6. From the list of choices displayed in the drop-down list, select Tanaka's diagnosis.
7. In the Allergies and Notes box, list the patient's allergies. Information on the patient's allergies is located in the Patient section of the patient information form (Source Document 1).
8. Save the changes. The Patient List dialog box is redisplayed.

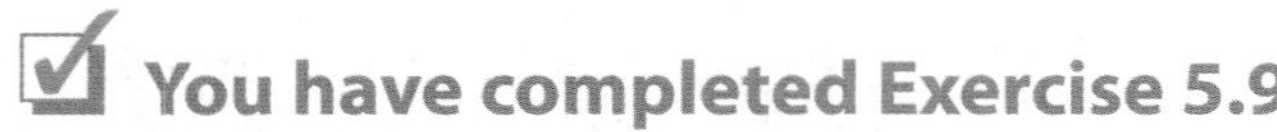

Condition Tab

The Condition tab stores data about a patient's illness, accident, disability, and hospitalization (see Figure 5.33). This information is used by insurance carriers to process claims.

Injury/Illness/LMP Date The date of a patient's injury, illness, or last menstrual period (LMP) is entered in the Injury/Illness/LMP Date box. (For an illness, the date when the symptoms first appeared is entered.)

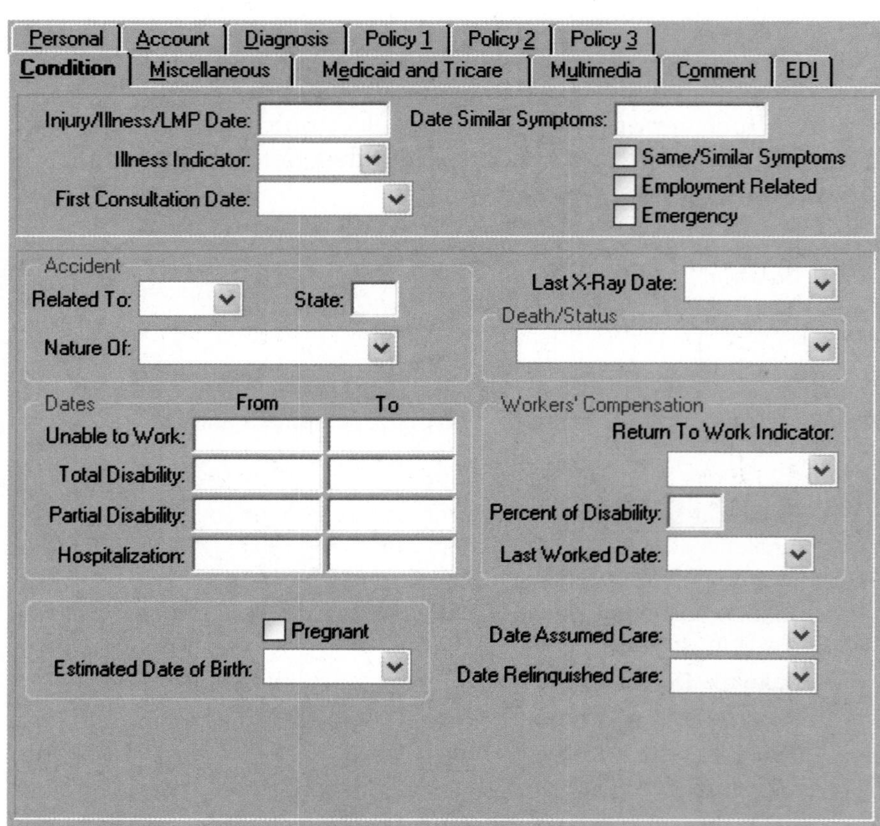

Figure 5.33 Condition Tab

Illness Indicator The Illness Indicator box specifies whether a patient's condition is an illness, a last menstrual period in the case of a pregnancy, or an injury.

First Consultation Date The date of a patient's first visit for a particular condition is entered in the First Consultation Date box. The actual date can be entered, or the pop-up calendar can be activated and dates selected.

Date Similar Symptoms If a patient has had similar symptoms in the past, enter the date of those symptoms in the Date Similar Symptoms box.

Same/Similar Symptoms A check mark in the Same/Similar Symptoms box indicates that a patient has had the same or similar symptoms in the past.

Employment Related If the Employment Related box is checked, it means that the illness or accident is in some way related to a patient's employment.

Emergency If a patient sees the provider on an emergency visit, a check mark is entered in the Emergency box.

Accident—Related To The Accident—Related To box indicates whether a patient's condition is related to an accident. The drop-down list offers three choices: Auto, if an automobile accident is involved; No, if it is not accident-related; and Yes, if it is accident-related but not related to an auto accident. If a patient's condition is accident-related, the State and Nature Of boxes should also be completed.

Accident—State The abbreviation for the state in which the accident occurred is entered in this box.

Accident—Nature Of This box provides additional information about the type of accident. The following choices can be selected from the drop-down list: Injured at home, Injured at school, Injured during recreation, Work injury/Self employed, Work injury/Non-collision, Work injury/Collision, and Motorcycle injury.

Last X-Ray Date The date of the last X-rays for the current condition are entered in this box.

Death/Status The Death/Status box indicates a patient's condition according to the Karnofsky Performance Status Scale. There are eleven options: Moribund (a terminal condition near death), Very sick, Severely disabled, Disabled, Requires considerable assistance, Requires occasional assistance, Cares for self, Normal activity with effort, Able to carry on normal activity, Dead, and Normal. If this information is not provided by the physician, the box should be left blank.

Dates—Unable to Work If a patient is unable to work, the dates of the absence from work are listed in these boxes.

Dates—Total Disability If a patient is totally disabled, the dates of the total disability are entered in these boxes.

Dates—Partial Disability If a patient is partially disabled, the dates of the partial disability are listed in these boxes.

Dates—Hospitalization If a patient is hospitalized, the dates of the hospitalization are entered in these boxes.

Workers' Compensation—Return to Work Indicator If a patient has been out of work on workers' compensation, the patient's return to work status is selected from the drop-down list of choices: Limited, Normal, or Conditional. If the status is Conditional or Limited, the Percent of Disability box should also be completed.

Workers' Compensation—Percent of Disability This box indicates a patient's percentage of disability upon returning to work.

Last Worked Date The last day the patient worked is listed in this box.

Pregnant This box is checked if a woman is pregnant.

Estimated Date of Birth If the patient is pregnant, enter the date the baby is due.

Date Assumed Care This field is used when providers share postoperative care. Enter the date the provider assumed care for this patient.

Date Relinquished Care This field is used when providers share postoperative care. Enter the date the provider relinquished care of the patient.

EXERCISE 5.10

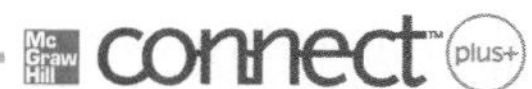

ENTERING DATA IN THE CONDITION TAB

Complete the Condition tab for Hiro Tanaka. The information needed to complete this exercise is found on Source Document 2.

Date: October 3, 2016

1. Verify that Medisoft Network Professional is open, that Hiro Tanaka is still listed in the Patient List dialog box, and that the Case radio button is selected.
2. Double click Hiro Tanaka's case in the Case window to edit it.
3. Make the Condition tab active.
4. Enter the date of the injury in the Injury/Illness/LMP Date box, using the MMDDCCYY or M/D/CCYY format.

5. Select Injury in the Illness Indicator box.
6. In the First Consultation Date box, enter the date Tanaka first saw Dr. Yan for this condition, which is 10/3/2016. Press Tab.
7. Since this visit resulted from a non-work-related accident, leave the Date Similar Symptoms box, the Same/Similar Symptoms box, and the Employment Related box blank.
8. Since this was an emergency visit, place a check mark in the Emergency box by clicking it.
9. In the Accident—Related To box, choose Auto.
10. In the Accident—State box, enter the two-letter abbreviation for the state in which the accident occurred.
11. Tanaka was injured while driving home from a softball game. Complete the Accident—Nature Of box regarding the type of accident with Injured during recreation.
12. Enter the dates Tanaka was unable to work in the Dates—Unable to Work boxes.
13. Enter the dates Tanaka was totally disabled in the Dates—Total Disability boxes.
14. Enter the dates Tanaka was partially disabled in the Dates—Partial Disability boxes.
15. Enter the dates Tanaka was hospitalized in the Dates—Hospitalization boxes.
16. Leave the remaining fields blank.
17. Save the changes. The Patient List dialog box is redisplayed.
18. Close the Patient List dialog box.

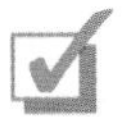
You have completed Exercise 5.10

5.13 Entering Other Information

Miscellaneous Tab

The Miscellaneous tab records a variety of miscellaneous information about the patient and his or her treatment (see Figure 5.34).

Outside Lab Work If the Outside Lab Work box is checked, the lab work was performed by a lab other than the physician office. If the lab bills the provider rather than the patient, then the provider bills the patient for the lab work even though it was performed by an outside lab.

Lab Charges The charges for lab work, whether performed inside or outside the practice, are entered in the Lab Charges box.

Local Use A and B These boxes may be used by some medical practices to record information specific to the local office.

Indicator If an indicator code is used to categorize patients or services, it is entered in the Indicator box. For example, patients might

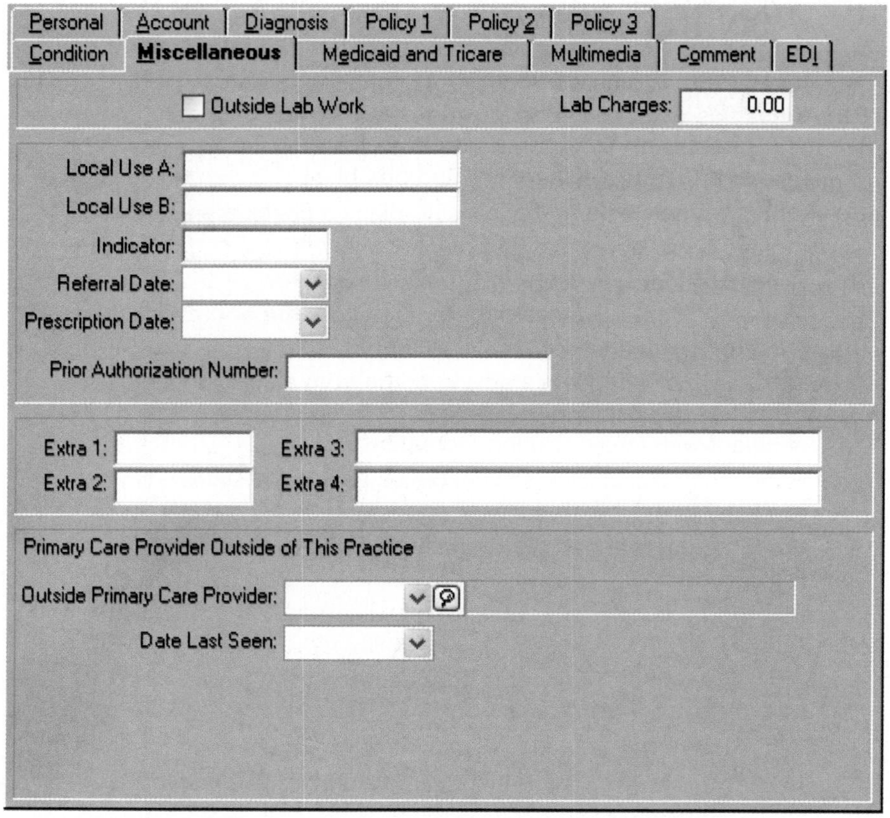

Figure 5.34 Miscellaneous Tab

be categorized according to the primary diagnosis. Services might be divided into such categories as lab work, consultations, and hospital visits.

Referral Date If the patient was referred to the provider, enter the date of the referral.

Prescription Date This field is required for hearing and vision claims.

Prior Authorization Number Before some services are performed, prior authorization must be obtained from the appropriate insurance carrier. If an insurance carrier has issued an authorization number for treatment that has not yet occurred, the number is entered in the Prior Authorization Number box.

Extra 1, 2, 3, and 4 The Extra 1, 2, 3, and 4 boxes are used for different purposes depending on the medical practice.

Outside Primary Care Provider If a patient is covered by a managed care plan and the patient's primary care provider is outside the medical practice, the name of the provider is selected from the drop-down list in this box.

Date Last Seen The Date Last Seen box lists the date a patient was last seen by the outside primary care provider.

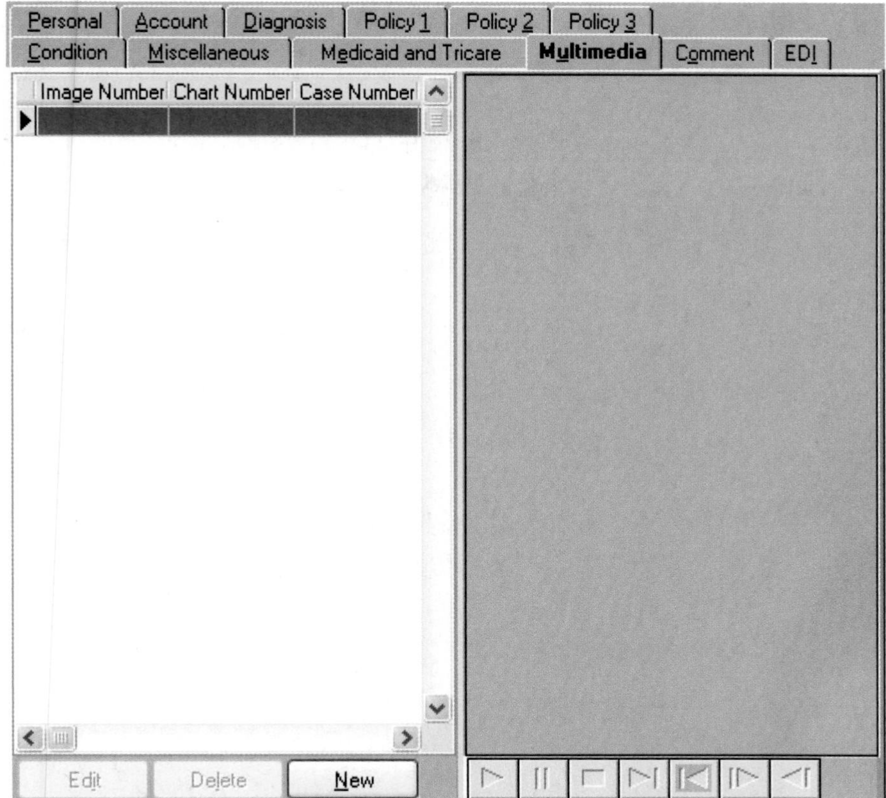

Figure 5.35 Multimedia Tab

Multimedia Tab

The Multimedia tab is used to save a multimedia file, such as a picture file or a sound file, to a patient's case (see Figure 5.35)

When the New button is clicked, a Multimedia Entry window displays that can be used to browse to an image or sound file to attach to the case. If an image file is selected, such as a patient's photo ID, the picture appears in the right panel of the Multimedia tab. If a sound file is selected, the sound control buttons at the bottom of the panel are enabled. If the Show on Patient Window box is selected in the Multimedia Entry window, the image displays in the Name, Address tab of the Patient/Guarantor dialog box along with the patient's demographic information.

Comment Tab

The Comment tab is used to enter case notes (see Figure 5.36). Notes entered in this box will print on statements if statements are formatted to include case comments.

EDI Tab

The EDI tab is used to enter information for electronic claims specific to this case (see Figure 5.37). Only fields that are relevant for the particular case need to be completed.

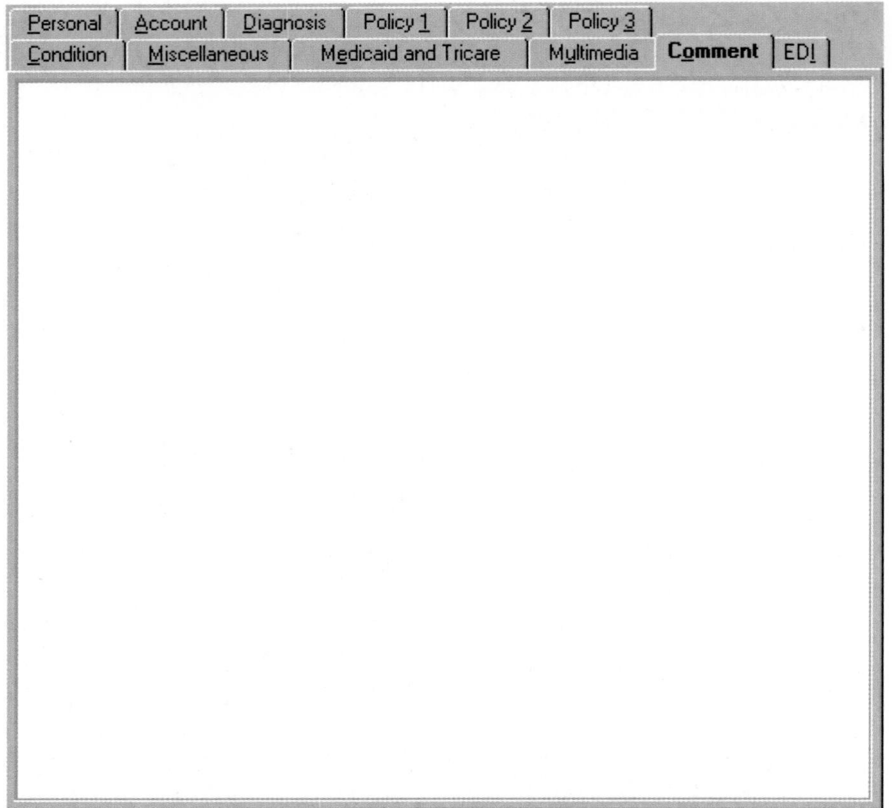

Figure 5.36 Comment Tab

Personal | Account | Diagnosis | Policy 1 | Policy 2 | Policy 3
Condition | Miscellaneous | Medicaid and Tricare | Multimedia | Comment | **EDI**

Care Plan Oversight #:
Hospice Number:
CLIA Number:
Mammography Certification:
Medicaid Referral Access #:
Demo Code: 0
IDE Number:

Assignment Indicator:
Insurance Type Code: 0
Timely Filing Indicator:
EPSDT Referral Code:
Homebound:

Vision Claims
Condition Indicator:
Code Category:
Certification Code Applies:

Home Health Claims
Total Visits Rendered: 0
Total Visits Projected: 0
Number of Visits: 0
Duration: 0
Number of Units: 0
Discipline Type Code:
Ship/Delivery Pattern Code:
Ship/Delivery Time Code:
Frequency Period:
Frequency Count: 0

Figure 5.37 EDI Tab

Care Plan Oversight # If a physician is billing for home health and hospice care plan oversight (CPO), enter the care plan oversight number.

Assignment Indicator The entry in this field is the assignment indicator for this case. Valid codes are:

A Assigned

B Assignment accepted on clinical lab services only

C Not assigned

P Patient refuses to assign benefits

Hospice Number If a physician is billing for hospice care, enter the hospice number.

Insurance Type Code The type of insurance that the patient has is selected in the Insurance Type Code field. This is required when sending Medicare secondary claims. Valid codes are:

12 Medicare secondary working-aged beneficiary or spouse with employer group health plan

13 Medicare secondary end-stage renal disease beneficiary in the twelve-month coordination period with an employer's group health plan

14 Medicare secondary, no-fault insurance including auto is primary

15 Medicare secondary workers' compensation

16 Medicare secondary public health service (PHS) or other federal agency

41 Medicare secondary black lung

42 Medicare secondary Veterans Administration

43 Medicare secondary disabled beneficiary under age sixty-five with large-group health plan (LGHP)

47 Medicare secondary, other liability insurance is primary

CLIA Number When laboratory claims are billed electronically, the Clinical Laboratory Improvement Act (CLIA) number must be included in the claim. This number is assigned to labs and required on all laboratory claims billed to Medicare.

Timely Filing Indicator If a response to a request for information from an insurance carrier was delayed, the reason for the delay is entered. Valid entries are:

1 Proof of eligibility unknown or unavailable

2 Litigation

3 Authorization delays

4 Delay in certifying provider

5 Delay in supplying billing forms
6 Delay in delivery of custom-made appliances
7 Third-party processing delay
8 Delay in eligibility determination
9 Original claim rejected or denied due to a reason unrelated to the billing limitation rules
10 Administration delay in the prior approval process
11 Other

Mammography Certification This box lists the provider's or facility's mammography certification number.

EPSDT Referral Code The patient's referral code for the EPSDT program is entered in this field.

Medicaid Referral Access # The referring physician's Medicaid referral access number for the patient is entered in this field.

Homebound If the patient is under homebound care, this box should be checked.

Demo Code This field is used when filing claims for the patient under demonstration projects.

IDE Number The IDE number is required when there is an investigational device exemption on the claim. This is usually for vision claims but can also be assigned for other types of claims.

Vision Claims

If a provider submits vision claims, entries are made in the following fields.

Condition Indicator The code indicator is entered in this field.

Code Category The code category for the vision device is entered in this field.

Certification Code Applies This box is checked if a certification code is applicable.

Home Health Claims

If a provider submits home health claims, these fields are filled in.

Total Visits Rendered This field indicates the total number of visits.

Discipline Type Code The provider's discipline type code is entered.

Total Visits Projected This field lists the total number of visits projected.

Ship/Delivery Pattern Code Enter the pattern code for the home visits.

Number of Visits The total number of visits is entered in this field.

Ship/Delivery Time Code This field records the time code for the home visits.

Duration The duration of the home health visits is recorded in this field.

Frequency Period The frequency period for the home visits is listed.

Number of Units This field contains the number of units for the home visits.

Frequency Count The frequency count for the home visits is entered.

chapter 5 summary

LEARNING OUTCOME	KEY CONCEPTS/EXAMPLES
5.1 List the six types of information that are gathered as part of the registration process for new patients. Pages 216–224	The six types of information are: 1. Medical history form 2. Patient information form 3. Insurance card 4. Assignment of benefits 5. Financial agreement and authorization for treatment 6. Acknowledgment of Receipt of Notice of Privacy Practices (NPP)
5.2 Determine which health plan is primary when there is more than one. Pages 224–226	The primary health plan is determined by following the coordination of benefits rules: - The plan that has been in effect for the patient for the longest period of time is primary. - If the patient is also covered as a dependent under another insurance policy, the patient's plan is primary. - If an employed patient has coverage under the employer's plan and additional coverage under a government-sponsored plan, the employer's plan is primary. - If the patient is a dependent child covered by both parents' plans and the parents are not separated or divorced or if the parents have joint custody of the child, the primary plan is determined by the birthday rule. - If two or more plans cover a dependent child of separated or divorced parents who do not have joint custody of their child, the child's primary plan is determined in this order (or by court order): (1) the plan of the custodial parent; (2) the plan of the spouse of the custodial parent if remarried; (3) the plan of the parent without custody.
5.3 Describe the purpose of a practice's financial policy. Pages 226–227	The financial policy explains what is required of the patient and when payment is due.

LEARNING OUTCOME	KEY CONCEPTS/EXAMPLES
5.4 List the types of payments that may be collected from patients at check-in. Pages 228–229	These payments may be collected at check-in: - Copayments - Balances - Partial payments
5.5 Discuss the advantages of tracking patients electronically during a visit. Pages 229–231	Tracking allows the staff to know patients' whereabouts. Tracking reports can be used to improve day-to-day functioning of the office. Tracking information also creates a record of a patient's appointment history.
5.6 In Medisoft Network Professional, describe the organization of patient data. Pages 232–233	- The Patient List window is divided into two primary sections: Patient information (left panel) and Case information (right panel). - When the Patient radio button in the upper-right corner of the window is selected, patient information is active and Edit Patient, New Patient, and Delete Patient command buttons become available. - When the Case radio button is selected, Case information and command buttons becomes active. - Either panel can be sized, or the scroll bar can be used to display the full range of data in the panel.
5.7 Discuss how a new patient is added to the database. Pages 233–241	Information on a new patient is entered by clicking the New Patient button at the bottom of the Patient List dialog box to open the Patient/Guarantor dialog box. The Patient/Guarantor dialog box contains three tabs: the Name, Address tab; the Other Information tab; and the Payment Plan tab. The information entered in the first two tabs is obtained from the patient information form. The third tab is used if the practice sets up a payment plan for the patient.
5.8 Name the two options used to conduct searches. Pages 241–245	The two options for searching in Medisoft Network Professional are the Search for and Field boxes and the Locate button.
5.9 Describe when it is necessary to create a new case or to utilize an existing case. Pages 245–250	A new case must be created when the patient has a new or unrelated condition, changes insurance plans, or is treated under workers' compensation. Otherwise, an existing case is utilized.

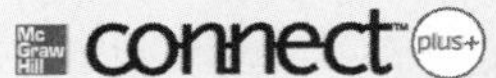

Enhance your learning at **mcgrawhillconnect.com**!
- *Practice Exercises*
- *Worksheets*
- *Activities*
- *Integrated eBook*

LEARNING OUTCOME	KEY CONCEPTS/EXAMPLES
5.10 Analyze the information contained in the Personal and Account tabs. Pages 250–256	The Personal tab contains the following basic information about a patient and his or her employment: case number, case closed, description, cash case, global coverage until, print patient statement, guarantor, marital status, student status, employer, employment status, retirement date, work phone, location, and extension. The Account tab includes information on a patient's assigned provider, referring provider, and referral source, as well as the following information that may be used in some medical practices but not others: supervising provider, attorney, facility, case billing code, price code, other arrangements, treatment authorized through, and visit series.
5.11 Discuss the information recorded in the Policy 1, 2, 3, and Medicaid and Tricare tabs. Pages 256–262	The Policy 1 tab is where information about a patient's primary insurance carrier and coverage is recorded, including the policyholder, policy and group numbers, copayment and deductible amounts, and whether the plan is capitated. The boxes in the Policy 2 tab are the same as those in the Policy 1 tab, with the exception of Capitated Plan, Deductible Met, Annual Deductible, and Copayment Amount boxes. Only the Policy 2 tab has a Crossover Claim box. The Policy 3 tab does not contain the Capitated Plan, Deductible Met, Annual Deductible, Copayment Amount, or Crossover Claim boxes. Otherwise, the boxes are the same as those in the Policy 1 and Policy 2 tabs. The Medicaid tab has information on EPSDT and family planning, among other data. The Tricare tab includes information on the nonavailability indicator, the service branch, and the sponsor status and grade.
5.12 Describe the information contained in the Diagnosis and Condition tabs. Pages 262–267	The Diagnosis tab contains a patient's diagnosis, information about allergies, and EDI notes. The Condition tab stores data about a patient's illness, accident, disability, and hospitalization. Insurance carriers use this information to process claims.
5.13 Discuss the purpose of the Miscellaneous, Multimedia, Comment, and EDI tabs. Pages 267–273	The Miscellaneous tab records a variety of miscellaneous information about the patient and his or her treatment, including information on outside lab work and lab charges as well the prior authorization number. The Multimedia tab is used to save a multimedia file, such as a picture file or a sound file, to a patient's case. The Comment tab is used to enter case notes that can be printed on statements if desired. The EDI tab is used to enter information for electronic claims specific to the case, such as for claims for home health care, hospice care, and vision services, as well as an insurance type code and various referral numbers.

chapter review

MATCHING QUESTIONS

Match the key terms with their definitions.

_____ 1. ***[LO 5.2]*** coordination of benefits

_____ 2. ***[LO 5.3]*** financial policy

_____ 3. ***[LO 5.2]*** birthday rule

_____ 4. ***[LO 5.1]*** guarantor

_____ 5. ***[LO 5.1]*** assignment of benefits

_____ 6. ***[LO 5.7]*** chart number

_____ 7. ***[LO 5.6]*** case

_____ 8. ***[LO 5.2]*** primary insurance plan

_____ 9. ***[LO 5.1]*** patient information form

_____ 10. ***[LO 5.1]*** registration

a. A unique alphanumeric code that identifies a patient.

b. Guidelines that ensure that when a patient has more than one policy, maximum appropriate benefits are paid, but without duplication.

c. Patient registration form.

d. Explains who is responsible for charges not paid by the carrier.

e. Subscriber.

f. A grouping of transactions that relate to a specific medical condition.

g. Authorization to allow benefits to be paid directly to a provider.

h. Process of gathering personal and insurance information about a patient at check-in.

i. First plan to be billed.

j. The parent whose day of birth is earlier in the calendar year holds the primary plan.

TRUE-FALSE QUESTIONS

Decide whether each statement is true or false.

_____ 1. ***[LO 5.1]*** On the patient registration form, the patient and the insured must always refer to the same person.

_____ 2. ***[LO 5.10]*** The Account tab contains basic information about a patient and his or her employment.

_____ 3. ***[LO 5.1]*** The Acknowledgment of Receipt of Notice of Privacy Practices states that the patient has received the document that states how the provider intends to protect the patient's rights to privacy under HIPAA.

_____ 4. ***[LO 5.1]*** Under the HIPAA Privacy Rule, providers do not need specific authorization to release patients' PHI for treatment, payment, and health care operations purposes.

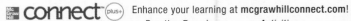

Enhance your learning at **mcgrawhillconnect.com**!
- *Practice Exercises*
- *Worksheets*
- *Activities*
- *Integrated eBook*

_____ 5. ***[LO 5.13]*** When laboratory claims are billed electronically, the Clinical Laboratory Improvement Act (CLIA) number must be included in the claim.

_____ 6. ***[LO 5.4]*** Some medical offices are now asking patients for partial payment of the office visit charges during check-in to increase cash flow.

_____ 7. ***[LO 5.11]*** Primary and secondary insurance claims are filed simultaneously to ensure prompt payment to the medical practice.

_____ 8. ***[LO 5.2]*** If a patient qualifies for Medicaid and Medicare, Medicaid is always considered the primary carrier and is billed accordingly.

_____ 9. ***[LO 5.7]*** An insurance carrier will not accept and process insurance claims for patients whose signatures are not on file with the medical practice.

_____ 10. ***[LO 5.12]*** Information about a patient's health is recorded in the Diagnosis and Condition tabs in Medisoft Network Professional.

MULTIPLE-CHOICE QUESTIONS

Select the letter that best completes the statement or answers the question.

1. ***[LO 5.5]*** _________ are used during patient encounters to track where patients are during the different steps of the encounter.
   a. patient information forms
   b. records of treatment and progress
   c. patient tracking features
   d. capitated plans

2. ***[LO 5.1]*** The medical history form contains all of the following EXCEPT _________.
   a. lifestyle factors, such as exercise and alcohol use
   b. medical conditions of family members
   c. details of prior surgeries, if any
   d. previous occupations held

3. ***[LO 5.1]*** The _________ form is used to collect basic demographic information about the patient.
   a. encounter
   b. patient information
   c. authorization
   d. coordination of benefits

4. ***[LO 5.1]*** Each of the terms below refers to the insured EXCEPT _________.
   a. guarantor
   b. policyholder
   c. subscriber
   d. preferred provider

5. ***[LO 5.1]*** The policyholder authorizes the physician to submit insurance claims for patients and receive payments directly by signing the ________ statement.
   a. assignment of benefits
   b. release authorization
   c. participating provider
   d. indemnity

6. ***[LO 5.1]*** If a provider thinks that a procedure will not be covered by Medicare, the patient is notified of this before the treatment by means of the ________ form.
   a. assignment of benefits
   b. advance beneficiary notice of noncoverage
   c. release authorization
   d. nonparticipating provider

7. ***[LO 5.2]*** ________ ensure that when patients have more than one policy, maximum appropriate benefits are paid.
   a. prior authorization numbers
   b. guarantors
   c. coordination of benefits guidelines
   d. walkout receipts

8. ***[LO 5.2]*** The process used to determine the primary insurance carrier if both parents cover dependents on their health insurance plans is called the ________.
   a. schedule of referrals
   b. birthday rule
   c. gender rule
   d. schedule of benefits

9. ***[LO 5.3]*** The financial policy of the practice addresses all of the following topics EXCEPT ________.
   a. assigned claims
   b. unassigned claims
   c. copayments
   d. referred claims

10. ***[LO 5.8]*** Which of the following options is *not* used for conducting searches in Medisoft Network Professional?
    a. Search for box
    b. Field box
    c. Locate buttons
    d. Quick Search button

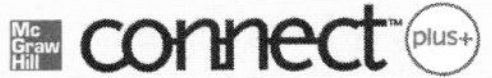

SHORT-ANSWER QUESTIONS

Define the following abbreviations.

1. ***[LO 5.1]*** ABN ________________________
2. ***[LO 5.2]*** COB ________________________
3. ***[LO 5.1]*** LCD ________________________

Create chart numbers for the following patients.

4. ***[LO 5.6]*** Phillip McKenzie ________________________
5. ***[LO 5.6]*** Sally T. Kim ____________________________

APPLYING YOUR KNOWLEDGE

Gathering Information

5.1 ***[LO 5.1]*** In the following list, put a *Y* (for *Yes*) before an item if it is routinely collected at registration and an *N* (for *No*) if it is not.

_____ Notice of Privacy Practices

_____ medical history

_____ insurance information

_____ copy of last bank statement

_____ copy of insurance card

_____ copy of living will

_____ advance beneficiary notice

_____ financial agreement and authorization for treatment

_____ assignment of benefits statement

_____ National Provider Identifier (NPI)

_____ Acknowledgment of Receipt of Notice of Privacy Practices

_____ HIPAA X12 837 transaction

_____ assignment of health care proxy

5.2 ***[LO 5.1]*** Refer to Tom Bridgewater's insurance card, and answer the following questions.

Insurance card

PROTECTION PLUS
HEALTH CARE OF NEW JERSEY
www.protectionplusnj.com

Tomas Bridgewater

2003.4916

OFC: **$15**
ER: **$50**
Rx: **$5/10**

Group: **6804 15**
Rel: **00**
Health Plan: **HMO Standard**
Effective Date: **05/01/2016**

a. What is the member's name? ________

b. What is the member's ID number? ________

c. What is the amount of the copayment due when the patient goes to the emergency room? ________

d. What is the date on which the coverage became effective? ________

e. What is the copayment for generic prescriptions? ________

f. What type of insurance plan does the patient have? ________

Evaluating Information

Consider the following situations.

5.3 ***[LO 5.2]*** Maria is twelve years old and is an established patient. She has flu symptoms and is checking in for an appointment. Her family has gone through a number of changes since Maria's last visit. Her parents are divorced, and her mother has recently remarried. Maria now lives full time with her mother and stepfather. Her mother is no longer working and does not have an independent health plan. However, her father and stepfather both have health insurance plans that include her.

____

Which plan is Maria's primary health plan? Why?

5.4 ***[LO 5.3]*** Brian's medical bills are quite large. He would like to make a financial arrangement that would allow him to make monthly payments. What steps do you need to take to facilitate this?

____

5.5 ***[LO 5.2]*** Tasha Maritski is enrolled in an indemnity plan through her employment. She is also a Medicare beneficiary. Who is her primary payer, the indemnity plan or Medicare, and why?

____

chapter 6

Office Visit: Patient Intake

KEY TERMS

family history (FH)
history of present illness (HPI)
past, family, and social history (PFSH)
past medical history (PMH)
patient flow
progress notes
review of systems (ROS)
social history (SH)

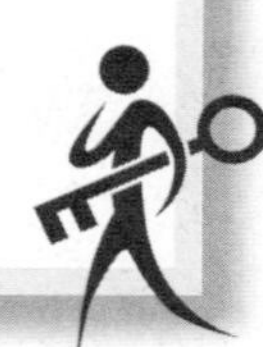

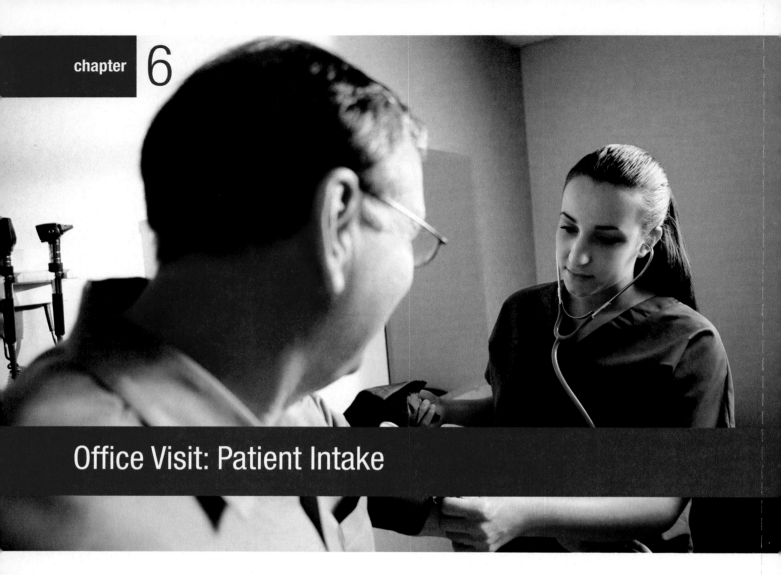

LEARNING OUTCOMES

When you finish this chapter, you will be able to:

6.1 Identify the four stages of patient flow.

6.2 Discuss the main sections of the patient chart.

6.3 Describe the procedures for recording a patient's past medical, family, and social history.

6.4 Explain how allergies and intolerances are entered in the patient chart.

6.5 Describe the procedure used to enter patient medications.

6.6 Explain how the chief complaint is recorded in a progress note.

6.7 Explain how a patient's vital signs are recorded in the patient chart.

6.8 Explain the uses of an intra-office messaging system in an EHR.

6.9 Describe how letters are created in an EHR.

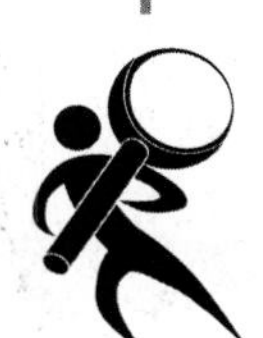

The Tradeoff...

The Family Care Clinic has had the new PM/EHR program for a little over a month.

Tiffany Patel, the consultant helping with the implementation, has come by to see how things are going. She finds out that Alex Horowitz, the medical assistant, has been writing down some of the patient information on paper during patient intake and entering it in the EHR later in the day. She catches up with Alex on his afternoon break and asks him about it.

"It's fine if they have one or two medications, but some of these patients have eight or ten," Alex responded. "How am I supposed to enter all those while in the exam room with the patient? I like to try and make the patient comfortable, especially when they are new to the practice. It's pretty hard to do that if you have your nose in the computer," said Alex.

As you read this chapter, think about the problem that Alex is experiencing. Is he doing the right thing by making notes on paper and entering them later? Do you see any possible consequences of not entering medications while in the exam room with the patient? Can you think of a solution to this problem?

WHEN YOU FINISH THIS CHAPTER, YOU WILL ALSO BE ABLE TO USE MEDISOFT CLINICAL TO:

1. Open a patient's chart.
2. Record a patient's past medical, family, and social history.
3. Record a patient's allergies and intolerances.
4. Record a patient's medications.
5. Create a progress note and record the chief complaint.
6. Record a patient's vital signs.
7. Create and retrieve intra-office messages.
8. Create letters to patients.

SOFTWARE SKILLS

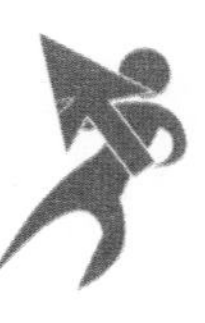

6.1 Patient Flow in the Physician Office

patient flow the progression of patients from the time they enter the office for a visit until they exit the system by leaving the office after a visit

Where does the information in a patient chart come from? Much of it comes from activities that occur during the stages of patient flow. The term **patient flow** refers to the progression of patients from the time they enter the office for a visit until they exit the system by leaving the office after a visit. A typical patient flow consists of four stages (see Figure 6.1).

Note: The term *medical assistant* is used frequently throughout this book to refer to the person performing clinical tasks. In actual practice, the person performing the task may also be a nurse or other health care professional.

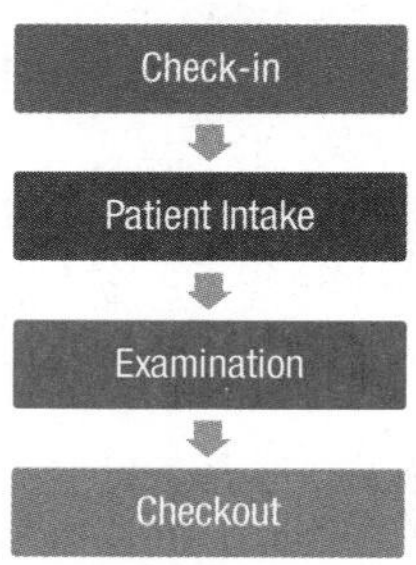

Figure 6.1 The Stages of Patient Flow

Check-in

During check-in, the patient arrives at the office and proceeds to the front desk. The front desk staff member checks the patient in, recording the time he or she arrived. This places the patient in the queue of patients waiting to see the provider. The staff member confers with the patient to determine whether any information, such as a change in insurance or employment, needs to be updated in the patient record. The patient may be asked for payment at the time of check-in. Once check-in is complete, the patient takes a seat in the waiting room.

Patient Intake

The patient is escorted to the exam room, where the medical assistant interviews him or her to obtain detailed information. The interview varies depending on the nature of the visit and whether the patient is new or established. Generally, the purpose of the interview is to:

- Obtain past medical, family, and social history
- Review allergies and medications
- Determine the chief complaint

Once the interview is complete, the medical assistant measures the patient's vital signs and prepares the patient for the examination. After the medical assistant has completed these tasks, the provider is notified that the patient is ready to be seen.

Examination

The provider reviews the patient's previous records, and then enters the room and examines the patient. During the encounter, the provider may order lab work or diagnostic tests. Medications may be prescribed. The provider develops a treatment plan and completes the examination. The details of the encounter must be documented. Some providers document the patient encounter during the visit, while others prefer to document the encounter later that same day.

Checkout

The patient leaves the exam room and proceeds to the checkout desk. During checkout, the office staff gives the patient any additional information required, such as patient education materials or lab work instructions. If necessary, a follow-up appointment is scheduled. Before the patient leaves, the staff member collects any payment that is due, if it was not collected during check-in.

This chapter provides detailed instructions on how to perform the steps that are completed by a medical assistant, nurse, or another member of the clinical staff. The steps completed by the physician or other health care provider are covered in Chapter 7.

Table 6.1 lists the steps of patient flow for a typical office visit. It shows both the tasks performed in a paper office and those performed in an office with an integrated practice management/electronic health record (PM/EHR) system.

Information Collected During Patient Flow

The clinical information collected during patient flow and recorded in the patient's chart includes the following:

- **Vital signs:** Measurements of a patient's temperature, respiratory rate, pulse, and blood pressure, height, and weight.
- **Chief complaint:** A brief description of the patient's current problem in his or her own words.
- **Progress notes:** **Progress notes** are notes documenting the care delivered to a patient, and the medical facts and clinical thinking relevant to diagnosis and treatment.
- **Past, family, and social history (PFSH): Past, family, and social history (PFSH)** is a commonly used abbreviation for past medical, family, and social history.
    - **Past medical history:** The **past medical history (PMH)** is the patient's history of medical problems, including chronic conditions, surgeries, and hospitalizations. This includes any illness (past or present) for which the patient has received treatment.
    - **Family history:** The **family history (FH)** details medical events among members of the patient's family, including the ages, living status, and diseases of siblings, children, parents, and grandparents. This includes diseases related to the chief complaint as well as any hereditary diseases.
    - **Social history:** The **social history (SH)** is information about the patient's tobacco use, alcohol and drug use, sexual history, relationship status, and other significant social facts that may contribute to the care of the patient.
- **Allergies:** A list of the patient's known allergies, including reactions to each one.

progress note note documenting the care delivered to a patient, and the medical facts and clinical thinking relevant to diagnosis and treatment

past, family, and social history (PFSH) a commonly used abbreviation for past medical, family, and social history

past medical history (PMH) the patient's history of medical problems, including chronic conditions, surgeries, and hospitalizations

family history (FH) a detailed record of medical events among members of the patient's family, including the ages, living status, and diseases of siblings, children, parents, and grandparents

social history (SH) information about the patient's tobacco use, alcohol and drug use, sexual history, relationship status, and other significant social facts that may contribute to the care of the patient

TABLE 6.1 Patient Flow in a Paper Office and an Office with a PM/EHR

Step	Paper Office	PM/EHR Office
Pre-Visit	Charts pulled for patients with appointments.	Daily schedule viewed in EHR.
Check-in	Patient completes or updates patient information form and HIPAA forms.	Patient completes or updates patient information form and HIPAA forms, which are scanned and stored in EHR.
	Insurance card and driver's license are photocopied.	Insurance card and driver's license are scanned and stored in EHR.
	Front desk looks in patient chart to see notes about overdue balance.	System alerts front desk if patient has overdue balance.
	Encounter form is placed in patient chart.	No paper encounter form is needed (now electronic).
	Chart is placed in bin for medical assistant (MA) or nurse; light turned on to notify MA or nurse that patient is checked in and ready for exam.	Message is sent in EHR to notify MA or nurse that patient has checked in and is ready for exam.
	Patient is escorted to exam room.	Patient is escorted to exam room.
Patient Intake	If new patient, MA or nurse interviews patient and writes past medical, family, and social history in patient chart.	If new patient, MA or nurse interviews patient and records past medical, family, and social history in EHR.
	MA or nurse reviews and updates medications and allergies in paper chart.	MA or nurse reviews and updates medications and allergies in EHR.
	MA or nurse records chief complaint in paper chart.	MA or nurse records chief complaint in EHR.
	MA or nurse takes vital signs and records them on paper form.	MA or nurse takes vital signs and enters them directly into patient chart in EHR.
	MA or nurse uses flag or light to notify physician that patient is ready; patient chart is placed in bin for physician.	MA or nurse sends electronic message in EHR to notify physician that patient is ready.
Examination	Physician picks up chart from bin, enters exam room, and reviews information in the chart.	Physician reviews patient chart in EHR, including today's vital signs and chief complaint.
	Physician examines patient.	Physician examines patient.
	Physician documents exam in paper chart during visit or later in the day. May use dictation.	Physician documents exam in EHR. May use templates.
	If prescription is required, physician writes it and gives it to patient.	If prescription is required, physician enters electronic prescription and transmits it to patient's pharmacy.
	If follow-up, referral, or tests are required, physician writes information on encounter form.	If follow-up, referral, or tests are required, physician enters orders in EHR.
	If patient education materials are required, physician notes that on encounter form, and checkout staff member locates paper materials to give to patient.	If patient education materials are required, physician prints them directly from EHR and hands them to patient.
	If additional procedures are required, physician uses flag or light system to alert medical assistant or nurse.	If additional procedures are required, physician sends electronic message to medical assistant or nurse.
	Medical assistant or nurse performs procedures.	Medical assistant or nurse performs procedures.
	If labs are required, MA or nurse locates paper form to write lab orders.	If labs are required, MA or nurse enters lab orders in EHR; order is transmitted electronically to lab.

(continued)

TABLE 6.1 *(continued)*

Step	Paper Office	PM/EHR Office
	MA or nurse records additional procedures on encounter form.	MA or nurse records additional procedures in EHR.
	Patient leaves exam room and proceeds to checkout desk.	Patient leaves exam room and proceeds to checkout desk.
Checkout	Coder reviews documentation in paper chart, assigns codes, and records them on encounter form.	Coder reviews documentation in EHR and assigns codes on electronic encounter form in EHR.
	Patient chart with instructions for follow-up, referral, tests, and so on and encounter form arrive at checkout desk.	Electronic message is sent to checkout desk with instructions for follow-up, referral, tests, and so on and link to electronic encounter form.
	Checkout staff member writes instructions for referral, tests, and so on; schedules follow-up appointment; and completes appointment card for patient.	Checkout staff member prints instructions for referral, tests, and so on from EHR; schedules follow-up appointment; and prints appointment reminder for patient.
	Checkout staff reviews encounter form to see whether payment is due.	Encounter information is transmitted electronically from EHR to PM.
	Payment is collected and recorded on encounter form; patient is given handwritten receipt.	Billing staff member reviews charges and payments in PM, and clicks button to electronically post charges in PM.
	Billing staff member reviews charges and payments on encounter form.	Checkout staff member views patient account in PM to see whether payment is due.
	Billing staff member enters charges and payments in PM.	Payment is collected and entered in PM; receipt is printed.

- **Medication list:** Includes all currently prescribed medications as well as over-the-counter medications and nontraditional therapies. Dosage and frequency should be noted.
- **History of present illness (HPI):** The **history of present illness (HPI)** is a description of the course of the present illness, including how and when the problem began, up to the present time. The HPI includes everything related to the illness or condition, including aggravating and alleviating factors, associated symptoms, previous treatment and diagnostic tests, related illnesses, and risk factors.
- **Review of systems (ROS):** The **review of systems (ROS)** is an inventory of body systems in which the patient reports signs or symptoms he or she is currently having or has had in the past.
- **Diagnosis and assessment:** The physician's thinking about the cause of the patient's problem as well as any tests performed to come to this determination.
- **Plan and treatment:** The physician's thinking about the intervention that will be necessary to cure or manage the patient's condition, including medications, procedures, and lifestyle changes.

history of present illness (HPI) a description of the course of the present illness, including how and when the problem began, up to the present time

review of systems (ROS) an inventory of body systems in which the patient reports signs or symptoms he or she is currently having or has had in the past

THINKING IT THROUGH 6.1

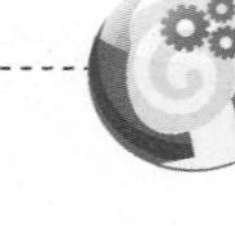

Table 6.1 compares the patient flow performed in an office using paper records with an office using computerized records. Explain why an office with computerized records is likely to have fewer medical errors.

6.2 The Patient Chart in Medisoft Clinical Patient Records

Most of the information in an electronic health record program such as Medisoft Clinical Patient Records (MCPR) is stored in the electronic version of the patient chart. The first step in opening a patient chart is to select Open Chart on the File menu or to click the chart button on the toolbar, which opens the Patient Lookup dialog box (see Figure 6.2).

The Patient Lookup Dialog Box

The Patient Lookup dialog box is used to select a patient (see Figure 6.2). There are three tabs in the Patient Lookup dialog box: General, Name, and ID.

The General Tab

The search options on the General tab include:

Patient Name Enter the patient's last name, first name, and middle initial. The Sounds Like box is used to search for names that sound similar to the name entered, even though the spelling may be different. The practice name, provider name, and birth date may also be added as additional search filters.

Patient ID Enter the patient's chart number.

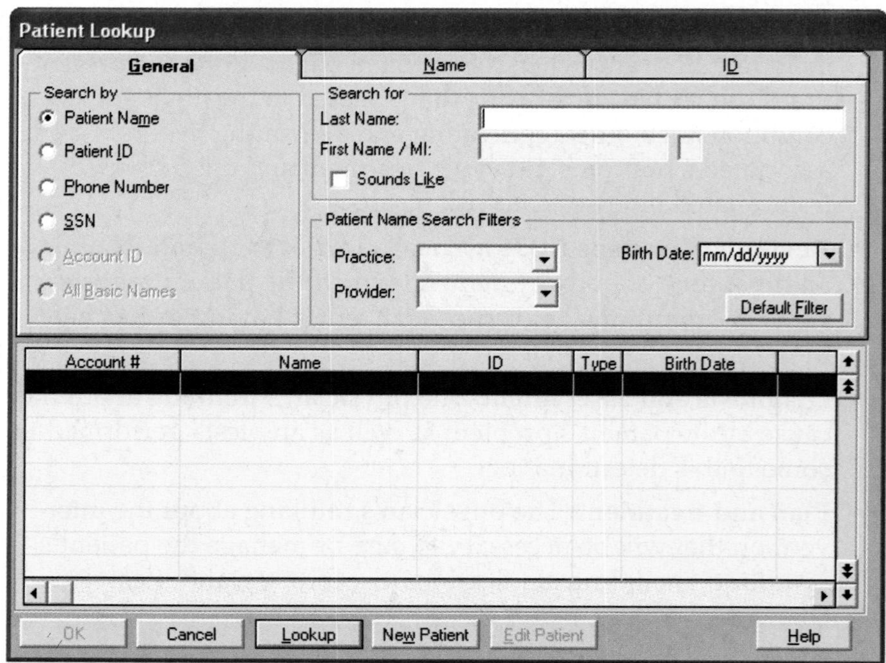

Figure 6.2 The Patient Lookup Dialog Box

Phone Number Enter the patient's home telephone number.

SSN Enter the patient's Social Security number.

The Account ID and All Basic Names options are not available.

The Name tab and the ID tab provide additional search capability. Once the search parameters are set, clicking the Lookup button begins the search.

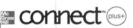

connect plus+ **EXERCISE 6.1**

USING THE PATIENT LOOKUP DIALOG BOX TO OPEN A PATIENT CHART

Log in as the medical assistant, Alex Horowitz, and use the Patient Lookup dialog box to open Jorge Barrett's patient chart.

1. Start Medisoft Clinical Patient Records.
2. On the Medisoft Clinical Sign In screen, enter ***MEDASST*** in the User ID field and ***master1$*** in the Password field. Click OK. When the disclaimer notice appears, click OK again.
3. Select Open Chart on the File menu, or click the Chart toolbar button. The Patient Lookup dialog box appears.
4. Select the radio button to search by patient name.
5. Enter ***BA*** in the Last Name field, and click the Lookup button. A list of patients with last names beginning with the letters *BA* is displayed.
6. Notice that Jorge Barrett's name is already selected. Click the OK button. The patient's chart is displayed.

 **You have completed Exercise 6.1**

Organization of the Patient Chart in Medisoft Clinical Patient Records

In MCPR, the chart is organized in much the same way as most paper-based medical records systems. The chart contains a collection of folders. Folders that do not have labels are available for custom use by the practice.

The main sections of the patient chart window, displayed in Figure 6.3, include:

- Patient identifying information (at the top and the bottom of the window)
- Chart folders (similar to paper folders)
- Notes area (used to enter notes about the patient)

A folder that contains information has a blue rectangle in the upper-right corner. Folders without information have empty yellow rectangles in the upper-right corner (see Figure 6.4).

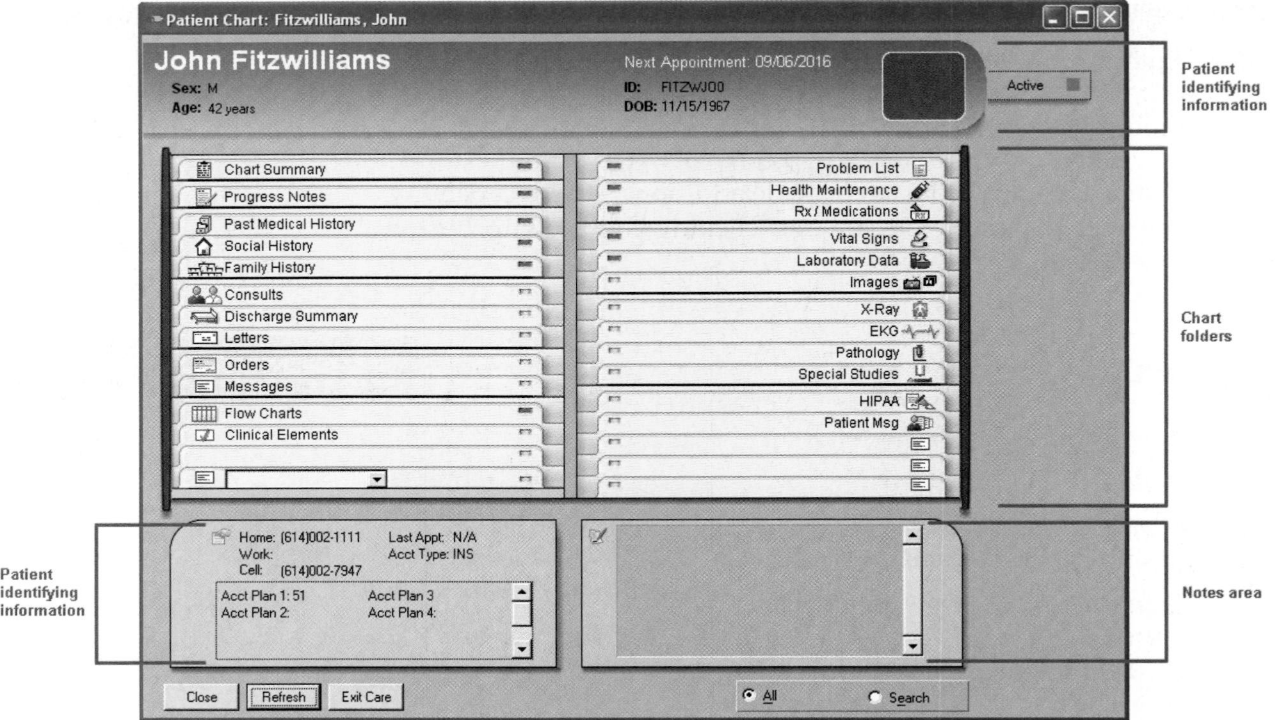

Figure 6.3 The Patient Chart in Medisoft Clinical Patient Records

Not all sections of the Patient Chart screen are discussed in this chapter. The focus is on providing an overall understanding of the features of an EHR system, and a closer look at the tasks often performed by allied health professionals. Chapter 7 discusses the sections of the chart used by physicians and other health care providers. The chart folders discussed in this chapter include:

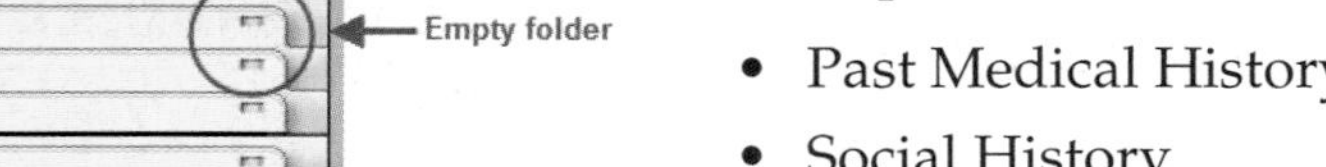

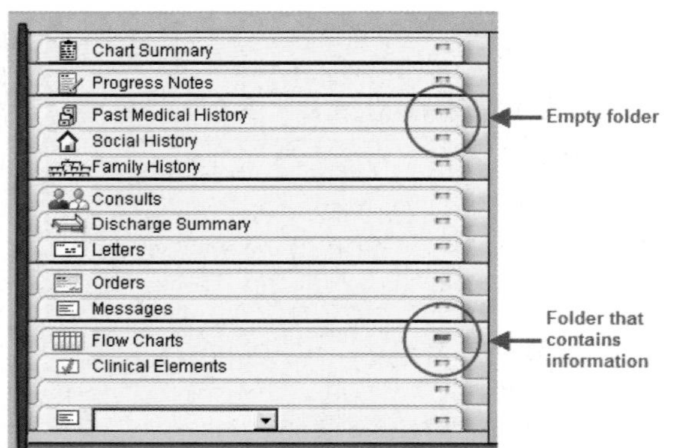

Figure 6.4 Folders in the Patient Chart

- Past Medical History
- Social History
- Family History
- Rx/Medications
- Progress Notes
- Vital Signs
- Messages
- Letters

6.3 Medical History

The medical history section of the patient chart includes three folders:

- **Past Medical History** Chronic illnesses, hospitalizations, and other health information
- **Social History** Medically relevant information about the patient's life, such as marital status, tobacco and alcohol use, habits, and work

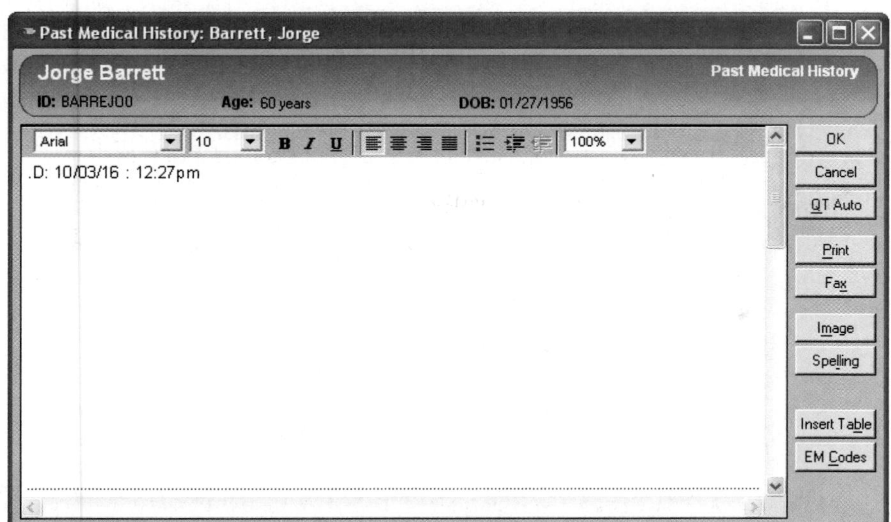

Figure 6.5 The Past Medical History Dialog Box

- **Family History** Medically relevant information about the patient's family, including major diseases and chronic conditions

The History Dialog Boxes

Each history section of the chart consists of a single note. There is no limit on the length of the note. The information recorded in the history folders of the patient chart can be completed by typing in the note or with the aid of templates. The exercises in this chapter use typing; the use of templates is covered in Chapter 7.

To enter a patient's history, open a patient's chart, and click the appropriate history folder. If no history note exists, a message appears asking whether you would like to create a new note. Clicking the Yes button causes a new note window to appear (see Figure 6.5).

In Medisoft Clinical Patient Records, a history note always contains a heading with the date and time. To enter information in the note, click in the body of the note below the date and time and begin typing. When finished, click the OK button to save the note.

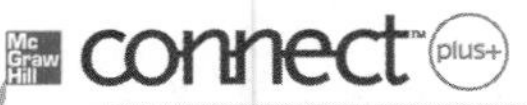

EXERCISE 6.2

ENTERING A PATIENT'S PAST MEDICAL HISTORY

Using Source Document 3, enter Jorge Barrett's past medical history.

1. Select Open Chart on the File menu, or click the Chart button on the toolbar. The Patient Lookup dialog box appears.
2. Confirm that the Search by selection is Patient Name, and enter ***BA*** in the Last Name field.
3. Click the Lookup button. When the list of patients appears, confirm that Jorge Barrett is selected, and click OK to open his chart. The patient's chart is displayed.
4. Click the Past Medical History folder. A message box appears stating that no past medical history exists for the patient and asking whether you want to create a new note. Click the Yes button to continue. The Past Medical History window appears.

(continued)

(Continued)

5. Enter the patient's medical history from Source Document 3.
6. When you are finished, click the OK button to save the note. The window closes, and you are returned to the chart.
7. Notice that the Past Medical History folder does not have a blue rectangle indicating that it contains data. Press the Refresh button to update the screen. The blue rectangle appears.
8. Now click the Past Medical History folder to review the note you just entered.

You have completed Exercise 6.2

EXERCISE 6.3

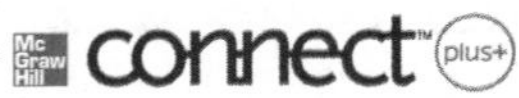

ENTERING A PATIENT'S SOCIAL HISTORY

Using Source Document 3, enter Jorge Barrett's social history.

1. Click the Social History folder. A message box appears stating that no social history exists for the patient and asking whether you want to create a new note. Click the Yes button to continue. The Social History window appears.
2. Enter the patient's social history using Source Document 3.
3. When you are finished, click OK.
4. Open the Social History folder, and review your work.

You have completed Exercise 6.3

EXERCISE 6.4

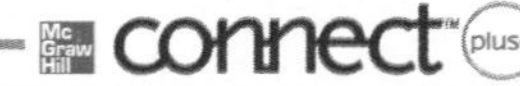

ENTERING A PATIENT'S FAMILY HISTORY

Using Source Document 3, enter Jorge Barrett's family history.

1. Click the Family History folder. A message box appears stating that no family history exists for the patient and asking whether you want to create a new note. Click the Yes button to continue. The Family History window appears.
2. Enter the patient's family history from Source Document 3.
3. Click the OK button to save the note. The window closes, and you are returned to the chart.
4. Open the Family History folder to review the note you just entered.

You have completed Exercise 6.4

6.4 Allergies

When a new medication is prescribed for a patient, MCPR checks whether the patient has any allergies or intolerances. While an allergy is a relative rare condition in which the immune system responds to a medication and causes adverse effects, an intolerance is generally a milder reaction, and does not involve the immune system. For example, an antibiotic may cause stomach upset, which is considered an intolerance and not an allergy. Intolerance can sometimes be eliminated by taking medication with food or by lowering the dosage.

Patient allergies are recorded and stored in the Rx/Medications folder of the patient chart. When the folder is clicked, the Rx/Medications dialog box is displayed. The top section of the Rx/Medications dialog box lists information about allergies or intolerances (see Figure 6.6).

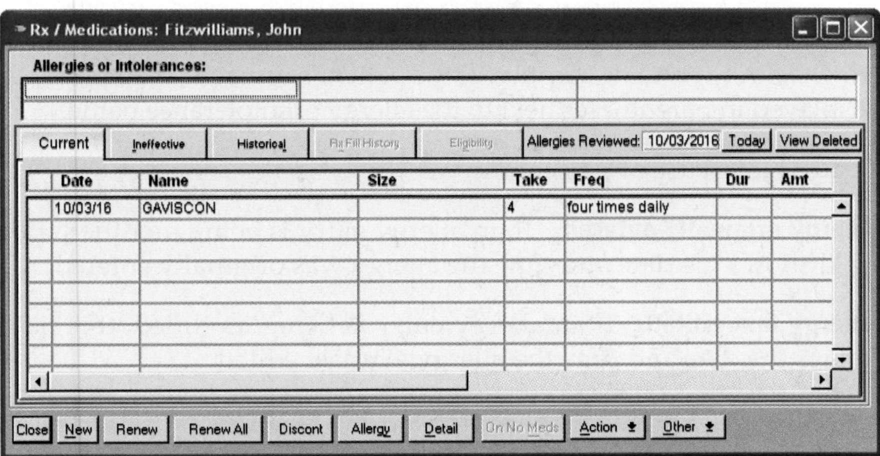

Figure 6.6 The Rx/Medications Dialog Box with Allergies or Intolerances Highlighted

In addition to adding, editing, or deleting allergies and intolerances, the program also records the date the allergies were last reviewed. This information is displayed in the box to the right of the Allergies Reviewed label. When the Today button is clicked, the program automatically enters today's date in the field. The View Deleted button allows you to see any allergies or intolerances that were deleted in the past.

The Allergy Dialog Box

To add a patient's allergies and intolerances, click the Allergy button in the bottom row of the Rx/Medications dialog box. When the button is clicked, the Allergy dialog box is displayed (see Figure 6.7). When an allergy or intolerance is added, it is displayed in the Allergies or Intolerances list at the top of the Rx/Medications dialog box.

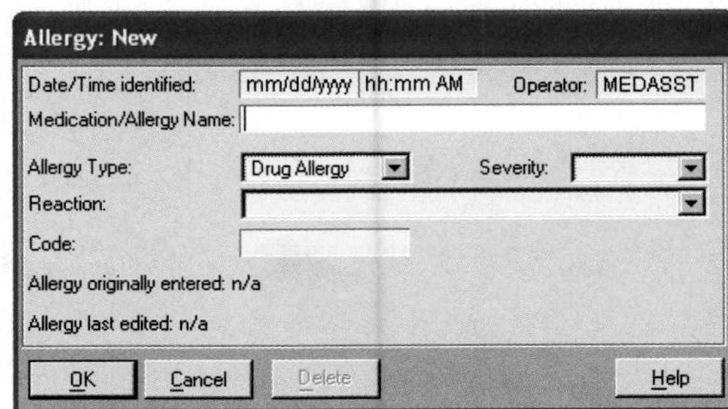

Figure 6.7 The Allergy Dialog Box

The fields in the Allergy dialog box include:

Date/Time identified Enter the date and time (if known) the patient's first allergic reaction occurred.

Operator Identifies the operator who is logged in to the program.

Medication/Allergy Name Enter the medication or allergy name. If the allergy is to a medication, to save time you can type the first few letters of the drug name and press the Help button. The Select Drug Name dialog box opens with a list of possible drugs. To select a drug, click the drug name and then click OK. The program inserts the drug into the Medication/Allergy Name field.

Allergy Type Select the allergy type—Drug Allergy, Drug Intolerance, Miscellaneous, Food Allergy—from the drop-down list.

Severity Select the severity of the allergy—Severe, Moderate, Mild—from the drop-down list.

Reaction Select the patient's reaction to the medication from the drop-down list, or type a description of the patient's reaction. The reaction is displayed in parentheses next to the allergy or intolerance name.

Code Not in use at present.

Allergy originally entered If an allergy entry is being modified, this field shows the date and time the allergy was originally entered.

Allergy last edited If an allergy entry is being modified, this field shows the date and time the allergy was last edited.

Once these fields have been completed, clicking the OK button saves the allergy information and adds it to the list at the top of the Rx/Medications dialog box. *Note:* If the medical assistant does not have enough information to complete any of the fields, those fields should remain blank.

EXERCISE 6.5

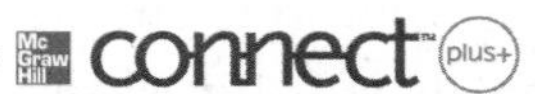

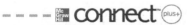

ENTERING A PATIENT ALLERGY AND AN INTOLERANCE

Using Source Document 3, enter Jorge Barrett's allergies and intolerances.

1. Click the Rx/Medications folder. The Rx/Medications dialog box appears.
2. Click the Allergy button. The Allergy dialog box opens.
3. Review the information in Source Document 3.
4. Since the patient cannot remember when the allergy was first identified, leave the Date/Time fields blank.
5. In the Medication/Allergy Name field, enter ***SULFA***.
6. In the Allergy Type field, select Drug Allergy.
7. Select Mild in the Severity field.

8. In the Reaction field, select Skin Rash.
9. Click the OK button. Notice that sulfa is now listed in the Allergies or Intolerances section at the top of the Rx/Medications dialog box.
10. Click the Allergy button again.
11. Review the information in Source Document 3.
12. Since the patient cannot remember when the intolerance was first identified, leave the Date/Time fields blank.
13. In the Medication/Allergy Name field, enter ***CODEINE.***
14. In the Allergy Type field, select Drug Intolerance.
15. Select Mild in the Severity field.
16. In the Reaction field, select Nausea/Vomiting/Diarrhea.
17. Click the OK button to save your work. Notice that codeine is listed in the Allergies or Intolerances section of the Rx/Medications dialog box.
18. Click the Close button to close the Rx/Medications dialog box

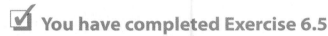

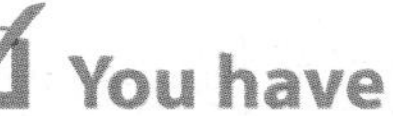 **You have completed Exercise 6.5**

6.5 Medications

In many medical offices, a medical assistant is responsible for reviewing medication lists with patients when they come in for an office visit. The patient or a family member is asked to look at the list of current medications and indicate whether anything has changed. Medications that have been added, discontinued, or changed are noted in the patient chart.

This section covers how to record patient medications in the patient chart. Creating and refilling prescriptions are covered in Chapter 7.

The Rx/Medications Dialog Box

Figure 6.8 shows the Rx/Medications dialog box for a patient. There are three tabs in the Rx/Medications dialog box:

1. **Current** Lists current medications
2. **Ineffective** Lists discontinued medications that were ineffective
3. **Historical** Lists discontinued medications that were effective

Note: The Rx Fill History and Eligibility tabs are active only when the ePrescribing feature is active. Since the exercises in this book do not permit the transmission of prescriptions, this feature is not active.

The Current Tab

The Current tab lists a patient's current medications, including information about the dose and frequency. The process of recording a patient's current medications begins with clicking the New button

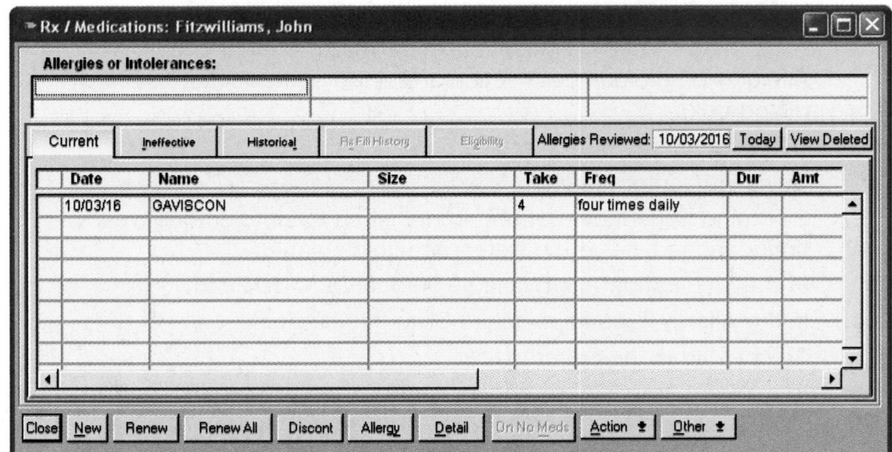

Figure 6.8 The Rx/Medications Dialog Box with the Medications Area Highlighted

Prescription: Fitzwilliams, John <New>

Rx Template Code: Lookup by Template Code by Indication(s)

Date Medication Size

10/03/16

Take Frequency PRN Route ORAL

Duration Amount Refills

Print: Print locally immediately Prov: Outside

Indication 1: Lookup 1

Indication 2: Lookup 2

Note:

Pharmacy:

Formulary:

Plan:

Details Alternatives

Extended Sig:

Code: Lookup

Create Sig Template

Use Extended Sig Limit Refills Drug Interaction Check New Rx Template

Use Extended Sig Only Substitution OK Allergy Check

Use Patient Instructions Update Progress Note OTC

Wholesale: per unit. Total: Generic: per unit. Total:

Actual Total:

OK Cancel Alternative... Dose Advisor Help

Figure 6.9 The Prescription Dialog Box

in the Current tab of the Rx/Medications folder. When the New button is clicked, the Prescription dialog box appears (see Figure 6.9). This is the same dialog box that is used by a physician to prescribe a new medication. In this chapter, the dialog box is used to record the patient's current medications, not to create a new prescription. As a result, only the fields used to record a patient's current medications are discussed in this section. The remaining fields are covered in Chapter 7.

The fields in the Prescription dialog box include:

Rx Template Code To find a specific medication, enter a template code or drug name in this field.

Date The date the medication is recorded in the program. The default value is today's date.

Medication Enter the medication name. To save time and reduce errors, it is possible to enter one or more letters of the drug name, click the Help button, and select the drug from a list of medications in the program.

Size Enter the size of the pill, such as 20 mg. The maximum length of an entry in this box is 25 characters.

Take Enter the number of doses the patient is taking.

Frequency Enter how often the medication is taken.

PRN Select this box if the medication is taken as needed.

Route Select the route of medication administration from a drop-down list, or type in the field. The maximum entry length is 20 characters.

Duration Specify how long the patient is taking the medication. Either type the number in days, enter "PRN," or leave blank if the medication is taken continuously, such as for a chronic condition.

Prov If the prescription has been written by a provider in the current practice, enter the prescribing physician's code.

Outside If the prescription has been written by a physician other than a provider in this practice, click this box.

Note Enter a note if appropriate.

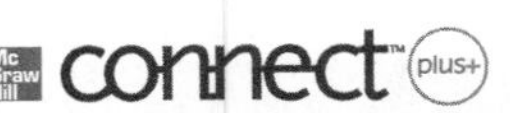

EXERCISE 6.6

ENTERING A PATIENT'S MEDICATIONS

Using Source Document 3, enter Jorge Barrett's medications.

1. Click the Rx/Medications folder. The Rx/Medications dialog box appears.
2. Click the New button. The Prescription dialog box opens.
3. Accept the default entry in the Date field.
4. Enter ***MAX*** in the Rx Template Code field, and click the Lookup button. The Select Rx Template dialog box is displayed.
5. Locate MAXALT10 on the list, and click the line to select it. Click the OK button. The Select Rx Template dialog box closes, and MAXALT appears in the Medication field.
6. Notice that some of the fields have been completed by the program.

(continued)

(Continued)

7. Click the Outside box to indicate that the medication has been prescribed by a physician who is not in the practice.
8. Click the OK button to save the entries. The Prescription dialog box closes, and you are returned to the Rx/Medications folder.
9. Confirm that MAXALT appears in the Current tab.

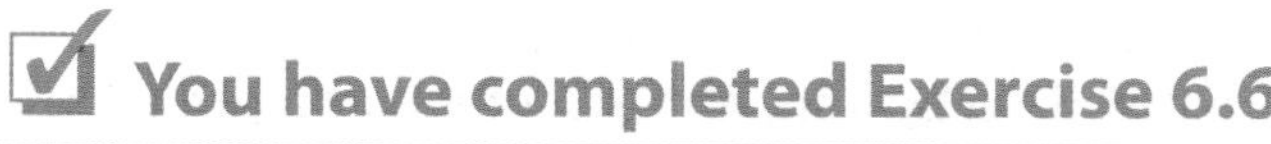

6.6 The Chief Complaint

In most practices, the chief complaint is entered as the title of the progress note for the patient's visit. Progress notes can be created only when a patient chart is open. To create a new note, click the Note button on the toolbar. To open an existing note, click the Progress Notes folder in the patient chart.

The progress note always contains a heading with the date and time and a placeholder for a note title (see Figure 6.10). The date line begins with.Date:, followed by the date and time. The note title line begins with.Title:, followed by a blue placeholder label. The title line is used to record the chief complaint or title of the patient visit. Text is entered to the right of the placeholder label. If more than one title is needed, a colon must be entered between each entry. Up to five titles can be entered on the title line. Once the title has been entered, click the OK button to save the note.

While the creation of progress notes is introduced in this section, Chapter 7 covers progress notes in detail.

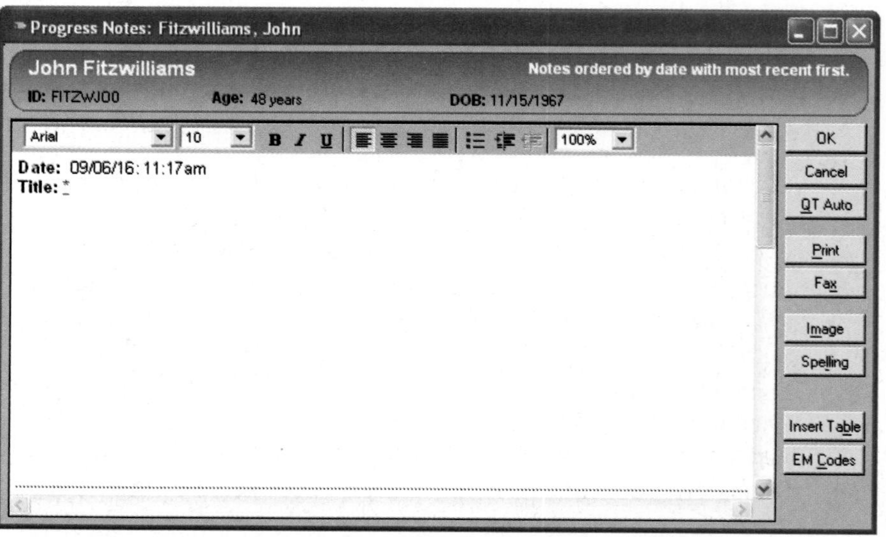

Figure 6.10 The Progress Notes Dialog Box

Shared Progress Notes

In Medisoft Clinical Patient Records, progress notes can be written by more than one person. A shared note is commonly needed when a medical assistant or nurse begins a note, and a physician completes the note. If a progress note has been started but is not complete, it can be saved as an incomplete note by clicking No when asked whether you are permanently finished with the note (see Figure 6.11).

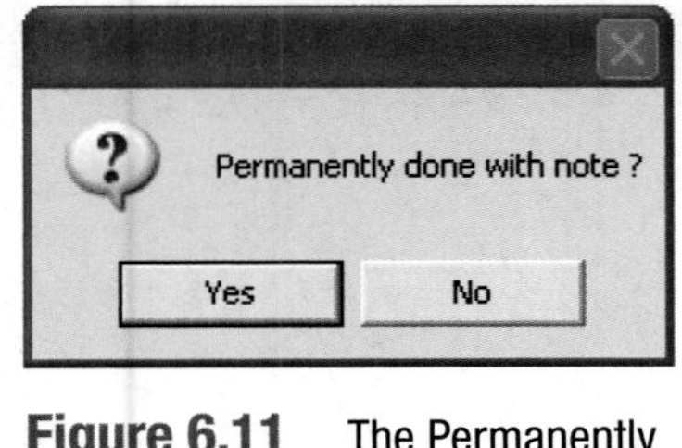

Figure 6.11 The Permanently Done with Note Message Box

Signing Shared Progress Notes

A feature in Medisoft Clinical Patient Records allows a shared note to be signed by each person who contributes to the note. To sign an incomplete note, "^Shared_Note_Signature" is entered into the progress note. The program then prompts the user for his or her signature PIN. Once the PIN is entered, the signature is added to the note. Figure 6.12 shows a partially complete note signed by the medical assistant.

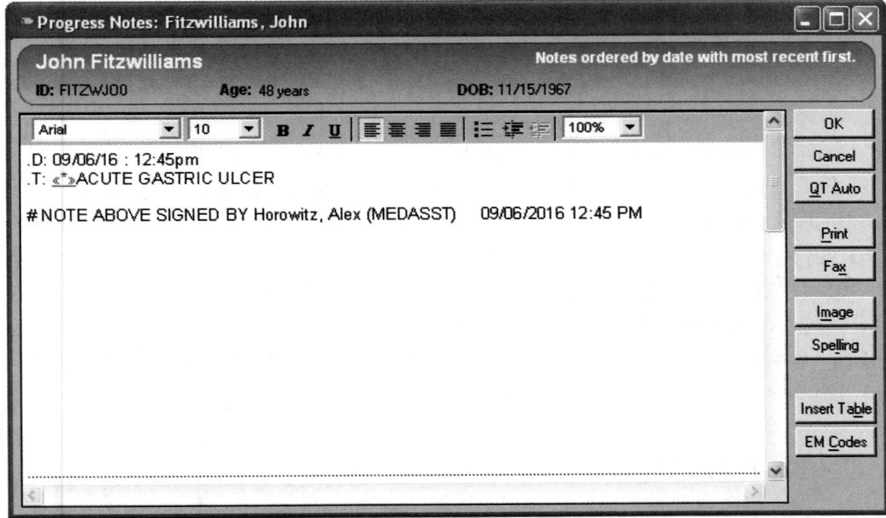

Figure 6.12 A Signature in an Incomplete Shared Note

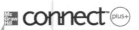

EXERCISE 6.7

CREATING A PROGRESS NOTE AND RECORDING A CHIEF COMPLAINT

Using Source Document 3, create a progress note for Jorge Barrett, and enter the chief complaint for today's visit on the title line of the note.

1. Click the Note button on the toolbar.
2. Click just to the right of the * symbol, and enter ***HYPERTENSION.***
3. Press Enter twice to move down two lines in the note.

(continued)

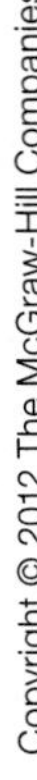

(Continued)

4. To sign the note, enter ***^Shared_Note_Signature.***
5. Click the OK button to save the note. A dialog box appears asking whether you are permanently done with the note. Since the physician will complete the note, click the No button.
6. The Enter Signature dialog box appears. Enter ***1234,*** in the Signature field, which is the medical assistant's signature PIN.
7. Press the OK button. The Progress Notes dialog box closes.
8. To view the progress note with the medical assistant's signature, click the Note button on the toolbar.
9. In response to the question about opening a shared note, click Yes.
10. The note opens, listing the medical assistant's signature, including the time and date of the signature.
11. Click Cancel to close the note. In response to the question about leaving without saving changes, click Yes. The note is closed.

 **You have completed Exercise 6.7**

6.7 Vital Signs

Patients' vital sign measurements are entered in the Vital Signs folder in the patient chart. The dialog box displayed in Figure 6.13 lists a patient's vital signs, including height, weight, temperature, pulse, systolic blood pressure, and diastolic blood pressure, among others. Vital signs taken over a period of time can be viewed in a table or a graph. Abnormal values are highlighted in red (high) or blue (low) on the Vital Signs screen. Blood pressure readings can be entered manually or imported from a digital monitor.

The Vital Signs (New) Dialog Box

To enter a new set of vital signs, click the New button. The Vital Signs (New) dialog box is displayed (see Figure 6.14).

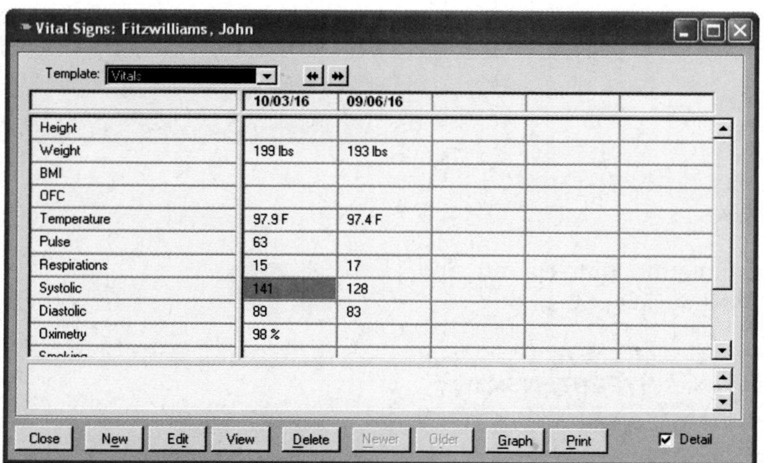

Figure 6.13 The Vital Signs Dialog Box

The fields in the Vital Signs dialog box that require numeric entry, such as weight, height, temperature, OFC, pulse, and blood pressure, contain a numeric keypad feature that is accessed via a drop-down list. Numeric entries can be entered by using this keypad, or they can be typed directly in the field.

The fields in the Vital Signs (New) dialog box include:

Date The current date is automatically displayed.

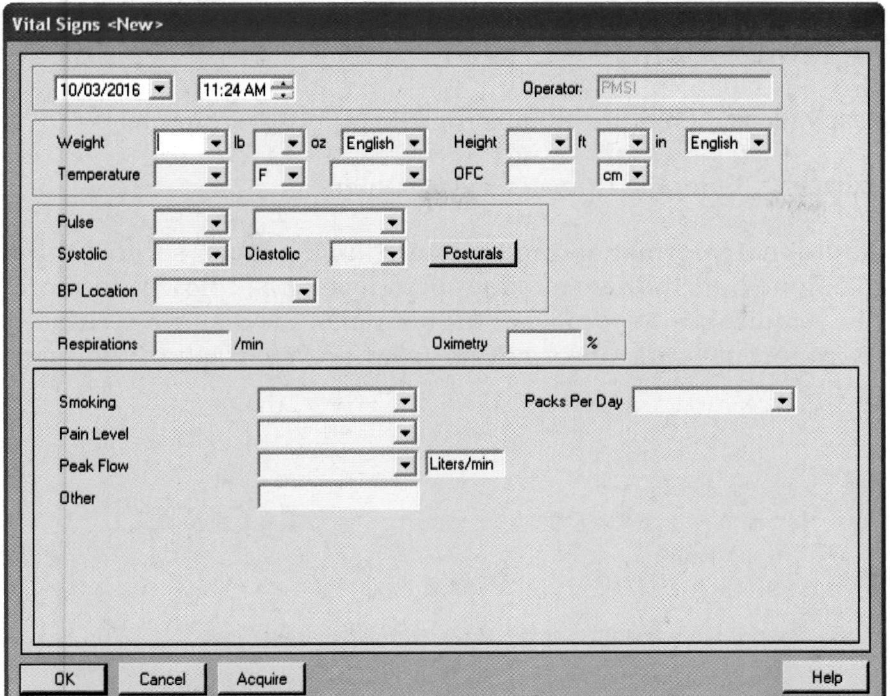

Figure 6.14 The Vital Signs (New) Dialog Box

Time The current time is automatically displayed.

Operator The current operator is displayed.

Weight Enter the patient's weight. A drop-down list is used to indicate whether the weight is in pounds and ounces or kilograms.

Height Enter the patient's height. A drop-down list is used to indicate whether the height is in feet and inches or in meters.

Temperature Enter the patient's temperature. A drop-down list is used to indicate whether the temperature in Fahrenheit (F) or Celsius (C). Another drop-down list indicates the route by which the temperature was measured.

OFC Enter the patient's occipito-frontal circumference (OFC) in inches or centimeters. (This is used to monitor growth in children.)

Pulse Enter the patient's pulse. A drop-down list next to the Pulse field can be used to indicate whether the patient's pulse was regular or irregular.

Systolic Enter the patient's systolic blood pressure.

Diastolic Enter the patient's diastolic blood pressure.

Posturals The Posturals button is used to record the patient's pulse, systolic blood pressure, and diastolic blood pressure while the patient is in different positions.

BP Location Enter the location where the blood pressure was measured.

Respirations Enter the number of respirations per minute.

Oximetry Enter the oximetry measurement.

Additional information can be entered in the lower section of the dialog box, including smoking, pain level, peak flow, and more. The Acquire button located at the bottom of the dialog box, is used to import postural information from a Welch Allyn vital sign device.

EXERCISE 6.8

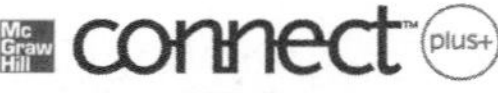

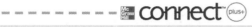

ENTERING A PATIENT'S VITAL SIGNS

Using Source Document 3, enter Jorge Barrett's vital signs.

1. Click the Vital Signs folder. The Vital Signs dialog box appears.
2. Click the New button. The Vital Signs (New) dialog box opens.
3. Review the information in Source Document 3.
4. Locate the Weight fields.
5. Click in the first Weight field, and enter ***153,*** the patient's weight.
6. Enter the patient's height: ***6*** in the ft field and ***1*** in the in field.
7. Enter ***98.6*** in the Temperature field. Confirm that *F* is selected for Fahrenheit. In the next field, select Oral.
8. The patient's pulse is 88 and regular. Enter this information in the two Pulse fields.
9. The patient's blood pressure is 184/104. Enter ***184*** in the Systolic field and enter ***104*** in the Diastolic field.
10. Enter the patient's respirations: ***14.***
11. Click the OK button to save your entries. You are returned to the Vital Signs dialog box. Notice that the entries for the patient's blood pressure are highlighted in red to indicate that the readings are above the normal range.
12. Click the Close button.

 **You have completed Exercise 6.8**

6.8 Messages

Using Medisoft Clinical Patient Records, staff members can send intra-office messages. The messaging feature works like an internal e-mail system. It is used to send messages to other staff members or providers, and it can also be used as a reminder system or to-do list. A message can contain attachments and can include a link to the

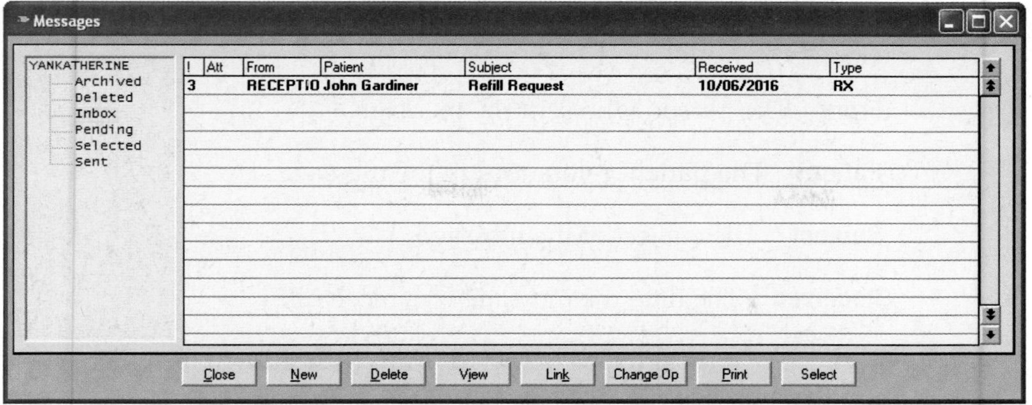

Figure 6.15 The Messages Dialog Box with the Inbox Folder Selected

relevant portion of a patient's chart. For example, if the message is about a prescription refill request, the program automatically opens the Rx/Medications folder in the patient's chart.

The Messages Dialog Box

To access the messaging feature, select Messaging on the Task menu, or click the Msg button on the toolbar. The Messages dialog box appears (see Figure 6.15). By default, the Messages box opens with the Inbox displayed. A list of messaging folders is displayed on the left side of the dialog box.

The yellow column on the left in the Messages dialog box lists the message folders:

Archived Archived messages are listed in order by date received and priority.

Deleted Deleted messages are listed in order by date received and priority.

Inbox Inbox messages are listed in order by date received and priority.

Pending The Pending messages folder is similar to a drafts folder in an e-mail program. Pending messages are stored here until they are sent, and they may be revised before being sent. Pending messages are listed in order by date to activate and priority.

Selected If multiple messages are selected in the Inbox for viewing, they are displayed here.

Sent Sent messages are listed in order by date sent and priority.

To the right of the folder list is the message area, where the messages in the selected folder are listed. The columns in the main section of the dialog box include:

! The message's priority, from zero (the lowest priority) to nine (the highest).

Att If there is an attachment to the message, a paper clip symbol appears.

From The person who sent the message.

Patient The patient referenced in the message.

Subject The subject of the message.

Received The date the message was received.

Type The message type (selected from a drop-down list when creating the message).

Below the message there are a series of buttons used to perform messaging tasks:

Close Close the messaging system.

New Create a new message.

Delete Move the selected message to the Deleted folder.

View Open the selected message.

Link Open the relevant section of the patient's chart (if a patient is referenced in the message). If the selection in the Type field corresponds to a chart folder, that folder will be displayed.

Change Op Allows a staff member to access another staff member's messaging account. If a message is sent while in another staff member's messages, the message shows as having been sent by the original staff member. Permission must be set in the program for this feature to be activated.

Print Prints the message.

Select Provides filters to control which messages are displayed in the message area.

When there is a new message in the inbox, the Msg button on the toolbar is blue. If the message has been marked as urgent by the sender, the Msg button is red. To open a message, click the Msg button. The Messages dialog box appears, with the Inbox displayed. To read the message, either double click the message itself, or click the message once and click the View button.

The New Message Dialog Box

To create a new message from within the Messages dialog box, click the New button. The New Message dialog box opens (see Figure 6.16). If the Messages dialog box is not open, click the Msg button on the toolbar to open the Messages dialog box, and then click the New button. The New Message dialog box appears.

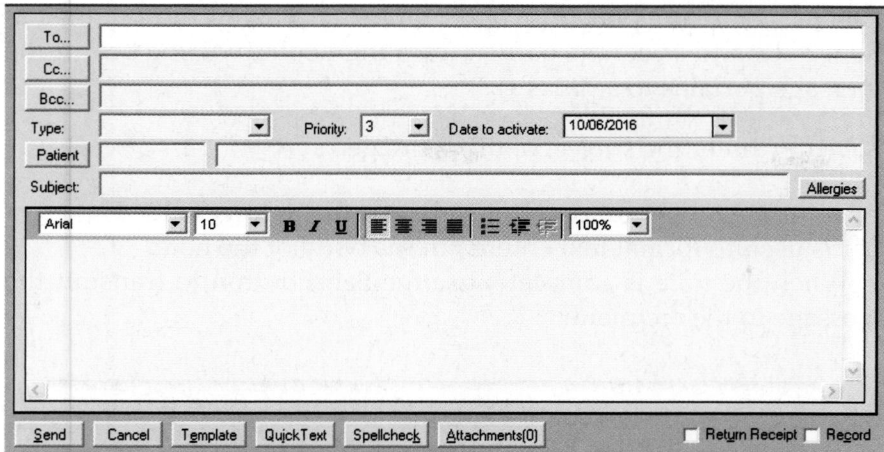

Figure 6.16 The New Message Dialog Box

The fields in the New Message dialog box include:

To... Enter the names or IDs of the recipients. To view a list of names, click the To... button. The Select Destination dialog box with a list of system operators appears (see Figure 6.17). To select a recipient, click the ID and name in the list displayed, and click the OK button. The recipient's ID is listed in the To... field.

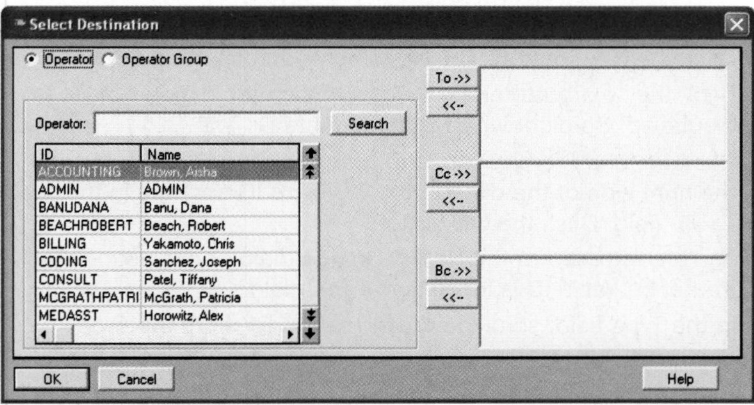

Figure 6.17 The Select Destination Dialog Box

Cc... Enter the names or IDs of anyone who should receive a copy of the message.

Bcc... Enter the names or IDs of anyone who should receive a blind copy of the message.

Type Select a message type from the drop-down list.

Priority Select a message priority from the drop-down list. The range is from zero to nine, with zero being the lowest priority and nine the highest. If a priority of nine is selected, the message is marked as urgent, and the Msg button on the recipient's toolbar turns red.

Date to activate Delays sending of the message until the date specified.

Patient Enter the patient's chart number and name, or click the Patient button to select the patient from the Lookup dialog box (if the message pertains to a patient).

Subject Enter the subject of the message.

A formatting toolbar appears just below the Subject field. This toolbar is used to format text entered in the body of the note.

When the note is complete, use the Send button to transmit the message to the recipient.

EXERCISE 6.9

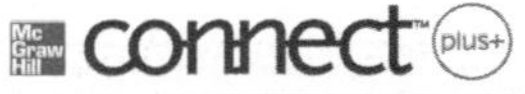

CREATING AND SENDING A MESSAGE

Send a message to a patient's provider about a prescription refill request.

1. Click Park on the toolbar to log out of Medisoft Clinical Patient Records. When the message appears asking whether you want to Park, click the Yes button. The Sign In—Park screen is displayed.
2. Log in as the receptionist by entering ***RECEPTION*** in the User ID field and ***master1$*** in the Password field. Click the OK button. You are now logged in as the practice's receptionist.
3. Click the Msg button on the toolbar. The Messages dialog box appears.
4. Click the New button. The New Message dialog box opens.
5. Click the To... button. The Select Destination dialog box is displayed. Scroll down the list to locate Dr. Yan.
6. Click the entry for Dr. Yan, and then click the To->> button on the right side of the dialog box. Dr. Yan's ID appears in the To->> field. Click the OK button.
7. You are returned to the New Message dialog box. Notice that Katherine Yan's ID is listed in the To... field.
8. In the Type field, scroll down and select RX from the drop-down list.
9. Accept the default entries in the Priority and Date to Activate fields.
10. Click the Patient button. The Patient Lookup dialog box is displayed.
11. Enter ***GA*** in the last name field, and press Enter. The list of patients is displayed, with John Gardiner at the top of the list. Click the OK button to select John Gardiner. The Lookup dialog box closes, and John Gardiner's chart number and name are listed in the Patient fields in the New Message dialog box.
12. Click in the Subject field, and enter ***Refill Request***.
13. Click in the body of the message, and enter ***Patient called and requested a refill of amlodipine***.
14. Click the Send button to send the message.
15. Click the Close button to close the Messages dialog box.

You have completed Exercise 6.9

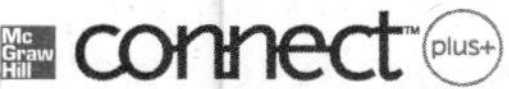

EXERCISE 6.10

READING A MESSAGE AND VIEWING A PATIENT CHART

Retrieve a message, and use the Link button to open the relevant section of the patient's chart.

1. Click Park on the toolbar to log out of Medisoft Clinical Patient Records. When the message appears asking whether you want to Park, click the Yes button. The Sign In—Park screen is displayed.
2. Log in as Dr. Katherine Yan by entering ***YANKATHERINE*** in the User ID field and ***master1$*** in the Password field. Click the OK button. You are now logged in as Dr. Yan.
3. Notice that the Msg button on the toolbar is blue, indicating that Dr. Yan has a new message. Click the Msg button. The Messages dialog box opens, with the Inbox folder selected. The new message is listed at the top of the Inbox message list.
4. Double click on the new message to view it. The message is displayed.
5. Click the Link button to view the relevant section of the patient's chart. The Rx/Medications dialog box from the patient's chart is displayed, with the patient's current medications listed.
6. Click the Close button to close the Rx/Medications dialog box.
7. Click the Close button to close the patient's chart. You are returned to the message.
8. Click the Record button to record this message in the Messages folder of the patient's chart. The Messages folder appears. The system has created a note containing the content of the message. A box appears asking whether to delete the original message. Click the Yes button. The message will be removed from the Inbox the next time Dr. Yan closes and reopens the Messages dialog box.
9. Click OK to save the message in the patient's chart. The Messages dialog box closes.
10. Click the Messages folder to verify that the message has been saved to the patient's chart.
11. Click the Close button on the toolbar to close the patient's chart.
12. Click the Close button to close the Messages dialog box.

You have completed Exercise 6.10

6.9 Letters

Creating and mailing letters are standard activities in medical practices. Letters are sent to patients, other providers, employers, insurance companies, and others. Patients are informed of test results and reminded about annual exams. Other providers, such as specialists, are asked to provide care to patients. Letters are sent to employers to document patients' absence from work. Insurance

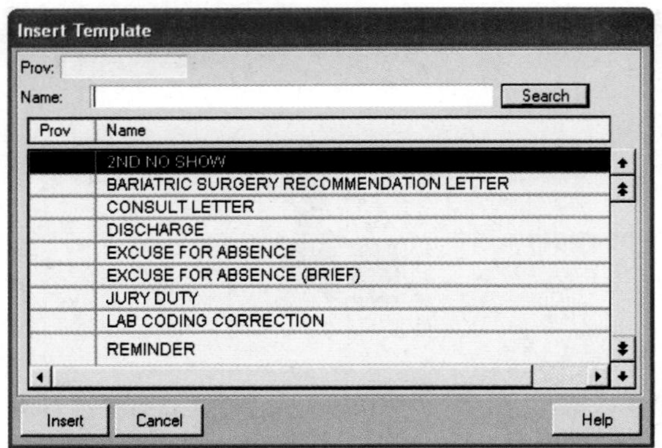

Figure 6.18 The Insert Template Dialog Box

companies receive letters that state the medical necessity of care or follow up on denied insurance claims. The Letters feature in Medisoft Clinical Patient Records makes it easy for providers to create letters about their patients.

In MCPR, letters are note-based in the same manner as patient histories and progress notes. Information can be entered by typing in the dialog box without the use of a template, although many practices use templates to save time when creating letters. Templates can be set up to automatically insert information in letters, such as the patient's name and address, the date of the last office visit, the name of a test performed, and so on.

The Letters Dialog Box

Letters are created by clicking the Letter button on the toolbar, or by selecting Letters on the Task menu, which opens the Insert Template dialog box (see Figure 6.18). This dialog box contains a list of letter templates that exist in the program. Select the template from the list, and click the Insert button. The template is inserted into the body of the letter (see Figure 6.19).

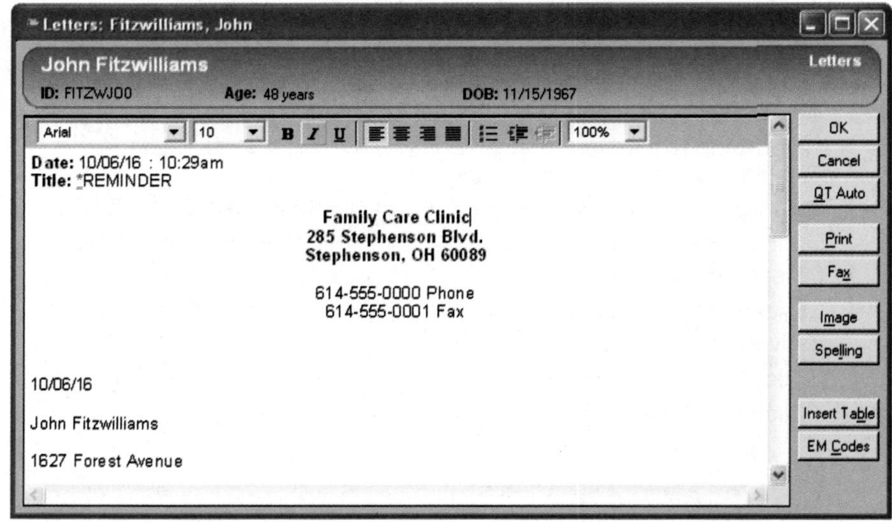

Figure 6.19 The Letters Dialog Box with a Template Inserted

connect plus+ EXERCISE 6.11

WRITING AN APPOINTMENT REMINDER LETTER

Create an appointment reminder letter using a letter template.

1. Click Park on the toolbar to log out of Medisoft Clinical Patient Records. When the message appears asking whether you want to Park, click the Yes button. The Sign In—Park screen is displayed.
2. Log in as the receptionist by entering ***RECEPTION*** in the User ID field and ***master1$*** in the Password field. Click the OK button. You are now logged in as the receptionist.
3. Click the Chart button on the toolbar, or select Open Chart on the File menu. The Patient Lookup dialog box appears.
4. Enter ***JO*** in the Last Name field, and press Enter. A list of patients is displayed, with Elizabeth Jones at the top. Click the OK button to open her chart.
5. Click the Letters button on the toolbar, or select Letters on the Task menu. The Insert Template dialog box appears, displaying a list of available templates.
6. Select the entry for a Reminder letter, and click the Insert button to insert the template into the note. The Letter dialog box appears with the reminder letter template inserted.
7. Notice that the program has automatically entered the practice name, the date, and the patient's name and address.
8. Scroll down the letter, and view the blue labels used to insert letter content. Since this is a reminder to schedule an appointment for an annual physical, click the blue label ANNUAL EXAM. The program inserts the words *annual physical exam*.
9. Scroll down the letter to see if any more fields need completion. Since no additional fields require data, the letter is finished. Click the OK button to save the letter.
10. When the Enter Signature dialog box appears, enter ***1*** (Dr. Yan's ID) in the Provider ID field. Enter ***1234*** in the Signature field. This is Dr. Yan's signature password. Click the OK button.
11. Click the Letters folder to view the letter you just created. Scroll down to view the rest of the letter. Notice that the program has marked the bottom of the letter with Dr. Yan's electronic signature.

 **You have completed Exercise 6.11**

chapter 6 summary

LEARNING OUTCOME	KEY CONCEPTS/EXAMPLES
6.1 Explain the four stages of patient flow. Pages 284–288	The four stages of patient flow are check-in, patient intake, examination, and checkout. 1. During check-in, the front desk staff member checks the patient in, recording the time he or she arrived; confers with the patient to determine whether any information, such as a change of insurance or employment, needs to be updated in the patient record; and may ask the patient for payment. 2. In the patient intake stage, the patient is escorted to the exam room, and the medical assistant obtains detailed information from him or her, including past medical, family, and social history; allergies and medications; and the chief complaint. The medical assistant measures the patient's vital signs and prepares the patient for the examination. 3. During the examination stage, the provider examines the patient. The provider may order lab work or diagnostic tests and may prescribe medications. The provider develops a treatment plan and completes the examination. 4. The patient leaves the exam room and proceeds to the checkout desk. During checkout, the office staff member gives the patient any additional information required, such as patient education materials or lab work instructions. If necessary, a follow-up appointment is scheduled. Before the patient leaves, the staff member collects any payment that is due, if it was not collected during check-in.
6.2 Discuss the main sections of the patient chart. Pages 288–290	1. Start Medisoft Clinical Patient Records, and log in. 2. Select Open Chart on the File menu, or click the Chart toolbar button. The Patient Lookup dialog box appears. 3. Select the radio button to search by patient name. 4. Enter one or more letters in the Last Name field, and click the Lookup button. A list of patients with last names beginning with the letters is displayed. 5. Click on the entry for the desired patient. Click the OK button. The patient's chart is displayed.
6.3 Describe the procedures for recording a patient's past medical, family, and social history. Pages 290–292	1. With a patient chart open, click the desired folder— Past Medical History, Family History, or Social History. 2. A message box appears stating that no history exists for the patient and asking whether you want to create a new note. Click the Yes button to continue. The appropriate history window appears.

LEARNING OUTCOME	KEY CONCEPTS/EXAMPLES
	3. Enter the appropriate information in the note. 4. When finished, click the OK button to save the note. The window closes, and you are returned to the chart.
6.4 Explain how allergies and intolerances are entered in the patient chart. Pages 293–295	1. Click the Rx/Medications folder. 2. Click the Allergy button. The Allergy dialog box opens. 3. If available, enter the date and time when the allergy was first identified. 4. In the Medication/Allergy Name field, enter the name of the medication or allergy. 5. Select the appropriate entry in the Allergy Type field—Drug Allergy, Drug Intolerance, Miscellaneous, or Food Allergy. 6. If known, select the level of severity in the Severity field. 7. Enter the reaction in the Reaction field. 8. Click the OK button to save the entry.
6.5 Describe the procedure used to enter patient medications. Pages 295–298	1. Click the Rx/Medications folder. The Rx/Medications dialog box appears. 2. Click the New button. The Prescription dialog box opens. 3. Accept the default entry in the Date field. 4. Enter a few letters of the drug name in the Rx Template Code field, and click the Lookup button. The Rx Template dialog box is displayed. 5. Locate the drug code on the list, and click the line to select it. Click the OK button. 6. Modify the information that was automatically entered by the program, if necessary. 7. Click the Outside box if the medication has been prescribed by a physician who is not in the practice. 8. Click the OK button to save the entries. The Prescription dialog box closes, and you are returned to the Rx/Medications folder. 9. Confirm that the drug name appears in the Current tab.

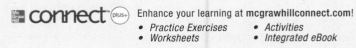

LEARNING OUTCOME	KEY CONCEPTS/EXAMPLES
6.6 Explain how the chief complaint is recorded in a progress note. Pages 298–300	Enter the chief complaint as the title of a new progress note: 1. Click the Chart button on the toolbar. 2. When the Patient Lookup dialog box appears, enter letters in the Last Name field and press Enter. 3. Select the patient from the list, and click the OK button to open the chart. 4. Click the Note button on the toolbar. 5. Click just to the right of the * symbol, and enter the chief complaint. 6. To sign the note, enter ***^Shared_Note_Signature.*** 7. Click the OK button to save the note. A dialog box appears asking whether you are permanently done with the note. Click the No button. The Enter Signature dialog box appears. 8. Enter the signature PIN in the Signature field. 9. Press the OK button. The Progress Notes dialog box closes.
6.7 Explain how a patient's vital signs are recorded in the patient chart. Pages 300–302	1. Click the Vital Signs folder. The Vital Signs dialog box appears. 2. Click the New button. The Vital Signs (New) dialog box opens. 3. Enter the patient's vital signs in the appropriate fields—Weight, Height, Temperature, OFC, Pulse, Systolic, Diastolic, Posturals, BP Location, Respirations, and Oximetry. For example, to enter a patient's height, click in the first Height field and enter the patient's height in feet. Then click in the second Height box to enter the inches measurement. 4. When finished, click the OK button to save your entries. 5. Click the Close button to close the Vital Signs (New) dialog box.
6.8 Explain the uses of an intra-office messaging system in an EHR. Pages 302–307	To send a message: 1. Click the Msg button on the toolbar. The Messages dialog box appears. 2. Click the New button. The New Message dialog box opens. 3. Click the To... button. The Select Destination dialog box is displayed. Locate the desired recipient's name. 4. Click the entry for the desired recipient, and then click the To->> button on the right side of the dialog box. When the individual's ID appears in the To->> field, click the OK button. 5. You are returned to the New Message dialog box. 6. In the Type field, scroll down and select the desired type of message from the drop-down list. 7. Either accept the default entries in the Priority and Date to Activate fields or make changes to them.

LEARNING OUTCOME	KEY CONCEPTS/EXAMPLES
	8. If the message is about a patient, click the Patient button. The Patient Lookup dialog box is displayed. 9. Enter several letters in the Last Name field, and press Enter. The list of patients is displayed. Select the appropriate patient, and click the OK button. 10. Click in the Subject field, and enter a subject. 11. Click in the body of the message, and enter the message. 12. Click the Send button to send the message. 13. Click the Close button to close the Messages dialog box. To retrieve a message: 1. Click the Msg button on the toolbar. The Messages dialog box opens, with the Inbox folder selected. The most recent message is listed at the top of the Inbox message list. 2. Double click the new message to view it. The message is displayed. 3. If appropriate, click the Link button to view the relevant section of the patient's chart. A dialog box from the patient's chart is displayed. 4. Click the Close button to close the dialog box. 5. Click the Close button to close the patient's chart. You are returned to the message. 6. Click the Record button to record this message in the Messages folder of the patient's chart. The Messages folder appears. A box appears asking whether to delete the original message. Click the Yes button. 7. Click OK to save the message in the patient's chart. The Messages dialog box closes.
6.9 Describe how letters are created in an EHR. Pages 307–309	1. Click the Letters button on the toolbar, or select Letters on the Task menu. The Insert Template dialog box appears, displaying a list of available templates. 2. Select the entry for the desired type of letter, and click the Insert button to insert the template into the letter. The Letter dialog box appears with the selected template inserted. 3. Notice that the program has automatically entered some information. 4. Scroll down the letter, and view the blue labels. Click the appropriate blue label(s) to enter content in the letter. 5. When the letter is finished, click the OK button to save the letter. 6. If the Enter Signature dialog box appears, enter the signature PIN number in the Signature field. Click the OK button.

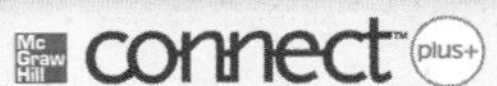

Enhance your learning at mcgrawhillconnect.com!
- *Practice Exercises*
- *Worksheets*
- *Activities*
- *Integrated eBook*

chapter review

MATCHING QUESTIONS

Match the key terms with their definitions.

_____ 1. ***[LO 6.1]*** past medical history (PMH)

_____ 2. ***[LO 6.1]*** progress note

_____ 3. ***[LO 6.1]*** patient flow

_____ 4. ***[LO 6.1]*** family history (FH)

_____ 5. ***[LO 6.1]*** social history (SH)

_____ 6. ***[LO 6.1]*** history of present illness (HPI)

_____ 7. ***[LO 6.1]*** review of systems (ROS)

_____ 8. ***[LO 6.1]*** past, family, and social history (PFSH)

a. Information about the patient's tobacco use, alcohol and drug use, sexual history, relationship status, and other significant social facts that may contribute to the care of the patient.

b. Note documenting the care delivered to a patient, and the medical facts and clinical thinking relevant to diagnosis and treatment.

c. Progression of patients from the time they enter the office for a visit until they exit the system by leaving the office after a visit.

d. Patient's history of medical problems, including chronic conditions, surgeries, and hospitalizations.

e. Detailed record of medical events among the patient's relatives, including the ages, living status, and diseases of siblings, children, parents, and grandparents.

f. A commonly used abbreviation for past medical, family, and social history.

g. An inventory of body systems in which the patient reports signs or symptoms he or she is currently having or has had in the past.

h. A description of the course of the present illness, including how and when the problem began, up to the present time.

TRUE-FALSE QUESTIONS

Decide whether each statement is true or false.

_____ 1. ***[LO 6.7]*** Patients' vital sign measurements are entered in the Progress Notes folder in the patient chart.

_____ 2. ***[LO 6.3]*** Each history section of a patient's chart consists of multiple notes.

_____ 3. ***[LO 6.4]*** Patient allergies are recorded and stored in the Rx/Medications folder of the patient chart.

_____ 4. ***[LO 6.1]*** A typical patient flow consists of check-in, patient intake, examination, and checkout.

_____ 5. ***[LO 6.2]*** The first step in opening a patient chart is to select Open Chart on the File menu or to click the Chart button on the toolbar.

_____ 6. ***[LO 6.3]*** The History dialog boxes are used to select a patient.

_____ 7. ***[LO 6.8]*** Using Medisoft Clinical Patient Records, staff members can send intra-office messages.

_____ 8. ***[LO 6.5]*** Medications that have been added, discontinued, or changed are noted in the patient chart.

_____ 9. ***[LO 6.1]*** The history of present illness (HPI) includes previous treatment and diagnostic tests.

_____ 10. ***[LO 6.2]*** A patient's chief complaint is recorded in the Medical History folder of the patient chart.

MULTIPLE-CHOICE QUESTIONS

Select the letter that best completes the statement or answers the question.

1. ***[LO 6.1]*** The __________ is the patient's history of medical problems, including chronic conditions, surgeries, and hospitalizations.
   a. past medical history (PMH)
   b. progress note
   c. family history (FH)
   d. social history (SH)

2. ***[LO 6.1]*** The __________ is information about the patient's tobacco use, alcohol and drug use, sexual history, relationship status, and other significant social facts that may contribute to the care of the patient.
   a. past medical history (PMH)
   b. progress note
   c. family history (FH)
   d. social history (SH)

3. ***[LO 6.1]*** The __________ details medical events among members of the patient's family, including the ages, living status, and diseases of siblings, children, parents, and grandparents.
   a. past medical history (PMH)
   b. progress note
   c. family history (FH)
   d. social history (SH)

4. ***[LO 6.1]*** The __________ documents the care delivered to a patient, and the medical facts and clinical thinking relevant to diagnosis and treatment.
   a. past medical history (PMH)
   b. progress note
   c. family history (FH)
   d. social history (SH)

5. ***[LO 6.9]*** __________ are sent to patients, other providers, employers, insurance companies, and others.
   a. letters
   b. templates
   c. progress notes
   d. all of the above
6. ***[LO 6.5]*** The __________ tab is in the Rx/Medications dialog box.
   a. Current
   b. Ineffective
   c. Historical
   d. all of the above
7. ***[LO 6.6]*** In most practices, the __________ is entered as the title of the progress note for the patient's visit.
   a. progress note
   b. template
   c. chief complaint
   d. past medical history (PMH)
8. ***[LO 6.4]*** A(n) __________ is a mild reaction to a medication and does not involve an immune system response.
   a. intolerance
   b. chief complaint
   c. skin rash
   d. allergy
9. ***[LO 6.7]*** Abnormally high blood pressure readings are highlighted in __________ in the Vital Signs dialog box.
   a. blue
   b. green
   c. red
   d. yellow
10. ***[LO 6.8]*** To open a new message in the inbox, select the __________ button on the toolbar.
    a. Messaging
    b. Msg
    c. Inbox
    d. Receive

SHORT-ANSWER QUESTIONS

Define the following abbreviations.

1. ***[LO 6.1]*** SH ____________________

2. ***[LO 6.1]*** PMH ____________________

3. ***[LO 6.1]*** FH ____________________

4. ***[LO 6.1]*** HPI ____________________

5. ***[LO 6.1]*** ROS ____________________

6. ***[LO 6.1]*** PFSH ____________________

APPLYING YOUR KNOWLEDGE

Answer the questions below in the space provided.

6.1. ***[LO 6.1]*** Why is it important for medical practices to collect information about a patient's family history (FH) and social history (SH)?

____

6.2. ***[LO 6.2]*** What advantages do you think the folder design of Medisoft's patient chart feature offers?

____

6.3. ***[LO 6.4]*** Why are patients' allergies and/or intolerances recorded in Medisoft?

____

chapter 7

Office Visit: Examination and Coding

KEY TERMS

Alphabetic Index
Category I codes
Category II codes
Category III codes
computer-assisted coding
Current Procedural Terminology (CPT)
dictation
digital dictation
electronic encounter form (EEF)
evaluation and management (E/M) codes
formulary
HCPCS
ICD-9-CM
ICD-9-CM Official Guidelines for Coding and Reporting
ICD-10-CM
key components
medical coding
primary diagnosis
SOAP
Tabular List
template
upcoding
voice recognition software

LEARNING OUTCOMES

When you finish this chapter, you will be able to:

7.1 Discuss the methods of entering documentation in an EHR.

7.2 Compare the process of entering a progress note with and without using a template.

7.3 Explain why e-prescribing reduces some medical errors.

7.4 List the steps required to enter a new prescription.

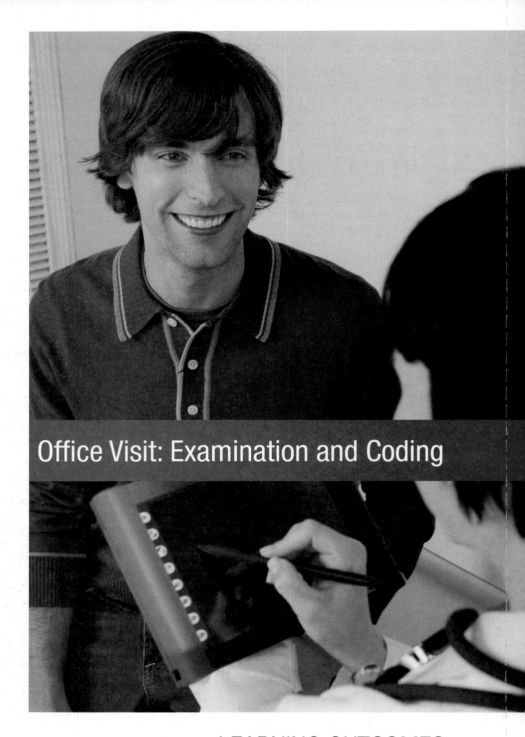

7.5 Explain why ordering and receiving test results electronically is more efficient than paper methods.

7.6 List the steps required to enter an electronic order.

7.7 Explain how orders are processed in an EHR.

7.8 Define medical coding.

7.9 Discuss the purpose of ICD-9-CM.

7.10 Discuss the purpose of the CPT/HCPCS code sets.

7.11 Demonstrate the process that is followed to select a correct evaluation and management code.

7.12 Compare coding in a paper-based office with coding in an office with an EHR.

7.13 Discuss the purpose of an electronic encounter form in an EHR.

Remember Alex Horowitz, the medical assistant who was wondering how to enter long lists of patient medications in the EHR? He is not the only one having difficulty adjusting to the new workflow. Dr. Katherine Yan uses the EHR to order medications and lab work, but still dictates her progress notes, and has Alex type them in the EHR. Dr. Patricia McGrath, on the other hand, finds that using the EHR's templates makes her more efficient. "I spend less time documenting visits," she said. "I had to spend time learning how to use the templates, but now I wouldn't go back to dictation."

Alex feels overwhelmed. In addition to learning how to use the EHR for recording medications and vital signs, he stays late each day to enter Dr. Yan's progress notes, something he never had to do before. He finds that since the EHR was installed, he has to spend more time on tasks, not less.

In this chapter, you will learn about the different methods of entering progress notes in an EHR. As you read the chapter and complete the exercises, think about how Dr. Yan and Dr. McGrath enter progress notes.

WHEN YOU FINISH THIS CHAPTER, YOU WILL ALSO BE ABLE TO USE MEDISOFT CLINICAL TO:

1. Enter a progress note in the SOAP format.
2. Use a template to enter a progress note in the SOAP format.
3. Sign a note using an electronic signature.
4. Enter an order for a new prescription.
5. Enter an order for a laboratory test.
6. Process an electronic order.
7. Use an electronic encounter form to code an office visit.

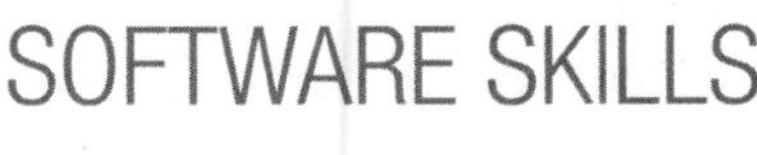

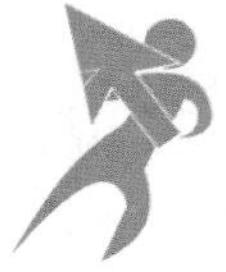

7.1 Methods of Entering Physician Documentation in an EHR

Every service submitted for payment, including medical care, diagnostic tests, consultations, surgeries, and other services eligible for payment, must be documented in the patient's medical record. Documentation is directly linked to the financial health of the practice. To be reimbursed, the provider must document each service provided to the patient. If a treatment is given to a patient and the provider fails to document it, the service will not be reimbursed. Incomplete or inaccurate records may result in claim denials or may even lead to an investigation of possible fraudulent and abusive actions.

Physicians in the United States create more than a billion clinical notes each year (Source: Health Level Seven International, "Health Story Project," Press Release, July 14, 2010). In the past, these notes were handwritten or were dictated and then transcribed. Electronic health records offer providers additional options, some of which totally eliminate the need for both written notes and dictated and transcribed notes. Each method has advantages and disadvantages, and many providers use a combination of methods. In this chapter, you will learn about the different documentation methods, and you will practice entering patient progress notes using both traditional and computerized techniques.

Dictation and Transcription

dictation the process of recording spoken words that will later be transcribed into written form

digital dictation the process of dictating using a microphone, a headset connected to a computer, a smart phone, or a PDA

Even after a successful transition to an EHR, some physicians prefer to continue using dictation as a means of entering progress notes. **Dictation** is the process of recording spoken words that will later be transcribed into written form. Dictation and transcription have been the traditional method of documenting patient encounters. The flow of dictation is illustrated in Figure 7.1. A medical provider dictates the medical note into a telephone or a recording device. A medical transcriptionist receives the dictation and transcribes it on a computer. After review, the final computerized word processing file is e-mailed to the health care provider, or the file is transferred to a website and is later downloaded by the provider. It is then reviewed and added to the patient's electronic record.

In **digital dictation,** physicians dictate using a microphone and/or a headset connected to a computer. Dictation can also be spoken into a smart phone or a personal digital assistant (PDA). The spoken words are saved as a digital audio file, which can be transferred to a transcriptionist via a secure website.

Dictation corresponds intuitively to the physician's usual way of working. It allows the physician to describe a patient's condition in his or her own words, reflecting both content and context. Physicians can dictate anytime, anywhere, using a telephone, a computer, or another recording device. By using this traditional method of documenting patient care, providers need not change the way they practice to accommodate an EHR system.

Figure 7.1 Flowchart of Traditional Dictation and Transcription

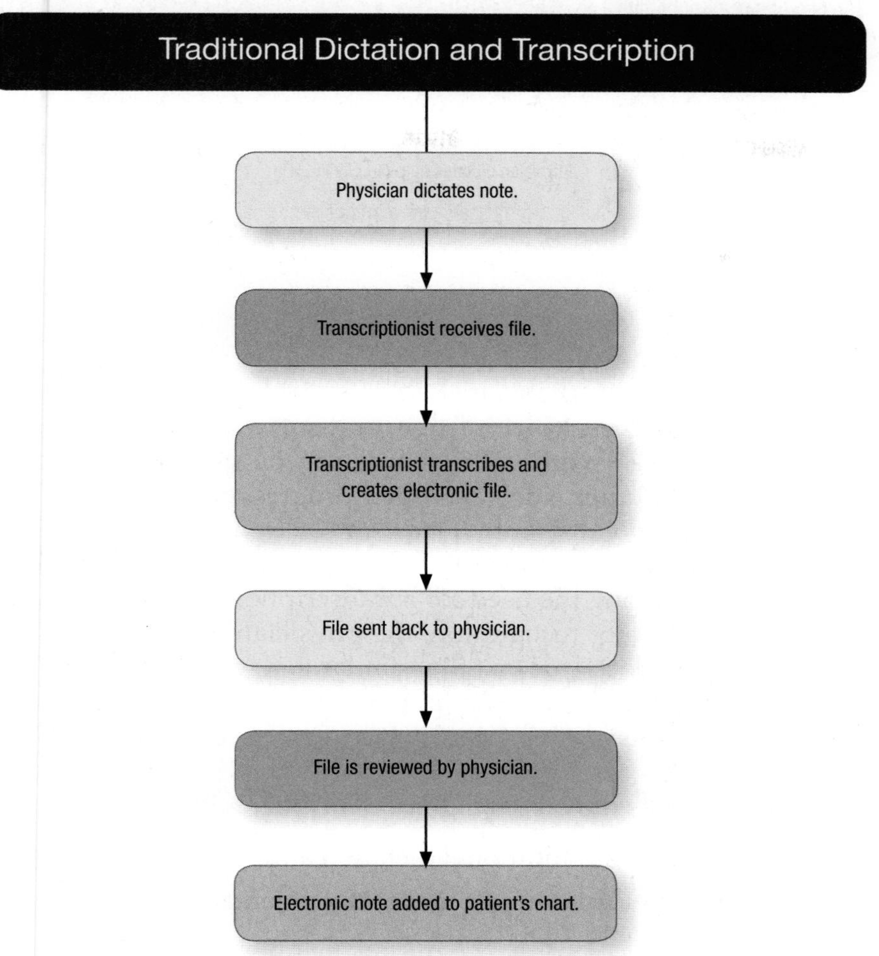

The benefits of dictation and transcription are as follows:

- Physicians who are uncomfortable with computers in the examination room can still use an EHR.
- Dictation retains the narrative form of documentation that promotes detail, context, and comprehensiveness.
- The method does not require additional training for physicians.

The drawbacks of dictation include these:

- Dictated reports are not immediately accessible.
- Dictation incurs transcription costs.
- The physician or an assistant must review and edit files.
- Detail is more likely to be omitted or forgotten if data are not captured at the point-of-care.

Voice Recognition Software

Even after a successful transition to an EHR, some physicians prefer to continue using dictation as a means of entering information.

Figure 7.2 Flowchart of Front-End Voice Recognition

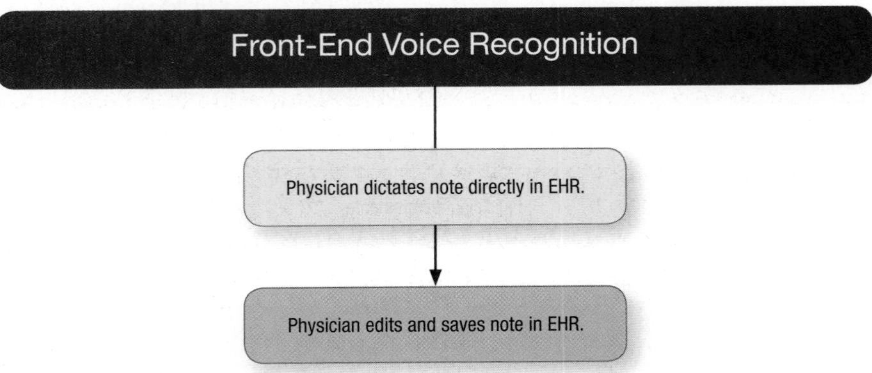
Front-End Voice Recognition
Physician dictates note directly in EHR.
Physician edits and saves note in EHR.

voice recognition software software that recognizes spoken words

Voice recognition programs make this a viable, cost-effective solution for some offices. **Voice recognition software** is software that recognizes spoken words. The words can be used to issue commands to a computer, such as "open progress note," or they can transcribe spoken words into text in an electronic file. In front-end voice recognition, the physician dictates and edits notes directly in the EHR, eliminating the need for a transcriptionist (see Figure 7.2). In background voice recognition, the physician dictates notes that are saved as an electronic text file, similar to a word processing file, which is then edited by a transcriptionist. After editing, it is uploaded to the EHR (see Figure 7.3). Most EHRs offer voice recognition as an add-on module.

The advantages of voice recognition include:

- Lower costs than traditional dictation and transcription
- Reduction of turnaround time for documentation

The disadvantages of voice recognition include:

- The possibility of an unacceptable accuracy rate if interference such as background noise is present
- The costs associated with purchasing voice recognition equipment and software

Figure 7.3 Flowchart of Background Voice Recognition

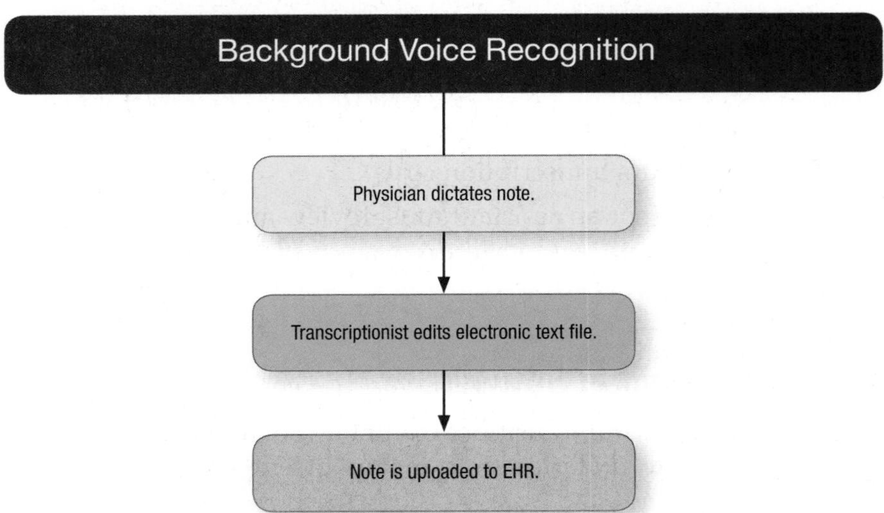
Background Voice Recognition
Physician dictates note.
Transcriptionist edits electronic text file.
Note is uploaded to EHR.

Templates

Another method of entering documentation in an EHR is through use of templates. A **template** is a preformatted file that serves as a starting point for a new document. When a template is used, only patient-specific information must be typed into the note. The rest of the information is entered by clicking on labels in the templates and making selections from a list of choices.

template preformatted file that serves as a starting point for a new document

Templates in an EHR are similar to macros in a word processing program. Macros automate repetitive tasks, such as inserting the current date at the beginning of every letter. In an EHR, a template presents the physician with the most common entries for a specific type of office visit. For example, a template for a fifty- to sixty-four-year-old well-woman examination would contain a list of common menopausal symptoms. Rather than typing in the entry "hot flashes" or "night sweats," the physician clicks Yes or No next to the entry for the condition. If more information is required, clicking a special label in the template causes a list of additional information to be displayed.

Offices commonly use a number of different templates, depending on patients' ages and illnesses and the purposes of the visits. For example, an office might use one template for a middle-aged well-woman checkup, another for a routine checkup of a two-year-old female, and another for a diabetes follow-up visit. Specialists commonly have a set of templates unique to their specialty. Most EHRs provide templates for text-heavy parts of the patient's chart, such as medical history, family history, social history, and progress notes.

Figures 7.4 illustrates sections of three different progress note templates: middle-aged well-woman exam, two-year-old female well-child exam, and type II diabetic follow-up examination.

The advantages of templates are as follows:

- Once learned, templates can be more efficient.
- Data can be searched and analyzed by computer.
- The physician is less likely to omit information.

The disadvantages of templates include these:

- It takes time to learn how to use them effectively.
- Standardized content may not apply to all patients.
- Entries may not capture the uniqueness of each patient.

THINKING IT THROUGH 7.1

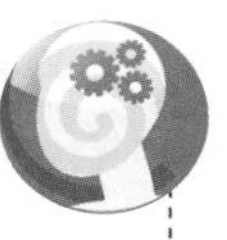

Most EHRs offer providers the option of using templates to enter progress notes, which can reduce the time it takes to enter notes. However, not all providers use templates. Given that over a billion notes are created each year, why do you think some providers have not switched to this method of documenting patient visits?

Figure 7.4
Sample Templates from an EHR

Well-woman template (excerpt)

GYN History: No concerns DELETE
Gravida 0 Past Pregnancies Post-Menopausal
Average interval between menses: DEL 28-31 days MenstrInt irregular P1
Length of menses: DEL DurDay P1
Flow: DEL MenstrFlo normal heavy light P1
Dysmenorrhea: DEL yes no controlled with NSAIDs controlled with OCPs H8
Post-coital bleeding: DEL yes no R7
Intermenstrual bleeding: DEL yes no R7
Pelvic pain: DEL yes no R7
Dyspareunia: DEL yes no R7
Vaginal discharge: DEL yes no VAG D/C DETAILS R7
GYN surgery: DEL GYNSURG none P1
Contraception: DEL Contracep P3 |

Menopausal Symptoms: none N/A DELETE
Hot flashes: DEL yes no tolerable intolerable R1
Night sweats: DEL yes no R1
Sleep disturbances: DEL yes no R11
Vaginal dryness: DEL yes no R7
Mood/cognitive disturbances: DEL yes no R11

Well-child template, female (excerpt)

Nutrition:
Milk: DEL Milktype MilkDrink
Table food: DEL TableFood varied diet

Developmental Milestones:
Knows 3-5 body parts: DEL yes no
Climbs stairs: DEL yes no
Scribbles spontaneously: DEL yes no
2 word sentences: DEL yes no
Points to named body parts: DEL yes no |
Removes clothing: DEL yes no
50 word vocabulary: DEL yes no

Objective:
Height Percentile DEL
Weight Percentile DEL
Complete Exam Girl 2-10 YO

Type 2 diabetic template (excerpt)

Glucose Monitoring: none DELETE
Accucheck frequency: DEL Not Checking QDay BID TID frequency
Fasting glucose: DEL blood sugars
Post prandial: DEL blood sugars

Most Recent HbA1C: DEL D1
Blood Pressure Range: DEL Not Checking Systolic / Diastolic * H3
Most Recent Lipid Panel:
DEL D1
Most Recent BMP:
DEL D1
Urine Microalbumin: DEL D1
Retinal Examination: DEL No Retinal Exam recorded in health maintenance unknown P1
Foot Exam: DEL No Foot Exam recorded in health maintenance unknown P1
Pneumovax Vaccine: DEL No Pneumovax vaccine recorded in health maintenance section UTD Not UTD Declines Pneumovax Postpones Pneumovax P1
Influenza Vaccine: DEL No Influenza vaccine recorded in health maintenance section UTD Not UTD Declines Influenza Postpones Influenza P1

Past Medical History/Complications of Diabetes: DELETE

7.2 Progress Notes in Medisoft Clinical Patient Records

In Medisoft Clinical Patient Records, progress notes can be entered using a variety of methods, including the methods described earlier—dictation and transcription, voice recognition software, and templates. A combination of techniques can also be used.

SOAP Format

In this chapter, progress notes are entered in the SOAP format. **SOAP** is a widely used format for documenting patient encounters. It stands for *subjective, objective, assessment,* and *plan*. A sample SOAP note is illustrated in Figure 7.5.

SOAP format used to enter progress notes; it stands for *subjective, objective, assessment,* and *plan*

HSU, EDWIN
#HSUEDWI
11/12/2016

SUBJECTIVE
Edwin says he recently had a cold, which seemed to resolve. He rolled over during the night and experienced acute facial pain and was aware that he had what he calls a "killer headache." He characterizes the pain as an 8 out of 10. Blowing his nose produces a thick, greenish-yellow mucous and bending over at all makes the pain intensify.

OBJECTIVE
Patient is a well-developed, well-nourished Asian male who is holding his head during the examination.
Vitals: 101.6º F P: 88 (reg) R: 14 BP: 124/84 WT: 208 lbs
HEENT: There is copious greenish-yellow drainage from the nose. Exquisite tenderness over the frontal sinuses, more marked on the right than on the left.
Chest: Clear to auscultation and percussion without wheezing, rales, or rhonchi.
Heart: Normal rate and rhythm without murmurs, gallops, or thrills.
Allergies: None.

ASSESSMENT
Acute sinusitis.

PLAN
He was given a prescription for erythromycin, 500 mg b.i.d. × 10 days (#20) and told he will need to take the medication until it is all gone, even if he begins to feel better. Also advised that he may use certrizine, 5 mg daily for decongestant relief, which is available over the counter, until the nasal congestion clears. To stay off work until his temperature returns to normal. Reminded to stay well hydrated. To call the office if his temperature is not down within 24 hours.

Patricia McGrath, MD

Figure 7.5 Sample SOAP Note

Subjective

The subjective section describes the patient's condition is his or her own words, including the degree of pain or discomfort, the presence of nausea or dizziness, when the problem first started, and any additional description that the patient provides.

Objective

The objective section of a note includes symptoms that can be measured, seen, heard, touched, felt, or smelled, including such vital signs as temperature, pulse, respiration, skin color, and swelling, and the results of diagnostic tests.

Assessment

The assessment section of a note contains the physician's diagnosis of the patient's condition.

Plan

The plan section of a note contains the provider's plan for treatment of the patient, such as laboratory, imaging, or radiological tests; medications; and procedures. The plan section may also include a referral to a specialist, patient directions, and follow-up care instructions.

Creating a New Progress Note

To create a new progress note, a patient's chart must be open. Clicking the Note button on the toolbar creates a new note (see Figure 7.6).

Every progress note starts with a date and a title. The program inserts the current date and time on the first line of the note, following the word *Date*.

The second line of the note contains the word *Title*, followed by a label marker. The title of the note, usually the chief complaint, is entered to the right of the marker.

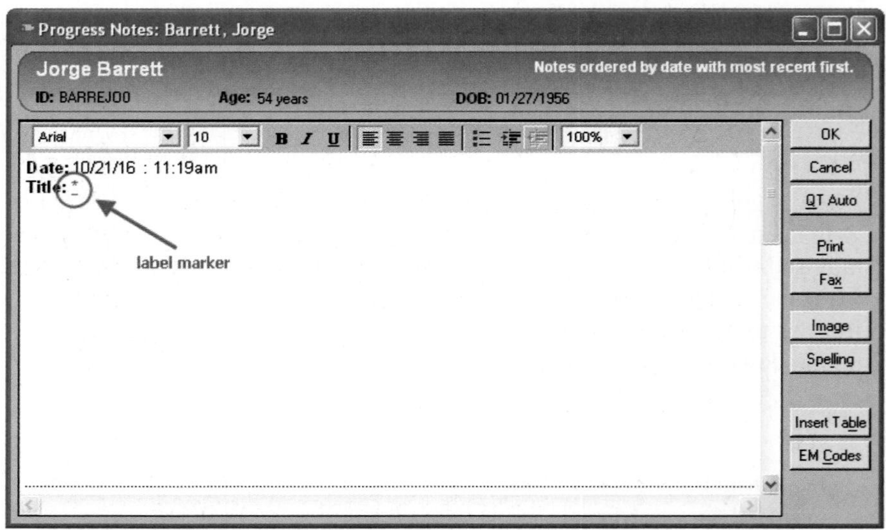

Figure 7.6 A New Progress Note in Medisoft Clinical Patient Records

The rest of the note is blank. This allows the physician to choose among the documentation entry methods described earlier in the chapter:

- If the note is being dictated, the rest of the note will be blank until the transcribed file is available for insertion.
- If the note is created using voice recognition software within the EHR, the spoken words will appear in the note window as the voice recognition software translates the speech into text.
- If the note is being typed without the use of a template, the physician types on the keyboard and enters text directly in the note.
- If a template is being used, the physician inserts the template in the note and responds to the labels in the template.

When the note is finished, the program prompts the provider to enter his or her PIN for an electronic signature. Once the PIN has been entered, the program inserts an electronic signature in the note (see Figure 7.7).

Entering a Progress Note Without a Template

A physician normally documents the office visit in a progress note. To gain an understanding of how patient visits are documented in an EHR, you will complete a note.

In the following four exercises, you will enter the information without the use of a template. Referring to Source Document 4, complete each exercise by typing the information in the appropriate section of the note. Later in the chapter, you will use a template to complete a progress note. The two sets of exercises will provide you with hands-on experience using different data-entry methods.

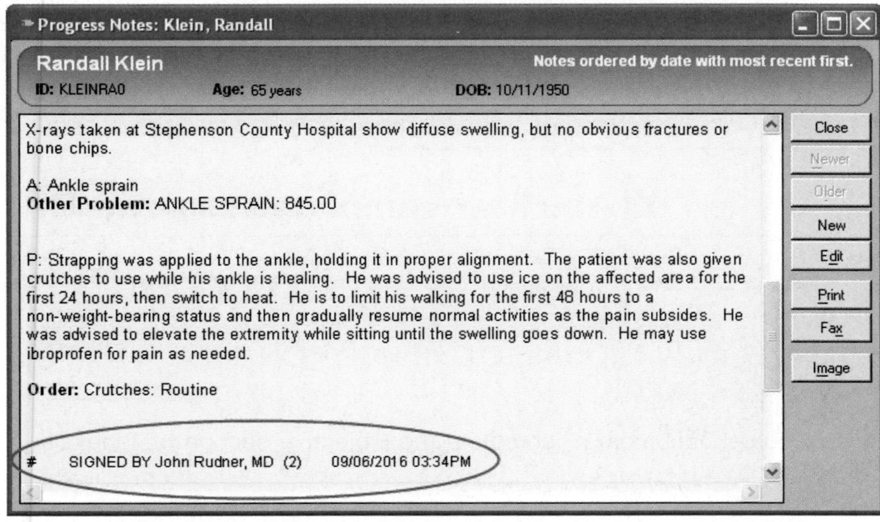

Figure 7.7 A Progress Note with an Electronic Signature

EXERCISE 7.1

OPENING A PROGRESS NOTE AND COMPLETING THE SUBJECTIVE SECTION

Log in as Dr. Katherine Yan. Open the progress note for Hiro Tanaka, and complete the Subjective section, using the information on Source Document 4.

Date: October 3, 2016

1. Start Medisoft Clinical Patient Records by clicking Start > All Programs > Medisoft Clinical—Client > Medisoft Clinical Client.
2. To log in as Dr. Yan, enter ***YANKATHERINE*** in the User ID field and ***master1$*** in the Password field.
3. Click the OK button.
4. When the disclaimer notice appears, click OK.
5. Click the Chart button on the toolbar.
6. When the Patient Lookup dialog box appears, enter ***TA*** in the Last Name field to locate Hiro Tanaka.
7. Click the Lookup button.
8. With Tanaka's line selected, click the OK button to open the chart.
9. Click the Note button on the toolbar. In response to the message about a shared note, click the Yes button to open the shared note. The note opens.
10. Click in the body of the note. The cursor is located on the title line, just after the words *BACK PAIN.* Press Enter twice to move down two lines in the note.
11. Enter ***Subjective:*** and press Enter.
12. Complete the Subjective section of the note by typing this information from Source Document 4:

    Patient is here today on referral from Dr. Bertram Brown. She was involved in a motor vehicle accident on 9/26/16, hit from behind. She was wearing her seat belt at the time, and the car's air bag deployed. The force of the impact caused a brief LOC, and she was admitted to the hospital for overnight observation. On release, she was still experiencing stiffness and pain in the lower back with difficulty ambulating. She has been attending physical therapy sessions daily since 9/27/16 and takes ibuprofen, 800 mg t.i.d. for pain. Patient states her pain is now a 2 on a scale of 10, easily managed with the ibuprofen as prescribed.

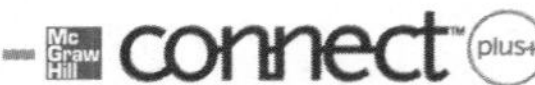

You have completed Exercise 7.1

EXERCISE 7.2

COMPLETING THE OBJECTIVE SECTION OF A PROGRESS NOTE

Using Source Document 4, complete the Objective section of Tanaka's progress note.

1. While still in the note, press Enter twice to move down two lines in the note.
2. Enter ***Objective:*** and press Enter.

3. Complete the Objective section of the note by typing this information from Source Document 4:

Allergies: Penicillin. [Press Enter.]

Past Medical History: Normal childhood immunizations. Denies surgeries or hospitalizations. [Press Enter.]

General: Patient is a well-developed, well-nourished 35-year-old Asian woman who appears to be in slight pain, and is alert and oriented in all spheres. [Press Enter.]

HEENT: Head: Normocephalic. Eyes: PERRLA. EOMI. [Press Enter.]

Neck: Supple; no thyromegaly. No limitation of range of motion. [Press Enter.]

Back and spine: No spinal tenderness. Lateral bending and forward bending within normal limits with little pain or stiffness. Gait is normal. [Press Enter.]

Neurological: DTRs are 2+ and equal bilaterally. [Press Enter.]

 You have completed Exercise 7.2

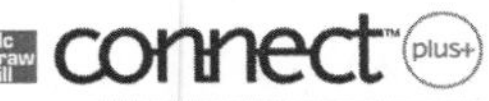

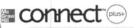

EXERCISE 7.3

COMPLETING THE ASSESSMENT SECTION OF A PROGRESS NOTE

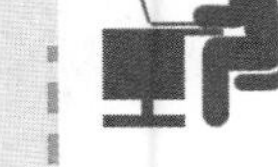

Using Source Document 4, complete the Assessment section of Tanaka's progress note.

1. While still in the note, press Enter twice to move down two lines in the note.
2. Enter ***Assessment:*** and press Enter.
3. Complete the Assessment section of the note by typing this information from Source Document 4:

Low back pain due to motor vehicle accident, resolving. [Press Enter.]

Allergy to penicillin.

 You have completed Exercise 7.3

EXERCISE 7.4

COMPLETING THE PLAN SECTION OF A PROGRESS NOTE

Using Source Document 4, complete the Plan section of Tanaka's progress note. (*Note:* In this exercise, you will use the Park feature that was discussed in Chapter 3.)

1. While still in the note, press Enter twice to move down two lines in the note.

(continued)

(Continued)

2. Enter ***Plan:*** and press Enter.

   Complete the Plan section of the note by typing this information from Source Document 4:

   Patient is released to return to work 10/5/2016. [Press Enter.]

   Continue with ibuprofen as needed. [Press Enter.]

   May discontinue physical therapy sessions. [Press Enter.]

   Return to clinic if any problems, otherwise for routine preventive care. [Press Enter.]

3. The note is complete. Click the OK button to save the note.
4. In response to the question about being permanently done with the note, click the Yes button.
5. The Enter Signature dialog box appears. Dr. Yan's provider ID, 1, is already listed in the Provider ID field.
6. To electronically sign the note, enter Dr. Yan's signature password, ***1234,*** in the Signature field.
7. Press the OK button. The progress note is saved.
8. Click the Progress Notes folder in the patient's chart to view the note again. Accept the default entry of Most Recent in the Progress Note Selection dialog box, and click OK.
9. The progress note opens. Scroll through the note to view the information that you entered. Notice that the program inserted Dr. Yan's electronic signature at the bottom of the note.
10. Click the Close button to close the note. You are returned to the patient's chart.
11. Click the Close button on the toolbar to close the patient's chart.
12. Click the Park button on the toolbar. In response to the question about whether you want to Park, click the Yes button.

 **You have completed Exercise 7.4**

Using a Template to Enter a Progress Note

In the following four exercises, you will use a template to enter information in a progress note. The information you need to complete the template is found in Source Document 3.

EXERCISE 7.5

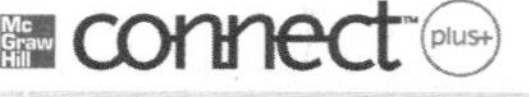

COMPLETING THE SUBJECTIVE SECTION OF A PROGRESS NOTE USING A TEMPLATE

Log in as Dr. Patricia McGrath. Open the progress note for Jorge Barrett, and complete the Subjective section, using the information in Source Document 3.

Date: October 3, 2016

1. To log in as Dr. McGrath, enter ***MCGRATHPATRICIA*** in the User ID field and ***master1$*** in the Password field.
2. Click the OK button.
3. Click the Chart button on the toolbar.

4. When the Patient Lookup dialog box appears, enter ***BA*** in the Last Name field to locate Jorge Barrett, and press Enter.
5. With Barrett's line selected, click the OK button to open the chart.
6. Click the Note button on the toolbar. In response to the message about a shared note, click the Yes button to open the shared note that you created in Chapter 6. The note opens.
7. Click in the body of the note. The cursor is located just after the word *Hypertension.* Press Enter twice to move down two lines in the note.
8. Select Template… on the Insert menu. The Insert Template dialog box is displayed with a list of templates.
9. The EASY SOAP template is selected. Press the Insert button to place the template in the note. Notice that the note contains a number of label markers.
10. Locate the Subjective section of the note. Notice that the program is alerting the physician about today's blood pressure readings, which were high.
11. Complete the line that begins "This 60 years old male presents…" by placing the cursor after the blue * label marker and entering ***with a series of elevated blood pressure readings.***
12. Click the PROBLEM 1 label. Two red labels appear.
13. Since this is a new problem, click the NewProb label. A list of Quick Text options is displayed.
14. Enter the letter ***E.*** The program moves down the list to the first entry that starts with the letter *E.* Scroll down the list and select ELEVATED BLOOD PRESSURE. Click the Insert button. Additional content is displayed below the heading ELEVATED BLOOD PRESSURE. Complete the list of entries as follows, based on the information in Source Document 3:

    Duration of elevated blood pressure: DEL DurWk chronic unknown
    Click the DurWk label. Scroll down the Quick Text list and select 4 weeks. Click the Insert button.

    Blood pressure monitoring frequency: DEL not checking Frequency rare
    Click the Frequency label. Select daily from the Quick text list. Click the Insert button.

    Blood pressure range: DEL Systolic / Diastolic
    Click the Systolic label. Select 170–180s from the list. Click the Insert button.
    Click the Diastolic label. Select 100–110s. Click Insert.

    Recent stressors: DEL yes no
    Click the no label.

    Family history of hypertension: DEL yes no
    Click the no label.

    Recurrent headaches: DEL yes no status HEADACHE DETAILS
    Click the no label.

    Visual changes: DEL yes no status
    Click the no label.

    Palpitations: DEL yes no status
    Click the no label.

(continued)

(Continued)

Dyspnea: DEL yes no status
Click the no label.

Chest pain: DEL yes no status
Click the no label.

Lower extremity edema: DEL yes no status
Click the no label.

Transient ischemic attacks: DEL yes no
Click the no label.

15. Since there is no other problem, skip the Problem 2 label.
16. Click the REVIEW OF SYSTEMS label. Additional text is inserted below the label.

Complete the Review of Systems entries as follows:

Constitutional: DEL neg ROSNEGGEN ROSGener
Click the ROSNEGGEN label to indicate that the patient reports no fevers, chills, or unexplained weight loss.

Eyes: DEL neg ROSNEGEYE ROSEyes
Click the ROSNEGEYE label to indicate that the patient reports no visual changes or eye pain.

Ears: DEL neg ROSNEGEARS
Click the ROSNEGEARS label to indicate that the patient reports no hearing loss, otorrhea or ear pain.

Nose/Mouth/Throat: DEL neg ROSNEGNMT ROSENMT
Skip this entry since it is not mentioned in the documentation in Source Document 3.

Cardiovascular: DEL neg ROSNEGCARDIO ROSCVS
Click the ROSNEGCARDIO label to indicate that the patient reports no chest pain or palpitations.

Respiratory: DEL neg ROSNEGRESP ROSResp
Skip this entry since it is not mentioned in the documentation in Source Document 3.

Gastrointestinal: DEL neg ROSNEGGI ROSGI
Click the ROSNEGGI label to indicate that the patient reports no diarrhea, constipation, blood in stools, abdominal pain, vomiting or heartburn

Genitourinary: DEL neg ROSNEGURINE ROSGU
Click the ROSGU label and select nocturia from the list. Click the Insert button.

Musculoskeletal: DEL neg ROSNEGMSK ROSMusc
Click the ROSNEGMSK label to indicate that the patient reports no arthralgias, myalgias or joint swelling

Skin: DEL neg ROSNEGSKIN ROSSkinBr
Click the ROSNEGSKIN label to indicate that the patient reports no rash or bothersome skin lesions.

Breast: DEL neg ROSNEGBREAST
Skip this entry since it is not mentioned in the documentation in Source Document 3.

Neurological: DEL neg ROSNEGNEURO ROSNeuro
Click the ROSNEGNEURO label to indicate that the patient reports no headaches, parasthesias, confusion, dysarthria or gait instability.

Psychiatric: DEL neg ROSNEGPSYCH ROSPsych
Skip this entry since it is not mentioned in the documentation in Source Document 3.

Hematologic/Lymphatic: DEL neg ROSNEGHEMELYMPH ROSHemeLy
Skip this entry since it is not mentioned in the documentation in Source Document 3.

Allergic/Immunologic: DEL neg ROSNEGALLERGIC ROSAllImm
Skip this entry since it is not mentioned in the documentation in Source Document 3.

17. Since there are no labs, skip the INSERT LABS label.
18. Since Dr. McGrath reviewed the patient's past medical, social, and family history before she came in the exam room, click the Reviewed PMH/SH/FH label.
19. Since the patient's current medications were entered in Chapter 6, they are automatically added to the note.
20. Click the OK button to save the note.
21. In response to the question about being permanently done with the note, click the No button.
22. The note closes, and you are returned to the patient's chart.

 **You have completed Exercise 7.5**

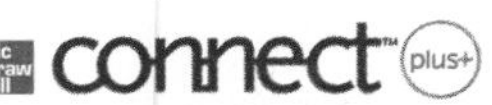

EXERCISE 7.6

COMPLETING THE OBJECTIVE SECTION OF A PROGRESS NOTE USING A TEMPLATE

Using Source Document 3, open the progress note for Jorge Barrett, and complete the Objective section.

1. With Barrett's chart open, click the Note button on the toolbar. In response to the message about a shared note, click the Yes button to open the shared note. The note opens.
2. Scroll down to the Objective section of the note.
3. Click the INSERT PHYSICAL EXAM label. Additional text is inserted below the label.
4. Complete the Review of Systems entries as follows:

General: DEL General ill GeneralCA
Click the General label to enter well appearing, well nourished, and in no distress.

Skin: DEL Skin SkinCA
Click the Skin label to enter no rash or prominent lesions.

Hair: DEL Hair HairCA
Skip this entry since it is not mentioned in the documentation in Source Document 3.

Nails: DEL Nails NailsCA
Skip this entry since it is not mentioned in the documentation in Source Document 3.

(continued)

(Continued)

Head: DEL Head HeadCA E1
Click the Head label to enter normocephalic, atraumatic.

Eyes: DEL Eyes EyesCA
Click the Eyes label to enter conjunctiva clear, EOM intact, PERRL.

Ears: DEL Ears Cerumen. EarsCA
Click the Ears label to enter ear canals clear, tympanic membranes clear, ossicles normal appearance.

Sinuses: DEL NT Rfront Lfront Rmax Lmax All Sinus TTP
Click the NT label to enter non-tender.

Nose: DEL Nose NoseCA
Click the Nose label to enter no external lesions, mucosa non-inflamed, septum and turbinates normal.

Mouth: DEL Mouth MouthCA
Click the Mouth label to enter mucous membranes moist, no mucosal lesions.

Teeth/gums: DEL Teeth TeethCA
Skip this entry since it is not mentioned in the documentation in Source Document 3.

Throat: DEL Throat ThroatCA
Click the Throat label to enter no erythema, exudates or lesions.

Neck: DEL Neck NeckNoBruit NeckCA
Click the Neck label to enter supple without lymphadenopathy.

Heart: DEL HeartBrief Heart HeartCA
Click the Heart label to enter RRR, no murmur or gallop. Normal S1, S2. No S3, S4.

Lungs: DEL Lungs LungsCA
Click the Lungs label to enter CTA bilaterally, no wheezes, rhonchi, rales. Breathing unlabored.

Chest wall: DEL NLinsp TTP No Crepitus No Masses O8
Click the NLinsp label to enter no swelling, ecchymosis, erythema or deformity.

Abdomen: DEL AbdomenBrief Abdomen AbdomenCA O6
Click the AbdomenBrief label to enter soft, NT/ND, no HSM, no masses.

Back: DEL Back BackCA E6
Skip this entry since it is not mentioned in the documentation in Source Document 3.

GU: DEL GUMale GUMaleCA O7
Skip this entry since it is not mentioned in the documentation in Source Document 3.

Rectal: DEL RectalMale RectalMaleCA E5
Skip this entry since it is not mentioned in the documentation in Source Document 3.

Extremities: DEL Extremitie ExtremitCA O8
Click the Extremitie label to enter no deformities, clubbing, cyanosis, or edema.

Musculoskeletal: DEL Musculoske MusculoCA MSK Exams O8
Click the Musculoske label to enter normal symmetry, tone, strength and ROM. No effusions, instability or tenderness to palpation.

Lymphatics: DEL LymphBrief Lymphatics LymphCA O12
Skip this entry since it is not mentioned in the documentation in Source Document 3.

Neurologic: DEL NeuroBrief Neuro NeuroCA O10
Click the NeuroBrief label to enter A/O x 3. No focal deficits. Gait WNL.

Psychiatric: DEL Psych PsychCA O11
Skip this entry since it is not mentioned in the documentation in Source Document 3.

5. Click the OK button to save the note.
6. In response to the question about being permanently done with the note, click the No button.
7. The note closes and you are returned to the patient's chart.

You have completed Exercise 7.6

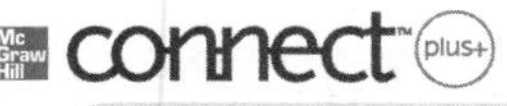

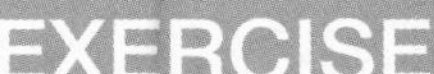

EXERCISE 7.7

COMPLETING THE ASSESSMENT SECTION OF A PROGRESS NOTE USING A TEMPLATE

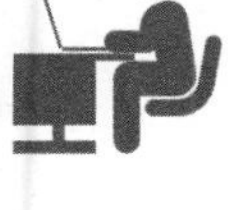

Using Source Document 3, open the progress note for Jorge Barrett, and complete the Assessment section.

1. With Barrett's chart open, click the Note button on the toolbar. In response to the message about a shared note, click the Yes button to open the shared note. The note opens.
2. Scroll down to the Assessment section of the note.
3. Click the label CHRONIC DISEASE DIAGNOSES. A list of chronic diseases is listed.
4. Click the entry for Hypertension Unspecified. The program enters the diagnosis code and description.
5. Click the Disease Status label. Select /-New Diagnosis from the list, and click Insert.
6. Click the OK button to save the note.
7. In response to the question about being permanently done with the note, click the No button.
8. The note closes and you are returned to the patient's chart.

You have completed Exercise 7.7

EXERCISE 7.8

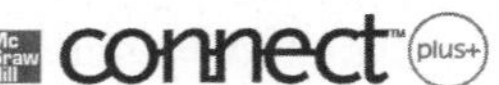

COMPLETING THE PLAN SECTION OF A PROGRESS NOTE USING A TEMPLATE

Using Source Document 3, open the progress note for Jorge Barrett, and complete the Plan section.

1. With Barrett's chart open, click the Note button on the toolbar. In response to the message about a shared note, click the Yes button to open the shared note. The note opens.
2. Scroll down to the Plan section of the note.
3. Dr. McGrath is going to order a hypertension medication for Mr. Barrett. Click the ePrescribe label. Additional labels appear.
4. Click the ePrescribe All Rx label. The program enters the following text: All prescriptions created during this encounter were generated using a qualified e-prescribing system. A procedure code and description for e-prescribing is also entered. (*Note:* This information is one of the requirements to receive a financial bonus as part of the Physician's Quality Reporting Initiative [PQRI] and the Meaningful Use portion of the HITECH Act.)
5. Enter follow-up information by clicking the red F/U label to the right of the word *Follow-up*. Select 1 month from the list that appears, and press the Insert button. The phrase "1 month" is inserted where the label had been.
6. The note is complete. Click the OK button to save the note.
7. In response to the question about being permanently done with the note, click the Yes button.
8. The Enter Signature dialog box appears. Dr. McGrath's provider ID, 4, is already listed in the Provider ID field.
9. To electronically sign the note, enter Dr. McGrath's signature password, ***4567,*** in the Signature field.
10. Press the OK button. The progress note closes.
11. Click the Progress Notes folder in the patient's chart to view the note again. Accept the default entry of Most Recent in the Progress Note Selection dialog box, and click OK.
12. The progress note opens. Scroll through the note to view the information that you entered. Notice that the program inserted Dr. McGrath's electronic signature at the bottom of the note.
13. Click the Close button to close the note. You are returned to the patient's chart.
14. Click the Close button on the toolbar to close the patient's chart.

You have completed Exercise 7.8

7.3 E-Prescribing and Electronic Health Records

Once a provider has finished examining a patient, he or she may decide to order a medication. In an electronic health record, this is known as e-prescribing. By writing prescriptions electronically, providers can avoid many of the mistakes that occur with handwritten prescriptions.

Safety Checks

E-prescribing also provides a number of built-in safety checks. For example, when a provider selects a drug for a patient, the EHR checks for drug allergies, drug–drug interactions, and other potential conflicts using information in the patient's medical record, including past history, allergies, and a complete medication list. Figure 7.8 shows a drug-diagnosis warning that appeared when lisinopril, a popular drug for high blood pressure, was prescribed for a woman with type II diabetes.

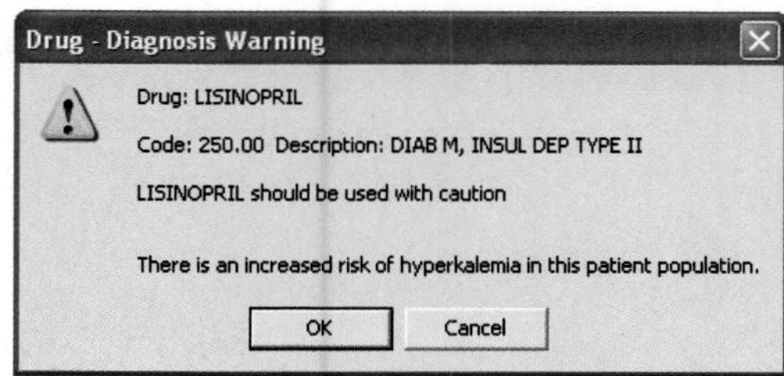

Figure 7.8 A Drug-Diagnosis Warning in an EHR

Formulary Check

The EHR also checks that the medication is in the formulary of the patient's health plan. A **formulary** is a list of pharmaceutical products and dosages deemed by a health care organization to be the best, most economical treatments for a condition or disease. Health plans reimburse patients for drugs listed in the formulary only, so it is essential for the provider to have this information before the patient leaves the office. If a medication is not in the formulary, the EHR can suggest an alternative drug. Since the medications in formularies change from time to time, the formulary data in the EHRs are updated regularly.

formulary list of a plan's selected drugs and their proper dosages

Some EHRs even check whether the medication is in stock at the patient's preferred pharmacy. It is much better to know that a drug is in stock before the patient goes to pick it up at the pharmacy. E-prescribing also gives the pharmacy time to prepare the prescription so the patient will not have to wait once he or she arrives.

The steps required to refill a patient prescription in a paper-based office and in an electronic office illustrate the advantages of e-prescribing (see Figures 7.9 and 7.10).

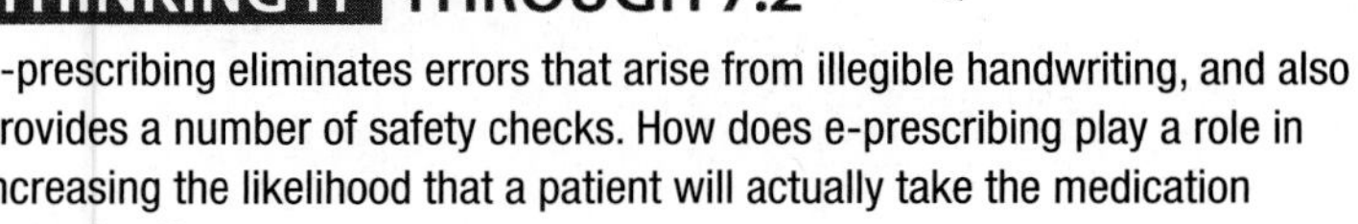

THINKING IT THROUGH 7.2

E-prescribing eliminates errors that arise from illegible handwriting, and also provides a number of safety checks. How does e-prescribing play a role in increasing the likelihood that a patient will actually take the medication prescribed?

Figure 7.9 Prescription Refill in a Paper-Based Office

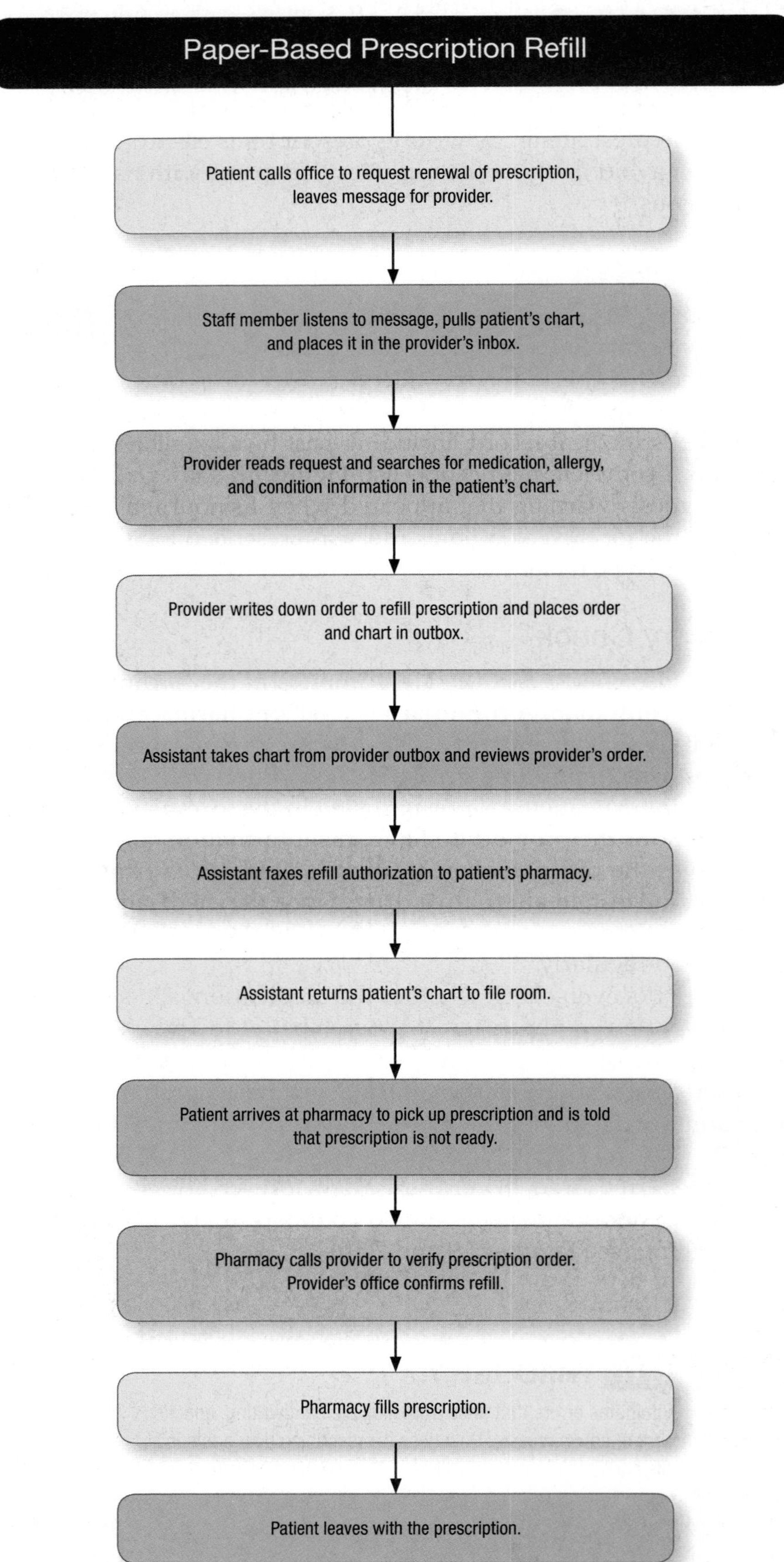

Paper-Based Prescription Refill
Patient calls office to request renewal of prescription, leaves message for provider.
Staff member listens to message, pulls patient's chart, and places it in the provider's inbox.
Provider reads request and searches for medication, allergy, and condition information in the patient's chart.
Provider writes down order to refill prescription and places order and chart in outbox.
Assistant takes chart from provider outbox and reviews provider's order.
Assistant faxes refill authorization to patient's pharmacy.
Assistant returns patient's chart to file room.
Patient arrives at pharmacy to pick up prescription and is told that prescription is not ready.
Pharmacy calls provider to verify prescription order. Provider's office confirms refill.
Pharmacy fills prescription.
Patient leaves with the prescription.

Figure 7.10 Prescription Refill in an Electronic Office

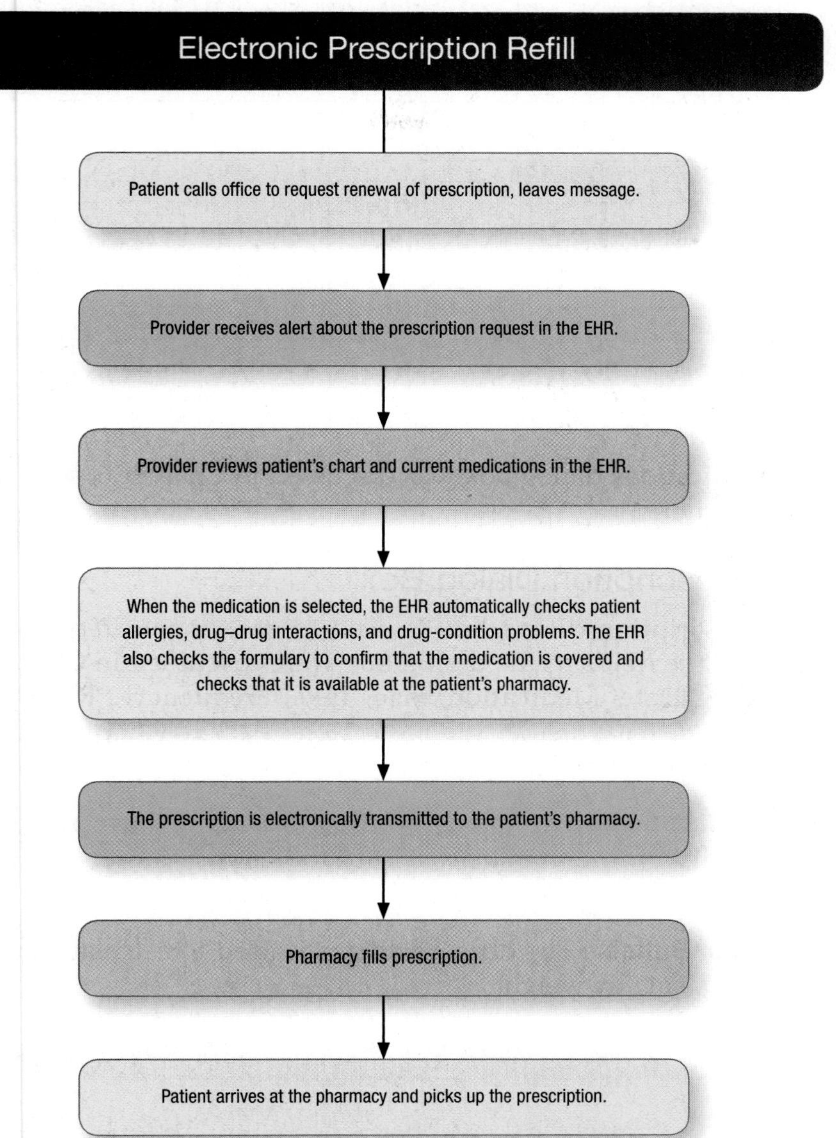

Electronic Prescription Refill
Patient calls office to request renewal of prescription, leaves message.
Provider receives alert about the prescription request in the EHR.
Provider reviews patient's chart and current medications in the EHR.
When the medication is selected, the EHR automatically checks patient allergies, drug–drug interactions, and drug-condition problems. The EHR also checks the formulary to confirm that the medication is covered and checks that it is available at the patient's pharmacy.
The prescription is electronically transmitted to the patient's pharmacy.
Pharmacy fills prescription.
Patient arrives at the pharmacy and picks up the prescription.

7.4 Entering Prescriptions in Medisoft Clinical Patient Records

In Medisoft Clinical Patient Records, the Rx/Medications folder in a patient's chart is used to order new medications and monitor current, historical, or ineffective medications. Figure 7.11 shows a patient's Rx/Medications dialog box listing current medications.

To prevent unauthorized personnel from writing prescriptions, a PIN that serves as a special electronic signature is required to transmit prescriptions. When a signature is required, the prescription cannot be transmitted until the PIN is provided.

New prescriptions can be entered from the Rx/Medications folder in a chart, or by clicking the Rx button on the toolbar. Much of the

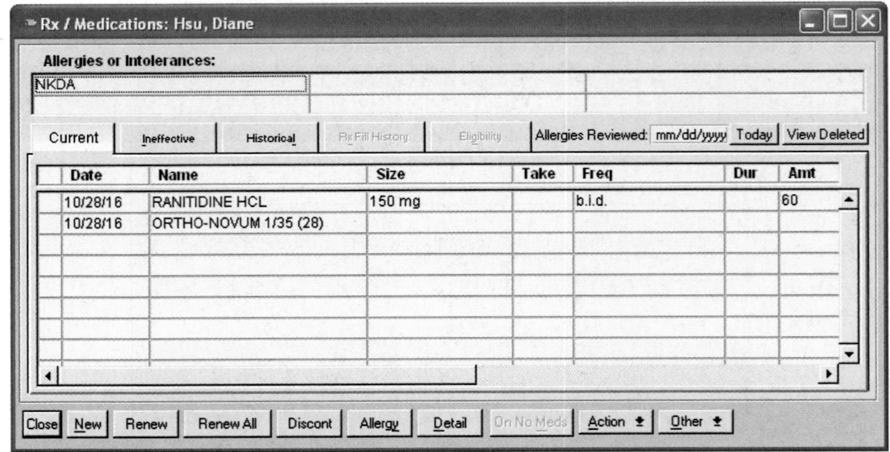

Figure 7.11 Rx/Medications Dialog Box Listing a Patient's Current Medications

Rx/Medications dialog box was discussed in Chapter 6, so it is not repeated here.

The Prescription Dialog Box

The Prescription dialog box is used to enter new prescriptions. Some of the fields in the dialog box were discussed in Chapter 6, including Date, Medication, Size, Take, Frequency, PRN, Route, Duration, Prov, Outside, and Note. Refer back to Chapter 6 for review, if necessary.

Rx Template Code To find a specific medication, enter a template code or drug name in this field. Click the Lookup button to display the Select Rx Template dialog box (see Figure 7.12).

Calculator Button The dose calculator is used to calculate patient-specific dosing by weight.

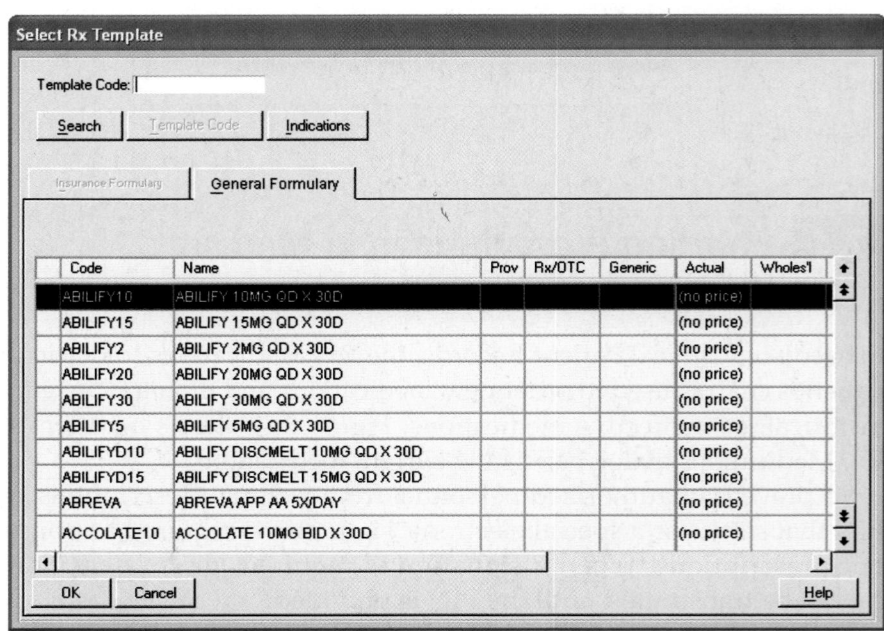

Figure 7.12 The Select Rx Template Dialog Box

Amount The amount of medication to be dispensed is entered here.

Refills Either type or select the number of refills. Use 0 (zero) for "no refills."

Print Click to indicate whether the prescription should be transmitted electronically, printed, or faxed.

Indication 1, Indication 2 The Indication fields list the condition for which the medication is being prescribed. Clicking the Lookup 1 or Lookup 2 button causes the Diagnosis Code Select dialog box to appear. Selections made in this dialog box will appear in the indications fields in the Prescription dialog box.

Note A note can be entered in the Note field.

Pharmacy Enter the name of the patient's pharmacy, or leave the box blank.

Formulary Area This area displays the result of the formulary check. It is used to determine the formulary status of a drug when writing a new prescription or renewing an existing prescription. Once the medication name, size, and route are entered, the program displays formulary data, if available, using the information from the most recent pharmacy benefits eligibility response.

Extended Sig Enter the instructions for prescriptions with complex instructions in this field. There is a limit of 250 characters.

Code Field If extended sig templates are used, one can be selected in the Code field.

Create Sig Template Clicking in this box saves the text entered in the Extended Sig field as a new template.

Check Boxes

The area near the bottom of the dialog box contains ten check boxes.

Use Extended Sig Enable the Extended Sig area.

Use Extended Sig Only Print the extended sig only.

Use Patient Instructions Print patient instructions.

Limit Refills Activate a warning approving a refill of the prescription.

Substitution OK Indicates to the pharmacist that substituting a generic medication is acceptable.

Update Progress Note Updates the progress note with the prescription information.

Drug Interaction Check Checks the new prescription against current medications for interactions.

Allergy Check Checks the new prescription against current allergies.

New Rx Template Creates a new template using this prescription.

OTC Indicates that this is an over-the-counter drug, so a prescription is not required.

Pricing

This bottom of the dialog box displays pricing information for the prescription, if available.

Buttons

The buttons at the bottom of the dialog box perform the following functions.

OK Saves the current prescription.

Cancel Cancels the current prescription.

Alternative Displays a list of alternative drugs of the same class and route as the one listed in the Medication field, with their cost information.

Dose Advisor Displays the dose advisor, which can be used to calculate a recommended dose for the patient.

EXERCISE 7.9

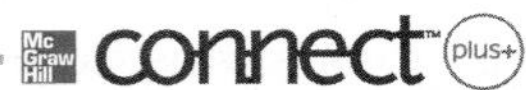

ENTERING AN ORDER FOR A NEW PRESCRIPTION

(*Note:* The intention of this exercise is to provide students with an understanding of how a prescription is written in an EHR. Students do not create a prescription that can actually be printed or transmitted.) Using Source Document 3, enter a new prescription order for Jorge Barrett.

1. Click the Chart button on the toolbar.
2. When the Patient Lookup dialog box appears, enter ***BA*** in the Last Name field to locate Jorge Barrett, and press Enter.
3. With Barrett's line selected, click the OK button to open his chart.
4. Click the Rx/Medications folder. The Rx/Medications dialog box opens, with the Current tab active.
5. Click the New button. The Prescription dialog box appears.
6. Enter ***LISINOPRIL*** in the Rx Template Code field.
7. Click the Lookup button. The Select Rx Template dialog box appears.
8. Scroll up to locate the entry for template LISINOPR10, for 10 mg of lisinopril to be taken once a day for thirty days.
9. Click the entry to select it, and then click the OK button. The Prescription dialog box reappears, with some of the fields completed based on the information in the template.
10. Leave the Duration field blank, since the patient is not taking the medication for a limited time.
11. Select 0 in the Refills field, since Dr. McGrath wants to see Mr. Barrett for a follow-up visit in one month, and this is a new medication for a newly diagnosed condition.

12. In the Print field, select Transmit as a Group.
13. Click the Lookup 1 button in the Indication 1 field. The Diagnosis Code Select dialog box opens.
14. Change the selection at the top of the dialog box to Office Code.
15. Click in the Search field and enter Barrett's diagnosis, ***401.9***. The program highlights the entry for 401.9.
16. Leave the Insert into Text and Insert As fields as they appear.
17. Click the OK button. The Prescription box reappears.
18. Leave the Note, Pharmacy, and Formulary fields blank.
19. Review the entries in the check box section of the Prescription dialog box. The Substitution OK, Update Progress Note, Drug Interaction Check, and Allergy Check boxes should be checked.
20. Click the OK button to save the new prescription. The Current tab of the Rx/Medications dialog box reappears with the new prescription listed.
21. Click the Close button to close the dialog box.
22. To confirm that the prescription was added to the progress note, click the Progress Notes folder and view the most recent note. Scroll down to the bottom of the note to view the prescription for lisinopril.
23. Click the Close button on the toolbar to close Barrett's chart.

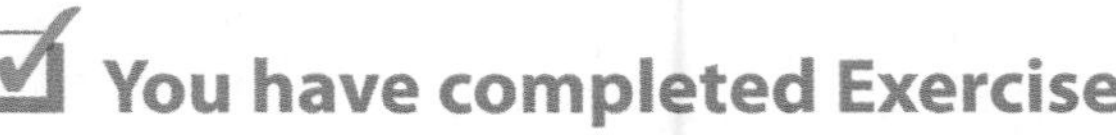
You have completed Exercise 7.9

7.5 Ordering Tests and Procedures in an EHR

Once a physician is finished examining a patient, it may be necessary to order tests or procedures as part of diagnosing or treating the patient's condition. EHRs allow doctors to order tests without the use of traditional paper forms. Some EHRs include built-in standard order sets based on the provider's specialty or on specific diseases.

Receiving Results

Physician practices vary in regard to whether tests and procedures are performed in-house or by an outside facility. Very small practices may use outside labs for almost all tests, while larger group practices may have their own in-house lab facilities. If an outside facility is used, an EHR can receive the results electronically.

Benefits of Electronic Order Entry

Electronic order entry is designed to reduce errors associated with handwritten and paper orders. It is, however, more than a replacement for a paper order system; it provides numerous safety and cost-control benefits. For example, the software can incorporate the rules of different insurance carriers, making it easy to determine whether a test requires preauthorization and whether it is limited to specified diagnoses. The software can delay sending out these orders until approval is received. In addition, Medisoft Clinical

Figure 7.13 Flowchart of Order Entry in a Paper-Based Office

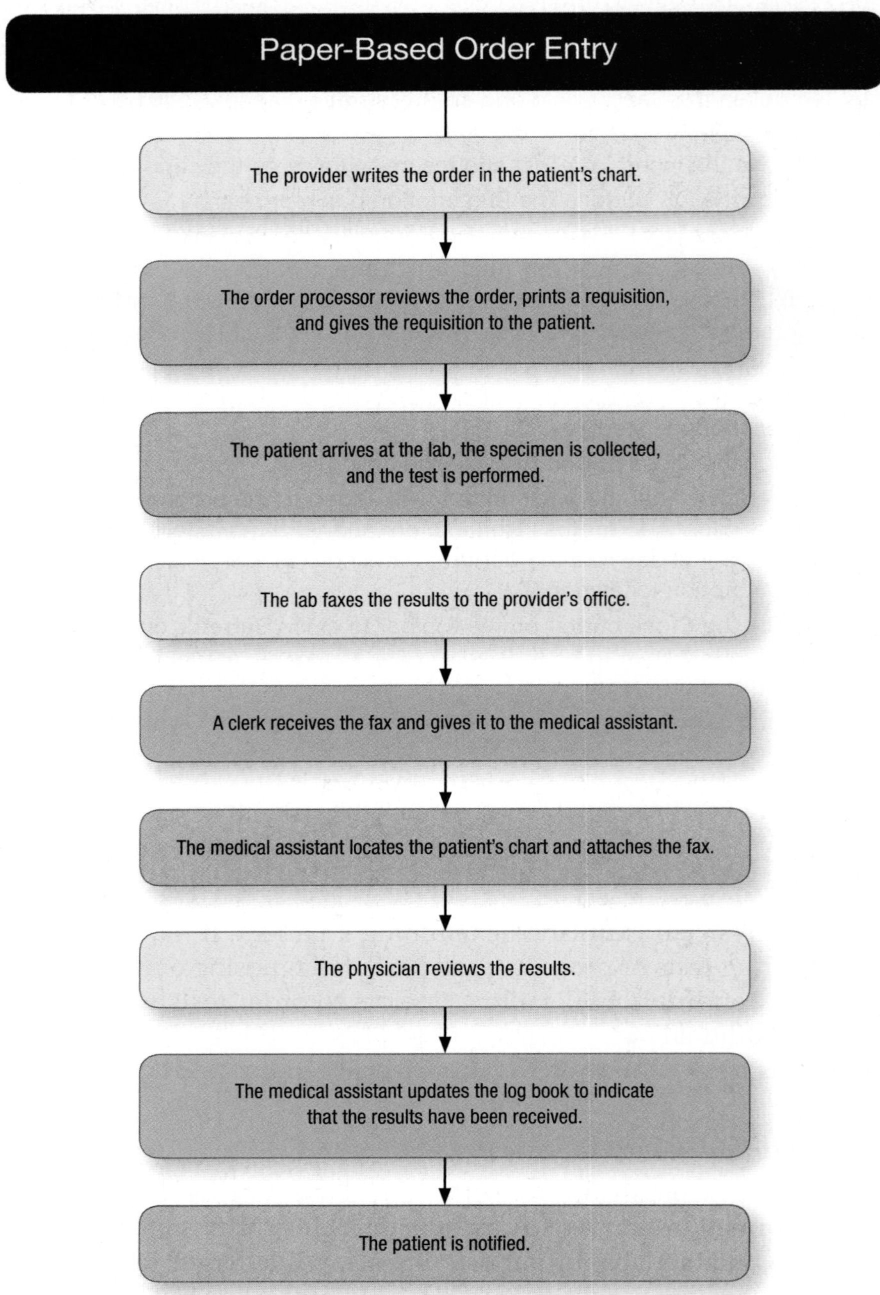

Patient Records is capable of checking orders against information specific to the patient, such as whether the order would be inappropriate based on a patient's medications, lab tests, diagnoses, allergies, or other factors.

In an office with an EHR, the provider enters the orders for a test directly in the program. Once the order has been entered, a staff member receives and processes the order. Orders can then be printed or transmitted electronically.

Figures 7.13 and 7.14 illustrate the steps required to send and receive a lab test in a paper-based office and in an office with an EHR.

THINKING IT THROUGH 7.3

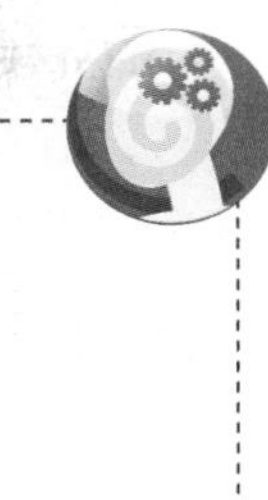

When an order is entered in an EHR, the program can check whether the test requires preauthorization and delay the order until that authorization is received. Obviously this is a benefit to the patient, who will not have to pay for a test that was performed prior to authorization. How does this also benefit the medical practice?

Figure 7.14 Flowchart of Order Entry in an Office with an EHR

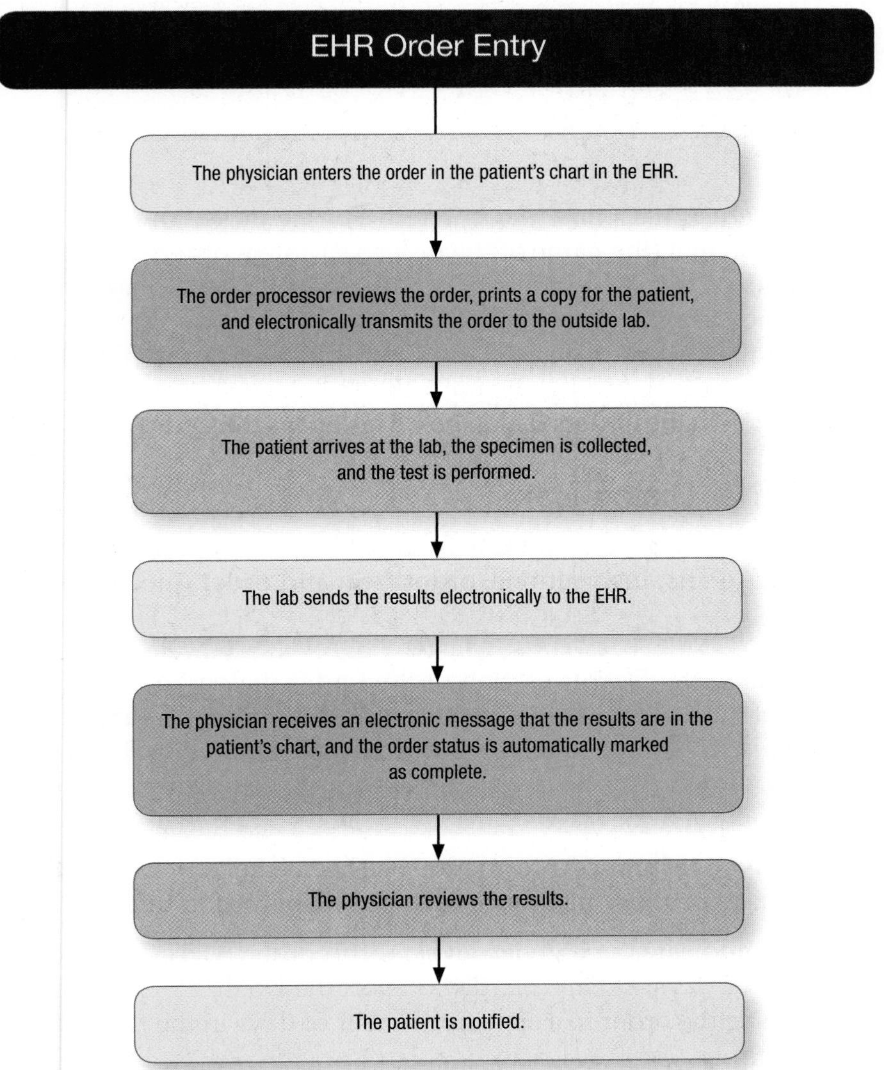

EHR Order Entry
The physician enters the order in the patient's chart in the EHR.
The order processor reviews the order, prints a copy for the patient, and electronically transmits the order to the outside lab.
The patient arrives at the lab, the specimen is collected, and the test is performed.
The lab sends the results electronically to the EHR.
The physician receives an electronic message that the results are in the patient's chart, and the order status is automatically marked as complete.
The physician reviews the results.
The patient is notified.

7.6 Order Entry in Medisoft Clinical Patient Records

In Medisoft Clinical Patient Records, a physician can enter orders for laboratory, radiology, pathology, and other diagnostic tests. If the physician has entered a progress note for the day that tests are ordered, the orders are automatically listed near the bottom of the note.

Most EHR programs permit orders to be grouped into sets, referred to as panels. When a panel is entered, the individual tests

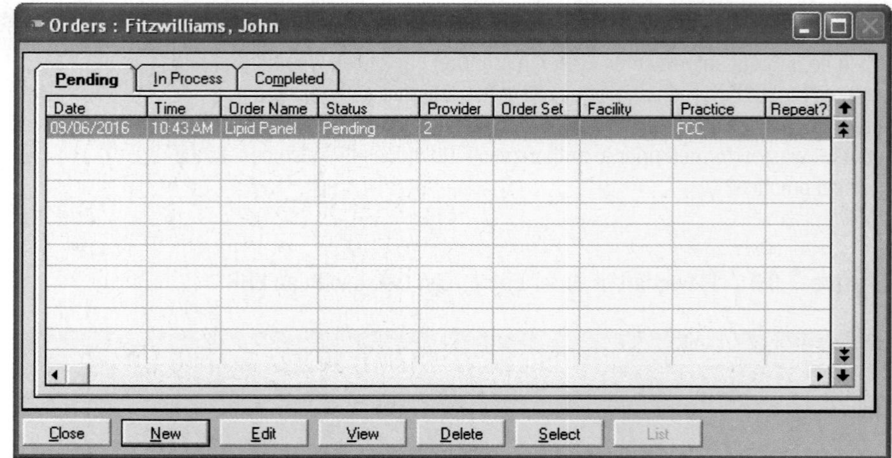

Figure 7.15 The Orders Dialog Box Listing a Pending Order

that make up that panel are entered. For example, an order for a metabolic panel (the name of the order set) enters orders for a group of individual tests (chloride, CO_2, creatinine, glucose, potassium, sodium, and urea nitrogen).

When the Orders folder is clicked in the patient's chart, the Orders dialog box is displayed (see Figure 7.15). To enter a new order, click the New button in the Orders dialog box. This opens the Order dialog box.

The Order Dialog Box

The Order dialog box contains four sections, as illustrated in Figure 7.16: details, instructions, order tree, and order queue.

Details

The fields in the Details section of the Order dialog box, located at the top of the screen, specify settings for orders. Some information in the details section are entered by the program, including Insurance, Urgency, Ordered by, Send Results to, and Practice. These fields can be modified as necessary.

Insurance If insurance information has been entered for the patient, the patient's primary insurance carrier is displayed in this field.

Urgency Indicate the urgency level for this order: STAT, Routine, Do within ____ days, Do in ____ days. Select the Do in ____ days check box to issue the order in a specific number of days in the future.

Ordered by Lists the provider who placed the order.

Facility Select the facility to be used for the order. If a facility is linked to the patient's insurance plan, it will be displayed in this field.

Practice If necessary, select the appropriate practice.

Send Results to Select one or more providers who should receive the results. The ordering provider is automatically entered in the first field.

Print Default Label If this box is checked, the default label will automatically print when the order is saved.

Encounter # Enter an encounter number for the order, if required.

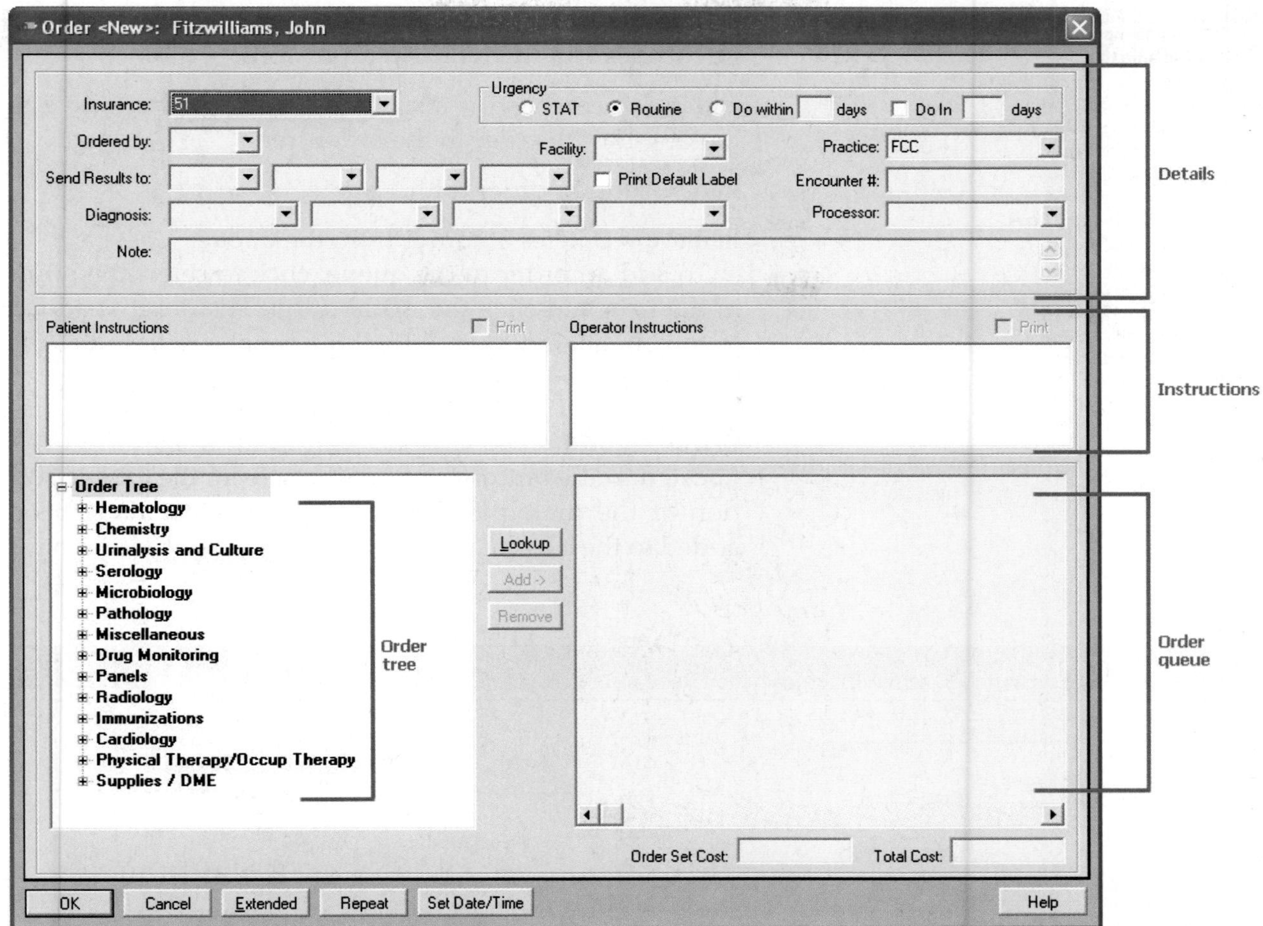

Figure 7.16 The Order Dialog Box

Diagnosis Select up to four diagnosis codes for the order. If the patient's insurance plan requires a specific diagnosis code, a message will display if this code is not selected.

Processor Selects the operator who will process the order.

Note Type a text note related to the order.

Instructions

Patient Instructions Instructions for the patient can be entered in this field. Instructions can be up to a thousand characters long. To print the instructions, select the Print check box above the instruction's box.

Operator Instructions Instructions for the order processor can be entered in this field. Instructions can be up to a thousand characters long. To print the instructions, select the Print check box above the instruction's box.

Order Tree

The order tree, displayed on the lower-left side of the dialog box, is used to select orders to add to the order queue. By clicking the plus sign next to each of the entries in the order tree, the tree expands to list orders within the set (see Figure 7.17).

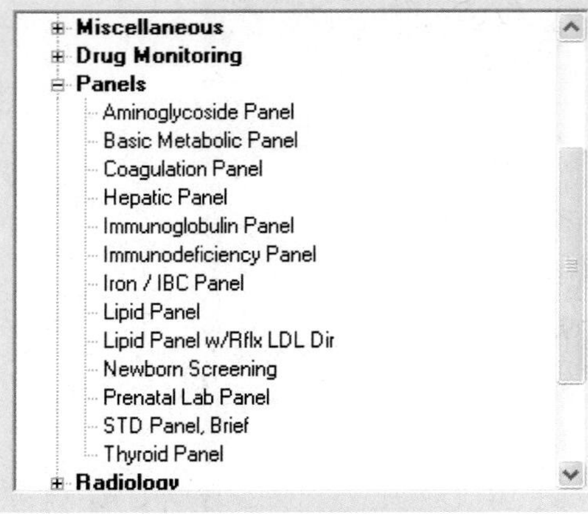

Figure 7.17 The Order Tree with the Panels Set Expanded

The three buttons between the order tree and the queue perform the following functions:

Lookup Searches for a specific order (an alternative to looking for the order in the order tree).

Add Adds an order to the queue.

Remove Deletes an order from the queue.

To add an order to the queue, click to select the order in the tree, and click the Add button. The order is added to the queue. In Figure 7.18, lipid panel is selected in the tree and has been added to the queue on the right.

Order Queue

Located in the bottom right of the screen, the Queue section of the dialog box lists the orders that have been added to the current order. If the costs of procedures have

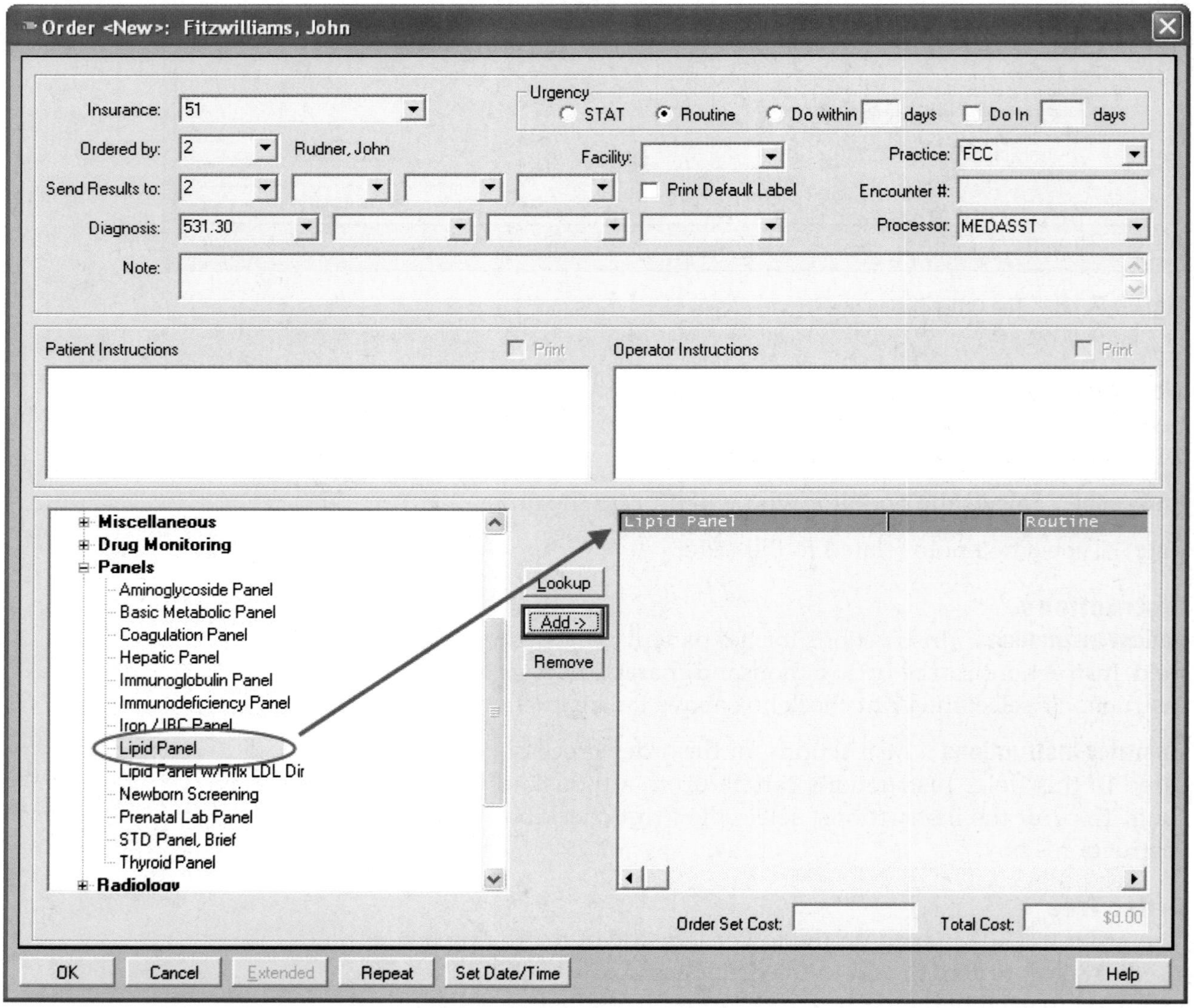

Figure 7.18 The Order Dialog Box with Lipid Panel Added to the Order Queue

been entered in the program, they will appear in the Order Set Cost and Total Cost fields.

Buttons

The buttons located at the bottom of the dialog box perform the following functions:

Extended This button accesses the Processing Extended Dialog feature, which is used to view and edit extended information about the order. Many labs require orders to have specific processing information, especially when samples are collected at the office.

Repeat Enters repeating or recurring orders.

Set Date/Time Used to backdate an order or to schedule a future order.

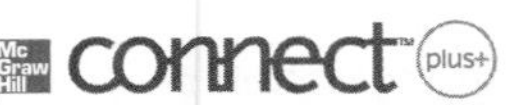

EXERCISE 7.10

ENTERING ORDERS FOR A PATIENT

Dr. McGrath decides to order some lab work for Jorge Barrett. Refer to Source Document 3, and enter the orders using the Orders folder in the patient's chart.

1. Click the Chart button on the toolbar.
2. When the Patient Lookup dialog box appears, enter ***BA*** in the Last Name field to locate Jorge Barrett, and press Enter.
3. With Barrett's line selected, click the OK button to open the chart.
4. Click the Orders folder. The Orders dialog box opens.
5. Click the New button to begin a new order. The Order dialog box opens.
6. Review the information already entered in the top of the dialog box:
   Insurance
   Urgency
   Ordered by
   Practice
   Send Results to
   Diagnosis
7. Click in the Processor field. In the Operator Select dialog box that appears, select MEDASST. Click the OK button.
8. In the Order Tree, click the plus sign next to Hematology. A list of orders within the category is displayed.
9. Click HEMATOCRIT, and then click the Add button. HEMATOCRIT is added to the order queue on the right side of the dialog box.
10. Scroll down the order tree, and locate the Chemistry category. Click the plus sign to open the list.
11. Select CALCIUM, and click the Add button. CALCIUM is added to the list of orders.
12. Select CREATININE CLEARANCE from the Chemistry list, and click Add.
13. Select GLUCOSE, FASTING from the Chemistry list, and click Add.
14. Select POTASSIUM from the Chemistry list, and click Add.

(continued)

(Continued)

15. Click the plus sign next to Urinalysis and Culture to display the list of tests available. Click DIP UA, and click Add.
16. Click the plus sign next to Panels to display the list of panels available. Select Lipid Panel, and click Add. With Lipid Panel selected (highlighted), enter the following text in the Patient Instructions field: ***No food or drink other than water for 12 hours before test.***
17. Click the plus sign next to Cardiology to display the list of procedures available. Select EKG with interpretation, and click Add.
18. There are now eight orders listed in the order queue on the right side of the dialog box.
19. Click OK to record the orders. The dialog box closes, and you are returned to the Orders dialog box. Notice that the tests ordered are now listed as pending.
20. Click the Close button to close the dialog box.
21. Click the Park button on the toolbar. In response to the question about whether you want to park, click the Yes button.

You have completed Exercise 7.10

7.7 Order Processing in Medisoft Clinical Patient Records

Once an order has been entered by a provider, it is received by the staff member responsible for processing orders. In Medisoft Clinical Patient Records, order processing begins with selecting Orders > Order Processing on the Task menu. The Order Processing Select screen appears, with the Select Orders dialog box on top.

The Select Orders Dialog Box

The Select Orders dialog box filters the orders that are displayed in the Order Processing Select dialog box (see Figure 7.19). The fields in the Select Orders dialog box include:

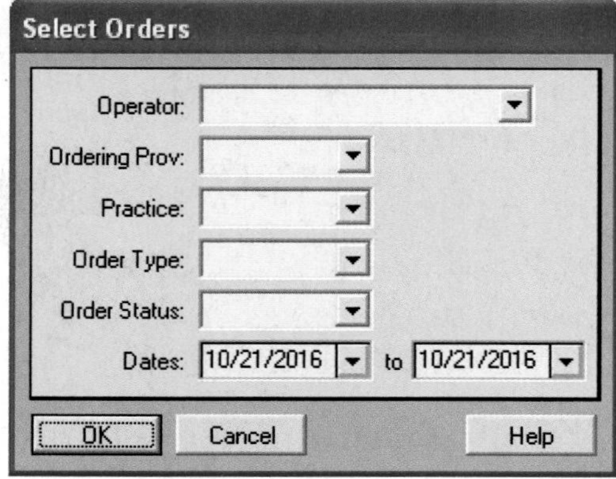

Figure 7.19 The Select Orders Dialog Box

Operator Select an operator. To view orders for all operators, leave this field blank.

Ordering Prov Select a provider. To view orders for all providers, leave this field blank.

Practice Select a practice. To view orders for all practices, leave this field blank.

Order Type Select the order type from the drop-down list. The options are cardiology, immunizations, laboratory, PT/OT, procedures, radiology, and supplies. To view orders for all order types, leave this field blank.

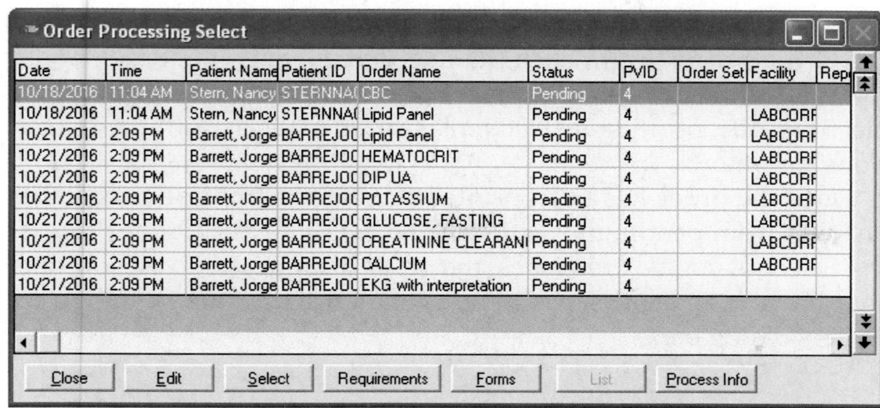

Date	Time	Patient Name	Patient ID	Order Name	Status	PVID	Order Set	Facility	Rep
10/18/2016	11:04 AM	Stern, Nancy	STERNNA(	CBC	Pending	4			
10/18/2016	11:04 AM	Stern, Nancy	STERNNA(	Lipid Panel	Pending	4		LABCORF	
10/21/2016	2:09 PM	Barrett, Jorge	BARREJOC	Lipid Panel	Pending	4		LABCORF	
10/21/2016	2:09 PM	Barrett, Jorge	BARREJOC	HEMATOCRIT	Pending	4		LABCORF	
10/21/2016	2:09 PM	Barrett, Jorge	BARREJOC	DIP UA	Pending	4		LABCORF	
10/21/2016	2:09 PM	Barrett, Jorge	BARREJOC	POTASSIUM	Pending	4		LABCORF	
10/21/2016	2:09 PM	Barrett, Jorge	BARREJOC	GLUCOSE, FASTING	Pending	4		LABCORF	
10/21/2016	2:09 PM	Barrett, Jorge	BARREJOC	CREATININE CLEARAN	Pending	4		LABCORF	
10/21/2016	2:09 PM	Barrett, Jorge	BARREJOC	CALCIUM	Pending	4		LABCORF	
10/21/2016	2:09 PM	Barrett, Jorge	BARREJOC	EKG with interpretation	Pending	4			

Figure 7.20 The Order Processing Select Dialog Box

Order Status Select the order status from the drop-down list. The options are Pending, Sent, Suspended, Partial, Approved, Denied, Cancelled, and Completed. If the field is left blank, all orders with a status of Pending or Approved will be displayed.

Dates The current date is displayed in both date boxes. The entries can be changed to select a range of dates. All orders that fall between the two dates will be selected.

When the selections have been made, clicking the OK button causes the program to list the orders that meet the specified criteria (see Figure 7.20).

The Order Processing Select Dialog Box

The Order Processing Select dialog box displays the orders that meet the criteria selected. The information listed about each order includes:

- Date the order was entered
- Time the order was entered
- Patient name
- Patient ID
- Order name
- Status
- PVID
- Order Set
- Facility
- Repeat (a Y in this column indicates that the order is recurrent/repeating)

To view an order before it is processed, click the Edit button. To print an order for a patient, click the Forms button. The Standard Orders Printing Select dialog box appears (see Figure 7.21). To print the order, click the OK button. Notice that the box at the bottom of the dialog box indicates that pending and approved orders are marked as sent when printed.

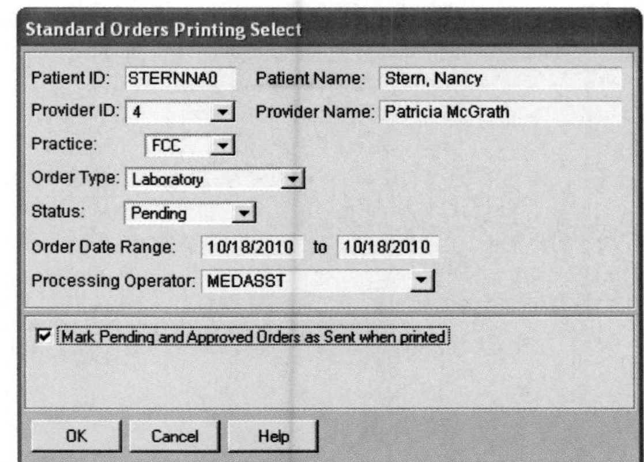

Figure 7.21 The Standard Orders Printing Select Dialog Box

To send an order electronically from within the Order Processing Select dialog box, right click the line that contains the order, and a menu appears. The menu includes options for sending the order electronically, printing instructions, printing labels, printing requisitions, and more.

Once the order has been printed or sent electronically, its status changes from pending to sent, and the next time the Order Processing Select dialog box refreshes, the order disappears. To view orders that have been sent, select Sent as the Order Status in the Select Orders dialog box.

EXERCISE 7.11

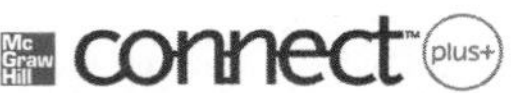

PROCESSING ORDERS

Log in as the medical assistant, and process the orders for Jorge Barrett entered by Dr. McGrath.

1. To log in as the medical assistant, enter ***MEDASST*** in the User ID field and ***master1$*** in the Password field. Click the OK button.
2. Select Orders > Order Processing on the Task menu. The Select Orders dialog box appears.
3. Click the drop-down triangle in the Operator field. The Operator Select dialog box is displayed.
4. Click on the entry for the medical assistant, MEDASST, and click the OK button. You are returned to the Select Orders dialog box.
5. Click the drop-down triangle in the Ordering Prov field. The Provider Select dialog box is displayed.
6. Click on the entry for 4 McGrath, Patricia, and click the OK button. You are returned to the Select Orders dialog box.
7. Select Family Care Clinic, FCC, in the Practice field.
8. Leave the Order Type and Order Status fields blank.
9. Accept the default entries in the Date fields.
10. Click the OK button. The orders placed by Dr. McGrath on that date display.
11. Right click the first entry in the list. Review the options on the pop-up menu that appears.
12. In an actual office, clicking the Send button would send the electronic order to the lab facility and change the order status to Sent.
13. Click the Close button to close the Order Processing Select dialog box.
14. Click the Park button on the toolbar. In response to the question about whether you want to park, click the Yes button.

 **You have completed Exercise 7.11**

7.8 Medical Coding Basics

Once the patient examination is complete, the information recorded in the visit documentation becomes the basis for medical billing in the practice management program. The procedures that were performed, as well as the patient's diagnosis, must be submitted to the patient's insurance carrier for reimbursement. Before the information is transmitted to the practice management program, it must be coded. **Medical coding** is the process of applying the HIPAA-mandated code sets (under the HIPAA Electronic Health Care Transactions and Code Sets Rule) to assign codes to diagnoses and procedures. In the physician practice coding environment, the required code sets are:

- CPT (*Current Procedural Terminology*)
- HCPCS (Healthcare Common Procedure Coding System)
- ICD-9-CM (*International Classification of Diseases*, Ninth Revision, *Clinical Modification*)

medical coding the process of applying the HIPAA-mandated code sets to assign codes to diagnoses and procedures

primary diagnosis the patient's major illness or condition for an encounter

These code sets are used to report the diagnostic and procedural information in the medical record on health care claims. Whether physicians are reimbursed for the services they provide is directly linked to the codes submitted to the payer on the insurance claim. When a payer receives a claim, the codes are reviewed. Payers want to know whether the service provided was appropriate for the patient's condition and whether the treatment was necessary. If an asthmatic patient diagnosed with an upper respiratory infection receives a chest X-ray to rule out pneumonia, the payer probably will not question the claim. If the same patient receives an ankle X-ray, the claim will probably be rejected, since there is not a clear relationship between the diagnosis and the service provided. And while a chest X-ray would be common for the asthmatic patient, its medical necessity might be questioned if it was performed on a twenty-year-old with the same symptoms but no asthma. Since the codes assigned to diagnoses and services play a major role in whether a physician is paid, it is important to document and code the information as accurately as possible.

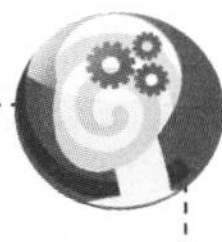

THINKING IT THROUGH 7.4

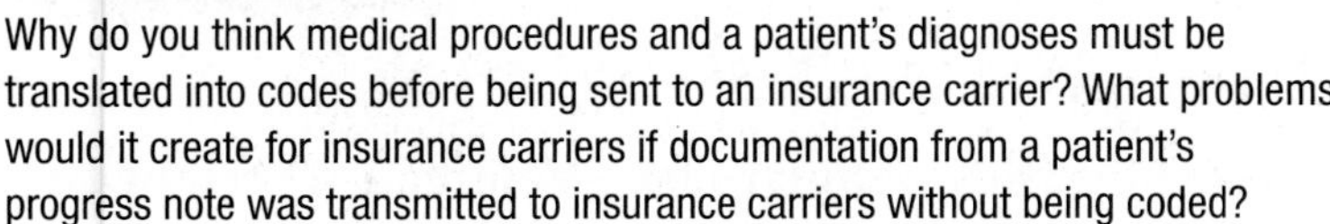

Why do you think medical procedures and a patient's diagnoses must be translated into codes before being sent to an insurance carrier? What problems would it create for insurance carriers if documentation from a patient's progress note was transmitted to insurance carriers without being coded?

7.9 Diagnostic Coding

In physicians' practices, diagnosis codes are used to report patients' conditions on claims. Physicians determine the diagnosis, both the **primary diagnosis**—the diagnosis that relates to the patient's stated reason for the visit—and secondary or additional

HIPAA/HITECH TIP

Mandated Use of ICD-9-CM

ICD-9-CM is the mandated code set for diagnoses under HIPAA's Electronic Health Care Transactions and Code Sets. Codes must be current as of the date of service.

problems. The physicians, medical coders, insurance/billing specialists, or medical assistants may be responsible for assigning the codes for those diagnoses. Expertise in diagnostic coding requires knowledge of medical terminology, pathophysiology, and anatomy, as well as experience in correctly applying the guidelines for assigning codes.

ICD-9-CM

ICD-9-CM abbreviated title of *International Classification of Diseases*, Ninth Revision, *Clinical Modification*, the source of the codes used for reporting diagnoses

The diagnosis codes used in the United States are based on the *International Classification of Diseases* (ICD). A U.S. version of the ninth revision of the ICD (ICD-9) was published in 1979. A committee of physicians from various organizations and specialties prepared this version, which is called the ICD-9's *Clinical Modification*, or **ICD-9-CM.** It is used to code and classify morbidity data from patient medical records, physician offices, and surveys conducted by the National Center for Health Statistics. Using these diagnosis codes in the health care industry is now law under the Health Insurance Portability and Accountability Act of 1996 (HIPAA).

An ICD-9-CM diagnosis code has either three, four, or five digits, plus a description. The system is built on categories for diseases, injuries, and symptoms. A category has three digits. Most categories have subcategories with four-digit codes. Some codes are further subclassified into five-digit codes.

EXAMPLE

Category 415: Acute pulmonary heart disease (three digits)
Subcategory 415.1: Pulmonary embolism and infarction (four digits)
Subclassification: 415.11: Iatrogenic pulmonary embolism and infarction (five digits)

The ICD-9-CM code set has three parts:

Tabular List section of ICD-9-CM listing diagnosis codes numerically

Alphabetic Index section of ICD-9-CM alphabetically listing diseases and injuries with corresponding diagnosis codes

1. **Diseases and Injuries: Tabular List—Volume 1** The **Tabular List** is made up of seventeen chapters of disease descriptions and codes, with two supplementary classifications (V codes and E codes) and five appendixes.
2. **Diseases and Injuries: Alphabetic Index—Volume 2** The **Alphabetic Index** provides (a) an index of the disease descriptions in the Tabular List, (b) an index in table format of drugs and chemicals that cause poisoning, and (c) an index of external causes of injury, such as accidents.

3. **Procedures: Tabular List and Alphabetic Index—Volume 3** This volume covers procedures performed by physicians and other practitioners, chiefly in hospitals.

Volumes 1 and 2 are used for physician practice (outpatient) diagnostic coding; Volume 3 is used only for hospital (inpatient) coding.

Official Guidelines and Coding Selection Process

Diagnosis coding in health care follows specific guidelines. These ***ICD-9-CM Official Guidelines for Coding and Reporting*** (known as the "Official Guidelines") are developed by a group known as the four cooperating parties. The group includes government advisers plus representatives of the American Hospital Association (AHA), the American Health Information Management Association (AHIMA), and the National Center for Health Statistics (NCHS). The Official Guidelines have sections for general rules as well as inpatient (hospital) and outpatient (physician office/clinic) coding.

ICD-9-CM Official Guidelines for Coding and Reporting American Hospital Association publication that provides rules for selecting and sequencing diagnosis codes

ICD-10-CM abbreviated title of *International Classification of Diseases*, Tenth Revision, *Clinical Modification*, which will be used beginning in 2013

The steps that are followed to select correct codes are indicated in the Official Guidelines, which note that although the Tabular List and the Alphabetic Index are labeled Volume 1 and Volume 2, they are related like the parts of a book. First, the Alphabetic Index is used to find a code for a patient's condition or symptom. The index entry provides a pointer to the correct code number in the Tabular List. Then, that code is located in the Tabular List so that its correct use can be checked. Table 7.1 shows the organization of the Tabular List.

The correct process for assigning accurate diagnosis codes has five steps, as shown in Figure 7.22.

Introducing ICD-10-CM

The tenth edition of the ICD was published by the World Health Organization in 1990. The new code set, which is already used in many other countries, was developed to provide many improvements to ICD-9-CM. The Department of Health and Human Services, under a HIPAA Final Rule on January 16, 2009, mandated the adoption of this diagnosis code set, called **ICD-10-CM,** as of 2013. (Note that the Final Rule also mandated a new code set to replace ICD-9-CM, Volume 3, for inpatient coding. That new code set is called ICD-PCS, for "procedural coding system.")

ICD-10-CM provides many more categories for disease and other health-related conditions and much greater flexibility for adding new codes in the future. It is a larger code set, having about 141,000 codes, as compared to ICD-9-CM's approximately 13,000 codes. It also offers a higher level of specificity and additional characters and extensions for expanded detail. There are also many more codes that combine etiology and manifestations, poisoning and external causes, or diagnoses and symptoms.

Although the adoption date is in the future, medical practices have begun planning the transition. In fact, although the code numbers look different, the basic systems are very much alike, and people who are familiar with the current codes will find that their training quickly applies to the new system.

TABLE 7.1 Tabular List Organization

Classification of Diseases and Injuries		
Chapter		**Categories**
1	Infectious and Parasitic Diseases	001–139
2	Neoplasms	140–239
3	Endocrine, Nutritional, and Metabolic Diseases, and Immunity Disorders	240–279
4	Diseases of the Blood and Blood-Forming Organs	280–289
5	Mental Disorders	290–319
6	Diseases of the Central Nervous System and Sense Organs	320–389
7	Diseases of the Circulatory System	390–459
8	Diseases of the Respiratory System	460–519
9	Diseases of the Digestive System	520–579
10	Diseases of the Genitourinary System	580–629
11	Complications of Pregnancy, Childbirth, and the Puerperium	630–677
12	Diseases of the Skin and Subcutaneous Tissue	680–709
13	Diseases of the Musculoskeletal System and Connective Tissue	710–739
14	Congenital Anomalies	740–759
15	Certain Conditions Originating in the Perinatal Period	760–779
16	Symptoms, Signs, and Ill-Defined Conditions	780–799
17	Injury and Poisoning	800–999
Supplementary Classifications		
V Codes	Supplementary Classification of Factors Influencing Health Status and Contact with Health Services	V01–V83
E Codes	Supplementary Classification of External Causes of Injury and Poisoning	E800–E999
Appendixes		
Appendix A	Morphology of Neoplasms	
Appendix B	Glossary of Mental Disorders [now deleted]	
Appendix C	Classification of Drugs by American Hospital Formulary Services List Number and Their ICD-9-CM Equivalents	
Appendix D	Classification of Industrial Accidents According to Agency	
Appendix E	List of Three-Digit Categories	

There are two major differences in the two code sets that are important to understand: the order of the chapters, and the structure of a code.

Different Chapter Order

ICD-10-CM chapters are not organized in the exact same order as ICD-9-CM chapters. Diseases of the skin and subcutaneous tissue (Chapter 12) and diseases of the musculoskeletal system and

HIPAA/HITECH TIP

HIPAA requires the use of ICD-10-CM beginning on October 1, 2013. The codes should not be used for coding and claims before that date, and they must be used as of that date, with no overlapping of old codes. Payers must accept the new codes for electronic transmission even if they convert them back to a previous code set internally.

Figure 7.22 Diagnosis Code Assignment Flowchart

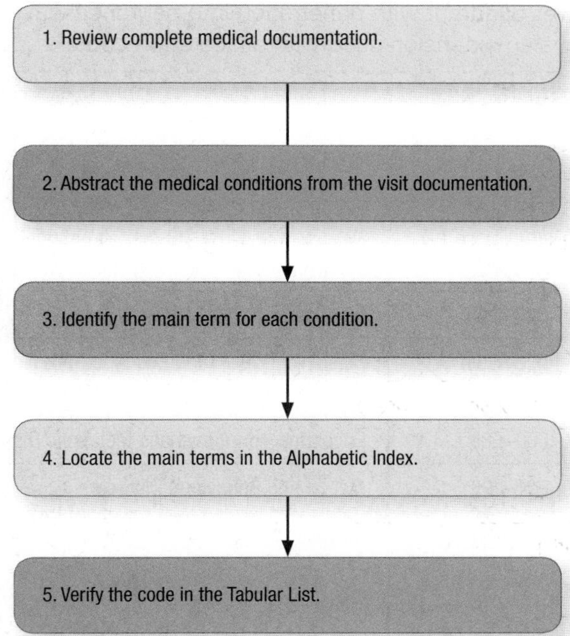

connective tissue (Chapter 13) follow the chapter on diseases of the digestive system. Next are chapters for diseases of the genitourinary system (Chapter 14), pregnancy, childbirth, and the puerperium (Chapter 15), certain conditions originating in the perinatal period (Chapter 16), and congenital malformations, deformations and chromosomal abnormalities (Chapter 17).

1. Review complete medical documentation.
2. Abstract the medical conditions from the visit documentation.
3. Identify the main term for each condition.
4. Locate the main terms in the Alphabetic Index.
5. Verify the code in the Tabular List.

Different Code Structure

ICD-10-CM codes are alphanumeric and have five, six, or seven digits, whereas ICD-9-CM codes have three to five characters. In ICD-10-CM the first digit is alpha, digits 2 and 3 are numeric, and digits 4 through 7 are alpha or numeric.

The code set contains full code titles for all codes, rather than referring back to common fourth and fifth digits, as is done in ICD-9-CM.

Most codes have either five or six digits; injury and fracture codes in Chapter 19 often need the seventh digit. For example, injury codes often allow for a seventh code to be added to capture the episode:

A for an initial encounter

D for a subsequent encounter

S for sequela

THINKING IT THROUGH 7.5

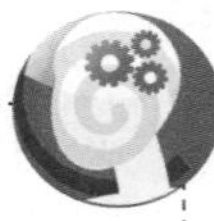

In October 2013, ICD-10-CM will replace ICD-9-CM. Why was it necessary to develop a new set of diagnosis codes? What are the advantages of ICD-10-CM as compared to ICD-9-CM?

EXAMPLE

ICD-10-CM code S31.623A, Laceration with foreign body of abdominal wall, right lower quadrant with penetration into peritoneal cavity, initial encounter, shows an extension used with a laceration code.

TABLE 7.2 ICD-10-CM Chapter Structure

Chapter	Code Range	Title
1	A00–B99	Certain Infectious and Parasitic Diseases
2	C00–D49	Neoplasms
3	D50–D89	Diseases of the Blood and Blood-Forming Organs and Certain Disorders Involving the Immune Mechanism
4	E00–E89	Endocrine, Nutritional and Metabolic Diseases
5	F01–F99	Mental and Behavioral Disorders
6	G00–G99	Diseases of the Nervous System
7	H00–H59	Diseases of the Eye and Adnexa
8	H60–H95	Diseases of the Ear and Mastoid Process
9	I00–I99	Diseases of the Circulatory System
10	J00–J99	Diseases of the Respiratory System
11	K00–K94	Diseases of the Digestive System
12	L00–L99	Diseases of the Skin and Subcutaneous Tissue
13	M00–M99	Diseases of the Musculoskeletal System and Connective Tissue
14	N00–N99	Diseases of the Genitourinary System
15	O00–O9A	Pregnancy, Childbirth and the Puerperium
16	P00–P96	Certain Conditions Originating in the Perinatal Period
17	Q00–Q99	Congenital Malformations, Deformations and Chromosomal Abnormalities
18	R00–R99	Symptoms, Signs and Abnormal Clinical and Laboratory Findings, Not Elsewhere Classified
19	S00–T88	Injury, Poisoning and Certain Other Consequences of External Causes
20	V01–Y95	External Causes of Morbidity
21	Z00–Z99	Factors Influencing Health Status and Contact with Health Services

7.10 Procedural Coding

Procedure codes, like diagnosis codes, are an important part of medical billing. Standard procedure codes are used by physicians in medical practices to report the medical, surgical, and diagnostic services they provide. These codes are used by payers to determine payments. Accurate procedural coding ensures that providers receive the maximum appropriate reimbursement for services.

Procedure codes are also used to establish guidelines for the delivery of the best possible care for patients. Medical researchers track various treatment plans for patients with similar diagnoses and evaluate patients' outcomes. The results are shared with physicians and payers so that best practices can be implemented. For example, this type of analysis has shown that patients who have had heart attacks can reduce the risk of another attack by taking a class of drugs called beta blockers.

CPT and HCPCS

The procedure codes for physicians' and other health care providers' services are selected from the ***Current Procedural Terminology*** data set, called **CPT,** which is owned and maintained by the American Medical Association (AMA).

CPT lists the procedures and services that are commonly performed by physicians across the country. There was also a need for codes for items that are used in medical practices but not listed in CPT, like supplies and equipment. These codes are found in the Healthcare Common Procedure Coding System, referred to as **HCPCS** and pronounced hick-picks. Officially, CPT is the first part (called Level I) of HCPCS, and the supply codes are the second part (Level II). Most people, though, call the codes in the CPT book "CPT codes" and the Level II codes "HCPCS codes."

***Current Procedural Terminology* (CPT)** the standardized classification system for reporting medical procedures and services

HCPCS procedure codes for Medicare claims

Category I codes procedure codes found in the main body of CPT

There are three categories of CPT codes:

1. Category I codes
2. Category II codes
3. Category III codes

Category I Codes

CPT **Category I codes** —which are the majority—have five digits (with no decimals) followed by a descriptor, which is a brief explanation of the procedure:

EXAMPLE

99204 Office visit for evaluation and management of a new patient
00730 Anesthesia for procedures on upper posterior abdominal wall
24006 Arthrotomy of the elbow, with capsular excision for capsular release
70100 Radiologic examination of the mandible
80400 ACTH stimulation panel; for adrenal insufficiency
93000 Electrocardiogram, routine ECG with at least 12 leads; with interpretation and report

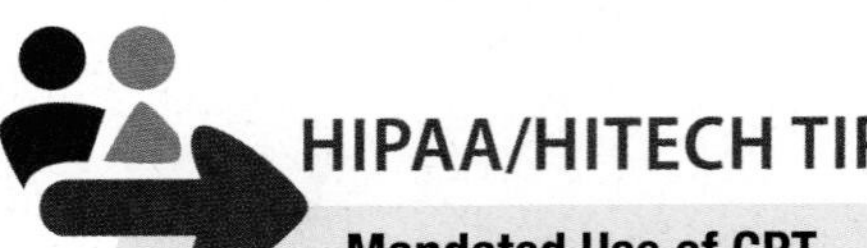

Mandated Use of CPT

CPT is the mandated code set for physicians' work under HIPAA's Electronic Health Care Transactions and Code Sets. Codes must be current as of the date of service.

Although the codes are grouped into sections, such as Surgery, codes from any section can be used by all types of physicians. For example, a family practitioner might use codes from the Surgery section to describe an office procedure such as the incision and drainage of an abscess.

Category II codes optional CPT codes that track performance measures

Category III codes temporary codes for emerging technology, services, and procedures

Category II Codes

Category II codes are used to track performance measures for a medical goal, such as reducing tobacco use. These codes are optional; they are not paid by insurance carriers. They help in the development of best practice care and improve documentation. These codes have an alphabetic character for the fifth digit:

EXAMPLE

0002F Tobacco use, smoking, assessed
0004F Tobacco use cessation intervention, counseling

Category III Codes

Category III codes are temporary codes for emerging technology, services, and procedures. These codes also have an alphabetic character for the fifth digit:

EXAMPLE

0001T Endovascular repair of infrarenal abdominal aortic aneurysm or dissection
0041T Urinalysis infectious agent detection

A temporary code may become permanent and part of the regular codes if the service it identifies proves effective and is widely performed.

THINKING IT THROUGH 7.6

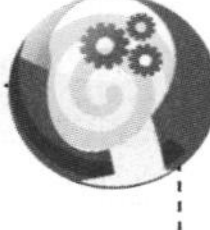

Which category of procedure codes—I, II, or III—do you think is most important for physician reimbursement? Why are three different categories necessary?

CPT Organization and Format

The CPT manual is made up of the main text—sections of codes—followed by appendixes and an index. The main text has the following six sections of Category I procedure codes:

1.	Evaluation and Management	Codes 99201–99499
2.	Anesthesia	Codes 00100–01999
3.	Surgery	Codes 10040–69990
4.	Radiology	Codes 70010–79999
5.	Pathology and Laboratory	Codes 80047–89398
6.	Medicine	Codes 90281–99607

Each section begins with section guidelines for the use of its codes. The guidelines also include special notes about the structure or rules for use. The guidelines must be carefully followed in order to correctly assign codes from the section. In general, the steps for assigning correct codes are shown in Figure 7.23:

Figure 7.23 Procedure Code Assignment Flowchart

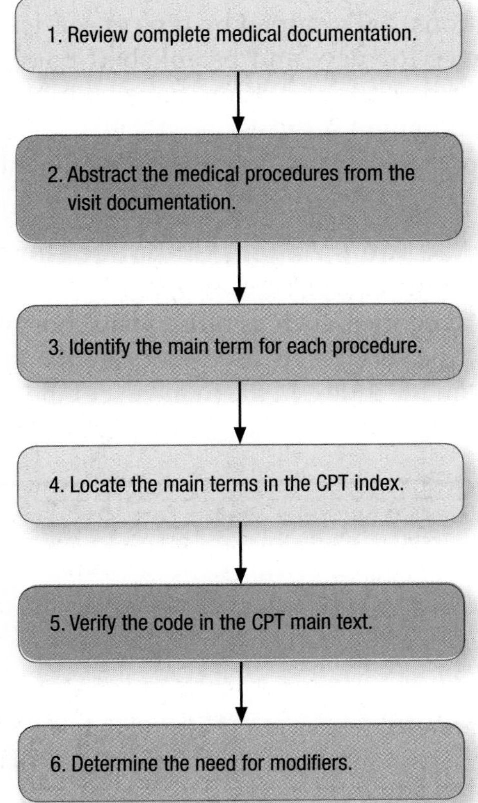

1. Review complete medical documentation.
2. Abstract the medical procedures from the visit documentation.
3. Identify the main term for each procedure.
4. Locate the main terms in the CPT index.
5. Verify the code in the CPT main text.
6. Determine the need for modifiers.

7.11 Evaluation and Management (E/M) Codes

evaluation and management (E/M) codes codes that cover physicians' services performed to determine the optimum course for patient care

When billing for a patient visit, the provider must submit a procedure code that represents the work done by the physician. Often, the service involves a process physicians use to collect and analyze information about a patient's condition and to make decisions about the best treatment, rather than surgery or a specialized service like X-rays or laboratory testing. The CPT codes that represent the thought process that the physician follows to determine the best course of care are known as **evaluation and management (E/M) codes.**

Patients' conditions require different levels of information gathering, analysis, and decision making by physicians. For example, a patient with a mild case of poison ivy might be on the low end of the range. On the opposite end is a patient with a life-threatening condition. The E/M codes reflect these different levels. For example, there are five codes for an office visit with a new patient, and another five for an office visit with an established patient. (New and established patients are defined in Chapter 4.) A financial value is assigned by payers to each code in a range. To justify the use of a higher-level code in the range—one that is tied to a higher value—physicians must perform and document specific clinical facts about patient encounters.

E/M Code Selection Process

Most codes in the E/M section are organized by the place of service, such as the office, the hospital, or a patient's home. A few (for example, consultations) are grouped by type of service. Some have different code ranges for new and established patients, such as the office visits described above. Others have a single range of codes, such as hospital inpatient services.

To select the correct E/M code, eight steps are followed (see Figure 7.24).

Step 1: Determine the Category and Subcategory of Service Based on the Place of Service and the Patient's Status

The list of E/M categories, such as office visits, hospital services, and preventive medicine services, is used to locate the appropriate place or type of service in the index. In the main text of the selected category, the subcategory—such as new or established patient—is then chosen.

EXAMPLE

Documentation: initial hospital visit to established patient
Index: Hospital Services
  Inpatient Services
    Initial Care, New or Established Patient
Code Ranges: 99221–99223

Figure 7.24 Selecting an Evaluation and Management Code

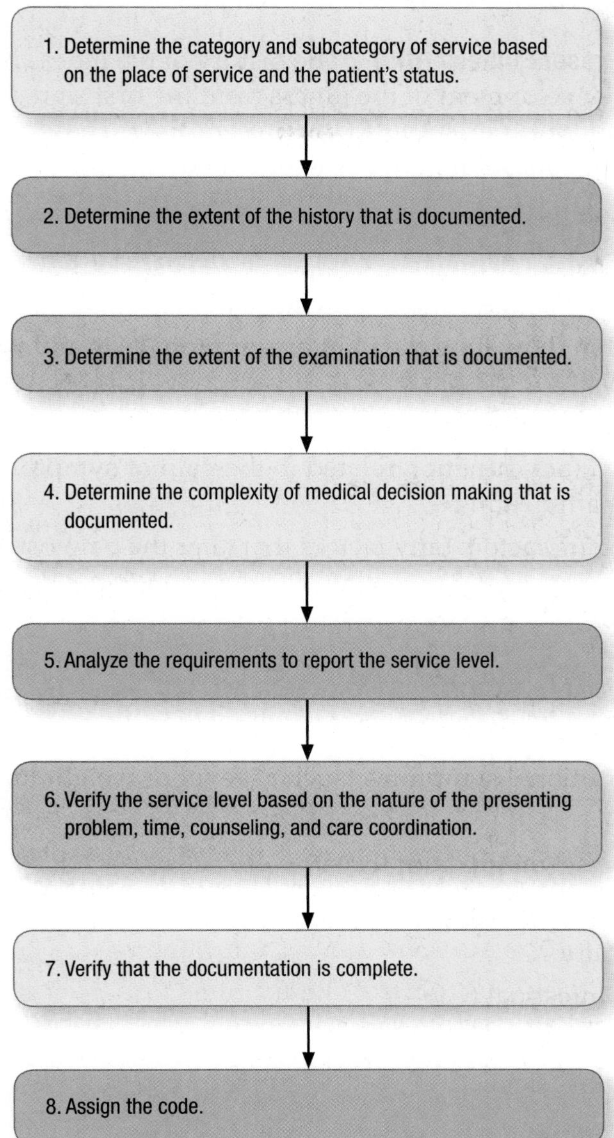

1. Determine the category and subcategory of service based on the place of service and the patient's status.
2. Determine the extent of the history that is documented.
3. Determine the extent of the examination that is documented.
4. Determine the complexity of medical decision making that is documented.
5. Analyze the requirements to report the service level.
6. Verify the service level based on the nature of the presenting problem, time, counseling, and care coordination.
7. Verify that the documentation is complete.
8. Assign the code.

For most types of service, from three to five codes are listed. To select an appropriate code from this range, consider three key components: (1) the history the physician documented, (2) the examination that was documented, and (3) the medical decisions the physician documented. (The exception to this guideline is selecting a code for counseling or coordination of care, where the amount of time the physician spends may be the only key component in some situations.)

Step 2: Determine the Extent of the History That Is Documented

History is the information the physician received by questioning the patient about the chief complaint and other signs or symptoms, about all or selected body systems, and about pertinent past history, family background, and other personal factors. The history is documented in the patient medical record as follows:

History of Present Illness (HPI) The history of the illness is a description of the development of the illness from the first sign or symptom that the patient experienced to the present time. These points about the illness or condition may be documented:

- Location (body area of the pain or symptom)
- Quality (type of pain or symptom, such as sudden or dull)
- Severity (degree of pain or symptom)
- Duration (how long the pain or symptom lasts and when it began)
- Timing (time of day pain or symptom occurs)
- Context (any situation related to the pain or symptom, such as occurs after eating)
- Modifying factors (any factors that alter the pain or symptom)
- Associated signs and symptoms (things that also happen when the pain or symptom occurs)

Review of Systems (ROS) The review of systems is an inventory of body systems. These systems are:

- Constitutional symptoms (such as fever or weight loss)
- Eyes
- Ears, nose, mouth, and throat
- Cardiovascular (CV)
- Respiratory
- Gastrointestinal (GI)
- Genitourinary (GU)
- Musculoskeletal
- Integumentary
- Neurological
- Psychiatric
- Endocrine
- Hematologic/lymphatic
- Allergic/immunologic

Past Medical, Family, and Social History (PFSH) As explained in Chapter 6, the past history of the patient's experiences with illnesses, injuries, and treatments contains data about other major illnesses and injuries, operations, and hospitalizations. It also covers current medications the patient is taking, allergies, immunization status, and diet. The family history reviews the medical events in the patient's family. It includes the health status or cause of death of parents, brothers and sisters, and children; specific diseases that are related to the patient's chief complaint or the patient's diagnosis;

and the presence of any known hereditary diseases. The social history, which depends on the patient's age, includes marital status, employment, and other factors.

This history is then categorized as one of four types on a scale from lesser to greater extent of amount of history obtained:

1. **Problem-focused** Determining the patient's chief complaint and obtaining a brief history of the present illness
2. **Expanded problem-focused** Determining the patient's chief complaint and obtaining a brief history of the present illness, plus a problem-pertinent system review of the particular body system that is involved
3. **Detailed** Determining the chief complaint; obtaining an extended history of the present illness; reviewing both the problem-pertinent system and additional systems; and taking pertinent past, family, and/or social histories
4. **Comprehensive** Determining the chief complaint and taking an extended history of the present illness, a complete review of systems, and complete past, family, and social histories

Step 3: Determine the Extent of the Examination That Is Documented

The physician may examine a particular body area or organ system or may conduct a multisystem examination. The body areas are divided into the head and face; chest, including breasts and axilla; abdomen; genitalia, groin, and buttocks; back; and each extremity.

The organ systems that may be examined are the eyes; the ears, nose, mouth, and throat; cardiovascular; respiratory; gastrointestinal; genitourinary; musculoskeletal; skin; neurologic; psychiatric; and hematologic/lymphatic/immunologic.

The examination that the physician documents is categorized as one of four types on a scale from lesser to greater extent:

1. **Problem-focused** A limited examination of the affected body area or system
2. **Expanded problem-focused** A limited examination of the affected body area or system and other related areas
3. **Detailed** An extended examination of the affected body area or system and other related areas
4. **Comprehensive** A general multisystem examination or a complete examination of a single organ system

Step 4: Determine the Complexity of Medical Decision Making That Is Documented

The complexity of the medical decisions that the physician makes involves how many possible diagnoses or treatment options were considered; how much information (such as test results or previous records) was considered in analyzing the patient's problem; and how serious the illness is, meaning how much risk there is for significant complications, advanced illness, or death.

The decision-making process that the physician documents is categorized as one of four types on a scale from lesser to greater complexity:

1. **Straightforward** Minimal diagnosis options, a minimal amount of data, and minimum risk
2. **Low complexity** Limited diagnosis options, a low amount of data, and low risk
3. **Moderate complexity** Multiple diagnosis options, a moderate amount of data, and moderate risk
4. **High complexity** Extensive diagnosis options, an extensive amount of data, and high risk

Step 5: Analyze the Requirements to Report the Service Level

The descriptor for each E/M code explains the standards for its selection. For office visits and most other services to new patients, and for initial care visits, all three of the **key components** must be documented. An example of how this is stated in CPT is:

key components factors documented for various levels of evaluation and management services

EXAMPLE

99203 **Office or other outpatient visit** for the evaluation and management of a new patient, which requires three key components: (1) a detailed history; (2) a detailed examination; and (3) medical decision making of low complexity

For most services for established patients and for subsequent care visits, two out of three of the key components must be met.

BILLING TIP

Key Components, 99203

This means that to select code 99203, the medical record must show that a detailed history and examination were taken, and that medical decision making was at least at the level of low complexity.

EXAMPLE

99232 **Subsequent hospital care,** per day, for the evaluation and management of a patient, which requires at least two of three key components: (1) an expanded problem-focused interval history; (2) an expanded problem-focused examination; and (3) medical decision making of moderate complexity

BILLING TIP

Key Components, 99232

This means that to select code 99232, the medical record must document two out of the three factors.

Step 6: Verify the Service Level Based on the Nature of the Presenting Problem, Time, Counseling, and Care Coordination

Many descriptors mention two additional components: (1) how severe the patient's condition is, referred to as the nature of the presenting problem, and (2) how much time the physician typically spends directly treating the patient. These factors, while not key components, help in selecting the correct E/M level.

Step 7: Verify That the Documentation Is Complete

Meeting the requirements means that the documentation must contain the record of the physician's work. When an E/M code is assigned, the patient's medical record must contain the clinical details to support it. The history, examination, and medical decision making must be sufficiently documented so that the medical necessity and appropriateness of the service can be determined.

Step 8: Assign the Code

The code that has been selected is assigned.

THINKING IT THROUGH 7.7

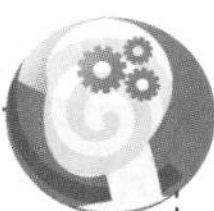

Evaluation and management (E/M) codes have separate codes for new and established patients. Most insurance carriers reimburse the codes for a new patient's visit at a higher level than a similar visit for an established patient. Why do you think there is a difference in reimbursement rates between new and established patient visits?

7.12 Coding Methods

In an office that does not use software in the coding process, codes are assigned by a member of the coding staff. The typical sequence of the paper-based coding process is as follows (see Figure 7.25).

Figure 7.25 Flowchart of Coding in a Paper-Based Office

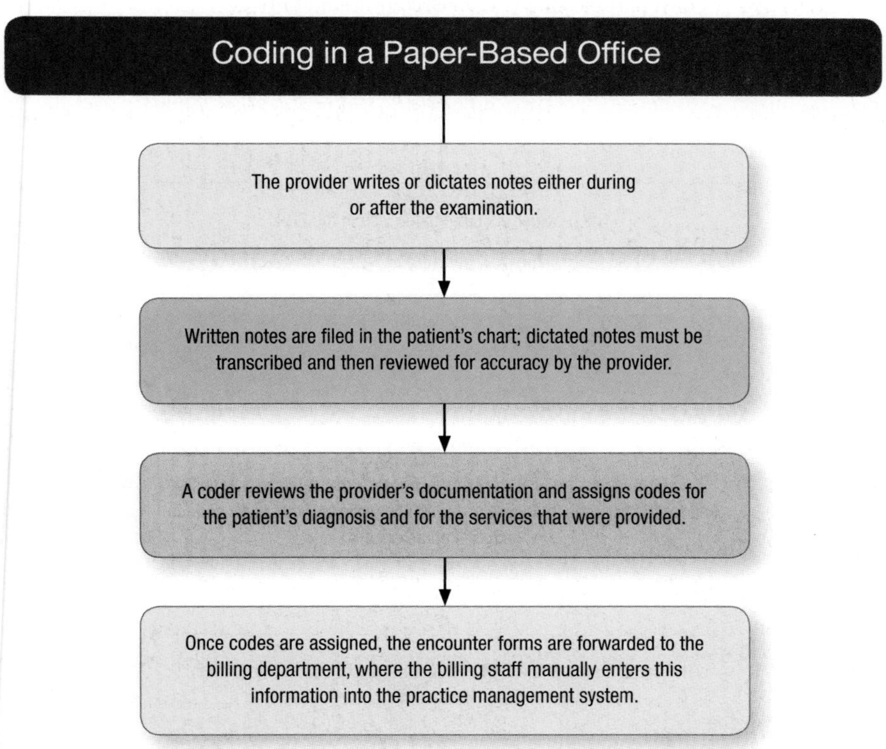

Coding in a Paper-Based Office

In a paper-based office, the coding, billing, and reimbursement cycle normally takes anywhere from three to fourteen days. As a result, there is an extra time lag between when the service was provided and when the provider receives reimbursement. Also, it has been estimated that physicians lose as much as 10 percent of potential revenue as a result of forgetting to bill for services, losing patients' paperwork, making errors when preparing claims, and other reasons.

Coding in an Electronic Health Record

computer-assisted coding assigning preliminary diagnosis and procedure codes using computer software

Most electronic health record programs automate some part of the coding process. The process of coding with software is known as **computer-assisted coding.** The methods of assigning codes vary from program to program. In Medisoft Clinical Patient Records, the program assigns codes based on keywords that are included in the progress note template.

The program analyzes information in the progress note and suggests the appropriate E/M code for the visit. If not enough information is available to calculate the code, the message "E/M code cannot be determined for new/established patient based on the following" is displayed, and additional information must be provided. The program automatically determines whether the patient is new or established, based on whether there are existing progress notes in the patient's chart. A patient is considered new if there are no existing progress notes for the patient or the last progress note is more than three years old. Otherwise the patient is considered an established patient.

Figure 7.26 Flowchart of Coding in an Office with an EHR

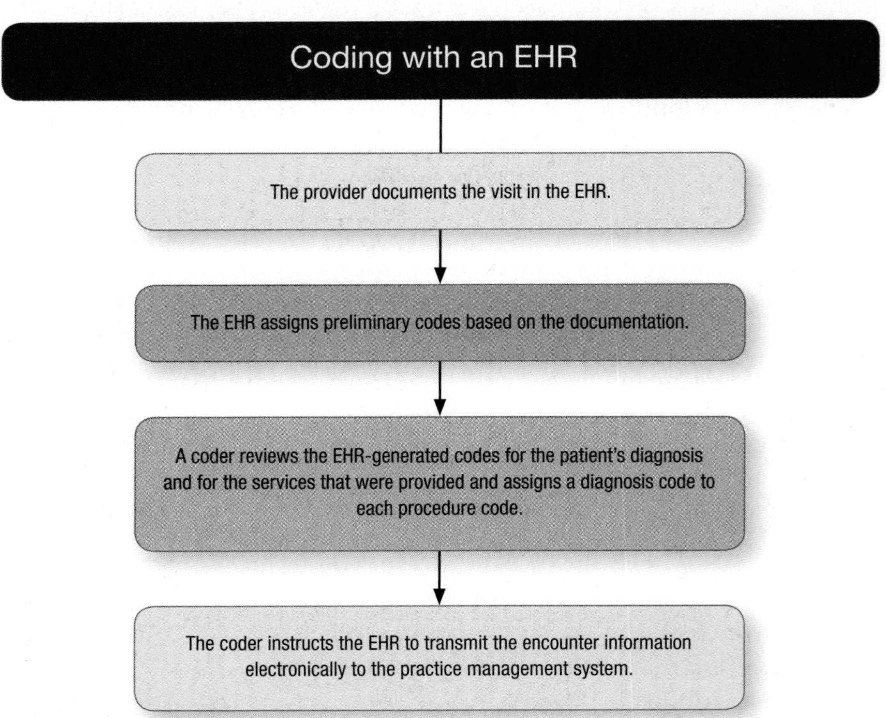

Once the codes have been suggested by the software, they are reviewed and verified by a professional coder. If the coder wants to review the documentation before finalizing the codes, the EHR provides easy access to the patient's chart. Once the codes are finalized, they are sent to the billing staff, who will verify the information and generate claims.

EHR coding tools, if used correctly, can improve charge capture and the accuracy of E/M coding. The coding tools:

- Ensure that documentation exists for services billed, since codes were assigned based on electronic documentation
- Aid in selection of appropriate codes
- Reduce the number of unbilled procedures due to lost or forgotten procedures
- Automatically enter codes in the practice management system or EHR
- Reduce the time between the patient visit and the submission of the claim for payment, leading to more timely reimbursement

On the other hand, if electronic coding tools are improperly used, there is a risk of submitting inaccurate codes or even committing fraud. It is important for the provider or medical coder to carefully audit the EHR-suggested codes and verify that they are accurate. For example, documentation stored in the form of templates may populate sections of the note, such as the review of systems, with information that may not be accurate for the current visit. Similarly, the EHR may allow providers to reuse some or all components of an old progress note as a template for a new visit. It is important to update the information that is pulled forward so that it accurately represents the visit.

Accepting entries that do not precisely match the information that was obtained during the encounter may be considered fraud, particularly if the default information is used to support the E/M code submitted via a claim or reflects procedures that were not performed. **Upcoding**—assigning a higher level E/M code, for example, than is supported by documentation—is looked at carefully by government and private payers when they examine claims for payment.

upcoding assigning a higher level code than is supported by documentation

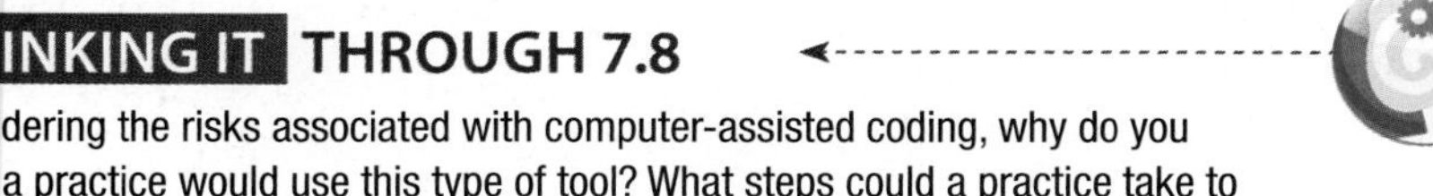

THINKING IT THROUGH 7.8

Considering the risks associated with computer-assisted coding, why do you think a practice would use this type of tool? What steps could a practice take to minimize the risks?

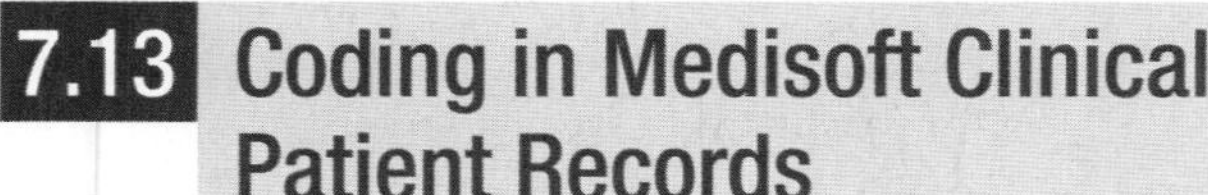

7.13 Coding in Medisoft Clinical Patient Records

Encounter forms are used to document patient encounter data for billing and claims. Most practices use a paper encounter form, also known as a superbill. When the office visit is finished, the procedures performed and the patient's diagnosis are marked on the form. The form then goes to the checkout desk, where patient charges are calculated. After checkout, the form is routed to the billing staff members, who input the codes on the form into the practice management program.

electronic encounter form (EEF) an electronic version of the form that lists procedures and charges for a patient's visit

Some electronic health records provide an electronic version of this form, which is referred to as an **electronic encounter form (EEF).** The EEF eliminates the need for paper encounter forms. The form is automatically populated with preliminary codes derived from information in the progress note in the EHR. These codes are reviewed by a coding specialist, any changes are made, and the electronic form is marked complete and transmitted to the practice management program.

The Electronic Encounter Select Dialog Box

The command for viewing electronic encounter forms in Medisoft Clinical Patient Records is located on the Task menu. Clicking Electronic Encounter forms on the Task menu causes the Electronic Encounter Select dialog box to display (see Figure 7.27). The information on the forms comes from the documentation entered by the medical assistant and the provider in the patient's chart. The encounter forms are listed by the date and time the encounter was created, with the most recent encounters at the bottom of the list.

The fields at the top of the dialog box are used to filter the encounter forms that appear in the list.

Practice Select a practice name to display encounter forms for that practice only. If the field is left blank, encounter forms for all practices will be listed.

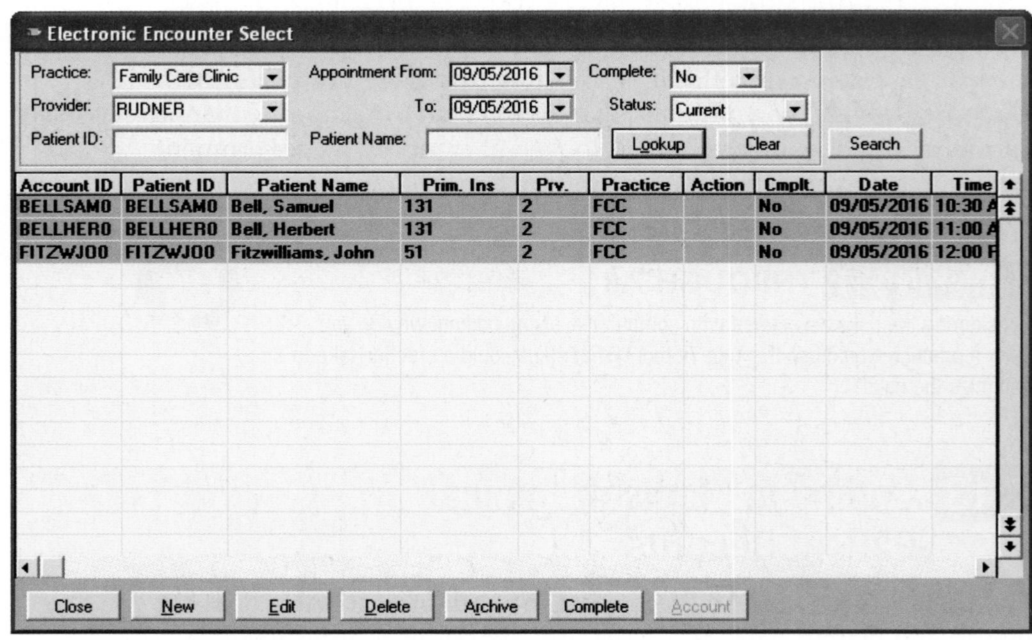

Figure 7.27 The Electronic Encounter Select Dialog Box

Provider Select a provider to display encounter forms for that provider only. If the field is left blank, encounter forms for all providers will be listed.

Appointment From/To Select from and to dates to display the electronic encounter forms within a range of specified dates. Clicking the drop-down list displays a calendar. If the field is left blank, encounter forms for all dates will be listed.

Complete Select whether encounter forms marked complete should be listed. If you do not want to see encounter forms marked complete, select No.

Status Select whether current or archived electronic encounter forms are displayed.

Patient ID/Patient Name Enter a patient name or ID to display electronic encounter forms for that patient only, or leave the field blank to display electronic encounter forms for all patients. If the field is left blank, encounter forms for all patients will be listed.

The Electronic Encounter Dialog Box

When an encounter is selected in the Electronic Encounter Select dialog box, clicking the Edit button causes the Electronic Encounter dialog box to open (see Figure 7.28). This dialog box is used to select or confirm the appropriate procedure and diagnosis codes for the encounter.

The Control # field displays a control number assigned by the program for tracking purposes. The number cannot be changed.

The dialog box contains three tabs: Procedures, Diagnoses, and Action Items. The Diagnoses tab is similar to the Procedures tab except that it lists diagnosis codes. The Action Items tab is used to attach a message to the encounter form. When an action item has been added, a red circle displays on the Action Items tab (see Figure 7.29). The message must be reviewed for the red circle

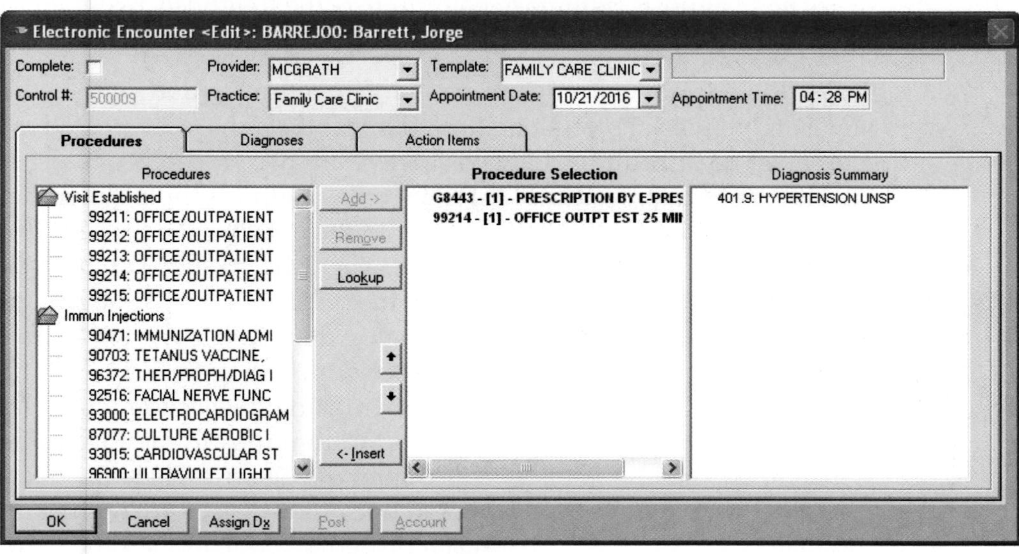

Figure 7.28 The Electronic Encounter Dialog Box

Figure 7.29 Electronic Encounter Dialog Box with Unresolved Action Item

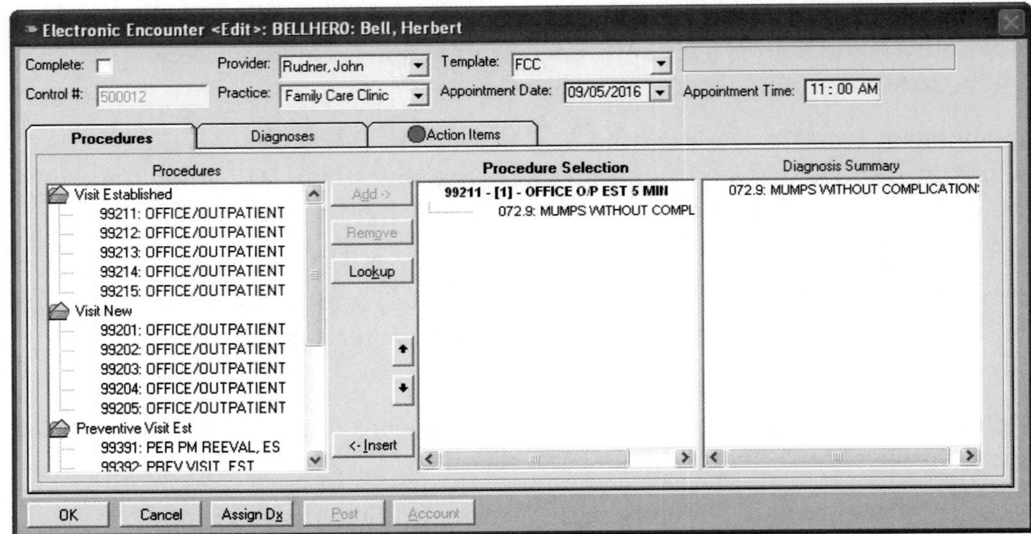

to disappear. When the red circle is present, the electronic encounter form cannot be transmitted to Medisoft Network Professional.

The Procedures Tab

The Procedures tab contains three columns:

1. The Procedures column lists the CPT and HCSPS codes on the encounter form used by the practice. In Figure 7.29, the codes are grouped into folders, including Visit Established, Visit New, and Preventive Visit Est, among others. This column is used when a code generated by the EHR needs to be changed or when a code needs to be added to the encounter form.
2. The Procedure Selection column lists the procedure codes for the services performed during the visit. These codes are generated from information entered in the progress note in the patient's chart.
3. The Diagnosis Summary column lists the diagnosis assigned by the physician in the progress note.

Before the encounter form can be marked complete and sent to the Medisoft Network Professional for billing and claims, each procedure code must be linked to a diagnosis. There are two methods of assigning diagnoses to procedures: (1) Click on a diagnosis, hold down the mouse button, and drag the diagnosis to the appropriate procedures; and (2) click the Assign DX button. When the button is clicked, the Assign Dx dialog box is displayed listing three options (see Figure 7.30).

After making a selection, click the OK button to return to the Electronic Encounter dialog box, where the diagnosis code is now listed on a line below each procedure code in the Procedure Selection column (see Figure 7.31).

Assign Dx
- Assign first 4 codes to all procedures.
- Assign first 4 codes to first procedure and first code to remaining procedures.
- Assign first 4 codes to currently selected procedure.

OK Cancel

Figure 7.30 The Assign Dx Dialog Box

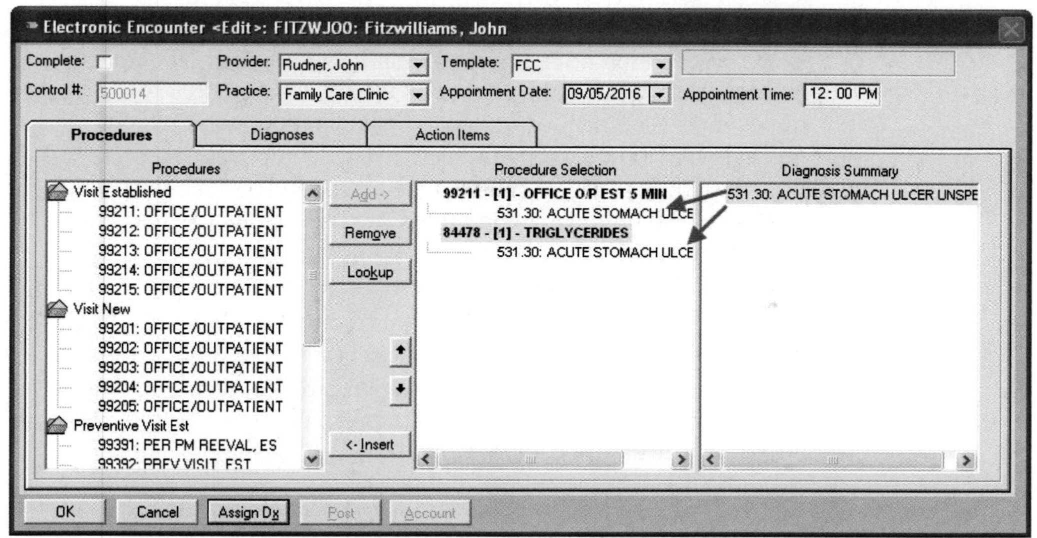

Figure 7.31 The Electronic Encounter Dialog Box with Diagnosis Codes Assigned to Procedure Codes

Once all procedure codes have been linked to a diagnosis, click the Complete check box in the top-left corner of the dialog box, and click OK. The dialog box closes, the encounter data are transmitted to the practice management application, and the encounter is no longer listed in the Electronic Encounter Select dialog box.

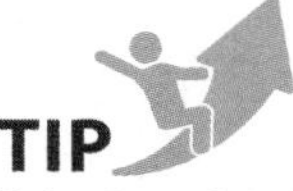

TIP
If the Complete box is not marked, the encounter information will not be transmitted to Medisoft Network Professional.

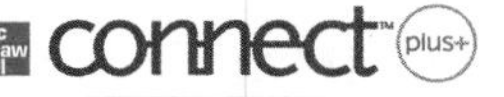

EXERCISE 7.12

CODING A PATIENT ENCOUNTER

Log in as Joseph Sanchez, the coding specialist at Family Care Clinic. Review the codes on the electronic encounter form for Jorge Barrett, and read the documentation to determine whether the codes are correct.

1. To log in as Joseph Sanchez, enter ***CODING*** in the User ID field and ***master1$*** in the Password field. Then click the OK button.
2. Select Electronic Encounter Forms on the Task menu. The Electronic Encounter Select dialog box is displayed.
3. Click on the line that contains the office visit for Jorge Barrett, and click the Edit button. The Electronic Encounter dialog box is displayed.
4. Review the information entered in the Procedure Selection and Diagnosis Summary columns.
5. To view the visit documentation while reviewing the encounter form, click the Chart button on the toolbar.
6. Enter ***BA*** in the Last Name field of the Patient Lookup dialog box, and click the Lookup button.
7. With Jorge Barrett selected, click the OK button. Barrett's chart opens.
8. Click the Progress Notes folder.
9. Accept the selection to search by most recent note, and click OK. The progress note for the visit is displayed.

(continued)

(Continued)

10. Scroll through the note, and determine whether there is documentation to support the E/M code 99203. Code 99203 requires a detailed history, a detailed examination, and medical decision making of low complexity.
11. Also note that CPT II code G8443 is listed in the Procedure section of the note, indicating that all prescriptions for this visit were created using a qualified e-prescribing system.
12. Click the Close button to close the note.
13. Click the Close button on the toolbar to close the patient's chart. The Electronic Encounter dialog box reappears.
14. To assign the diagnosis code to the two procedure codes, first click the diagnosis entry in the Diagnosis Summary column.
15. Click on the entry in the Diagnosis Summary column. Hold down the mouse button and drag the entry to the first entry in the Procedure Selection field. The diagnosis appears below the first procedure entry.
16. Click on the entry in the Diagnosis Summary column. Hold down the mouse button and drag the entry to the second entry in the Procedure Selection field. The diagnosis now appears below both procedure entries.
17. Click the Complete box in the top-left corner of the dialog box.
18. Click the OK button to save the encounter information.
19. You are returned to the Electronic Encounter Select dialog box, and the encounter you just completed no longer appears in the list of encounters. It has been transmitted to Medisoft Network Professional for billing.

 **You have completed Exercise 7.12**

chapter 7 summary

LEARNING OUTCOME	KEY CONCEPTS/EXAMPLES
7.1 Discuss the methods of entering documentation in an EHR. Pages 320–324	Progress notes may be entered by the following methods: - Dictation and transcription, in which a provider dictates the medical note into a telephone or a recording device and a medical transcriptionist transcribes it on a computer. After review, the final computerized word processing file is e-mailed to the health care provider, or the file is transferred to a website and is later downloaded by the provider. It is then reviewed and added to the patient's electronic record. - Digital dictation, in which the physician dictates using a microphone and/or a headset connected to a computer, a smart phone, or a PDA. The spoken words are saved as a digital audio file, which can be transferred to a transcriptionist via a secure website. - Voice recognition software, which transcribes spoken words into text in an electronic file. In front-end voice recognition, the physician dictates and edits notes directly in the EHR, eliminating the need for a transcriptionist. In background voice recognition, the physician dictates notes that are saved as an electronic text file, which is then edited by a transcriptionist. After editing, it is uploaded to the EHR. - Templates, which are preformatted notes that contain selections appropriate to the medical condition or type of visit. When a template is used, only patient-specific information must be typed into the note. The rest of the information is entered by clicking on labels in the templates and making selections from a list of choices. - Directly typing into the EHR.

LEARNING OUTCOME	KEY CONCEPTS/EXAMPLES
7.2 Compare the process of entering a progress note with and without using a template. Pages 325–337	To enter a progress note without a template, a note is opened. The program inserts the current date and time on the first line of the note. The title is typed in, and the rest of the note is entered by using one of the methods described in the first section of the chapter. To enter a note with a template, Template… is selected on the Insert menu, and one of the templates listed in the Insert Template dialog box is selected and inserted. The provider goes through the sections of the template, first reading any alerts. The provider clicks labels and chooses the relevant options, skipping any labels not covered during the encounter. Once learned, templates can be more efficient than other methods of entering information. Data can be searched and analyzed by computer. The physician is less likely to omit information. On the other hand, it takes time to learn how to use templates effectively. Standardized content may not apply to all patients, and entries may not capture the uniqueness of each patient.
7.3 Explain why e-prescribing reduces some medical errors. Pages 337–339	In e-prescribing, the EHR checks for drug allergies, drug–drug interactions, and other potential conflicts using information in the patient's medical record, including past history, allergies, and a complete medication list. The EHR also checks that the medication is in the formulary of the patient's health plan. If a medication is not in the formulary, the EHR can suggest an alternative drug. The EHR can also check to make sure the patient's pharmacy has the medication in stock.
7.4 List the steps required to create a new prescription. Pages 339–343	1. Open the patient's chart. 2. Click the Rx button on the toolbar, or open the Rx/Medications folder and click the New button. 3. In the new Prescription dialog box, enter the template code or perform a search to locate the drug template. 4. Complete the remaining fields as appropriate for the medication and the patient. Some fields may be left blank. 5. Click the OK button to save the new prescription. 6. When prompted for a signature, enter the provider's signature PIN in the Signature field.
7.5 Explain why ordering and receiving test results electronically is more efficient than paper methods. Pages 343–345	Electronic order entry is designed to reduce errors associated with handwriting and paper orders. It also provides numerous safety and cost-control benefits. It can incorporate the rules of different insurance carriers, making it easy to determine whether a test requires preauthorization and whether it is limited to specified diagnoses. It can delay sending orders until approval is received. In addition, it is capable of checking orders against information specific to the patient, such as whether the order would be inappropriate based on a patient's medications, lab tests, diagnoses, allergies, or other factors.

LEARNING OUTCOME	KEY CONCEPTS/EXAMPLES
7.6 List the steps required to enter an electronic order. Pages 345–350	1. Open the patient's chart. 2. Click the Orders folder. 3. In the Orders dialog box, click the New button to begin a new order. 4. In the new Order dialog box, review the information already entered in the top of the dialog box. 5. Select an order processor. 6. Use the Order Tree by clicking the plus signs next to the relevant order types, and select the appropriate orders from the list. 7. Click the Add button for each order chosen. 8. Click OK to record the orders.
7.7 Explain how orders are processed in an EHR. Pages 350–353	1. Select Orders > Order Processing on the Task menu. 2. In the Select Orders dialog box, click the drop-down triangle in the Operator field. 3. In the Operator Select dialog box, click the entry for the relevant operator, and click the OK button. 4. Also select the provider in the Ordering Prov field and the practice in the Practice field. 5. Change the dates or accept the default entries in the Date fields. 6. Click the OK button. 7. Right click entries in the list, and review the options on the pop-up menu that appears. 8. Select the appropriate option for sending the order.
7.8 Define medical coding. Page 353	Medical coding is the process of applying the HIPAA-mandated code sets to assign codes to diagnoses and procedures. In the physician practice coding environment, the required code sets are CPT (*Current Procedural Terminology*), HCPCS (Healthcare Common Procedure Coding System), and ICD-9-CM (*International Classification of Diseases*, Ninth Revision, *Clinical Modification*). They are used to report the diagnostic and procedural information in the medical record on health care claims.

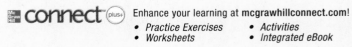

LEARNING OUTCOME	KEY CONCEPTS/EXAMPLES
7.9 Discuss the purpose of the ICD-9-CM. Pages 353–358	ICD-9-CM is used to code and classify morbidity data from patient medical records, physician offices, and surveys conducted by the National Center for Health Statistics. Under the Health Insurance Portability and Accountability Act of 1996 (HIPAA), the codes are required to be used in the health care industry.
7.10 Discuss the purpose of the CPT/HCPCS code sets. Pages 359–361	CPT is used to code the procedures and services that are commonly performed by physicians. Codes for items that are used in medical practices but not listed in CPT, like supplies and equipment, are found in the HCPCS code set. Officially, CPT is the first part (called Level I) of HCPCS, and the supply codes are the second part (Level II).
7.11 Demonstrate the process that is followed to select a correct evaluation and management code. Pages 362–367	To select a correct evaluation and management code: 1. Determine the category and subcategory of service based on the place of service and the patient's status. 2. Determine the extent of the history that is documented. 3. Determine the extent of the examination that is documented. 4. Determine the complexity of medical decision making that is documented. 5. Analyze the requirements to report the service level. 6. Verify the service level based on the nature of the presenting problem, time, counseling, and care coordination. 7. Verify that the documentation is complete. 8. Assign the code.

LEARNING OUTCOME	KEY CONCEPTS/EXAMPLES
7.12 Compare coding in a paper-based office with coding in an office with an EHR. Pages 367–369	In a paper-based office, the provider writes or dictates notes either during or after the examination. Written notes are filed in the patient's chart; dictated notes must be transcribed and then reviewed for accuracy by the provider. A coder reviews the provider's documentation and assigns codes for the patient's diagnosis and for the services that were provided. Once codes are assigned, the forms are forwarded to the billing department, where the billing staff member manually enters this information into the practice management system. The coding, billing, and reimbursement cycle normally takes anywhere from three to fourteen days. As a result, there is an extra time lag between when the service was provided and when the provider receives reimbursement. Also, physicians may lose as much as 10 percent of potential revenue as a result of forgetting to bill for services, losing patients' paperwork, making errors when preparing claims, and other reasons. In an office that uses an electronic health record program, the provider documents the visit in the EHR. The EHR assigns preliminary codes based on the documentation. A coder reviews the EHR-generated codes for the patient's diagnosis and for the services that were provided and assigns a diagnosis code to each procedure code. The EHR transmits the encounter information electronically to the practice management system.
7.13 Discuss the purpose of an electronic encounter form in an EHR. Pages 369–374	An electronic encounter form eliminates the need for a paper encounter form. The form is automatically populated with preliminary codes derived from information in the progress note in the EHR. These codes are reviewed by a coding specialist, necessary any changes are made, and the electronic form is marked complete and is transmitted to the practice management program.

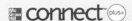

chapter review

MATCHING QUESTIONS

Match the key terms with their definitions.

_____ 1. ***[LO 7.3]*** formulary

_____ 2. ***[LO 7.11]*** evaluation and management (E/M) codes

_____ 3. ***[LO 7.9]*** ICD-9-CM

_____ 4. ***[LO 7.9]*** Tabular List

_____ 5. ***[LO 7.1]*** dictation

_____ 6. ***[LO 7.8]*** medical coding

_____ 7. ***[LO 7.12]*** computer-assisted coding

_____ 8. ***[LO 7.9]*** primary diagnosis

_____ 9. ***[LO 7.1]*** voice recognition software

_____ 10. ***[LO 7.1]*** template

a. The section of the ICD-9-CM in which diagnosis codes are presented in numerical order.

b. A computer program that can recognize spoken words.

c. The diagnosis that relates to the patient's stated reason for the visit.

d. The process of recording spoken words that will later be transcribed into written form.

e. A preformatted file that serves as a starting point for a new document.

f. The process of applying the HIPAA-mandated code sets to assign codes to diagnoses and procedures.

g. The CPT codes that represent the thought process that the physician follows to determine the best course of care.

h. A list of pharmaceutical products and dosages deemed by a health care organization to be the best, most economical treatments for a condition or disease.

i. The ninth revision of the *International Classification of Diseases*, which is used for diagnosis codes in the United States.

j. The process of coding with software.

TRUE/FALSE QUESTIONS

Decide whether each statement is true or false.

_____ 1. ***[LO 7.4]*** In Medisoft Clinical Patient Records, the Rx/Medications folder in a patient's chart is used to order new medications and monitor current, historical, or ineffective medications.

_____ 2. ***[LO 7.1]*** Many physicians prefer to use dictation and transcription because it is the most efficient method of entering documentation.

_____ 3. ***[LO 7.3]*** In Medisoft Clinical Patient Records, orders are checked to determine if they are inappropriate for a patient based on factors such as allergies.

_____ 4. ***[LO 7.1]*** When a template is used to create a progress note, it is not necessary to enter patient-specific information.

_____ 5. ***[LO 7.3]*** When an EHR is used for e-prescribing, a new prescription can be automatically checked for drug interactions, appropriate dosage levels, and patient allergies.

_____ 6. ***[LO 7.10]*** The procedure codes for physicians' and other health care providers' services are selected from the *Current Procedural Terminology* data set, called CPT.

_____ 7. ***[LO 7.13]*** When an electronic encounter form (EEF) is used to record a patient's procedures and diagnoses, it is not necessary to complete a paper form.

_____ 8. ***[LO 7.2]*** SOAP stands for Subjective, Objective, Assessment, and Procedure.

_____ 9. ***[LO 7.11]*** Most codes in the E/M section are organized by the place of service, such as the office, the hospital, or a patient's home.

_____ 10. ***[LO 7.7]*** In Medisoft Clinical Patient Records, order processing begins with selecting Orders > Order Processing on the Lists menu.

MULTIPLE-CHOICE QUESTIONS

Select the letter that best completes the statement or answers the question.

1. ***[LO 7.10]*** _________ are used to track performance measures for a medical goal such as reducing tobacco use.
   a. Category I codes
   b. Category II codes
   c. Category III codes
   d. Category IV codes

2. ***[LO 7.5]*** In Medisoft Clinical Patient Records, orders can be checked against insurance company rules to determine if a test requires preauthorization or is limited to certain _________.
   a. benefits
   b. ABNs
   c. procedure codes
   d. diagnoses

3. ***[LO 7.2]*** In Medisoft Clinical Patient Records, every progress note starts with a date and a _________.
   a. plan
   b. SOAP note
   c. title
   d. signature

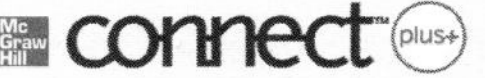

4. *[LO 7.1]* ________ transcribes spoken words into text in an electronic file.
   a. digital dictation
   b. dictation
   c. voice-recognition software
   d. all of the above

5. *[LO 7.13]* In the Electronic Encounter dialog box, the three tabs are Procedures, Diagnoses, and ________.
   a. Coding
   b. Action Items
   c. Lab Tests
   d. Orders

6. *[LO 7.8]* ________ is the process of applying the HIPAA-mandated code sets to assign codes to diagnoses and procedures.
   a. dictation
   b. medical coding
   c. digital dictation
   d. upcoding

7. *[LO 7.2]* In Medisoft Clinical Patient Records, progress notes can be entered through the use of ________.
   a. dictation and transcription
   b. voice recognition software
   c. a template
   d. all of the above

8. *[LO 7.9]* ICD-10-CM codes contain ________ characters, while ICD-9-CM codes consist of 3 to 5 characters.
   a. 3 to 9
   b. 5 to 13
   c. 5 to 9
   d. 5 to 7

9. *[LO 7.10]* The procedure codes for physicians' and other health care providers' services are selected from the ________.
   a. Alphabetic Index
   b. Tabular List
   c. CPT
   d. ICD

10. *[LO 7.1]* Which of the following is not an advantage of using a template to enter a progress note?
    a. efficiency
    b. computer search and analysis
    c. information less likely to be omitted
    d. easy to learn

SHORT-ANSWER QUESTIONS

Define the following abbreviations.

1. ***[LO 7.10]*** CPT ______________________________

2. ***[LO 7.13]*** EEF ______________________________

3. ***[LO 7.11]*** E/M ______________________________

4. ***[LO 7.9]*** ICD-9-CM ______________________________

5. ***[LO 7.9]*** ICD-10-CM ______________________________

6. ***[LO 7.2]*** SOAP ______________________________

7. ***[LO 7.10]*** HCPCS ______________________________

APPLYING YOUR KNOWLEDGE

Answer the questions below in the space provided.

7.1 ***[LO 7.1]*** In your own words, explain the advantages that voice recognition software can offer a provider.

____

____

7.2 ***[LO 7.3]*** Explain the advantages offered by electronic prescribing.

____

____

7.3 ***[LO 7.9]*** Do you think the implementation of the ICD-10-CM codes will help providers improve the quality of care they offer? If so, how?

____

____

7.4 ***[LO 7.12]*** How might computer-assisted coding be beneficial to a medical practice?

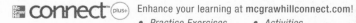

____

____

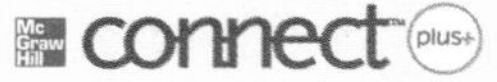

Enhance your learning at **mcgrawhillconnect.com**!
- *Practice Exercises*
- *Worksheets*
- *Activities*
- *Integrated eBook*

part three

Charge Capture and Billing Patient Encounters

chapter 8

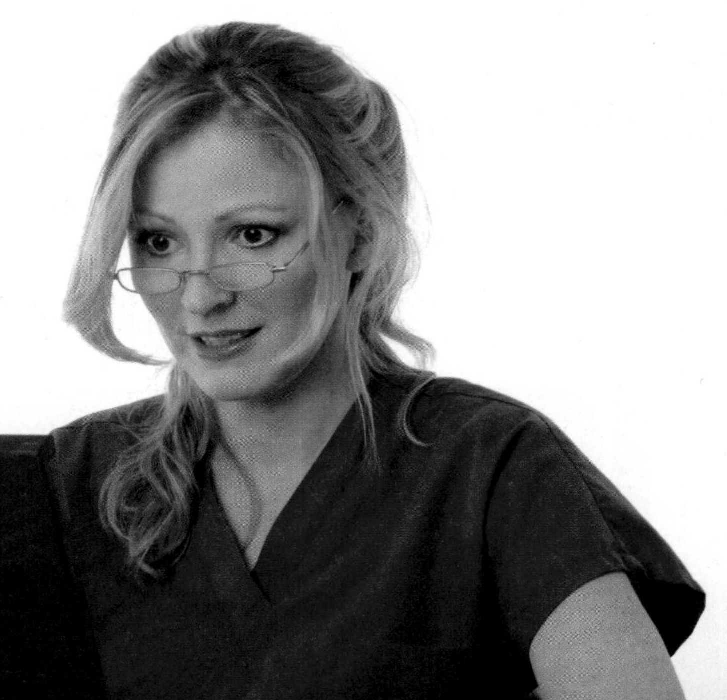

Third-Party Payers

KEY TERMS

allowed charge
balance billing
Blue Cross and Blue Shield Association (BCBS)
capitation (cap) rate
Civilian Health and Medical Program of the Department of Veterans Affairs (CHAMPVA)
consumer-driven (directed) health plan (CDHP)
disability compensation programs
discounted fee-for-service
dual-eligible
Employee Retirement Income Security Act of 1974 (ERISA)
Federal Employees Health Benefits (FEHB)
fee schedule
flexible savings account (FSA)
group health plan (GHP)
health maintenance organization (HMO)
health reimbursement account (HRA)
health savings account (HSA)
high-deductible health plan (HDHP)
individual health plan (IHP)
Medicaid
Medicare
Medicare Part A, Hospital Insurance (HI)
Medicare Part B, Supplementary Medical Insurance (SMI)
Medicare Part C, Medicare Advantage
Medicare Part D
Medicare Physician Fee Schedule (MPFS)
Medigap
Medi-Medi beneficiary
Original Medicare Plan
point-of-service (POS) plan
preferred provider organization (PPO)
primary care physician (PCP)
relative value scale (RVS)
resource-based relative value scale (RBRVS)
self-insured health plans
third-party payer
TRICARE
usual, customary, and reasonable (UCR)
usual fees
workers' compensation insurance
write off

LEARNING OUTCOMES

When you finish this chapter, you will be able to:

8.1 Compare the major features of PPO, HMO, and POS health plans.

8.2 Identify the two parts of CDHPs.

8.3 Discuss the organization and regulation of employer-sponsored group health plans and self-insured plans.

8.4 Explain the purpose of Medicare Parts A, B, C, and D.

8.5 Describe the fee structures that are used to set charges.

8.6 Identify the three methods most payers use to pay physicians.

8.7 Maintain insurance carrier information in the PM/EHR.

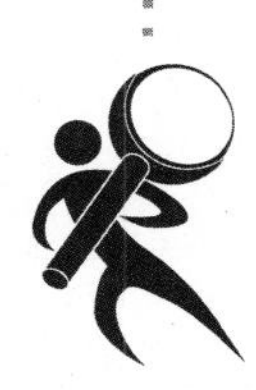

Beneficial Questions

"Good morning, Family Care Clinic. This is Laurie, how may I help you?" Leila Patterson is calling and wants to make an appointment for her annual physical examination. Leila also explains that she has just become a Medicare beneficiary and has selected the Original Medicare Plan. Laurie asks her to hold on for a moment, so she can double-check Medicare's coverage for new beneficiaries with Chris. She then explains that Medicare now covers the cost of one physical exam under "Welcome to Medicare" and since Dr. Banu participates in Medicare, there'll be no cost for the visit. Leila is delighted!

Reflect on the range of information the medical office staff deals with on a daily basis. What informational and organizational skills do medical administrative staff need to help patients, doctors, and insurance companies with regard to patients' health benefits?

WHEN YOU FINISH THIS CHAPTER, YOU WILL ALSO BE ABLE TO USE MEDISOFT CLINICAL TO:

1. Use MNP to enter a new insurance carrier.
2. Use MNP to update insurance carrier information.
3. Use MNP to enter a referral number.
4. Use MNP to enter a preauthorization number.

SOFTWARE SKILLS

8.1 Types of Health Plans

Insured patients have medical coverage under either managed care or indemnity (fee-for-service) plans. The type of health plan affects the payments that patients must make for medical services, so it is important for medical office administrative staff to understand the plans' key features.

Third-Party Relationship

There are three participants in the medical insurance relationship. The patient (policyholder) is the first party, and the physician is the second party. In legal terms, a patient–physician contract is created when a physician agrees to treat a patient who is seeking medical services. Through this unwritten contract, the patient is legally responsible for paying for services.

When the patient has a policy with a health plan, the plan is a third party. The plan agrees to carry some of the risk of paying for the services and therefore is called a **third-party payer.**

third-party payer private or government organization that insures or pays for health care on behalf of beneficiaries

preferred provider organization (PPO) managed care network of health care providers who agree to perform services for plan members at discounted fees

Preferred Provider Organizations

The most popular type of health plan, as shown in Figure 8.1, is the **preferred provider organization (PPO),** which contracts with physicians, hospitals, clinics, and pharmacies to provide a network of care providers for its beneficiaries.

Under a PPO, the policyholder pays an annual premium and a yearly deductible to pay out-of-pocket. A PPO plan may offer either a low deductible with a higher premium or a high deductible with a lower premium. The insured member typically pays a copayment at the time of each medical service, and coinsurance may also be charged for in-network providers. A patient may see an out-of-network doctor without a referral or preauthorization, but the deductible, copayment, and/or coinsurance for out-of-network services may be higher and the amount the plan will pay may be lower. In other words, the patient will be responsible for more of the fee. This encourages the people insured with a PPO to use the physicians, other medical providers, and hospitals in their network.

Advantages of a PPO include the flexibility of seeking care with an out-of-network provider if desired, even though doing so is more

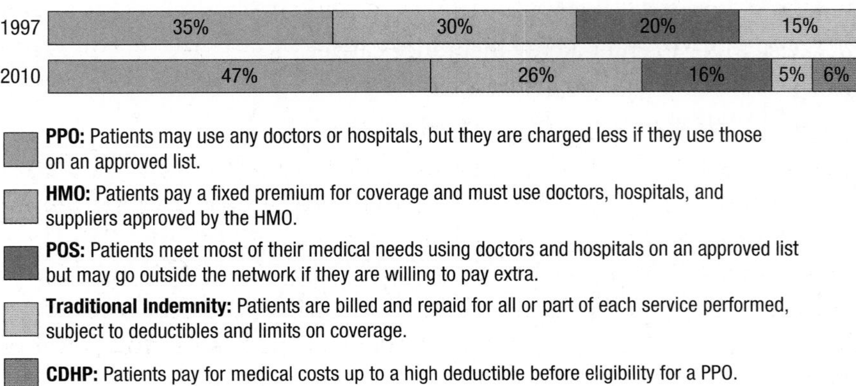

1997
35%
30%
20%
15%
2010
47%
26%
16%
5%
6%
PPO: Patients may use any doctors or hospitals, but they are charged less if they use those on an approved list.
HMO: Patients pay a fixed premium for coverage and must use doctors, hospitals, and suppliers approved by the HMO.
POS: Patients meet most of their medical needs using doctors and hospitals on an approved list but may go outside the network if they are willing to pay extra.
Traditional Indemnity: Patients are billed and repaid for all or part of each service performed, subject to deductibles and limits on coverage.
CDHP: Patients pay for medical costs up to a high deductible before eligibility for a PPO.

Figure 8.1 Employer-Sponsored Health Plans
Source: www.Kaiserhealthnews.org.

expensive for the patient. PPO networks also have prescription services that provide prescription drugs at a reduced cost. A PPO plan often includes more covered medical services than do other types of plans. PPOs have large networks of medical providers representing large geographic areas.

Health Maintenance Organizations

Health maintenance organizations (HMOs) are licensed by the state. They have the most stringent guidelines and the narrowest choice of providers. Their members are assigned to **primary care physicians (PCPs)** and must use the network except in emergencies or pay a penalty. HMOs have traditionally emphasized preventive and wellness services as well as disease management, although PPOs and other plans now also often include many of these services.

health maintenance organization (HMO) managed health care system in which providers offer health care to members for fixed periodic payments

primary care physician (PCP) physician in a managed care organization who directs all aspects of a patient's care

HMOs were originally designed to cover all basic services at a cost to patients of an annual premium and visit copayments. This arrangement is called "first-dollar coverage," because patients who received treatment were not required to pay deductibles before the plan started covering services. However, HMOs may now apply deductibles to family coverage, and employer-sponsored HMOs are also beginning to replace copayments with coinsurance for some services.

An HMO is organized around one of three business models: the staff model, the group or network model, and the independent practice association model. Each model is based on the way the terms of the agreement connect the provider and the plan. In all, however, enrollees must see HMO providers in order to be covered.

Staff Model

In a staff HMO, physicians are employed by the organization. All the premiums and other revenues come to the HMO, which in turn pays the physicians' salaries. For medical care, patients visit the clinics and health centers owned by the HMO.

Group (Network) Model

A group (network) HMO contracts with more than one physician group, creating a network of physicians. In some plans, HMO members receive medical services in HMO-owned facilities from providers who work only for that HMO. In others, members visit the providers' facilities, and the providers can also treat nonmember patients. The medical practices under contract are paid a per member per month (PMPM) capitated rate for each subscriber assigned to them for primary care services.

Independent Practice Association Model

An independent practice association (IPA) type of HMO is an association formed by physicians with separately owned practices who contract together to provide care for HMO members. An HMO pays negotiated fees for medical services to the IPA. The IPA, in turn, pays its physician members, either by a capitated rate or a fee. A provider may join more than one IPA and usually also sees nonmember patients.

THINKING IT THROUGH 8.1

If PPO patients use out-of-network rather than participating providers, what is the effect on the payments they are responsible for?

point-of-service (POS) plan managed care plan that permits patients to receive medical services from nonnetwork providers

consumer-driven (directed) health plan (CDHP) medical insurance that combines a high-deductible health plan with one or more tax-preferred savings accounts that the patient directs

high-deductible health plan (HDHP) health plan that combines high-deductible insurance and a funding option to pay for patients' out-of-pocket expenses up to the deductible

Point-of-Service (POS) Plans

A **point-of-service (POS) plan** is a hybrid of HMO and PPO networks. Members may choose from a primary or secondary network. The primary network is HMO-like, and the secondary network is often a PPO network. Like HMOs, POS plans charge annual premiums and copayments for office visits. Monthly premiums are slightly higher than for HMOs, but POS plans offer some coverage for visits to nonnetwork physicians for specialty care. A POS may be structured as a tiered plan, for example, with different rates for specially designated providers, regular participating providers, and out-of-network providers.

Indemnity Plans

Indemnity or fee-for-service plans require premium, deductible, and coinsurance payments. They typically cover 70 to 80 percent of the costs of covered benefits after the deductible is met. Some plans are structured with high deductibles, such as $5,000 to $10,000, in order to offer policyholders relatively lower premiums. Many have some managed care features, as payers compete for employers' contracts and try to control costs.

8.2 Consumer-Driven Health Plans

A recent type of managed care plan—the **consumer-driven (directed) health plan (CDHP)**—is increasingly popular. CDHPs combine a high-deductible health plan with one or more tax-preferred savings accounts that the patient (the "consumer") directs. The two plans work together; the high-deductible health plan covers catastrophic losses, while the savings account pays out-of-pocket or noncovered expenses.

The High-Deductible Health Plan

The first part of a CDHP is a **high-deductible health plan (HDHP),** usually a PPO. The annual deductible is over $1,000. Many of the plan's covered preventive care services, as well as coverage for accidents, disability, dental care, vision care, and long-term care, are not subject to this deductible.

The Funding Options

The second part is one of three types of CDHP funding options (see Table 8.1) that may be used with high-deductible health plans to form consumer-driven health plans: health reimbursement accounts, health savings accounts, and flexible savings accounts.

TABLE 8.1 CDHP Funding Options

Health Reimbursement Account	Health Savings Account	Flexible Savings Account
Contributions from employer	Contributions from individual (regardless of employment status), employer, or both	Contributions from employer and/or employee
Rollovers allowed within employer-set limits	Unused funds roll over indefinitely	Unused funds revert to employer
Portability allowed under employer's rules	Funds are portable (job change; retirement)	No portability
Tax-deductible deposits	Tax-deductible deposits	Tax-advantaged deposits
Tax-free withdrawals for qualified expenses	Tax-free withdrawals for qualified expenses	Tax-free withdrawals for qualified expenses
	Tax-free interest can be earned	

Health Reimbursement Accounts

A **health reimbursement account (HRA)** is a medical reimbursement plan set up and funded by an employer. HRAs are usually offered to employees with health plans that have high deductibles. Employees may submit claims to the HRA to be reimbursed for out-of-pocket medical expenses. For example, an employee may pay a health plan deductible, copayments, coinsurance, and any medical expenses not covered by the group health plan and then request reimbursement from the HRA. In some HRA plans, employers allow funds that remain in the account at the end of the benefit period to roll over to the next year's HRA.

health reimbursement account (HRA) consumer-driven health plan funding option where an employer sets aside an annual amount for health care costs

health savings account (HSA) consumer-driven health plan funding option under which funds are set aside to pay for certain health care costs

Health Savings Accounts

A **health savings account (HSA)** is a savings account created by an individual. Employers that wish to encourage employees to set up HSAs offer qualified high-deductible health plans to go with them. Both employee and employer can contribute to the HSA. The maximum amount that can be saved each year is set by the Internal Revenue Service (IRS). The IRS also sets the maximum out-of-pocket spending under HSA-compatible high-deductible health plans.

HSA money can be held in an account by an employer, a bank, or a health plan. This holder is referred to as the "custodian" for the account. The federal government decides the limits on the amount of the contribution that is tax-sheltered, just as it does for individual retirement accounts (IRAs).

HSAs do not have to be used up at the end of a benefit period. Instead, the account can roll over from year to year and go with an employee who changes jobs or retires. HSAs can earn tax-free interest and can be used for nonmedical purposes after age sixty-five.

flexible savings account (FSA) consumer-driven health plan funding option that has employer and employee contributions

Flexible Savings Accounts

Some companies offer a **flexible savings account (FSA)** that augments employees' other health insurance coverage. Employees can choose to put pretax dollars from their salaries in the FSA and use the fund to pay for certain medical and dependent care expenses. The permitted expenses include deductibles, copayments, coinsurance, medical expenses that are not covered under the regular insurance plan (such as routine physical examinations and eyeglasses), and child care. Employers may contribute to each employee's account.

The disadvantage of FSAs compared with HSAs is that at the end of the year, unused dollars in the account go back to the employer under the "use it or lose it" rule. Employees must try to calculate what their year's expenses are likely to be to avoid either over- or underfunding the account. For this reason, HSAs are becoming more popular than FSAs.

Billing Under Consumer-Driven Health Plans

A consumer-driven health plan operates as follows:

- The group health plan establishes a funding option (HRA, HSA, FSA, or some combination) designed to help pay out-of-pocket medical expenses.
- The patient uses the money in the account to pay for qualified medical services.
- The total deductible must be met before any benefits are paid by the high-deductible health plan.
- Once the deductible is met, the HDHP covers a portion of the benefits per the policy. The funding option can also be used to pay the uncovered portion.

Consumer-driven health plans may reduce cash flow to a practice. Under plans with visit copayments, cash is collected at the time of service. But if the plan instead has a high deductible, it may not be collected until after the claim is paid and the patient is sent a bill to pay. Physician reimbursement up to the amount of the deductible will come from the patient's funding option and, if there is not enough money there, out of the patient's pocket.

EXAMPLE

Following is an example of payments under a CDHP with an HSA fund of $1,000 and a deductible of $1,000. The HDHP has 80-20 coinsurance. The plan pays the visit charges as billed.

Patient's Visits	Charges	Amount Paid and Payer
First visit	$150	$150 paid from HSA.
Second visit	$450	$450 paid from HSA.
Third visit	$600	$400 paid from HSA and $160 paid by HDHP. Patient owes $40 coinsurance on account.
Total	$1,200	HSA pays $1,000; HDHP pays $160; patient pays $40 out-of-pocket.

BILLING TIP

Avoid Uncollectible Amounts from CDHPs

Educating patients about their financial responsibility before they leave their encounters, extending credit wisely, and improving collections are all key to avoiding uncollectible accounts under CDHPs.

THINKING IT THROUGH 8.2

Which of the three types of CDHP funding options would you choose? Why?

8.3 Private Insurance Payers and Blue Cross and Blue Shield

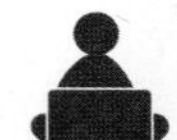

BILLING TIP

Know Your Terms!

Payers' rules and interpretations may vary. The definitions of basic terms (for example, the age range for "neonate") differ, as do preauthorization requirements. Billers must research each payer's rules for correct billing and reimbursement.

The major payers of medical insurance are either private payers or government-sponsored programs. Private insurance payers include:

- Employer-sponsored medical insurance
- The Federal Employees Health Benefits Program
- Self-insured health plans
- Individual health plans
- The Blue Cross and Blue Shield Association

Employer-Sponsored Medical Insurance

group health plan (GHP) plan of an employer or employee organization to provide health care to employees, former employees, and/or their families

Many employees have medical insurance coverage under **group health plans (GHPs)** that their employers sponsor. Human resource departments manage these health care benefits, negotiating with insurance carriers and managed care organizations and selecting one or more plans to offer employees. Both basic plans and riders that employees may buy and add to their policies may be offered. Riders, also called options, are often offered for vision and dental services. Another popular rider is for complementary health care, covering treatments such as chiropractic or manual manipulation, acupuncture, massage therapy, dietetic counseling, and vitamins and minerals.

During specified periods (usually once a year) called open enrollment periods, employees choose the plans they prefer for the coming benefit period. The employer provides tools (often Internet-based) and information to help employees match their personal and family needs with the best-priced plans. Employees can customize their policies by choosing to accept various levels of premiums, deductibles, and other costs.

Regulation and Eligibility for Benefits

Employer-sponsored group health plans must follow federal and state laws that mandate coverage of specific benefits or treatments and access to care. When a state law is more restrictive than the related federal law, the state law is followed.

The group health plan specifies the rules for eligibility and the process of enrolling and disenrolling members. Rules cover employment status, such a full-time, part-time, disabled employees, and laid-off or terminated employees, as well as the age and the conditions for enrolling a dependent.

- Many plans have a waiting period, an amount of time that must pass before a newly hired employee or a dependent is eligible to enroll. The waiting period usually begins on the date of hire and continues until the date the insurance is effective.

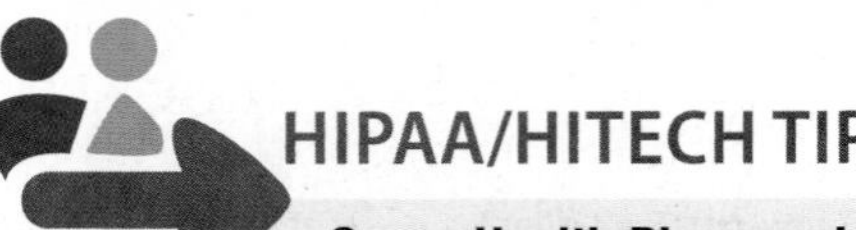

HIPAA/HITECH TIP

Group Health Plans and PHI

Both employer-sponsored health plans and self-insured health plans are group health plans (GHPs) under HIPAA and are subject to HIPAA regulations, including the use of HIPAA-compliant claims and provision of the Notice of Privacy Practices.

- The plan may impose different eligibility rules on a late enrollee, an individual who enrolls in a plan after the earliest possible enrollment date or other than on a special enrollment date. For example, special enrollment may occur when a person becomes a dependent of a covered employee through marriage.
- Most plans require annual premiums. Although employers used to pay the total premium as a benefit for employees, currently they pay an average 80 percent of the cost.
- Each health plan also has a deductible that is due per time period. Noncovered services under the plan that the patient must pay out-of-pocket do not count toward satisfying a deductible. Some plans require an individual deductible that must be met for each person—whether the policyholder or a covered dependent—who has an encounter. Others have a family deductible that can be met by the combined payments to providers for any and all covered members of the insured's family.

Federal Employees Health Benefits Program

Federal Employees Health Benefits (FEHB) health care program that covers federal employees

self-insured health plans health insurance plans paid for directly by the organization, which sets up a fund from which to pay

Employee Retirement Income Security Act of 1974 (ERISA) law providing incentives and protection for companies with employee health and pension plans

The largest employer-sponsored health program in the United States is the **Federal Employees Health Benefits (FEHB)** program, which covers more than 8 million federal employees, retirees, and their families through over 250 health plans from a number of carriers. FEHB is administered by the federal government's Office of Personnel Management (OPM), which receives and deposits premiums and remits payments to the carriers. Each carrier is responsible for furnishing identification cards and benefits brochures to enrollees, adjudicating claims, and maintaining records.

Self-Insured Health Plans

To save money, some large employers cover the costs of employee medical benefits themselves, rather than buying insurance from carriers or managed care organizations. They create **self-insured health plans** that do not pay premiums to insurance carriers or managed care organizations. Instead, employers with self-insured health plans "insure themselves" and assume the risk of paying directly for medical services, setting aside funds with which to pay benefits. The employer establishes the benefit levels and the plan types offered to employees.

Self-insured health plans may set up their own provider networks or, more often, lease the use of managed care organizations' networks. Self-insured health plans (in contrast to employer-sponsored fully insured plans) are regulated by the federal **Employee Retirement Income Security Act of 1974 (ERISA)** instead of by state laws.

Individual Health Plans

Individual health plans (IHPs) are also available for purchase; almost 10 percent of people with private health insurance have individual plans. People often elect to enroll in individual plans, although coverage is expensive, in order to continue their health insurance between jobs. Purchasers also include self-employed entrepreneurs, students, recent college graduates, and early retirees. Individual insurance plans have basic benefits without the riders or additional features associated with group health plans.

individual health plan (IHP) medical insurance plan purchased by an individual

Blue Cross and Blue Shield Association (BCBS) licensing agency of Blue Cross and Blue Shield plans

Major Private Payers and Blue Cross and Blue Shield

A small number of large insurance companies dominate the national market and offer all types of health plans to employers and to self-insured plans. Local or regional payers are often affiliated with national plans or with the Blue Cross and Blue Shield Association (discussed below). Some carriers offer health insurance to individuals and to small businesses. The law in a few states, such as Maryland, requires major insurance carriers to provide limited health plans that small businesses can afford.

BILLING TIP

Timely Payments

Group health plans must follow states' clean claims and/or prompt payment acts and pay claims they accept for processing on a timely basis. ERISA (self-insured) plans are obligated to follow similar rules from the federal Department of Labor.

Major Private Payers

Private payers supply complete insurance services, such as:

- Contracting with employers and with individuals to provide insurance benefits
- Setting up physician, hospital, and pharmacy networks
- Establishing fees
- Processing claims
- Managing the insurance risk

The leading national payers are:

- WellPoint, Inc.
- UnitedHealth Group
- Aetna
- CIGNA
- Kaiser Permanente
- Health Net
- Humana, Inc.
- Coventry

Blue Cross and Blue Shield

The **Blue Cross and Blue Shield Association (BCBS),** founded in the 1930s to provide low-cost medical insurance, is a national organization of independent companies called Member Plans that insure over 90 million people. About half of the plan subscribers (policyholders) join PPOs; a quarter are in indemnity plans; about 20 percent in HMOs; and 8 percent in point-of-service plans. All BCBS Member Plans offer a full range of health plans, including consumer-driven health plans, to individuals, small and large employer

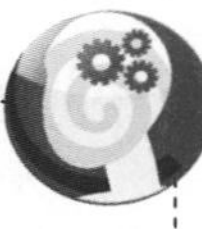

THINKING IT THROUGH 8.3

How would payments toward an individual deductible versus a family deductible be totaled, assuming a time period of one year? Do payments for noncovered services count toward meeting the deductible?

groups, senior citizens, federal government employees, and others. In addition to major medical and hospital insurance, the "Blues" also have freestanding plans for dental, vision, mental health, prescription, and hearing coverage.

8.4 Government-Sponsored Insurance Programs, Workers' Compensation, and Disability Plans

Many patients of medical practices are insured under one of the four major government-sponsored insurance programs:

- Medicare
- Medicaid
- TRICARE
- CHAMPVA

Two other types of coverage, workers' compensation and disability plans, help people pay for losses from accidents and lost wages.

Medicare

Medicare federal health insurance program for people sixty-five or older and some people with disabilities

Medicare is a federal medical insurance program established in 1965 under Title XVIII of the Social Security Act. The Medicare program is managed by the Centers for Medicare and Medicaid Services (CMS) under the Department of Health and Human Services (HHS). Although it has just four parts, it is arguably the most complex program that medical practices deal with, involving numerous rules and regulations that must be followed.

Medicare benefits are controlled by federal statute. To be covered, an item or service must be in a benefit category established by law and not otherwise excluded. To receive benefits, individuals must be eligible under one of six beneficiary categories:

1. **Individuals age sixty-five or older** Persons age sixty-five or older who have paid FICA taxes or Railroad Retirement taxes for at least forty calendar quarters (ten years).
2. **Disabled adults** Individuals who have been receiving Social Security disability benefits or Railroad Retirement Board disability benefits for more than two years. Coverage begins five months after the two years of entitlement.
3. **Individuals disabled before age eighteen** Individuals under age eighteen who meet the disability criteria of the Social Security Act.

4. **Spouses of entitled individuals** Spouses of deceased or disabled individuals who are or were entitled to Medicare benefits.
5. **Retired federal employees enrolled in the Civil Service Retirement System (CSRS)** Retired CSRS employees and their spouses.
6. **Individuals with end-stage renal disease (ESRD)** Individuals of any age who receive dialysis or renal transplants for ESRD. Coverage typically begins on the first day of the month following the start of dialysis treatments. In the case of a transplant, entitlement begins the month the individual is hospitalized for the transplant, and the transplant must be completed within two months. The donor is covered for services related to the donation of the organ only.

Medicare Part A

Medicare Part A, which is also called **Hospital Insurance (HI),** pays for inpatient hospital care, skilled nursing facility care, home health care, and hospice care. Anyone who paid Medicare taxes while working is eligible for Part A at age sixty-five. Those who are receiving Social Security benefits automatically receive Part A coverage; others have to enroll. Eligible beneficiaries do not pay premiums. Individuals age sixty-five or older who are not eligible for Social Security benefits may enroll in Part A, but they must pay premiums for the coverage, and most are also required to take and pay for Part B coverage.

Medicare Part A, Hospital Insurance (HI) program that pays for hospitalization, care in a skilled nursing facility, home health care, and hospice care

Medicare Part B, Supplementary Medical Insurance (SMI) program that pays for physician services, outpatient hospital services, durable medical equipment, and other services and supplies

Original Medicare Plan Medicare fee-for-service plan

Medicare Part B

Medicare Part B, which is also called **Supplementary Medical Insurance (SMI),** helps beneficiaries pay for physician services, outpatient hospital services, medical equipment, and other supplies and services. Individuals entitled to Part A benefits are automatically qualified to enroll in Part B. United States citizens and permanent residents over the age of sixty-five are also eligible. (People eligible for this coverage can choose either the Original Medicare Plan or a Medicare Advantage plan, also known as Medicare Part C, both of which are explained below.)

Part B is a voluntary program; eligible persons do not have to take part in it. People who are receiving Social Security benefits are automatically signed up for Part B and must opt out if they do not want to take part. Others desiring Part B coverage must enroll; coverage is not automatic. If enrollment takes place more than twelve months after a person's initial enrollment period, there is a permanent 10 percent increase in the premium for each year the beneficiary failed to enroll.

Beneficiaries pay monthly premiums for Part B. They are also subject to annual deductibles and coinsurance, which are established by federal law.

Original Medicare Plan

The Medicare fee-for-service plan, referred to by Medicare as the **Original Medicare Plan,** allows the beneficiary to choose any licensed physician certified by Medicare. Each time the beneficiary receives services, a fee is billable. Part of this fee is generally paid by Medicare, and part is paid by the beneficiary or sometimes by a secondary policy.

Original Medicare Plan patients are responsible for an annual deductible. They are also responsible for the portion of the bill that Medicare does not pay (coinsurance), typically 20 percent of allowed charges. Patients receive a Medicare Summary Notice (MSN) that details the services they were provided over a thirty-day period, the amounts charged, and the amounts they may be billed.

Medigap plan offered by a private insurance carrier to supplement Medicare coverage

Medicare Part C, Medicare Advantage managed care health plans under the Medicare program

Medicare Part D Medicare prescription drug reimbursement plans

Medicaid federal and state assistance program that pays for health care services for people who cannot afford them

Medigap Insurance

Medigap is private insurance that Original Medicare Plan beneficiaries may purchase to fill in some of the gaps—unpaid amounts—in Medicare coverage. These gaps include the annual deductible, any coinsurance that is required, and payment for some noncovered services. Even though private insurance carriers offer Medigap plans, coverage and standards are regulated by federal and state law.

Medicare Part C (Medicare Advantage Plans)

Medicare Part C (Medicare Advantage) is a program that permits private insurance carriers to contract with CMS to offer Medicare benefits under a managed care option. A Medicare Advantage organization (MAO) is responsible for providing all Medicare-covered services other than hospice care in return for a predetermined capitated payment. Medicare Advantage plans include fee-for-service and other types of plans, and some cover vision, dental, and other services.

Medicare Part D

Medicare Part D provides voluntary Medicare prescription drug plans that are open to people who are eligible for Medicare. All Medicare prescription drug plans are private insurance plans that are approved by Medicare, and most participants pay monthly premiums to access discounted prices. There are two types of plans. The prescription drug plan covers only drugs and can be used with an Original Medicare Plan and/or a Medicare supplement plan. The other type combines a prescription drug plan with a Medicare Advantage plan that includes medical coverage for doctor visits and hospital expenses. This kind of plan is called Medicare Advantage Plus Prescription Drug. A Medicare prescription drug plan has a list of drugs it covers, often structured in payment tiers.

Medicaid

The **Medicaid** program covers more than 50 million low-income people, pays for more than one-third of births, and finances care for two-thirds of nursing home residents. The program was established under Title XIX of the Social Security Act of 1965 to pay for the health care needs of individuals and families with low incomes and few resources.

Medicaid is jointly funded by the federal and state governments. The federal government makes payments to states under the Federal

Medicaid Assistance Percentage (FMAP). The amount of the payment is based on the state's average per capita income in relation to the national income average.

Because Medicaid is run by states rather than by the federal government, billers refer to the laws and regulations of their state Medicaid programs to correctly process claims for these patients. Although the federal government sets broad standards for Medicaid coverage, there is variation among the states. States establish their own eligibility standards; the type, amount, duration, and scope of services; and payments to providers. States' income limits usually consider the applicant's income relative to the federal poverty level (FPL), taking household size into account. Most states also provide Medicaid coverage to medically needy individuals—people with high medical expenses and low financial resources (but not low enough to receive cash assistance). States may choose their own names for these programs.

Medi-Medi

Some individuals, called **Medi-Medi beneficiaries** or **dual-eligibles,** are eligible for both Medicaid and Medicare benefits. In many instances, Medicare requires payment of a deductible or coinsurance. When an individual has Medi-Medi coverage, such payments are sometimes paid by Medicaid. The total amount paid by Medicare and Medicaid is subject to a maximum allowed limit. In most states, Medicaid plans do not pay if Medicare does not.

Medi-Medi beneficiary person eligible for both Medicare and Medicaid

dual-eligible Medicare-Medicaid beneficiary

TRICARE government health program serving dependents of active-duty service members, military retirees and their families, some former spouses, and survivors of deceased military members

TRICARE

TRICARE is the Department of Defense health insurance plan for military personnel and their families. TRICARE, which includes managed care options, replaced the program known as CHAMPUS, the Civilian Health and Medical Program of the Uniformed Services.

TRICARE is a regionally managed health care program that brings the resources of military hospitals together with a network of civilian facilities and providers to offer increased access to health care services. All military treatment facilities, including hospitals and clinics, are part of the TRICARE system. TRICARE also contracts with civilian facilities and physicians to provide more extensive services to beneficiaries.

TRICARE offers beneficiaries access to three different health care plans.

1. TRICARE Standard is a fee-for-service program that replaces the CHAMPUS program, which was also fee-for-service. The program covers medical services provided by a civilian physician when the individual cannot receive treatment from a military treatment facility (MTF). Military families may receive services at an MTF, but the services offered vary by facility, and first priority is given to service members on active duty. When service is not available, the individual seeks treatment from a civilian provider, and TRICARE Standard benefits go into effect.

2. TRICARE Prime is a managed care plan similar to an HMO. After enrolling in the plan, individuals are assigned a Primary Care Manager (PCM) who coordinates and manages their medical care. The PCM may be a single military or civilian provider or a group of providers. In addition to most of the benefits offered by TRICARE Standard, TRICARE Prime offers preventive care, including routine physical examinations. Active-duty service members are automatically enrolled in TRICARE Prime. TRICARE Prime enrollees receive the majority of their health care services from military treatment facilities and receive priority at these facilities.
3. TRICARE Extra is an alternative managed care plan for individuals who want to receive services primarily from civilian facilities and physicians rather than from military facilities. Since it is a managed care plan, individuals must receive health care services from a network of health care professionals. They may also seek treatment at military facilities, but active-duty personnel and other TRICARE Prime enrollees receive priority at those facilities, so care may not always be available. TRICARE Extra is more expensive than TRICARE Prime, but less costly than TRICARE Standard.

CHAMPVA

Civilian Health and Medical Program of the Department of Veterans Affairs (CHAMPVA) health care plan for families of veterans with 100 percent service-related disabilities and the surviving spouses and children of veterans who die from service-related disabilities

The **Civilian Health and Medical Program of the Department of Veterans Affairs (CHAMPVA)** is the government's health insurance program for veterans with a 100 percent service-related disability and their families. Under the program, health care expenses are shared between the Department of Veterans Affairs (VA) and the beneficiary.

The Veterans Health Care Eligibility Reform Act of 1996 requires veterans with a 100 percent disability to be enrolled in the program as CHAMPVA sponsors. The VA is responsible for determining eligibility for the CHAMPVA program. Eligible beneficiaries include:

- Dependents of a veteran who is totally and permanently disabled due to a service-connected injury
- Dependents of a veteran who was totally and permanently disabled due to a service-connected condition at the time of death
- Survivors of a veteran who died as a result of a service-related disability
- Survivors of a veteran who died in the line of duty

Note that an eligible CHAMPVA sponsor may be entitled to receive medical care through the VA health care system based on his or her own veteran status. Additionally, if the eligible CHAMPVA sponsor is the spouse of another eligible CHAMPVA sponsor, both may now be eligible for CHAMPVA benefits. In each instance where the eligible spouse requires medical attention, he or she may choose the VA health care system or coverage under CHAMPVA for his/her health care needs.

Workers' Compensation

When someone is injured accidentally in the course of performing work or a work-related duty or becomes ill as a result of the employment environment, the cost of medical care for the injury or illness is covered by a federal or state plan known as **workers' compensation insurance.** These plans also provide benefits for lost wages and permanent disabilities.

workers' compensation insurance state or federal plan that covers medical care and other benefits for employees who suffer accidental injury or become ill as a result of employment

disability compensation programs programs that provide partial reimbursement for lost income when a disability prevents an individual from working

Workers' compensation covers two kinds of situations that require medical care. A traumatic injury is caused by a specific event or series of events within a single workday or shift. An example is a broken leg caused by a fall from a catwalk in a warehouse. Occupational disease or illness (also known as nontraumatic injury) is caused by the work environment over a longer period of time. An example of an occupational disease is a lung condition caused by repeated exposure to fumes in the workplace.

Workers' compensation includes five types of payments for work-related illnesses and injuries:

1. For medical treatment
2. To replace lost wages (temporary disability)
3. As permanent disability payments (either partial or full disability)
4. As compensation for dependents of employees who are fatally injured
5. For vocational rehabilitation

Work-related illnesses or injuries suffered by civilian (nonmilitary) employees of most federal agencies are covered under the Federal Employees' Compensation Act (FECA) and administered by the Office of Workers' Compensation Programs (OWCP). Injured employees can choose a physician from among those who are authorized by the OWCP. When such a patient requests treatment, the biller should verify that the selected physician is authorized to administer medical care under the patient's workers' compensation coverage. If the patient later wants to change physicians, the OWCP must approve the change. A patient who seeks care from an unauthorized physician may be responsible for the cost of that treatment.

State programs cover traumatic and nontraumatic injuries to state and private business employees within each state, although there are some exceptions. Eligibility and exceptions vary from state to state. A state compensation board or commission administers workers' compensation laws for employees eligible under state laws. The state board or commission handles employee appeals and provides information to employers and health care providers about regulations. Compliance with state laws is important.

Disability

Most of the insurance and compensation plans pay for health care costs resulting from illnesses or injuries. By comparison, **disability compensation programs** pay benefits for lost income when an

THINKING IT THROUGH 8.4

Why is it important to understand which services are and are not covered under patients' insurance plans?

illness or injury prevents a person from working. Unlike workers' compensation programs, which also include compensation for lost income, the illness or injury does not have to be work-related.

The federal government, some states, and many private insurance companies offer disability compensation programs and policies. Eligibility and benefits vary. However, they all require the insured to provide convincing medical evidence that the condition resulting from the illness or injury satisfies the criteria of the program or policy.

8.5 Setting Fees

Given all the possible types of health plans and payers, billers must often handle questions from patients about their fees. The answers are based on knowledge of the practice's charges and on estimates of what patients' insurance plans will pay.

fee schedule document that specifies the amount the provider bills for services

usual fees normal fees charged by a provider

usual, customary, and reasonable (UCR) fees set by comparing usual fees, customary fees, and reasonable fees

relative value scale (RVS) system of assigning unit values to medical services based on their required skill and time

Physicians have **fee schedules,** lists of fees for the procedures and services they frequently perform. These fees are called **usual fees,** meaning that the physicians charge them to most of their patients most of the time under typical conditions. Payers, too, set the fees that they pay providers. Most payers use one of three methods to set the fees that the health plan will pay physicians: (1) usual, customary, and reasonable; (2) relative value scale; and (3) resource-based relative value scale.

Usual, Customary, and Reasonable Payment Structure

Some health plans take the physicians' usual charges into account when they set their fee structures. A plan studies what many physicians have charged for similar services over a period of time. The fee that is set for each service is an average of the usual fee an individual physician charges for the service, the customary fee charged by most physicians in the community, and the reasonable fee for the service. This approach is called **usual, customary, and reasonable (UCR).**

UCR fees, for the most part, accurately reflect the charges of most physicians. However, fees may not be available for new or rare procedures. Lacking better information, a payer may set too low a fee for such procedures.

Relative Value Scale

Another method payers use to establish fees is the **relative value scale (RVS)** approach. Based on nationwide research, the relative

THINKING IT THROUGH 8.5

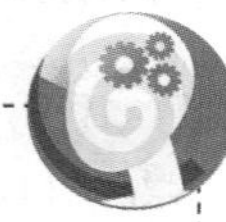

If a participating provider has two different fees for a particular CPT code for Medicare and a private payer, which should be lower?

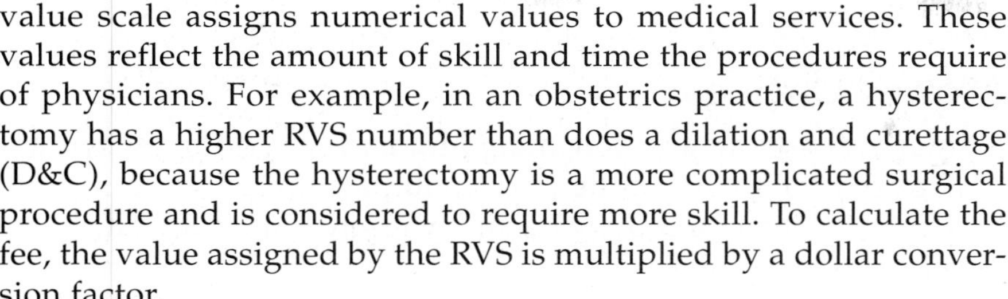

value scale assigns numerical values to medical services. These values reflect the amount of skill and time the procedures require of physicians. For example, in an obstetrics practice, a hysterectomy has a higher RVS number than does a dilation and curettage (D&C), because the hysterectomy is a more complicated surgical procedure and is considered to require more skill. To calculate the fee, the value assigned by the RVS is multiplied by a dollar conversion factor.

BILLING TIP

Setting Fees

Most practices set their fees slightly above those paid by the highest reimbursing plan in which they participate. Medicare rules state that the amount billed Medicare must not be higher) than the lowest fee billed any payer for the same service.

Resource-Based Relative Value Scale

The payment system used by Medicare is called the **resource-based relative value scale (RBRVS).** The RBRVS establishes relative value units for services. It replaces providers' consensus on fees—the historical charges—with a relative value that is based on resources—what each service really costs to provide.

There are three parts to an RBRVS fee:

1. **The nationally uniform relative value unit** The relative value is based on three cost elements: the physician's work, the practice cost (overhead), and the cost of malpractice insurance.
2. **A geographic adjustment factor** A geographic adjustment factor called the geographic practice cost index (GPCI) is a number that is used to multiply each relative value element so that it better reflects a geographic area's relative costs. For example, the cost of the provider's work is affected by average physician salaries in an area. The cost of the practice depends on things such as office rental prices and local taxes. Malpractice expense is also affected by where the work is done.
3. **A nationally uniform conversion factor** A uniform conversion factor is a dollar amount used to multiply the relative values to produce a payment amount. It is used by Medicare to make adjustments according to changes in the cost of living index.

resource-based relative value scale (RBRVS) relative value scale for establishing Medicare charges

Medicare Physician Fee Schedule (MPFS) RBRVS-based allowed fees that are the basis for Medicare reimbursements

BILLING TIP

Updating Fee Schedules

Fee schedules must be updated when new CPT codes are released. For example, if the definition of a surgical package changes, a surgeon's fees need to be altered to tie exactly to the revised elements of the package, or a new procedure may need to be included. Providers may refer to the national databases or, more likely, review those databases and the Medicare rate of pay to establish the new fees.

Medicare Physician Fee Schedule

Each part of the RBRVS—the relative values, the GPCI, and the conversion factor—is updated each year by CMS. The year's **Medicare Physician Fee Schedule (MPFS)** is published by CMS in the *Federal Register* and is available through the CMS website. Many private payers use the MPFS as the basis for the fees they pay as well.

8.6 Third-Party Payment Methods

Which entity is paying for the charges listed on a claim also affects the way physicians are paid for providing those services. Table 8.2 reviews the payment methods of the types of health plans. Payers use one of three main methods of paying providers: allowed charges, contracted fee schedules, and capitation.

Allowed Charges

allowed charge maximum charge a plan pays for a service or procedure

Many payers set an **allowed charge** for each procedure or service. This amount is the most the payer will pay any provider for that CPT code. Whether a provider actually receives the allowed charge depends on three things:

1. **The provider's usual charge for the procedure or service** The usual charge on the physician's fee schedule may be higher than, equal to, or lower than the allowed charge.
2. **The provider's status in the particular plan or program** The provider is either participating or nonparticipating (see Chapter 4). Participating (PAR) providers agree to accept allowed charges that are lower than their usual fees. In return, they are eligible for incentives, such as quicker payments of their claims and more patients.
3. **The payer's billing rules** These rules govern whether the provider can bill a patient for the part of the charge that the payer does not cover.

BILLING TIP

Other Terms for Allowed Charge

The allowed charge is also called a maximum allowable fee, maximum charge, allowed amount, allowed fee, and allowable charge.

When a payer uses an allowed charge method, it never pays more than the allowed charge to a provider. If a provider's usual fee is higher, only the allowed charge is paid. If a provider's usual fee is

TABLE 8.2 Health Plan Payment Methods

Plan Type	Participating Provider Payment Method
Preferred provider organization (PPO)	Discounted fee-for-service
Staff health maintenance organization (HMO)	Salary
Group HMO	Salary or contracted capitation rate Discounted fee-for-service
Independent practice association (IPA)	PCP: Contracted capitation rate Specialist: Fee-for-service
Point-of-service (POS) plan	Contracted capitation rate or discounted fee-for-service
Indemnity	Fee-for-service
Consumer-directed health plan (combined HDHP and funding option)	Up to deductible: Payment by patient After deductible: Discounted fee-for-service

lower, the payer reimburses that lower amount. The payer's payment is always the lower of the two amounts: the provider's charge or the allowed charge.

EXAMPLE

The payer's allowed charge for a new patient's evaluation and management (E/M) service (CPT 99204) is $160.

Provider	Usual Charge	Payment
A	$180	$160
B	$140	$140

Whether a participating provider can bill the patient for the difference between a higher physician fee and a lower allowed charge—called **balance billing**—depends on the terms of the contract with the payer. Payers' rules may prohibit participating providers from balance billing the patient. Instead, the provider must **write off** the difference, meaning that the amount of the difference is subtracted from the patient's bill and never collected.

balance billing collecting the difference between a provider's usual fee and a payer's lower allowed charge

write off to deduct an amount from a patient's account

For example, Medicare-participating providers may not receive an amount greater than the Medicare allowed charge from the Medicare Physician Fee Schedule. Medicare is responsible for paying 80 percent of this allowed charge (after patients have met their annual deductible; see Chapter 9). Patients are responsible for the other 20 percent.

EXAMPLE

A Medicare PAR provider reports a usual charge of $200 for a diagnostic flexible sigmoidoscopy (CPT 45330), and the Medicare allowed charge is $84. The provider must write off the difference between the two charges. The patient is responsible for 20 percent of the allowed charge, not of the provider's usual charge:

Provider's usual fee	$200.00
Medicare allowed charge	$ 84.00
Medicare pays 80 percent	$ 67.20
Patient pays 20 percent	$ 16.80

The total the provider can collect is $84. The provider must write off the difference between the usual fee and the allowed charge, $116.

A provider who does not participate in a private plan can usually balance bill patients. As shown in the example below, in this situation, if the provider's usual charge is higher than the allowed charge, the patient must pay the difference. (Note, however, that Medicare and other government-sponsored programs often have different rules for nonparticipating providers.)

EXAMPLE

Payer policy: There is an allowed charge for each procedure. The plan provides a benefit of 100 percent of the provider's usual charges, up to this maximum fee. Provider A is a participating provider; Provider B does not participate and can balance bill. Providers A and B both perform abdominal hysterectomies (CPT 58150). The policy's allowed charge for this procedure is $2,880.

Provider A (PAR)

Provider's usual charge	$3,100.00
Policy pays its allowed charge	$2,880.00
Provider writes off the difference	$ 220.00

Provider B (nonPAR)

Provider's usual charge	$3,000.00
Policy pays its allowed charge	$2,880.00
Provider bills patient for the difference	$ 120.00 ($3,000.00 − $2,880.00)
There is no write-off	

Coinsurance provisions in many private plans provide for patient cost-sharing. Rather than paying the provider the full allowed charge, for example, a plan may require the patient to pay 25 percent, while the plan pays 75 percent. In this case, if a provider's usual charges are higher than the plan's allowed charge, the patient owes more for a service from a nonparticipating provider than from a participating provider. The calculations are explained below.

EXAMPLE

Payer policy: A policy provides a benefit of 75 percent of the provider's usual charges, and there is a maximum allowed charge for each procedure. The patient is responsible for 25 percent of the maximum allowed charge. Balance billing is not permitted for plan participants.

Provider A is a participating provider, and Provider B is a nonparticipant in the plan. Providers A and B both perform total abdominal hysterectomies (CPT 58150). The policy's allowed charge for this procedure is $2,880.00.

Provider A (PAR)

Usual charge	$3,100.00
Policy pays 75 percent of its allowed charge	$2,160.00 (75% of $2,880.00)
Patient pays 25 percent of the allowed charge	$ 720.00 (25% of $2,880.00)
Provider writes off the difference	$ 220.00

Provider B (nonPAR)

Usual charge	$3,000.00
Policy pays 75 percent of its allowed charge	$2,160.00 (75% of $2,880.00)
Patient pays for:	
(1) 25 percent of the allowed charge +	$ 720.00 (25% of $2,880.00)
(2) the difference between the usual charge and the allowed charge	$ 120.00 ($3,000.00 − $2,880.00)
Patient pays	$ 840.00 ($720.00 + $120.00)
The provider has no write-off	

THINKING IT THROUGH 8.6

In a CDHP, why is the patient's payment after meeting the deductible based on a discounted fee?

Contracted Fee Schedule

Some payers, particularly those that contract directly with providers, establish fixed fee schedules with participating providers. They first decide what they will pay in particular geographic areas and then offer participation contracts with those fees to physician practices. If the practice chooses to join, it agrees by contract to accept the plan's fees for its member patients.

The plan's contract states what percentage of the charges, if any, its patients owe, and what percentage the payer covers. These fee schedules are often called **discounted fee-for-service** arrangements, since they are based on a reduction from the physician's usual fee schedule. Participating providers can typically bill patients their usual charges for procedures and services that are not covered by the plan.

discounted fee-for-service payment schedule for services based on a reduced percentage of usual charges

capitation (cap) rate periodic prepayment to a provider for specified services to each plan member

Capitation

The fixed prepayment for each plan member in capitation plans, called the **capitation rate** or **cap rate,** is determined by the managed care organization that contracts with providers. To determine the cap rate, the plan first decides on the allowed charges for the contracted services and then analyzes the health-related characteristics of the plan's members. The plan calculates the number of times each age group and gender group of members is likely to use each of the covered services. For example, if the primary care provider (PCP) contract covers obstetrics and a large percentage of the group's members are young women who are likely to require services related to childbirth, the cap rate is higher than for a group of members containing a greater percentage of men or of women in their forties or fifties who are not as likely to require obstetrics services.

8.7 Maintaining Insurance Information in the PM/EHR

Setting up the insurance carriers correctly in the PM/EHR is essential to getting claims paid in a timely manner. Insurance carriers must be entered in Medisoft before they can be assigned to patients in the Policy 1, 2, and 3 tabs in the Case folders, which you learned about in Chapter 5.

Insurance carrier information is accessed by selecting Insurance on the Lists menu, and then selecting Carriers or Classes on the submenu that appears (see Figure 8.2). The Carriers option on the submenu is used to enter, edit, or delete insurance carriers. The Classes option is used to group carriers for the purposes of reporting.

Figure 8.2 Lists Menu with the Insurance Submenu Displayed

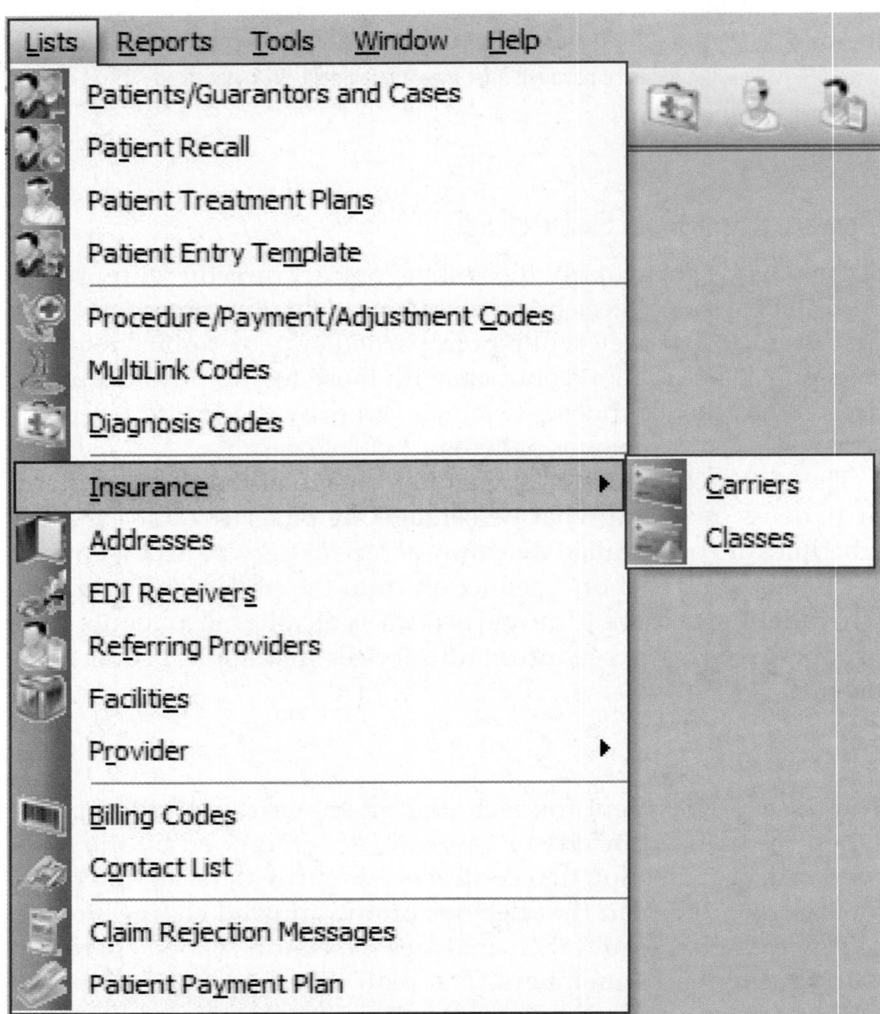

When the Carriers option is selected from the submenu, the Insurance Carrier List dialog box is displayed (see Figure 8.3). This dialog box lists all insurance carriers in the database. The Edit, New, and Delete buttons are used to change, create, and delete insurance carriers. The Print Grid button is used to print the information in the dialog box. The Close button closes the dialog box.

Figure 8.3 Insurance Carrier List Dialog Box

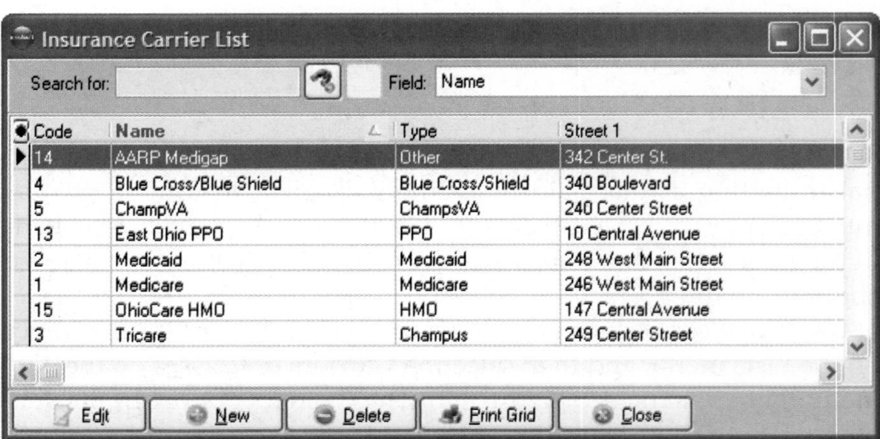

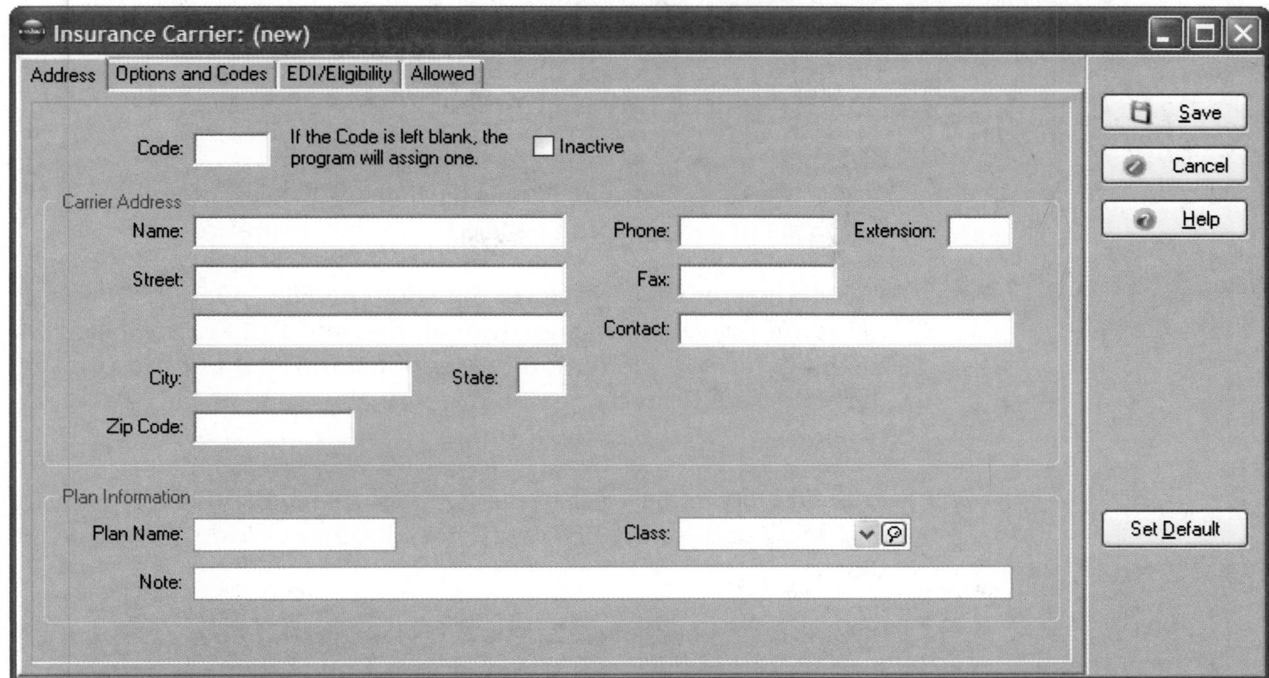

Figure 8.4 Insurance Carrier: (new) Dialog Box

Detailed information about an insurance carrier is stored in the Insurance Carrier dialog box for each carrier. To view information on a carrier already in the database, select the carrier in the Insurance Carrier List dialog box, and click the Edit button. To enter a carrier not already in the database, click the New button. The Insurance Carrier: (new) dialog box appears (see Figure 8.4). The Insurance Carrier: (new) dialog box contains four tabs: Address, Options and Codes, EDI/Eligibility, and Allowed.

Address Tab

The Address tab contains basic information such as the plan name, address, and contact information. Refer to Figure 8.4 to view the Address tab.

Code A unique code is assigned to the carrier. If the field is left blank, the program will assign a code.

Inactive This box is checked if the carrier is no longer active.

Carrier Address

The Carrier Address section of the tab contains the Name, Street, City, State, Zip Code, Phone, Extension, Fax, and Contact fields.

Plan Information

Plan Name The Plan Name field lists the name of the plan.

Class The Class field contains the insurance class for the carrier.

Note This is an optional field for additional plan information (for internal use).

Options and Codes Tab

The Options and Codes tab stores a carrier's billing options and default payment and adjustment codes (see Figure 8.5).

Options

Procedure Code Set and Diagnosis Code Set These codes specify which set of codes should be used with this insurance plan.

Patient, Insured, and Physician Signature on File Options for these fields are Leave blank, Signature on file, and Print name. Selecting the Signature on file option causes "Signature on File" to print on the form. The Print name option prints the name of the patient, insured, or physician on the form.

Print PINs on Forms Select PIN Only or Leave Blank. For Medicare and Medicaid, select PIN Only; for all other carriers, select Leave Blank.

Default Billing Method 1, 2, and 3 Select either Paper or Electronic for handling primary (1), secondary (2), and tertiary (3) claims.

Default Payment Application Codes

The default payment and adjustment codes are set up in the database using the Procedure/Payment/Adjustment Codes option on the Lists menu. Once the codes are set up in the database, they can be selected from the drop-down lists in the Options and Codes tab.

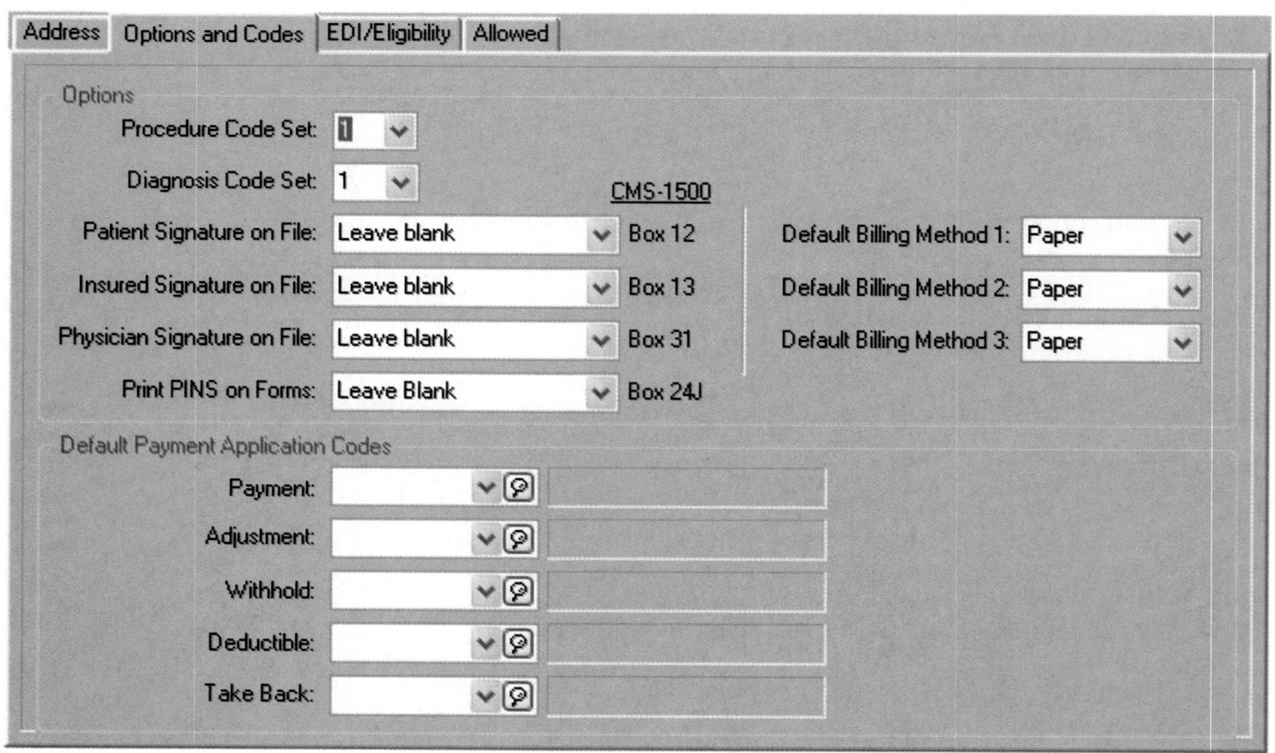

Figure 8.5 Options and Codes Tab

Payment Select a default payment code from the drop-down list.

Adjustment Select a default adjustment code from the drop-down list.

Withhold Select a default withhold code from the drop-down list.

Deductible Select a default deductible code from the drop-down list.

Take Back Select a default take back code from the drop-down list.

EDI/Eligibility Tab

The EDI/Eligibility tab contains information used for electronic claims and online eligibility verification (see Figure 8.6).

Primary Receiver

EDI Receiver This lists the EDI receiver used to send electronic claims for primary insurance plans.

Claims Payer ID This lists the claims payer ID for the insurance carrier—the commercial identification number/submitter identification number assigned to the insurance carrier by the clearinghouse that processes the claim.

Eligibility Payer ID This lists the eligibility payer ID for the insurance carrier. In some cases this number is the same as the claims payer ID; in other cases it is a separate number.

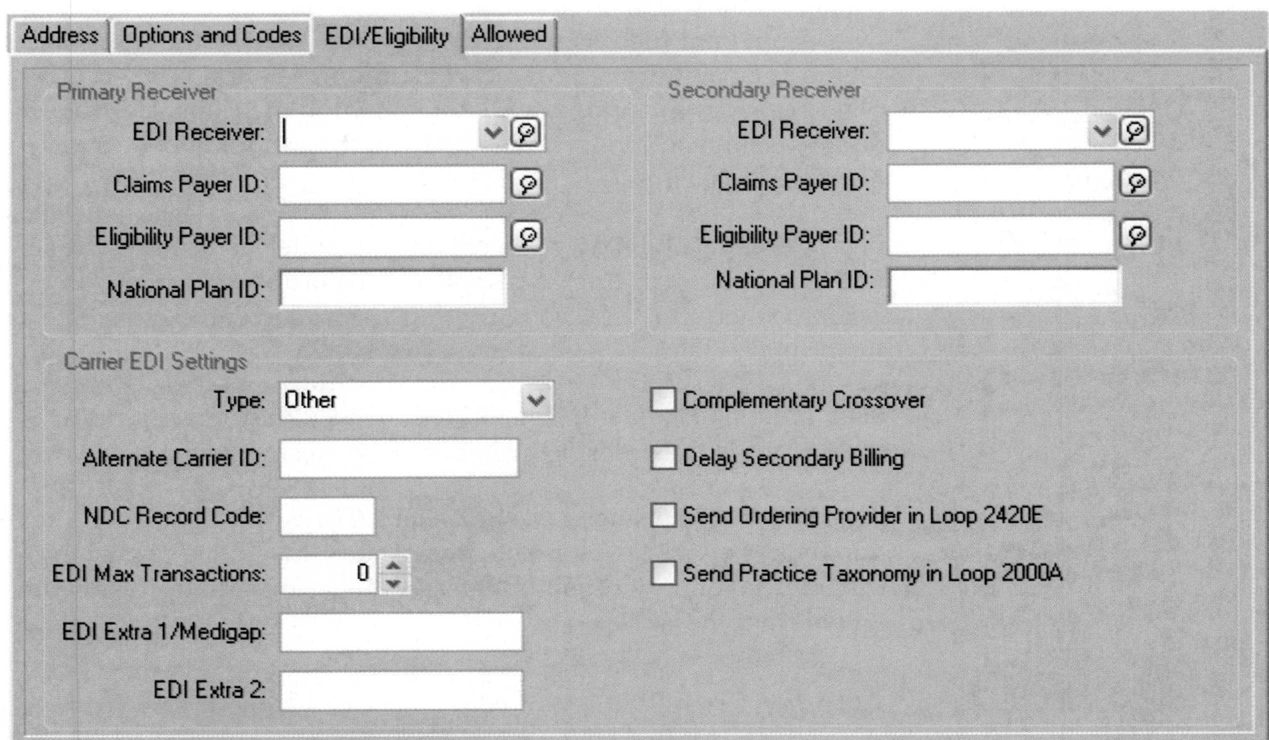

Figure 8.6 EDI/Eligibility Tab

National Plan ID The unique identification number assigned to insurance plans is currently not in use for most carriers. It is expected to be implemented by October 1, 2012.

Secondary Receiver

These fields are used if the plan is also a secondary receiver. The fields are identical to the Primary Receiver fields.

Carrier EDI Settings

Type Select the insurance plan type from the drop-down list. Choices include Other, Medicare, Medicaid, Tricare/Champus, ChampVA, Group, FECA, Blue Cross/Shield, Worker's Comp, HMO, and PPO.

Alternate Carrier ID This field should be left blank. The program will complete the field automatically if it is required.

NDC Record Code This field should be left blank. The program will complete the field automatically if it is required.

EDI Max Transactions Optional; it is used only for carriers that limit the maximum number of transactions per claim.

EDI Extra 1/Medigap If the insurance carrier is used as a primary insurer and a Medigap insurer, enter the Medigap number in this field.

EDI Extra 2 This field should be left blank. The program will complete the field automatically if it is required.

Complementary Crossover Check this box if complementary crossover claims are filed. Complementary crossover is the transfer by Medicare of adjudicated Medicare claim information to a secondary plan. Secondary insurance will not be sent in the claim file, but secondary claim will be marked as sent. This box should not be checked for Medigap claims.

Delay Secondary Billing A check in this box delays printing the secondary claim form until a response is recorded from the primary carrier. Otherwise, the secondary claim is printed at the same time as the primary claim.

Send Ordering Provider in Loop 2420E Check this box to send information about the ordering provider on an electronic claim.

Send Practice Taxonomy in Loop 2000A Check this box to send taxonomy in Loop 2000A for electronic claims. Insurance carriers have different taxonomy requirements, so this information must be obtained from the carrier.

Allowed Tab

This tab lists procedure codes in the database and the amounts allowed by the payer for the procedures (see Figure 8.7). The allowed

Address | Options and Codes | EDI/Eligibility | Allowed

Code	Procedure	Allowed
12011	Simple suture--face--local anes.	0.00
29125	Application of short arm splint; static	0.00
29425	Application of short leg cast, walking	0.00
29540	Strapping, ankle	0.00
50390	Aspiration of renal cyst by needle	0.00
71010	Chest x-ray, single view, frontal	0.00
71020	Chest x-ray, two views, frontal & lat...	0.00
71030	Chest x-ray, complete, four views	0.00
73070	Elbow x-ray, AP and lateral views	0.00
73090	Forearm x-ray, AP and lateral views	0.00
73100	Wrist x-ray, AP and lateral views	0.00
73510	Hip x-ray, complete, two views	0.00
73600	Ankle x-ray, AP and lateral views	0.00
80048	Basic metabolic panel	0.00
80061	Lipid panel	0.00
82270	Blood screening, occult; feces	0.00
82947	Glucose screening--quantitative	0.00
82951	Glucose tolerance test, three specimens	0.00
83718	HDL cholesterol	0.00

Figure 8.7 Allowed Tab

amount is used to calculate an estimate of the patient's responsibility for a procedure. Values entered in the Allowed Tab of the Insurance Carrier dialog box appear simultaneously in the Allowed Amounts tab of the Procedure/Payment/Adjustment dialog box, accessed via the Procedure/Payment/Adjustment Codes option on the Lists menu. Allowed amounts, which can be entered in either dialog box, can be entered manually, or, if an amount is not entered, the program uses actual transactions from the carrier to calculate an amount. The allowed amounts feature is covered in Chapter 9. Figure 8.8 shows the allowed amounts for procedure code 12011 in the Allowed Amounts tab of the Procedure/Payment/Adjustment dialog box.

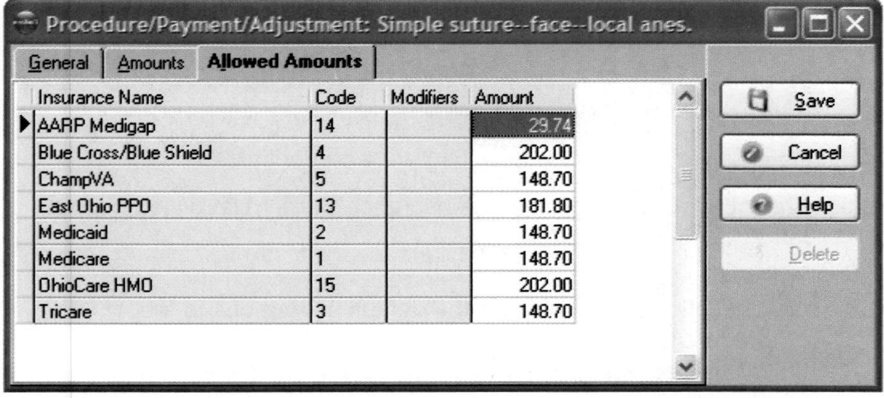
Procedure/Payment/Adjustment: Simple suture--face--local anes.

General | Amounts | Allowed Amounts

Insurance Name	Code	Modifiers	Amount
AARP Medigap	14		29.74
Blue Cross/Blue Shield	4		202.00
ChampVA	5		148.70
East Ohio PPO	13		181.80
Medicaid	2		148.70
Medicare	1		148.70
OhioCare HMO	15		202.00
Tricare	3		148.70

Save
Cancel
Help
Delete

Figure 8.8 Allowed Amounts Tab for Procedure Code 12011, Simple Suture—Face—Local Anes.

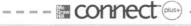

EXERCISE 8.1

SETTING UP A NEW INSURANCE CARRIER RECORD: ADDRESS TAB

Enter a new insurance carrier in Medisoft using the Address tab.

Date: October 17, 2016

1. Verify that Medisoft Network Professional is open, that the practice name in the title bar at the top of the screen is Family Care Clinic, and that the Medisoft Program Date is set to October 17, 2016.
2. Select Insurance, and then Carriers on the Lists menu. The Insurance Carrier List dialog box is displayed.
3. Click the New button. The Insurance Carrier: (new) dialog box appears.
4. Enter ***16*** in the Code field, and then press Tab twice.
5. In the Carrier Address section, enter the following information, pressing Tab to move from box to box:
   Name: ***Midwest Choice***
   Street: ***3700 East 9th Street***
   City: ***Cleveland***
   State: ***OH***
   Zip Code: ***44119***
   Phone: ***216-555-5555***
   Extension: ***42***
   Fax: ***216-555-5556***
   Contact: ***Denise Rodriguez***
6. In the Plan Information section, enter the following information:
   Plan Name: ***Midwest Choice PPO***
   Leave the Class and Note boxes blank.
7. Click the Save button. The Insurance Carrier: (new) dialog box closes.
8. Locate the new carrier, Midwest Choice, in the Insurance Carrier List dialog box.

You have completed Exercise 8.1

EXERCISE 8.2

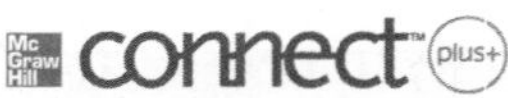

SETTING UP A NEW INSURANCE CARRIER RECORD: OPTIONS AND CODES TAB

Continue entering data for the new insurance carrier in Medisoft.

1. Select Midwest Choice in the Insurance Carrier List dialog box, and click the Edit button.
2. Click the Options and Codes tab.
3. In the Options section, keep the default setting of 1 in the Procedure Code Set and Diagnosis Code Set boxes. Select the following settings for the remaining boxes, using the drop-down lists:
   Patient Signature on File: Signature on file
   Insured Signature on File: Signature on file

Physician Signature on File: Signature on file
Print PINS on Forms: keep the default setting, Leave Blank
Default Billing Method 1: Electronic
Default Billing Method 2: keep the default setting, Paper
Default Billing Method 3: keep the default setting, Paper

4. In the Default Payment Application Codes section, select the following codes, using the drop-down lists:
   Payment: MIDPAY
   Adjustment: MIDADJ
   Withhold: MIDWIT
   Deductible: MIDDED
   Take Back: MIDTBK
5. Do not click the Save button yet, as you will continue to enter data in the remaining tabs of the Insurance Carrier: Midwest Choice dialog box in the next exercise.

You have completed Exercise 8.2

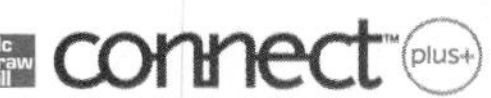

EXERCISE 8.3

SETTING UP A NEW INSURANCE CARRIER RECORD: EDI ELIGIBILITY AND ALLOWED TABS

Finish entering data on the new insurance carrier in Medisoft.

1. Click the EDI/Eligibility tab to make it active.
2. In the Primary Receiver section, enter the following information:
   EDI Receiver: from the drop-down list, select 0000 - National Data Corporation
   Claims Payer ID: ***1234***
   Eligibility Payer ID: ***MIDWCH***

   Leave the Secondary Receiver section blank.

   In the Carrier EDI Settings section, enter the following information:
   Type: scroll down the drop-down list to select PPO
   NDC Record Code: ***09***
3. Click the Allowed tab.
4. To practice using this tab, enter the following amounts for the first three procedures. Use the Tab key to move from box to box. These amounts represent the fee schedule currently used with managed care payers in contract with the Family Care Clinic.
   12011 (Simple suture—face—local anes.) ***181.80***
   29125 (Application of short arm splint; static) ***89.10***
   29425 (Application of short leg cast, walking) ***206.10***
   For the purposes of this exercise, you do not need to fill in the rest of the amounts.
5. Click the Save button to save the information you have entered in the last three tabs of the Insurance Carrier: Midwest Choice dialog box.

(continued)

(Continued)

6. The Insurance Carrier dialog box closes, and you are returned to the Insurance Carrier List dialog box.
7. Click the Close button to close the Insurance Carrier List dialog box. You have successfully set up a new insurance carrier record in Medisoft.

 **You have completed Exercise 8.3**

EXERCISE 8.4

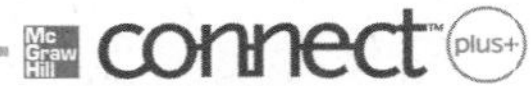

UPDATING INSURANCE CARRIER INFORMATION

One of the insurance carriers in the database has moved and has a new address, phone number, fax number, and contact name.

Date: October 17, 2016

1. Select Insurance, and then Carriers on the Lists menu. The Insurance Carrier List dialog box is displayed.
2. Select East Ohio PPO from the list of carriers, and click the Edit button. The Insurance Carrier: East Ohio PPO dialog box is displayed.
3. In the following boxes, enter the updated information as follows:
   Street: ***3000 Prairie Parkway***
   City: ***Cincinnati***
   State: ***OH***
   Zip Code: ***45202***
   Phone: ***513-555-5555***
   Fax: ***513-555-1111***
   Contact: ***James Spera***
4. Click the Save button to save your work. The Insurance Carrier dialog box closes, and you are returned to the Insurance Carrier List dialog box.
5. Click the Close button to close the Insurance Carrier List dialog box.

 **You have completed Exercise 8.4**

Referral Numbers and Preauthorization Numbers

As explained in Chapter 4, under various payer policies, patients may need a referral to see a specialist, and prior authorization for particular procedures. The referral and the preauthorization are both assigned a number by the payer, which must be logged into the patient's record.

Entering Referral Information

In Medisoft Network Professional, referrals are entered in the Account tab within the patient's Case dialog box (see Figure 8.9). The provider referral is entered by selecting the physician from the

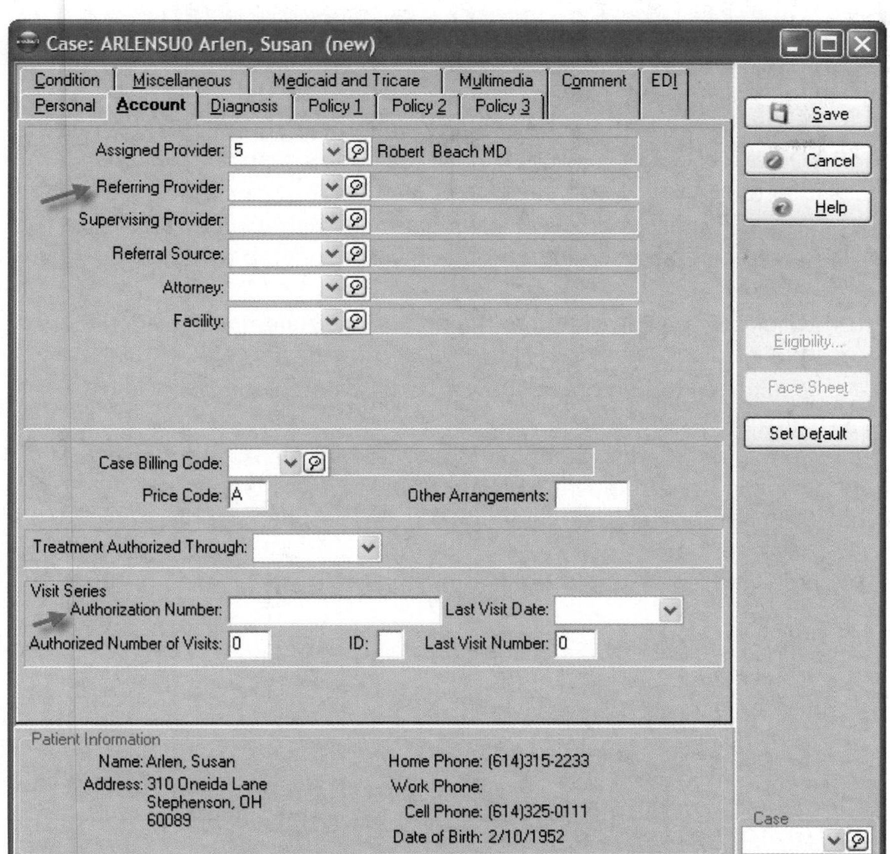

Figure 8.9 Account Tab of the Case Dialog Box with Referral Boxes

list of choices in the Referring Provider drop-down list at the top of the Account tab. A provider who is not listed in the Referring Provider drop-down list needs to be added to the database by selecting Referring Providers on the Lists menu and then clicking the New button. Referral numbers are entered in the Visit Series: Authorization Number box located toward the bottom of the Account tab.

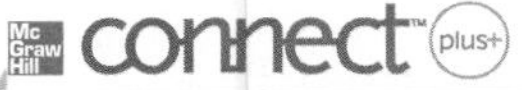

EXERCISE 8.5

ENTERING A REFERRAL NUMBER

Hector Valaquez, a new patient, has been referred to Dr. Patricia McGrath at Family Care Clinic for treatment of carpal tunnel syndrome. Hector's patient and case information have already been entered in the Family Care Clinic database. Hector's health plan requires a referral number for the visit. His primary care physician has obtained this information from the insurance carrier and faxed it to the Family Care Clinic. Enter the new information in Hector's case.

Date: October 17, 2016

1. Verify that Medisoft Network Professional is open and that the Medisoft Program Date is set to October 17, 2016.
2. On the Lists menu, click Patients/Guarantors and Cases, or click the corresponding shortcut button on the toolbar, to display the Patient List dialog box.

(continued)

(Continued)

3. Enter the first letter of the patient's last name, ***V***, in the Search for box. The entry line for Hector Valaquez should be selected in the left pane of the Patient List dialog box.
4. Double click the line with Hector Valaquez's case description in the right pane to edit the case information.
5. The Case dialog box is displayed. Since referral information is entered in the Account tab, click the Account tab to make it active.
6. Click the triangle button to the right of the Referring Provider box to display the drop-down list of providers.
7. Hector's referring provider is Dr. Janet Wood. Select this provider from the list.
8. In the Visit Series section at the bottom of the Account tab, click in the Authorization Number box. Enter the referral number for Hector's visit, ***489002***, in the Authorization Number box.
9. Click the Save button to store the information you have entered.
10. Close the Patient List dialog box.

You have completed Exercise 8.5

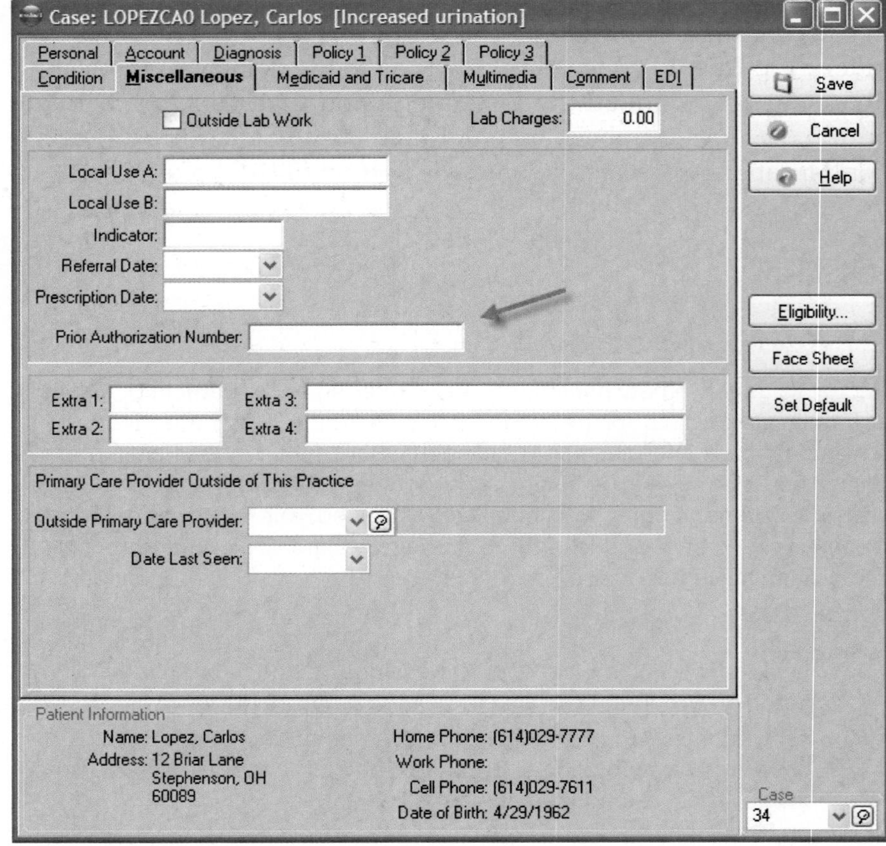

Figure 8.10 Miscellaneous Tab of the Case Dialog Box with Prior Authorization Number Box

Entering Preauthorization Numbers

Sometimes insurance carriers require services to be authorized before they are performed. If preauthorization is not given, the claim will not be paid. Once preauthorization numbers are obtained from the insurance carrier, they are entered in Medisoft Network Professional in the Prior Authorization Number box, which is located in the Miscellaneous tab of the Case dialog box (see Figure 8.10). From one to fifteen characters can be entered in the Prior Authorization Number box.

connect plus+ EXERCISE 8.6

ENTERING A PREAUTHORIZATION NUMBER

Tyrone Jackson, a five-year-old patient of Dr. Dana Banu, sprained his ankle two days ago and is still complaining of pain. Dr. Dana Banu decides Tyrone should go to the radiology department of the hospital for an X-ray. He obtains a preauthorization number for the procedure from Tyrone's insurance carrier. Enter the preauthorization number in Tyrone's case information.

Date: October 17, 2016

1. Verify that Medisoft Network Professional is open and that the Medisoft Program Date is set to October 17, 2016.
2. On the Lists menu, click Patients/Guarantors and Cases to display the Patient List dialog box.
3. Enter the first two letters of the patient's last name, ***JA***, in the Search for box. Click on Tyrone Jackson's name in the list of names displayed.
4. When you click on Tyrone's name, his case description, Ankle sprain, appears in the Case window on the right. Double click the case description to open the case.
5. The Case dialog box with Tyrone's case is displayed. Make the Miscellaneous tab active.
6. Click inside the Prior Authorization Number box.
7. Enter the preauthorization number for Tyrone's procedure, ***9200BA5,*** in the Prior Authorization Number box.
8. Click the Save button to store the information you have entered. The Miscellaneous tab of the Case dialog box closes, and you are returned to the Patient List dialog box.
9. Click the Close button to close the Patient List dialog box.

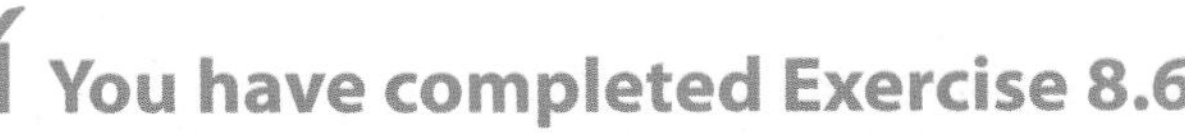
You have completed Exercise 8.6

chapter 8 summary

LEARNING OUTCOME	KEY CONCEPTS/EXAMPLES
8.1 Compare the major features of PPO, HMO, and POS health plans. Pages 388–390	A PPO offers patients lower fees in exchange for receiving services from plan providers, but does not usually require care coordination or referrals. An HMO locks patients into receiving services from providers with whom it has contracts; sometimes a primary care physician coordinates care and makes required referrals to specialists. A POS offers more flexibility to choose providers, but at an increased cost to the patient.
8.2 Identify the two parts of CDHPs. Pages 390–393	A consumer-driven health plan combines a high-deductible health plan (HDHP) that is usually a PPO for catastrophic coverage with one or more employer or employee funding options for out-of-pocket medical expenses.
8.3 Discuss the organization and regulation of employer-sponsored group health plans and self-insured plans. Pages 393–396	Employer-sponsored group health plans are organized by employers to provide heath care benefits to employees. The insurance coverage is purchased from an insurance carrier or managed care organization. Group health plans are subject to state laws for coverage and payment. Self-insured plans are also organized by employers, but the employers insure the plan's members themselves rather than buying insurance coverage. These plans are controlled by federal ERISA law rather than by state laws.
8.4 Explain the purpose of Medicare Parts A, B, C, and D. Pages 396–402	Medicare Part A provides coverage for care in hospitals and skilled nursing facilities, home health care, and hospice care. Part B provides outpatient medical coverage. Part C offers managed care plans called Medicare Advantage as an option to the traditional fee-for-service coverage under the Original Medicare Plan. Part D is a prescription drug benefit.

LEARNING OUTCOME	KEY CONCEPTS/EXAMPLES
8.5 Describe the fee structures that are used to set charges. Pages 402–403	Fee structures for providers' services are either charge-based or resource-based. Charge-based structures, such as UCR (usual, customary, and reasonable), are based on the fees that many providers have charged for similar services. Relative value scale (RVS) systems account for the relative difficulty of procedures by comparing the skill involved in each of a group of procedures. An RVS is charge-based if the charges that are attached to the relative values are based on historical fees. Resource-based relative value scale (RBRVS) structures, such as the Medicare Physician Fee Schedule (MPFS), are built by comparing three cost factors: (a) how difficult it is for the provider to do the procedure, (b) how much office overhead the procedure involves, and (c) the relative risk that the procedure presents to the patient and the provider. Both charge-based and resource-based fee structures are affected by the geographic area in which the service is provided.
8.6 Identify the three methods most payers use to pay physicians. Pages 404–407	Most payers use one of three provider payment methods: allowed charges, contracted fee schedules, and capitation. When a maximum allowed charge is set by a payer for each service, if a provider's usual fee is greater, the provider does not receive the difference from the payer. If the provider participates in the patient's plan, the difference is written off; if the provider does not participate, the plan's rules on balance billing determine whether the patient is responsible for the amount. Under a contracted fee schedule, the allowed charge for each service is all that the payer or the patient pays; no additional charges can be collected. Under capitation, the health care plan sets a capitation rate that pays for all contracted services to enrolled members for a given period.
8.7 Maintain insurance carrier information in the PM/EHR. Pages 407–419	Insurance carrier information is accessed by selecting Insurance > Carriers or Insurance > Classes on the Lists menu. The Insurance > Carriers option is used to enter, edit, or delete insurance carriers. The Insurance > Classes option is used to group carriers for the purposes of reporting. Detailed information about an insurance carrier is stored in the Insurance Carrier dialog box. To view information on a carrier already in the database, select the carrier in the Insurance Carrier List dialog box, and click the Edit button. To enter a carrier not already in the database, click the New button.

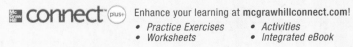

Enhance your learning at mcgrawhillconnect.com!
- *Practice Exercises*
- *Worksheets*
- *Activities*
- *Integrated eBook*

chapter review

MATCHING QUESTIONS

Match the key terms with their definitions.

_____ 1. ***[LO 8.6]*** allowed charge

_____ 2. ***[LO 8.1]*** third-party payer

_____ 3. ***[LO 8.2]*** consumer-driven health plan (CDHP)

_____ 4. ***[LO 8.4]*** Medicare

_____ 5. ***[LO 8.5]*** fee schedule

_____ 6. ***[LO 8.1]*** point-of-service (POS) plan

_____ 7. ***[LO 8.4]*** Medicaid

_____ 8. ***[LO 8.1]*** preferred provider organization (PPO)

_____ 9. ***[LO 8.3]*** group health plan (GHP)

_____ 10. ***[LO 8.1]*** health maintenance organization (HMO)

a. Managed health care system in which providers offer health care to members for fixed periodic payments.

b. Managed care network of health care providers who agree to perform services for plan members at discounted fees.

c. Maximum charge a plan pays for a service or procedure.

d. Federal and state assistance program that pays for health care services for people who cannot afford them.

e. Federal health insurance program for people sixty-five or older and some people with disabilities.

f. Managed care plan that permits patients to receive medical services from nonnetwork providers.

g. Plan of an employer or employee organization to provide health care to employees, former employees, and/or their families.

h. Medical insurance that combines a high-deductible health plan with one or more tax-preferred savings accounts that the patient directs.

i. Document that specifies the amount the provider bills for services.

j. Private or government organization that insures or pays for health care on behalf of beneficiaries.

TRUE-FALSE QUESTIONS

Decide whether each statement is true or false.

_____ 1. ***[LO 8.2]*** A health savings account (HSA) is a medical reimbursement plan set up and funded by an employer.

_____ 2. ***[LO 8.3]*** Almost 10 percent of people with private health insurance have individual health plans.

_____ 3. ***[LO 8.1]*** Health maintenance organizations (HMOs) are licensed by the federal government.

_____ 4. ***[LO 8.5]*** The payment system used by Medicare is called the resource-based relative value scale (RBRVS).

_____ 5. ***[LO 8.6]*** A provider who does not participate in a private plan can usually balance bill patients.

_____ 6. ***[LO 8.1]*** A PPO plan may offer either a low deductible with a higher premium or a high deductible with a lower premium.

_____ 7. ***[LO 8.4]*** Medicare Part B pays for inpatient hospital care, skilled nursing facility care, home health care, and hospice care.

_____ 8. ***[LO 8.3]*** The largest employer-sponsored health program in the United States is the Federal Employees Health Benefits (FEHB).

_____ 9. ***[LO 8.1]*** A point-of-service (POS) plan is a hybrid of HMO and PPO networks.

_____ 10. ***[LO 8.7]*** Insurance carriers cannot be entered in Medisoft until they are assigned to patients in the Policy 1, 2, and 3 tabs in the Case folders.

MULTIPLE-CHOICE QUESTIONS

Select the letter that best completes the statement or answers the question.

1. ***[LO 8.4]*** _________ helps beneficiaries pay for physician services, outpatient hospital services, medical equipment, and other supplies and services.
   a. Medicare Part A
   b. Medicare Part B
   c. Medicare Part C
   d. Medicare Part D

2. ***[LO 8.1]*** _________ have the most stringent guidelines and the narrowest choice of providers.
   a. health maintenance organizations (HMOs)
   b. preferred provider organizations (PPOs)
   c. point-of-service (POS) plans
   d. indemnity plans

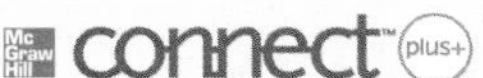

3. ***[LO 8.2]*** What type(s) of CDHP funding options may be used with high-deductible health plans to form consumer-driven health plans?
   a. health reimbursement account (HRA)
   b. health savings account (HSA)
   c. flexible savings account (FSA)
   d. all of the above
4. ***[LO 8.6]*** This amount is the most the payer will pay any provider for that CPT code.
   a. usual fee
   b. usual charge
   c. allowed charge
   d. capitation (cap) rate
5. ***[LO 8.4]*** The Medicare program is managed by the ________ under the Department of Health and Human Services (HHS).
   a. Centers for Medicare and Medicaid Services (CMS)
   b. Blue Cross and Blue Shield Association (BCBS)
   c. Federal Employees Health Benefits (FEHB) program
   d. Civilian Health and Medical Program of the Department of Veterans Affairs (CHAMPVA)
6. ***[LO 8.5]*** The payment system used by Medicare is called the ________.
   a. relative value scale (RVS)
   b. usual, customary, and reasonable (UCR) approach
   c. resource-based relative value scale (RBRVS)
   d. all of the above
7. ***[LO 8.1]*** The most popular type of health plan is the ________, which contracts with physicians, hospitals, clinics, and pharmacies to provide a network of care providers for its beneficiaries.
   a. health maintenance organization (HMO)
   b. preferred provider organization (PPO)
   c. point-of-service (POS) plan
   d. indemnity plan
8. ***[LO 8.1]*** ________ or fee-for-service plans require premium, deductible, and coinsurance payments.
   a. health maintenance organizations (HMOs)
   b. preferred provider organizations (PPOs)
   c. point-of-service (POS) plans
   d. indemnity plans
9. ***[LO 8.4]*** Workers' compensation covers what kind(s) of situations that require medical care?
   a. traumatic injury
   b. occupational disease or illness
   c. veterans with service-related disabilities
   d. both a and b

10. ***[LO 8.3]*** The largest employer-sponsored health program in the United States is the ________.
    a. Blue Cross and Blue Shield Association (BCBS)
    b. Medicare program
    c. Federal Employees Health Benefits (FEHB) program
    d. Medicaid program

SHORT-ANSWER QUESTIONS

Define the following abbreviations.

1. ***[LO 8.2]*** FSA ________________________
2. ***[LO 8.4]*** CMS ________________________
3. ***[LO 8.3]*** ERISA ________________________
4. ***[LO 8.2]*** HDHP ________________________
5. ***[LO 8.5]*** MPFS ________________________
6. ***[LO 8.4]*** CHAMPVA ________________________
7. ***[LO 8.1]*** PCP ________________________
8. ***[LO 8.3]*** BCBS ________________________
9. ***[LO 8.3]*** FEHB ________________________
10. ***[LO 8.5]*** UCR ________________________

APPLYING YOUR KNOWLEDGE

8.1 ***[LO 8.1, 8.2]*** An out-of-state vacationer with a broken ankle has a high-deductible consumer-driven health plan. The patient has already met half of the $1,000 annual deductible. The PPO is a 80-20 plan in network and a 60-40 plan out-of-network. The out-of-network physician's bill is $4,500. How much does the patient owe? How much should the PPO pay?

____

____

8.2 ***[LO 8.1, 8.2]*** Read this information from a medical insurance policy and answer the questions that follow.

Policy Number: 054351278
Insured: Jane Hellman Brandeis
Premium Due Quarterly: $1,414.98

AMOUNT PAYABLE
Maximum Benefit Limit, per *covered person* $2,000,000
Stated Deductible per *covered person*, per *calendar year*..................... $2,500

EMERGENCY ROOM DEDUCTIBLE (for each visit for *illness* to an emergency room when not directly admitted to the hospital) $50
Note: After satisfaction of the emergency room deductible, *covered expenses* are subject to any applicable *deductible amounts* and coinsurance provisions.

PREFERRED PROVIDER BENEFITS, per *calendar year*
For *covered expenses* in excess of the applicable stated deductible 100%

NON-PREFERRED PROVIDER BENEFITS
If *covered expenses* are incurred at a non-Preferred Provider, benefits will be reduced to 80% of Preferred Provider plan benefits. This reduction is limited to a *calendar year* maximum amount of $5,000 per *covered person.*

a. What type of health plan is described, an HMO, a PPO, or an indemnity plan?

____

____

b. What is the annual premium?

____

____

c. What is the annual deductible?

____

____

d. What percentage of preferred provider charges does the patient owe after meeting the deductible each year?

____

____

e. After the annual deductible has been met, the insured incurs a $6,000 out-of-network medical bill. How much will the health plan pay?

8.3 ***[LO 8.5]*** A physician's usual fee for a routine eye examination is $80. Under the discounted fee-for-service arrangement the doctor has with Plan A, the fee is discounted 15 percent for Plan A members. This month, the doctor has seen five Plan A members for routine eye exams.

a. What is the physician's usual fee for five patients?

b. What will the physician be paid for one Plan A member's exam?

c. What will the physician be paid for the five Plan A eye exams?

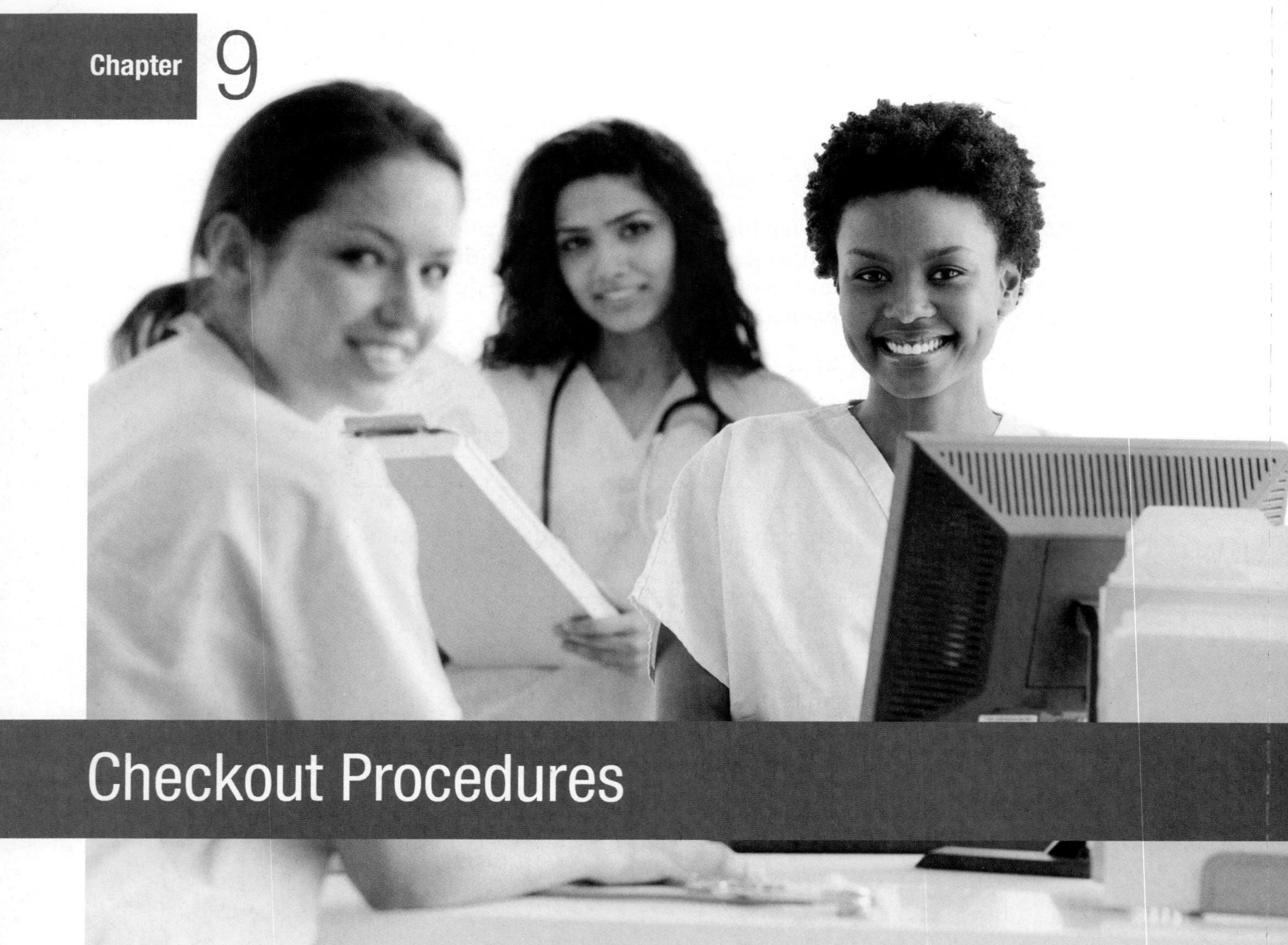

Chapter 9

Checkout Procedures

KEY TERMS

accept assignment
addenda
adjustments
bundled code
CCI column 1/column 2 code pair edits
CCI edits
CCI modifier indicator
CCI mutually exclusive code (MEC) edits
charge capture
charges
claim scrubbing
code linkage
compliant billing
Correct Coding Initiative (CCI)
global period
medically unlikely edits (MUEs)
modifier
MultiLink codes
package
payments
place of service (POS) code
query
real-time claim adjudication (RTCA)
self-pay patients
unbundling
walkout receipt

LEARNING OUTCOMES

When you finish this chapter, you will be able to:

9.1 List the six steps in the charge capture process.

9.2 Explain the purpose of auditing diagnosis and procedure code assignment.

9.3 Discuss the effect of health plans' rules on billing.

9.4 Describe the use of CPT/HCPCS modifiers to communicate billing information to health plans.

9.5 Discuss strategies to avoid common coding/billing errors.

9.6 Explain the difference between posting charges from a paper encounter form and posting charges from an electronic encounter form.

9.7 Identify the types of payments that may be collected following a patient's visit.

9.8 Identify the steps needed to create walkout receipts.

9.9 Describe use of a patient education feature in an electronic health record.

Smart Machines, Smarter People

Six weeks after the practice switched to a PM/EHR, Chris Yakamoto and Joseph Sanchez meet up at the coffee station. "Hey Chris, how's it going," asked Joseph. "Good, actually," replied Chris. "This EHR—I was worried I'd lose my job because of it, but it's actually made it more interesting. I don't spend all day entering charges from encounter forms anymore. Now I review the charges from the EHR, make any changes, and click the post button! I actually have time to read all those payer rule update notices now," said Chris. "Same here," replied Joseph. "I used to get stressed about how many records I could code and still be accurate. Now I do a lot more reviewing and editing, applying what I know about guidelines and rules." "I guess there are still some things that we can do that computers can't do," said Chris as he finished his last sip of coffee and headed back to his desk.

As you read this chapter, think about how the job of the billing specialist and the coder have changed as a result of technology. What skills do you think are important for today's billing specialist? For today's coders?

WHEN YOU FINISH THIS CHAPTER, YOU WILL ALSO BE ABLE TO USE MEDISOFT CLINICAL TO:

1. Add a procedure code to the procedure code database in MNP.
2. Add a diagnosis code to the diagnosis code database in MNP.
3. Post charges from a paper encounter form in MNP.
4. Post charges from an electronic encounter form in MNP.
5. Add a modifier to a procedure code in MNP.
6. Use MNP to enter a copayment made at checkout.
7. Use MNP to print a walkout receipt.
8. Print patient education materials in MCPR.

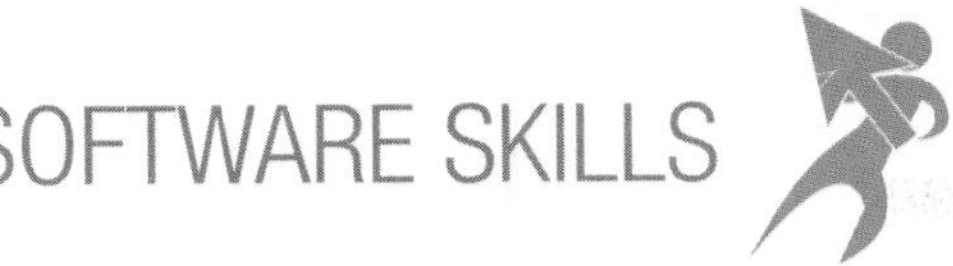

9.1 Overview: Charge Capture Process

Chapters 6 and 7 outlined the standard flow of an office visit from check-in until the completion of the patient examination. This chapter describes many of the steps that take place during checkout, including reviewing coding compliance, reviewing billing compliance, posting charges, posting payments made at the time of the visit, printing payment receipts, and printing patient education handouts.

When the patient examination is complete, the physician and the medical coder sign the visit documentation, review procedure codes for the visit, and assign diagnosis codes. The **charge capture** process, as shown in Figure 9.1, involves itemizing each medical treatment and service that was provided to determine the amounts to bill health plans and patients. The charges are also checked for accuracy. If all the information is correct, the transaction data are posted in Medisoft Clinical. If it is incorrect, the data are edited and then posted.

charge capture process of recording billable services

Step 1: Access Encounter Data

In the first step of the charge capture process, the procedure and diagnosis data from the patient visit are located.

Electronic Method

In a PM/EHR such as Medisoft Clinical, visit data are accessed by selecting Unprocessed Charges on the Activities menu. The Unprocessed Charges dialog box appears, as shown in Figure 9.2.

Clicking the Edit button brings up the Unprocessed Transactions Edit dialog box, as shown in Figure 9.3. This dialog box provides detailed information about the visit, including the procedure codes, the diagnosis codes, and the standard fees for the procedures.

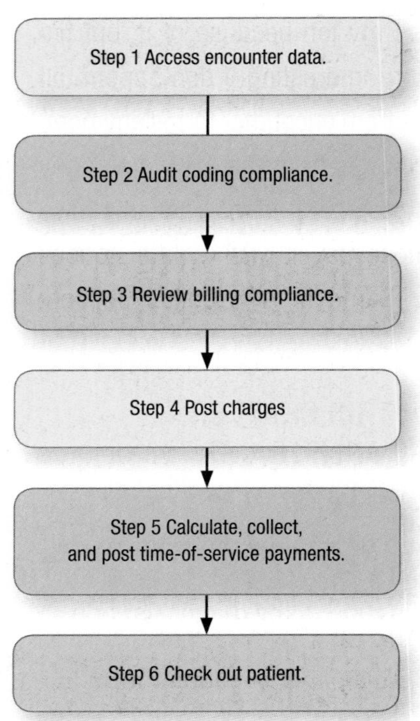
Step 1 Access encounter data.
Step 2 Audit coding compliance.
Step 3 Review billing compliance.
Step 4 Post charges
Step 5 Calculate, collect, and post time-of-service payments.
Step 6 Check out patient.

Figure 9.1 Electronic Charge Capture Process Flowchart

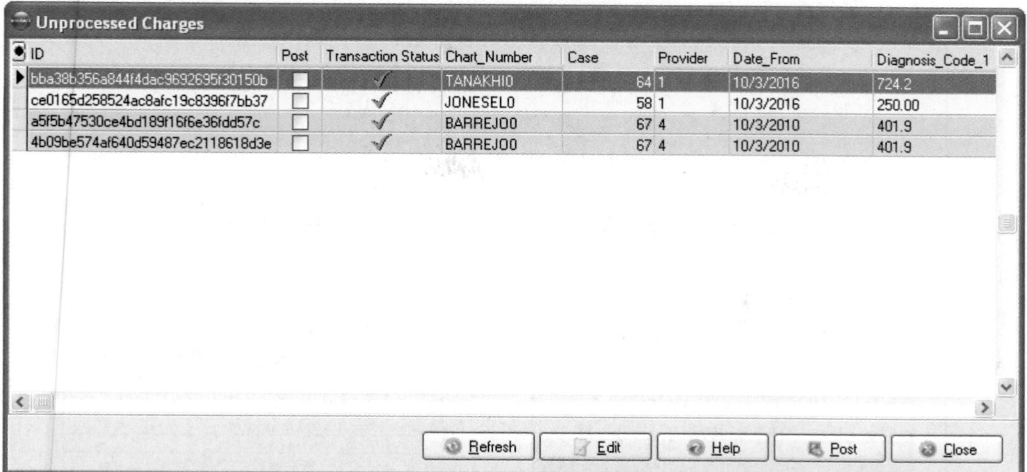

Figure 9.2 Unprocessed Charges Dialog Box

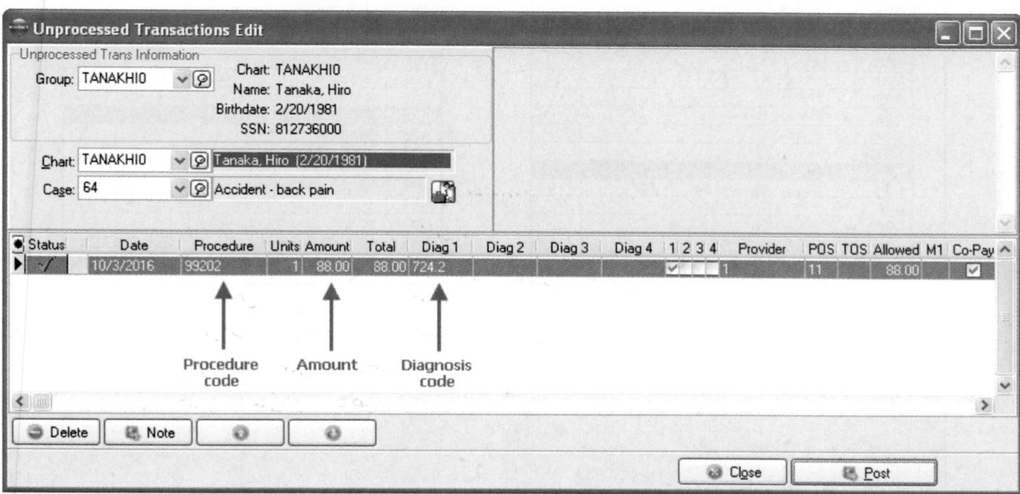

Figure 9.3 Unprocessed Transactions Edit Dialog Box

Paper Method

In practices without an integrated PM/EHR, a paper encounter form (see Figure 9.4) is marked by the physician or medical coder based on the visit documentation, and then given to the biller to use in the charge capture process.

Step 2: Audit Coding Compliance

In the second step of the charge capture process, all listed codes are checked to be sure that they are current and correct and that they are correctly linked to establish the medical necessity of the services the patient received. It is often necessary to also review and check documentation to be sure it supports the codes being reported.

Electronic Method

In a PM/EHR, codes can be checked in the EHR before they are transmitted to the PM, or, they can be reviewed in the PM before

ENCOUNTER FORM

DATE	TIME
PATIENT NAME	CHART #

OFFICE VISITS - SYMPTOMATIC		
NEW		
99201	OF--New Patient Minimal	
99202	OF--New Patient Low	
99203	OF--New Patient Detailed	
99204	OF--New Patient Moderate	
99205	OF--New Patient High	
ESTABLISHED		
99211	OF--Established Patient Minimal	
99212	OF--Established Patient Low	
99213	OF--Established Patient Detailed	
99214	OF--Established Patient Moderate	
99215	OF--Established Patient High	
PREVENTIVE VISITS		
NEW		
99381	Under 1 Year	
99382	1 - 4 Years	
99383	5 - 11 Years	
99384	12 - 17 Years	
99385	18 - 39 Years	
99386	40 - 64 Years	
99387	65 Years & Up	
ESTABLISHED		
99391	Under 1 Year	
99392	1 - 4 Years	
99393	5 - 11 Years	
99394	12 - 17 Years	
99395	18 - 39 Years	
99396	40 - 64 Years	
99397	65 Years & Up	
PROCEDURES		
12011	Simple suture--face--local anes.	
29125	App. of short arm splint; static	
29540	Strapping, ankle	
50390	Aspiration of renal cyst by needle	
71010	Chest x-ray, single view, frontal	

PROCEDURES		
71020	Chest x-ray, two views, frontal & lateral	
71030	Chest x-ray, complete, four views	
73070	Elbow x-ray, AP & lateral views	
73090	Forearm x-ray, AP & lateral views	
73100	Wrist x-ray, AP & lateral views	
73510	Hip x-ray, complete, two views	
73600	Ankle x-ray, AP & lateral views	
LABORATORY		
80019	19 clinical chemistry tests	
80048	Basic metabolic panel	
80061	Lipid panel	
82270	Blood screening, occult; feces	
82947	Glucose screening--quantitative	
82951	Glucose tolerance test, three specimens	
83718	HDL cholesterol	
84478	Triglycerides test	
85007	Manual differential WBC	
85018	Hemoglobin	
85651	Erythrocyte sedimentation rate--non-auto	
86580	TB Mantoux test	
87072	Culture by commercial kit, nonurine...	
87076	Culture, anerobic isolate	
87077	Bacterial culture, aerobic isolate	
87086	Urine culture and colony count	
87430	Strep test	
87880	Direct streptococcus screen	
INJECTIONS		
90471	Immunization administration	
90703	Tetanus injection	
96372	Injection	
92516	Facial nerve function studies	
93000	Electrocardiogram--ECG with interpretation	
93015	Treadmill stress test, with physician...	
96900	Ultraviolet light treatment	
99070	Supplies and materials provided	

FAMILY CARE CLINIC
285 Stephenson Blvd.
Stephenson, OH 60089
614-555-0000

☐ DANA BANU, MD
☐ ROBERT BEACH, MD
☐ PATRICIA MCGRATH, MD
☐ JESSICA RUDNER, MD
☐ JOHN RUDNER, MD
☐ KATHERINE YAN, MD

NOTES

REFERRING PHYSICIAN	NPI	AUTHORIZATION #
DIAGNOSIS		
PAYMENT AMOUNT		

Figure 9.4 Sample Encounter Form

they are posted to a patient's account. If necessary, the patient's chart can be viewed from within the EHR.

Paper Method

In practices that use paper encounter forms, the coder reviews the form and, if necessary, locates the patient's chart folder to review the visit documentation.

Step 3: Review Billing Compliance

In the third step of the charge capture process, the billing rules of the particular health plan providing primary coverage for the visit are reviewed. This process is similar in electronic and paper offices. Although the codes themselves may be current, correct, and properly linked, each service is not necessarily billable. For example, Medicare generally does not cover procedures considered experimental, and some private payers do not pay for two similar procedures on the same date of service. Following such rules when calculating charges results in billing compliance.

Step 4: Post Charges

In the fourth step of the charge capture process, the biller posts the visit charges in the PM. Three types of transactions are recorded in the PM/EHR: charges, payments, and adjustments. **Charges** are the amounts a provider bills for the services performed. **Payments** are monies received from patients and insurance carriers. **Adjustments** are changes to patients' accounts. Examples of adjustments include returned checks, refunds of overpayments, and differences between the amount billed and the amount allowed per contract.

charges amount a provider bills for performed health care services

payments money paid by patients and health plans

adjustments changes to a patient's account

Electronic Method

In a PM/EHR, after codes and charges are reviewed, they are electronically posted to a patient's account.

Paper Method

In practices that use paper encounter forms, the coder manually enters each procedure code listed on the encounter form into the PM.

Step 5: Calculate, Collect, and Post Time-of-Service (TOS) Payments

The fifth step of the charge capture process is to calculate the amounts that patients owe for their visits and to post the payments they make in the PM. Whether the office uses paper or electronic encounter forms, payments are calculated and posted in the PM.

Step 6: Check Out Patient

The final step of the charge capture process is patient checkout, which involves:

- Providing receipts to the patient for all payments made
- Scheduling any follow-up appointments, such as return office visits, laboratory tests, or radiology services ordered by the provider
- Providing referrals as required
- Providing patient education materials ordered by the provider

Electronic Method

In a PM/EHR, many of the checkout activities are completed electronically, such as printing receipts for payments and printing patient education handouts.

Paper Method

Practices that use paper encounter forms use the PM to print patient receipts, but other activities, such as providing the patient with education handouts, must be completed without the aid of technology.

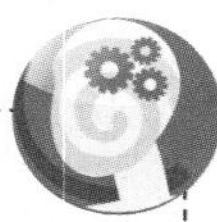

THINKING IT THROUGH 9.1

Assign the step number of the charge capture process to each of the following actions:

- ________ Provide patient with a booklet on controlling type II diabetes.
- ________ Receive the unprocessed transactions for yesterday's appointments.
- ________ Validate the connection between the diagnosis of a splinter and an incision/drainage procedure.
- ________ Send an e-mail message to a payer to clarify the rule for billing out-of-network visits.
- ________ Answer the patient who asks, "How much do I owe for this visit?"
- ________ Post a patient's copayment of $5 to the appropriate account.

9.2 Coding Compliance

Although physicians are ultimately responsible for proper documentation and correct coding, administrative staff members help ensure maximum appropriate reimbursement by auditing medical coding. The staff member must work with the physician to ensure that the codes that have been assigned are current and correct. This process takes place after a patient encounter, but before the charges are billed.

Current, Correct Diagnosis Codes

addenda updates to ICD-9-CM

The ICD-9-CM code set is revised annually. The National Center for Health Statistics and the Centers for Medicare and Medicaid Services (CMS) release ICD-9-CM updates called the **addenda** twice a year. The changes take effect on October 1 and April 1. The October 1 changes are the major updates; April 1 is used to catch up on codes that were not included in the major changes. The major new, invalid, and revised codes are posted on the CDC website (www.cdc.gov/nchs/icd.htm, and also on the CMS website), usually in June for use as of October 1.

Current codes must be used for reporting encounters as of the date they go into effect, and invalid (deleted) codes must not be used. Practices must ensure that the current reference is available and that the current codes are in use.

Current, Correct Procedure Codes

CPT is a proprietary code set, meaning that it is not available for free to the public. Rather, the information must be purchased, either in print or electronic format, from the American Medical Association (AMA), which issues revised CPT codes each year.

During the year, practicing physicians, medical specialty societies, and state medical associations send their suggestions for revision to the AMA. This input is reviewed by the AMA's Editorial Panel, which includes physicians as well as representatives from the Health Insurance Association of America, CMS, the American Health Information Management Association (AHIMA), the American Hospital Association (AHA), and Blue Cross and Blue Shield. The panel decides what changes will be made in the annual revision.

The annual changes are released by the AMA on October 1 and are in effect for procedures and services provided after January 1 of the following year. The AMA also reports the new codes on its website. Like the ICD-9-CM codes, the new CPT code set has to be used for dates of service starting January 1.

Claim Scrubbing

PM/EHRs typically include a software feature known as a **claim scrubber.** This term comes from the phrase "clean claim," meaning a claim submitted to a health plan that the health plan accepts for processing. (This topic is covered in Chapter 10.) The data reported in a claim can be made clean by scrubbing with the PM/EHR scrubber. This software tool analyzes medical codes for patient encounters and reports those that appear to be outdated or otherwise problematic. Reviewing this report gives billers an opportunity to research and revise the codes. If necessary, the PM/EHR must be updated to reflect code changes based on the scrubber's report before the claim is submitted.

claim scrubber software that checks claims to permit error correction

code linkage clinically appropriate connection between a provided service and a patient's condition or illness

Code Linkage and Medical Necessity

As explained in Chapter 1, the diagnosis and the medical services that are documented in the patient's medical record should be logically connected so that the medical necessity of the charges is clear to the health plan. Health plans require reported services to be consistent with the diagnosis and meet generally accepted professional medical standards of care. The term **code linkage** describes the connection between a procedure code and the related diagnosis code. Procedures must be:

- In accordance with generally accepted standards of medical practice
- Clinically appropriate in terms of type, frequency, extent, site, and duration
- Not primarily for the convenience of the patient, physician, or other health care provider

If medical necessity is not met, the physician will not receive payment from the health plan. In general, codes that support medical necessity meet these conditions:

- The CPT procedure codes match the ICD-9-CM diagnosis codes.

EXAMPLE

A procedure to drain an abscess of the external ear or auditory canal should be supported by a diagnosis of disorders of the external ear or an ear carbuncle or cyst.

- The procedures are not elective, experimental, or nonessential.

EXAMPLE

Cosmetic nasal surgery performed to improve a patient's appearance is typically excluded. However, a cosmetic procedure may be considered medically necessary when it is performed to repair an accidental injury or to improve the functioning of a malformed body member. A diagnosis of deviated septum, nasal obstruction, acquired facial deformity, or late effects of facial bone fracture supports medical necessity for cosmetic nasal surgery.

- The procedures are furnished at an appropriate level.

EXAMPLE

A high-level evaluation and management code for an office visit (such as 99204/99205 and 99214/99215) must be matched by a serious, complex condition such as a sudden, unexplained large loss of weight.

THINKING IT THROUGH 9.2

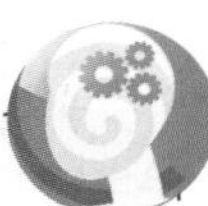

In your opinion, is each of the following procedures likely to be considered medically necessary by a payer's health care claim examiner? Why?

- Diagnosis: deviated septum; procedure: nasal surgery ________
- Diagnosis: mole on a female patient's cheek, questionable nature; procedure: surgical removal and biopsy ________
- Diagnosis: male syndrome hair loss; procedure: implant hair plugs on scalp ________
- Diagnosis: probable broken wrist; procedure: comprehensive full-body examination, with complete set of lab tests, chest X-ray, and ECG ________

The Procedure/Payment/Adjustment List Dialog Box

Procedure and diagnosis codes must be entered in Medisoft Network Professional before they can be used to enter transactions. The process of adding new procedure codes to the database begins with selecting Procedure/Payment/Adjustment Codes on the Lists menu. (The process for adding new diagnosis codes is described in the next section.)

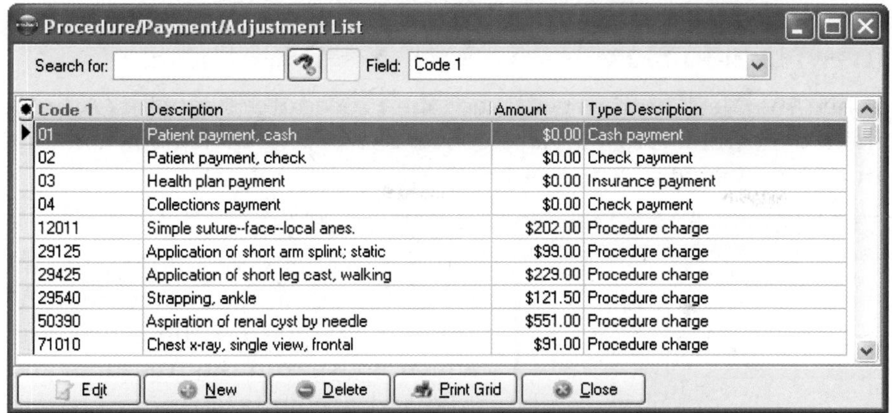
Procedure/Payment/Adjustment List
Search for:
Field: Code 1
Code 1
Description
Amount
Type Description
01 Patient payment, cash $0.00 Cash payment
02 Patient payment, check $0.00 Check payment
03 Health plan payment $0.00 Insurance payment
04 Collections payment $0.00 Check payment
12011 Simple suture--face--local anes. $202.00 Procedure charge
29125 Application of short arm splint; static $99.00 Procedure charge
29425 Application of short leg cast, walking $229.00 Procedure charge
29540 Strapping, ankle $121.50 Procedure charge
50390 Aspiration of renal cyst by needle $551.00 Procedure charge
71010 Chest x-ray, single view, frontal $91.00 Procedure charge
Edit
New
Delete
Print Grid
Close

Figure 9.5 The Procedure/Payment/Adjustment List Dialog Box

The Procedure/Payment/Adjustment List dialog box lists codes already in the database (see Figure 9.5).

At the top of the dialog box are two fields used to search for a procedure code: Search for and Field. To locate a code, enter the first few letters or numbers in the Search for field. As characters are typed, the list automatically filters to display records that match. Figure 9.6 shows the list after "99" is entered in the Search for field.

The columns in the dialog box include the following:

Code 1 The actual code for the procedure, payment, or adjustment

Description The description entered for the code

Amount The standard amount charged for the procedure

Type Description The type of code (procedure, payment, adjustment, and so on)

The buttons at the bottom of the dialog box are used to edit an existing code, add a new code, delete a code, print the information in the list, and close the dialog box.

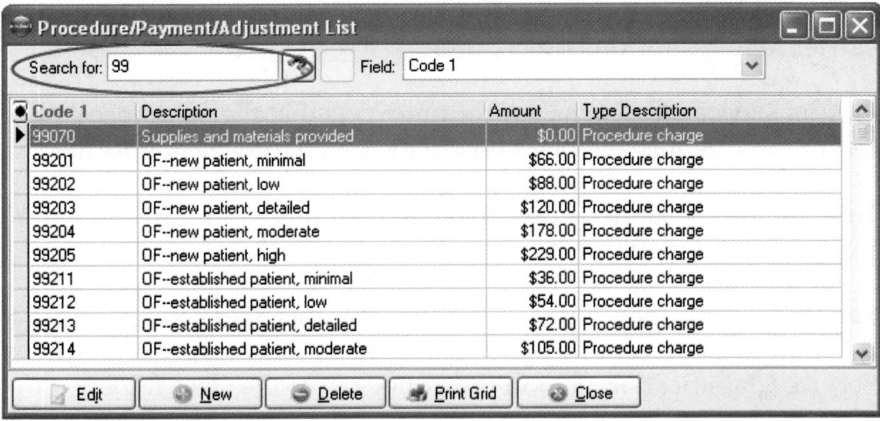

Figure 9.6 The Procedure/Payment/Adjustment List Dialog Box with "99" Entered in the Search for Field

The Procedure/Payment/Adjustment (new) Dialog Box

When the New button is clicked, the Procedure/Payment/Adjustment dialog box is displayed (see Figure 9.7). The dialog box contains three tabs: General, Amounts, and Allowed Amounts.

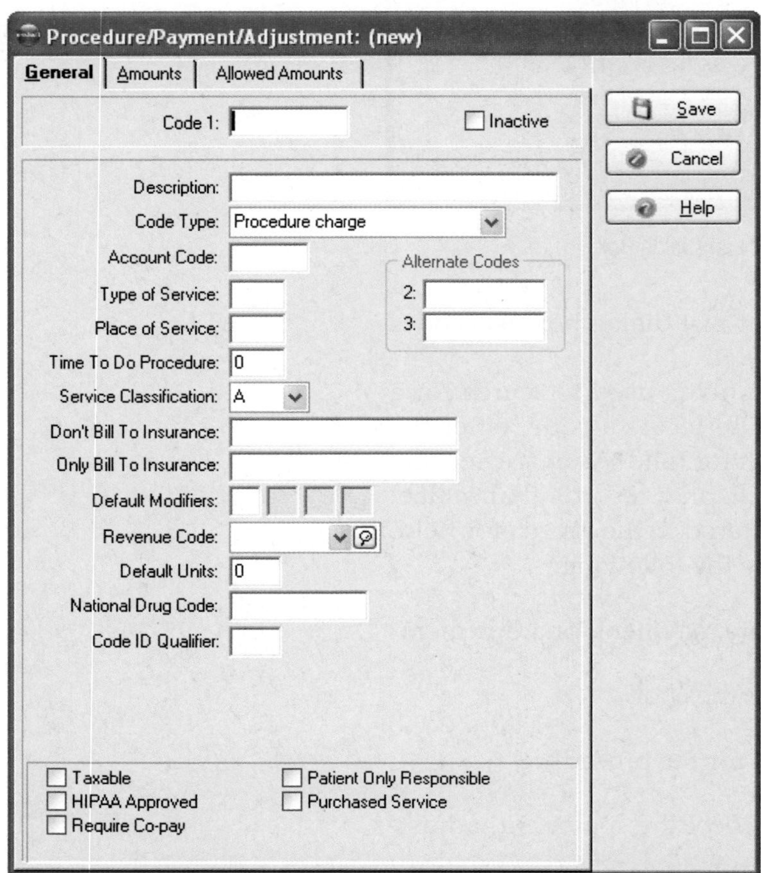

Figure 9.7 The Procedure/Payment/Adjustment List (new) Dialog Box

The General Tab

The General tab contains all the information about the code except the amount charged for the procedure, which is listed in the Amounts and Allowed Amounts tabs.

Code 1 Enter the code itself.

Inactive Click this box to indicate that the code is not active.

Description Enter a description for the code.

Code Type Select the type of code you are creating from the list of choices. The list includes different types of procedures, payments, and adjustments.

Account Code This is an internal code used by the practice to group procedures for reporting purposes.

Alternate Codes If desired, alternate codes for the same procedure can be entered. Some offices use internal "shorthand" codes that contain one or two numbers or letters in addition to the HIPAA-mandated code sets.

Type of Service Enter the appropriate code that the insurance carrier requires for this procedure.

Place of Service Enter the appropriate code that the insurance carrier requires to identify the place where the procedure was performed.

Time To Do Procedure Enter the average time, in minutes, required to perform this procedure.

Service Classification The code entered in this field—a letter from *A* through *H*—corresponds to the Insurance Coverage Percents by Service Classification field in the Policy tab of the Case folder.

Don't Bill To Insurance If the code is not to be billed to specific insurance carriers, enter the codes for those carriers in this field.

Only Bill To Insurance If the code is for specific insurance carriers, enter the codes for those carriers in this field.

Default Modifiers Enter up to four modifiers for the procedure code.

Revenue Code Enter the revenue code for this procedure (used on UB-04 claims).

Default Units Enter the common number of units associated with the procedure code.

National Drug Code Enter the code assigned to this procedure (used in reporting prescribed drugs and biologics when sending electronic claims).

Code ID Qualifier Enter the qualifier for the code (used to communicate the type of code that is being sent).

Taxable Click this box if the code needs a tax charge.

HIPAA Approved Click this box to indicate that the code is HIPAA compliant.

Require Co-pay Select this if a copayment should be applied to the code.

Patient Only Responsible Click this box if the code is billed to the patient only (not to the insurance carrier).

Purchased Service Check this box to indicate that the procedure is a service purchased from a third party, such as an outside laboratory.

The Amounts Tab

The Amounts tab shows the amount charged for the procedure as listed in the practice's fee schedule (see Figure 9.8). The amount entered in field A is the normal charge for the selected procedure. Additional charges (B through Z) may be used to record special pricing, such as a discount for cash patients or a negotiated charge for a managed care plan. Medisoft Network Professional includes space for up to twenty-six different charges for each procedure code. The amount entered in this field corresponds to the code entered in the Price Code field in the Account tab of the Case folder.

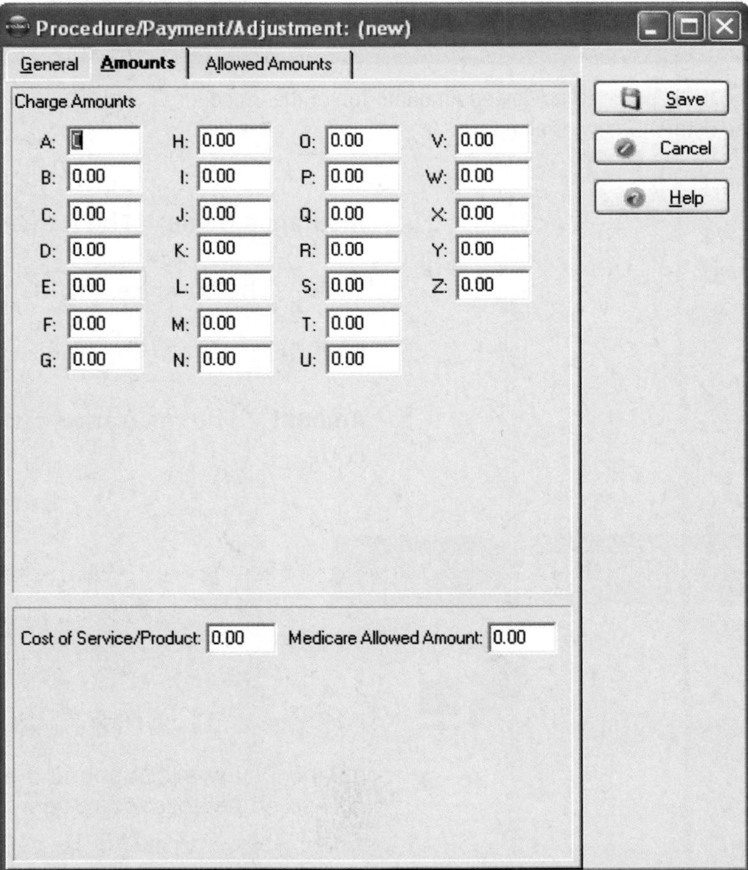

Figure 9.8 The Amounts Tab of the Procedure/Payment/Adjustment (new) Dialog Box

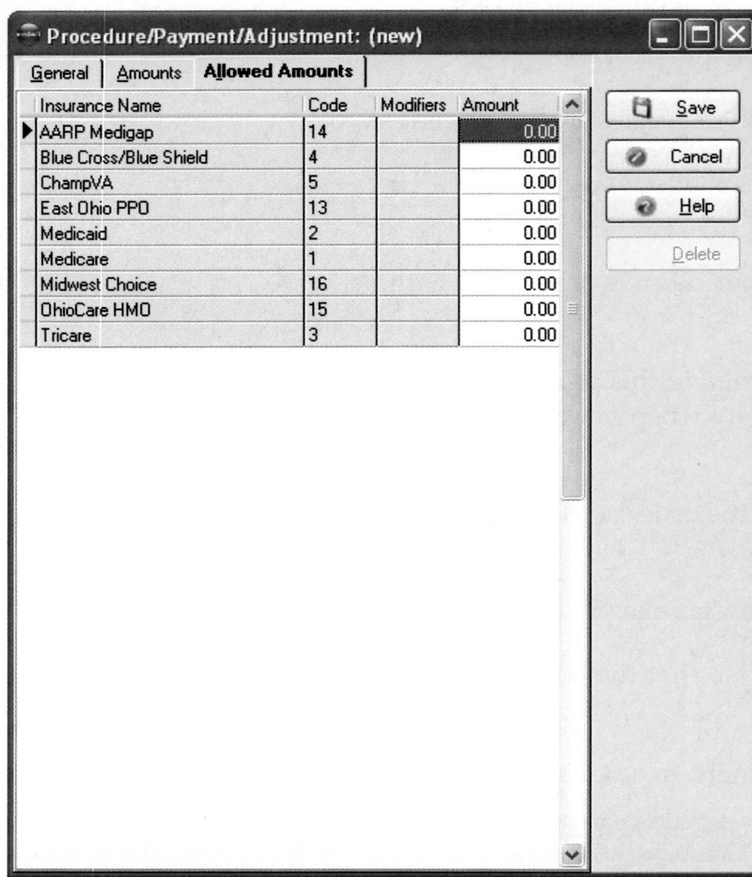

Figure 9.9 The Allowed Amounts Tab of the Procedure/Payment/Adjustment (new) Dialog Box

Cost of Service/Product Enter the actual cost of the service or product.

Medicare Allowed Amount Enter Medicare's allowed amount for the procedure. *Note*: Providers who are not Medicare participating should enter the limiting charge provided by Medicare. This field calculates the difference between the standard charge and the allowed amount. It is also used to calculate the patient's responsibility for the charge. If the field is left blank, the program will enter a value the first time an allowed amount is calculated for the procedure.

The Allowed Amounts Tab

The Allowed Amounts tab lists the amount each insurance carrier pays for a particular code (see Figure 9.9). If the fields in this tab are left blank, the program calculates the allowed amount based on the amount paid, any applicable deductible, and the service classification.

The columns in this dialog box list the following:

Insurance Name The name of the insurance carrier

Code The code for the insurance carrier code

Modifiers Modifiers that have been added to the procedure code

Amount The insurance carrier's allowed amount for the procedure code

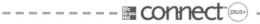

EXERCISE 9.1

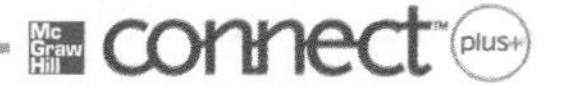

ADDING PROCEDURE CODES TO THE PROCEDURE CODE DATABASE

In 2010 the AMA added the following new code to CPT:

99444 Online evaluation and management service provided by a physician to an established patient . . . using the Internet or similar electronic communications network.

This code reflects the increasing use of online patient communications by providers. It is a non-face-to-face service in response to a patient's online inquiry, and it includes related work such as telephone calls and providing prescriptions or laboratory orders. The physician is required to permanently store an electronic or hard-copy record of the encounter.

1. Start Medisoft Network Professional by clicking Start > All Programs > Medisoft > Medisoft Network Professional.
2. Click the Lists menu. Click Procedure/Payment/Adjustment Codes. The Procedure/Payment/Adjustment List dialog box opens.
3. Click the New button. The Procedure/Payment/Adjustment dialog box is displayed.
4. Click in the Code 1 field. Enter 99444.
5. Click in the Description field and enter ***Online E/M, established.***
6. Click the HIPAA Approved box at the bottom of the dialog box.
7. Click the Require Co-pay box.
8. Click the Amounts tab.
9. Click in the A field. Enter ***30***.
10. Click the Save button. You are returned to the Procedure/Payment/Adjustment List dialog box.
11. Click the Close button to close the Procedure/Payment/Adjustment dialog box.

You have completed Exercise 9.1

The Diagnosis List Dialog Box

A similar procedure must be followed to update diagnosis codes in Medisoft Network Professional. The process of adding new diagnosis codes to the database begins with selecting Diagnosis Codes on the Lists menu.

The Diagnosis List dialog box lists the codes already in the database (see Figure 9.10).

At the top of the dialog box, the same two fields used to search for a procedure code are available.

The columns contain the following information:

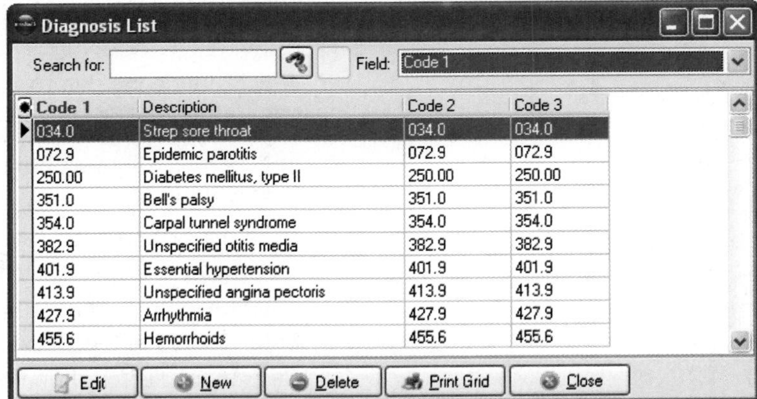

Figure 9.10 The Diagnosis List Dialog Box

Code 1 Enter the code itself.

Description Enter a description for the code.

Code 2, 3 If desired, alternate codes for the diagnosis can be entered. Some offices use internal codes in addition to the HIPAA-mandated codes.

The buttons at the bottom of the dialog box are also the same as those in the Procedure/Payment/Adjustment List dialog box.

The Diagnosis (new) Dialog Box

When the New button is clicked, the Diagnosis (new) dialog box is displayed (see Figure 9.11).

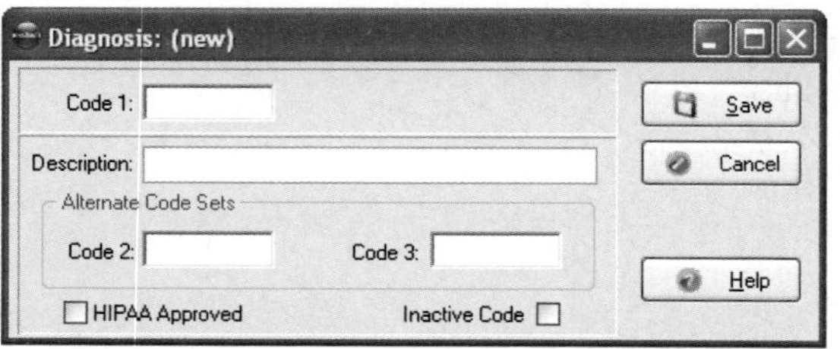

Figure 9.11 The Diagnosis (new) Dialog Box

The fields in the dialog box include the following:

Code 1 Enter the code itself.

Description Enter a description of the diagnosis (limited to one hundred characters).

Code 2, Code 3 The Code 2 and Code 3 fields are used when insurance carriers require that a set of diagnosis codes be associated with a particular procedure.

HIPAA Approved A check indicates that the code is HIPAA approved.

Inactive Code A check indicates that the code is inactive.

EXERCISE 9.2

connect plus+

ADDING DIAGNOSIS CODES TO THE DIAGNOSIS CODE DATABASE

In 2009 the United States had a widespread occurrence of swine flu (the popular name for H1N1 influenza), which was often accompanied by serious illnesses. As a result, the single ICD-9-CM code for this type of virus (ICD-9-CM 488.1, Influenza due to identified novel H1N1 influenza virus) was replaced by three codes, which were activated on October 1, 2010, to report more information about its complications:

488.11 Influenza due to identified novel H1N1 influenza with pneumonia

488.12 Influenza due to identified novel H1N1 influenza with other respiratory manifestations

488.13 Influenza due to identified novel H1N1 influenza with other manifestations

1. Click the Lists menu. Select Diagnosis Codes. The Diagnosis List dialog box is displayed.
2. Click the New button. The Diagnosis dialog box appears.
3. Enter ***488.11*** in the Code 1 field.
4. Click in the Description field. Enter ***Influenza H1N1 w/ pneumonia.***
5. Click the HIPAA Approved box, since this is a HIPAA-approved code.
6. Click the Save button.
7. Click the New button to enter the second new code.
8. Enter ***488.12*** in the Code 1 field.
9. Click in the Description field. Enter ***Influenza H1N1 w/other respiratory.***
10. Click the HIPAA Approved box, since this is a HIPAA-approved code.

11. Click the Save button.
12. Click the New button to enter the third new code.
13. Enter ***488.13*** in the Code 1 field.
14. Click in the Description field. Enter ***Influenza H1N1 w/other manifestations.***
15. Click the HIPAA Approved box, since this is a HIPAA-approved code.
16. Click the Save button.
17. Click the Close button to close the Diagnosis List dialog box.

 **You have completed Exercise 9.2**

9.3 Billing Compliance

Medical practices bill numerous health plans and government payers. The provider's fees for services are listed on the medical practice's fee schedule. Most medical practices have standard fee schedules listing their usual fees. Each charge, or fee, is related to a specific procedure code. The fee schedule for the practice used in the exercises in this text/workbook are listed on Source Document 14.

However, the fees listed on the master fee schedule are not necessarily the amount the provider will be paid. Instead, each health plan and government payer reimburses the practice according to its own negotiated or government-mandated fee schedule. For example, many providers enter into contracts with health plans that require a discount from standard fees. A single fee may be set for a number of related services, as is often done for obstetrical packages that set a fee that covers all of the mother's prenatal and birth services.

As a result, although there is a separate fee associated with each code, each code is not necessarily billable. Listing the correct individual codes on claims does not mean that each will be paid. Health plans issues many billing rules that govern what will and will not be covered. The term **compliant billing** refers to following these rules so that the practice and the health plan have the same expectations for the payment that will be made. Noncompliant billing, because it may appear to be intentional fraud, may have serious consequences:

compliant billing billing actions that satisfy official requirements

- Delays in processing claims and receiving payments
- Reduced payments
- Denied claims
- Fines and other sanctions
- Loss of hospital privileges
- Exclusion from health plans' programs
- Loss of the physician's license to practice medicine
- Prison sentences

Health plans' billing rules are stated in patients' medical insurance policies and in providers' participation contracts. Because contracts change and rules are updated, administrative staff members also rely on health plan bulletins, online billing manuals, websites, and regular communications with health plan representatives to stay current.

Package Codes and Global Periods

package combination of services included in a single procedure code

bundled code two or more related procedure codes combined into one

global period days surrounding a surgical procedure when all services relating to the procedure are considered part of the surgical package

Correct Coding Initiative (CCI) computerized Medicare system that prevents overpayment

CCI edits CPT code combinations that are used by computers to check Medicare claims

Many payer rules address typical surgical procedures that routinely involve a number of related procedural steps. A **package** is a group of related procedures and/or services included under a single code. As defined in CPT, a surgical package includes the operation itself, local anesthesia (injection of a metacarpal/digital block or topical anesthesia), and all routine follow-up services. The single code is called a **bundled code.** For example, in the musculoskeletal subsection, surgical package codes include the application and removal of the first cast or traction device. Health plans often add some preoperative services to their definition of a package.

Health plans set a **global period**—a certain length of time in which the expected services are to be provided—for each package. During a global period, no service that is part of the package is reimbursed in addition to the reimbursement for the package code. After the global period ends, all services that are provided can be reported.

Some types of services are not considered to be routine follow-up and are reported during the global period. For example, complications or recurrences that arise after therapeutic surgical procedures are reported with appropriate modifiers (such as for repeat or related surgical procedures). Care for other illnesses, injuries, or conditions that are unrelated to the surgical procedure are also separately reported. Following a diagnostic procedure, services not related to the recovery from that procedure may be reported, even though the care may be related to the patient's underlying condition.

Medicare National Correct Coding Initiative

The rules from CMS about billing Medicare often set the standard for the industry. Other health plans watch what CMS is doing and adopt similar rules. For this reason, two major Medicare reimbursement initiatives are discussed; other health plans can be expected to have similar programs in place that guide the practice's billing.

Especially important for billing is Medicare's national policy on correct coding, which is called the Medicare National **Correct Coding Initiative (CCI).** CCI controls improper coding that would lead to inappropriate payment for Medicare claims. It has coding policies that are based on:

- Coding conventions in CPT
- Medicare's national and local coverage and payment policies
- National medical societies' coding guidelines
- Medicare's analysis of standard medical and surgical practice

CCI, updated every quarter, has many thousands of CPT code combinations called **CCI edits** that are used by computers in the Medicare system to check claims. Examples of the CCI edits, which are available on a CMS website, are shown in Figure 9.12. CCI edits apply to claims that bill for more than one procedure performed on the same patient (Medicare beneficiary), on the same date of service, by the same performing provider. Claims are denied when codes reported together do not pass an edit.

CCI prevents billing two procedures that, according to Medicare, could not possibly have been performed together, such as reporting the removal of an organ both through an open incision and with laparoscopy, and reporting female-specific and male-specific codes for the same patient.

Column 1/Column 2 Edits

Column 1	Column 2	* = In existence prior to 1996	Effective Date	Deletion Date * = no data	Modifier 0 = not allowed 1 = allowed 9 = not applicable
10021	19290		20020101	*	1
10021	36000		20021001	*	1
10021	36410		20021001	*	1
10021	37202		20021001	*	1
10021	62318		20021001	*	1
10021	62319		20021001	*	1
10021	64415		20021001	*	1
10021	64416		20030101	*	1
10021	64417		20021001	*	1
10021	64450		20021001	*	1
10021	64470		20021001	*	1
10021	64475		20021001	*	1
10021	76000		20030701	*	1
10021	76003		20030101	*	1
10021	76360		20030101	*	1
10021	76393		20030101	*	1
10021	76942		20030101	*	1

Mutually Exclusive Edits

Column 1	Column 2	* = In existence prior to 1996	Effective Date	Deletion Date * = no data	Modifier 0 = not allowed 1 = allowed 9 = not applicable
11010	21240		19980101	*	1
11010	21242		19980101	*	1
11010	21243		19980101	*	1
11010	21244		19980101	*	1
11010	21245		19980101	*	1
11010	21246		19980101	*	1
11010	21247		19980101	*	1
11010	21248		19980101	*	1
11010	21249		19980101	*	1
11010	21255		19980101	*	1
11010	21256		19980101	*	1
11010	21260		19980101	*	1
11010	21261		19980101	*	1
11010	21263		19980101	*	1
11010	21267		19980101	*	1
11010	21268		19980101	*	1
11010	21270		19980101	*	1

Figure 9.12 Examples of Medicare CCI Edits: Column 1/Column 2 Edits and Mutually Exclusive Edits

unbundling incorrect billing practice of breaking a panel or package of services/procedures into component parts

CCI column 1/column 2 code pair edits Medicare code edit in which CPT codes in column 2 will not be paid if reported for same day of service, for the same patient, and by the same provider as the column 1 code

CCI mutually exclusive code (MEC) edits edits for codes for services that could not have reasonably been done during one encounter

CCI edits also test for **unbundling.** That is, a claim should report a bundled procedure code instead of multiple codes that describe parts of the complete procedure. For example, since a single code is available to describe removal of the uterus, ovaries, and fallopian tubes, physicians should not use separate codes to report the removal of the uterus, ovaries, and fallopian tubes individually. CCI requires physicians to report only the more extensive version of the procedure performed and disallows reporting of both extensive and limited procedures. For example, only a deep biopsy should be reported if both a deep biopsy and a superficial biopsy are performed at the same location.

Organization of the CCI Edits

CCI edits are organized into the following categories:

- Column 1/column 2 code pair edits
- Mutually exclusive code edits
- Modifier indicators

Column 1/Column 2 Code Pairs Two columns of codes are listed in the **CCI column 1/column 2 code pair edits.** Most often, one code is a component of the other. This means that the column 1 code includes all the services described by the column 2 code, so the column 2 code cannot be billed together with the column 1 code for the same patient on the same day of service. Medicare pays for the column 1 code only; the column 2 code is considered bundled into the column 1 code.

EXAMPLE

Column 1	*Column 2*
27370	20610, 76000, 76003

If 27370 is billed, neither 20610, 76000, nor 76003 should be billed with it, because the payment for each of these codes is already included in the column 1 code.

Mutually Exclusive Code Edits **CCI mutually exclusive code (MEC) edits** also list codes in two columns. According to CMS regulations, both services represented by these codes could not have reasonably been done during a single patient encounter, so they cannot be billed together. If the provider reports both codes from both columns for a patient on the same day, Medicare pays only the lower-paid code.

EXAMPLE

Column 1	*Column 2*
50021	49061, 50020

This means that a biller cannot report either 49061 or 50020 when reporting 50021.

THINKING IT THROUGH 9.3

What type of code edit could be used for the following rule?

Medicare Part B covers a screening Pap smear for women for the early detection of cervical cancer, but will not pay for an E/M service for the patient on the same day.

Medicare Medically Unlikely Edits

Also important for Medicare billing and compliance, and thus for other health plans as well, are the unit of service (UOS) edits CMS uses, which are called **medically unlikely edits (MUEs).** A MUE is related to a specific CPT or HCPCS code and applies to the services that a single provider (or supplier, for supplies such as durable medical equipment) provides for a single patient on the same date of service. The MUE value is based on the maximum units of service that would be reported for a code on the vast majority of correct claims.

medically unlikely edits (MUEs) units of service edits used to lower the Medicare fee-for-service paid claims error rate

modifier number appended to a code to report particular facts

MUEs are designed to reduce errors on claims due to clerical entries, and scrubbers store these rules to check encounter data before claims are transmitted. MUEs check for correct coding mistakes based on anatomic considerations, CPT/HCPCS code descriptors, CPT coding instructions, Medicare policies, or unlikely services. An example is a MUE edit that rejects a claim for a hysterectomy on a male patient. The goal is to reduce the number of health care claims that are sent back simply because of data-entry errors. The MUE system is set up to allow reporting of appropriate extra units of services when the situation warrants it.

9.4 Modifiers

A CPT/HCPCS **modifier** is a two-digit number that may be attached to most five-digit procedure codes. Modifiers are used to communicate special circumstances involved with procedures; a modifier tells the health plan that the physician considers the procedure to have been altered in some way. A modifier usually affects the normal level of reimbursement for the code to which it is attached.

CPT Modifiers

A CPT modifier indicates that a procedure was different from the standard description, but not in a way that changed the definition or required a different code. Table 9.1 lists the modifiers that can be used with the various sections of CPT codes. Modifiers are needed mainly when:

- A service or procedure was performed more than once or by more than one physician.
- A service or procedure has been increased or reduced.
- Only part of a procedure was done. For example, some procedures have two parts—a technical component performed by a technician, and a professional component that the physician performs, usually the interpretation and reporting of the results. A modifier is used to show that just one of the parts was done.
- Unusual difficulties occurred during the procedure.

TABLE 9.1	CPT Modifiers: Description and Common Use in Main Text Sections						
Code	**Description**	**E/M**	**Anesthesia**	**Surgery**	**Radiology**	**Pathology**	**Medicine**
–22	Increased Procedural Services	Never	Yes	Yes	Yes	Yes	Yes
–23	Unusual Anesthesia	Never	Yes				Never
–24	Unrelated E/M Service by the Same Physician During a Postoperative Period	Yes	Never	Never	Never	Never	Never
–25	Significant, Separately Identifiable E/M Service by the Same Physician on the Same Day of the Procedure or Other Service	Yes	Never	Never	Never	Never	Never
–26	Professional Component	—	—	Yes	Yes	Yes	Yes
–32	Mandated Services	Yes	Yes	Yes	Yes	Yes	Yes
–47	Anesthesia by Surgeon	Never	Never	Yes	Never	Never	Never
–50	Bilateral Procedure	—	—	Yes	—	—	—
–51	Multiple Procedures	—	Yes	Yes	Yes	Never	Yes
–52	Reduced Services	Yes	—	Yes	Yes	Yes	Yes
–53	Discontinued Procedure	Never	Yes	Yes	Yes	Yes	Yes
–54	Surgical Care Only	—	—	Yes	—	—	—
–55	Postoperative Management Only	—	—	Yes	—	—	Yes
–56	Preoperative Management Only	—	—	Yes	—	—	Yes
–57	Decision for Surgery	Yes	—	—	—	—	Yes
–58	Staged or Related Procedure/ Service by the Same Physician During the Postoperative Period	—	—	Yes	Yes	—	Yes
–59	Distinct Procedural Service	—	Yes	Yes	Yes	Yes	Yes
–62	Two Surgeons	Never	Never	Yes	Yes	Never	—
–63	Procedure Performed on Infants	—	—	Yes	Yes	—	Yes
–66	Surgical Team	Never	Never	Yes	Yes	Never	—
–76	Repeat Procedure by Same Physician	—	—	Yes	Yes	—	Yes
–77	Repeat Procedure by Another Physician	—	—	Yes	Yes	—	Yes
–78	Return to the Operating Room for a Related Procedure During the Postoperative Period	—	—	Yes	Yes	—	Yes
–79	Unrelated Procedure/Service by the Same Physician During the Postoperative Period	—	—	Yes	Yes	—	Yes
–80	Assistant Surgeon	Never	—	Yes	Yes	—	—

(continued)

TABLE 9.1 *(continued)*							
Code	**Description**	**E/M**	**Anesthesia**	**Surgery**	**Radiology**	**Pathology**	**Medicine**
–81	Minimum Assistant Surgeon	Never	—	Yes	—	—	—
–82	Assistant Surgeon (when qualified resident surgeon not available)	Never	—	Yes	—	—	—
–90	Reference (Outside) Laboratory	—	—	Yes	Yes	Yes	Yes
–91	Repeat Clinical Diagnostic Laboratory Test	—	—	Yes	Yes	Yes	Yes
–92	Alternative Laboratory Platform Testing	—	—	Yes	Yes	Yes	Yes
–99	Multiple Modifiers	—	—	Yes	Yes	—	Yes

Source: CPT 2011
Key:
Yes = commonly used
— = not usually used with the codes in that section
Never = not used with the codes in that section

EXAMPLE

The modifier –76, Repeat Procedure by Same Physician, is used when the reporting physician repeats a procedure or service after doing the first one. A situation requiring this modifier to show the extra procedure might be:

Procedural Statement: Physician performed a chest X-ray before placing a chest tube and then, after the chest tube was placed, performed a second chest X-ray to verify its position.

Code: 71020–76 Radiologic examination, chest, two views, frontal and lateral; repeat procedure or service by same physician

The modifiers are listed in Appendix A of CPT and on the inside cover of the code book. However, not all CPT modifiers are available for use with every section's codes. Some modifiers apply only to certain sections. Health plans require the hyphen and the two-digit modifier to be appended to the CPT code. Two or more modifiers may be used with one code to give the most accurate description possible.

HCPCS Modifiers

HCPCS (Level II) modifiers—also two-digit units appended to procedure codes—add some element of additional description relating to the procedure. They may be two letters (such as –HS, family/couple without client present) or a letter and a number (such as –F5, right hand, thumb). These modifiers do not impact billing, but they may answer a payer's question about the details of a procedure.

Like the HCPCS codes themselves, the related modifiers address situations not covered by CPT modifiers. They are especially useful for indicating anatomical details. The most commonly used modifiers are listed in Table 9.2.

TABLE 9.2	Selected HCPCS Level II (National) Modifiers
Modifier	**Description**
–CA	Procedure payable in the inpatient setting only when performed emergently on an outpatient who expires prior to admission
–E1	Upper left, eyelid
–E2	Lower left, eyelid
–E3	Upper right, eyelid
–E4	Lower right, eyelid
–FA	Left hand, thumb
–F1	Left hand, second digit
–F2	Left hand, third digit
–F3	Left hand, fourth digit
–F4	Left hand, fifth digit
–F5	Right hand, thumb
–F6	Right hand, second digit
–F7	Right hand, third digit
–F8	Right hand, fourth digit
–F9	Right hand, fifth digit
–LC	Left circumflex coronary artery
–LD	Left anterior descending coronary artery
–RC	Right coronary artery
–LT	Left side (identifies procedures performed on the left side of the body)
–RT	Right side (identifies procedures performed on the right side of the body)
–TC	Technical component

Overriding Payer Edits

CCI modifier indicator number showing whether the use of a modifier can bypass a CCI edit

A common use of CPT modifiers is to override the CCI edits when circumstances warrant it and the documentation supports their use. The **CCI modifier indicators,** as shown in the last column in Figure 9.12, govern modifier use to "break," or avoid, CCI edits. CCI modifier indicators appear next to items in both the CCI column 1/column 2 code pair list and the mutually exclusive code list. A CCI modifier indicator of 1 means that a CPT modifier may be used to bypass an edit (if the circumstances are appropriate). A CCI modifier indicator of 0 means that use of a CPT modifier will not change the edit, so the column 2 codes or mutually exclusive code edits will not be bypassed.

For example, flu vaccine code 90656 includes bundled flu vaccine codes 90655 and 90657–90660. It has a CCI indicator of 0. No modifier will be effective in bypassing these edits, so only CPT 90656 will be paid in every case.

THINKING IT THROUGH 9.4

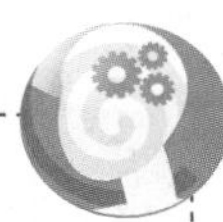

Based on Table 9.1, which CPT modifier would be assigned to each of these billing scenarios?

- Multiple modifiers ____________________
- Distinct procedural service ____________________
- Unrelated evaluation and management service by same physician during a postoperative period ____________________
- Staged procedure ____________________

However, when two procedures, such as CPT codes 10021 (fine needle aspiration without imaging guidance) and 19290 (preoperative placement of needle localization wire, breast), as shown in Figure 9.12, are both done and the modifier indicator is 1, the –59 modifier that means "distinct procedural service" can be attached to override the CCI edit.

The purpose of the modifier is to report both services and to be paid for both, rather than receiving no payment or reduced payment for the second procedure. However, the situation must warrant the modifier use. Based on the definition of –59, the two procedures must have been done in different anatomical areas. In this case, if both were breast procedures, the modifier cannot be attached.

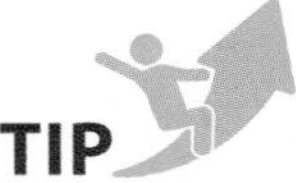

TIP

If a provider reports two codes of an edit pair (see Figure 9.12), the payer will deny the column 2 code and pay the column 1 code. When appropriate, attach modifier –59 to the applicable column 2 procedure rather than to the column 1 code.

9.5 Strategies to Avoid Common Coding/Billing Problems

Health plans often base their decisions to pay or deny claims only on the diagnosis and procedure codes. The integrity of the request for payment rests on the accuracy and honesty of the coding and billing. Incorrect work may simply be an error, or it may represent a deliberate effort to obtain fraudulent payment. Compliance errors can result from incorrect code selection or billing practices.

Errors Relating to the Coding Process

These coding problems may cause rejected claims:

- Truncated coding—using diagnosis codes that are not as specific as possible
- Mismatching between the gender or age of the patient and the selected code when the code involves selection for either criterion
- Assumption coding—reporting items or services that are not actually documented, but that the coder assumes were performed
- Altering documentation after services are reported
- Coding without proper documentation
- Reporting services provided by unlicensed or unqualified clinical personnel

- Failing to satisfy the conditions of coverage for a particular service, such as the physician's direct supervision of a radiologist's work
- Coding conditions that are present but were not addressed during the visit

Errors Relating to the Billing Process

A number of errors are related to the billing process. These are the most frequent errors:

- Billing noncovered services.
- Billing overlimit services.
- Unbundling.
- Using an inappropriate modifier or no modifier when one is required.
- Always assigning the same level of E/M service.
- Billing a consultation instead of an office visit.
- Billing invalid/outdated codes.
- Either upcoding—using a procedure code that provides a higher reimbursement rate than the correct code—or downcoding—using a lower-level code. Some physicians downcode to be "safe," especially E/M codes.
- Billing without proper signatures on file.
- Billing a service with the incorrect **place of service (POS) code.** The POS indicates where services were performed. Since some places of service are paid at higher rates than others because more equipment and supplies have to be available, it is important to correctly assign POS codes. The standard numerical codes used for physician practices are:

  11 Provider's office

  21 Inpatient hospital

  22 Outpatient hospital

  23 Hospital emergency room

place of service (POS) code location where medical services were provided

Strategies for Compliance

Compliant billing can be difficult and complex; the strategies discussed in this section are helpful.

- **Carefully define bundled codes and know global periods** To avoid unbundling, coders and medical insurance specialists must be clear on which individual procedures are contained in bundled codes and what the global periods are for surgical procedures. Many practices use Medicare's CCI list of bundling rules and global periods for deciding what is included in a procedure code; they inform their other health plans that they are following this system of edits. If the health plan has a unique set of edits, coders and billers need access to it.

- **Use modifiers appropriately** CPT modifiers can eliminate the impression of duplicate billing or unbundling.
- **Follow the practice's compliance plan, especially the guidelines about physician queries** A **query** is a question transmitted to a provider to obtain additional clarifying documentation to improve the specificity and completeness of the data used to assign diagnosis and procedure codes in the patient's health record. Queries are used when there is conflicting, incomplete, or ambiguous information in the health record regarding a significant condition or procedure. For example, two treating providers of a hospitalized patient might disagree with respect to a diagnosis, as in the case of a patient who has shortness of breath that a pulmonologist documents as caused by pneumonia but the attending physician documents as congestive heart failure.

  Practices' compliance plans often provide for a query process. EHRs often provide electronic templates to generate and respond to electronic queries. Query guidelines must be followed in order to avoid leading the provider in any way.

query request for more information from a provider

THINKING IT THROUGH 9.5

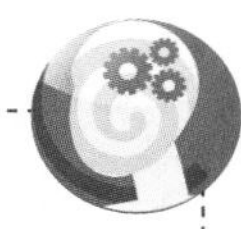

Botox injections have been approved by the Food and Drug Administration (FDA) to treat spasms of the flexor muscles of the elbow, wrist, and fingers. Should a payer reject a claim for this use of Botox based on lack of medical necessity?

9.6 Posting Charges in Medisoft Network Professional

As you learned earlier in the chapter, the methods of posting charges in an office that uses an electronic encounter form in a PM/EHR differ from the method used in an office that uses a paper encounter form. Some offices begin using electronic encounter forms right after they switch to a PM/EHR, while other offices continue to use paper encounter forms for posting charges. In this section, you will learn how to post charges from a paper encounter form, and then how to post charges that have been electronically transmitted from an EHR using an electronic encounter form.

In Medisoft Network Professional, transactions that are posted (whether from a paper or electronic form) appear in the Transaction Entry dialog box. The Transaction Entry dialog box consists of three main sections, each consuming about a third of the window (see Figure 9.13):

1. **Patient/Account Information** The top third contains information about the patient, the insurance coverage, and the patient's account.
2. **Charge Transactions** The middle section is where charge transactions are shown.

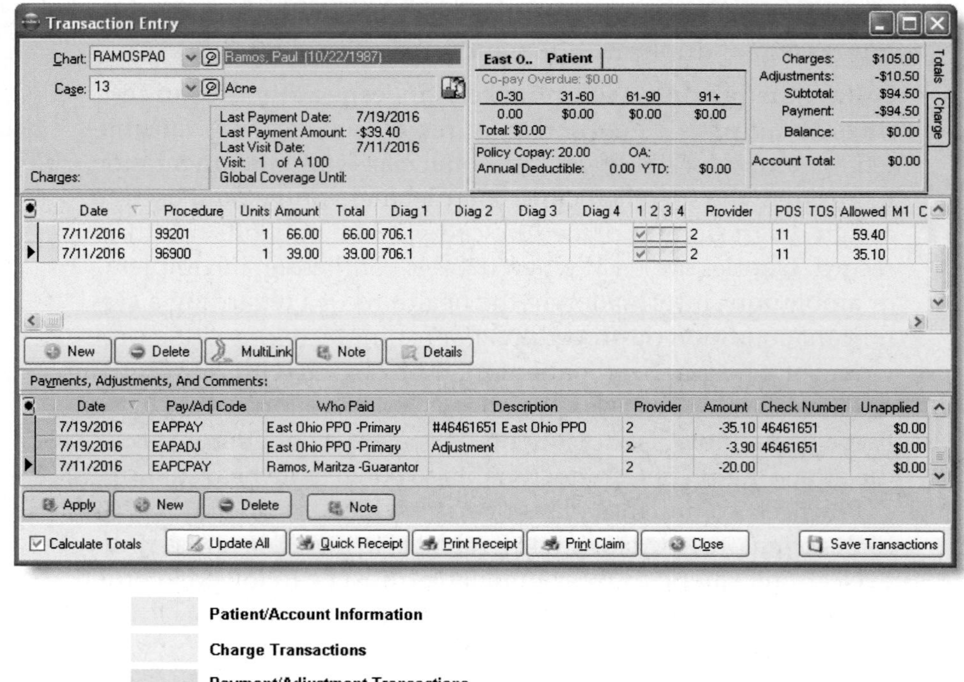

Figure 9.13 Transaction Entry Dialog Box with Three Sections Highlighted

3. **Payment/Adjustment Transactions** The bottom third is where patient payments and different types of adjustments are posted and applied. The topic of posting payments from insurance carriers is discussed in Chapter 11.

Patient/Account Information

The Patient/Account Information section of the Transaction Entry dialog box consists of the top third of the Transaction Entry dialog box (see Figure 9.14). It contains two critical pieces of information: chart number and case number.

Chart

The Chart drop-down list includes all patients in the practice. In large practices, the list of chart numbers could be very long, so it is

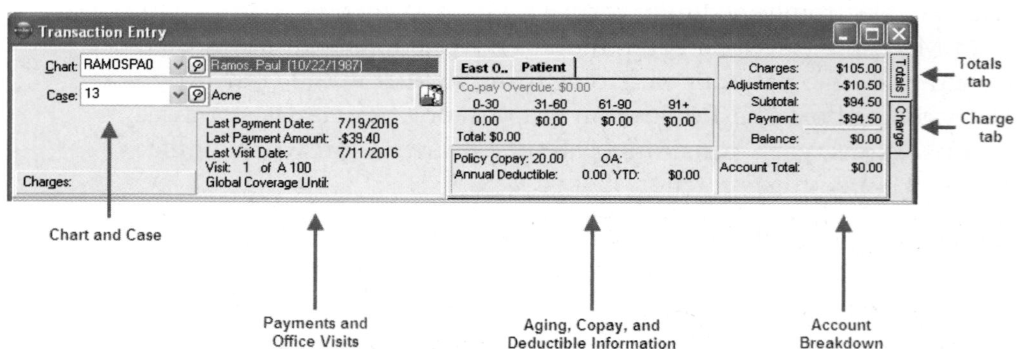

Figure 9.14 The Patient/Account Information Section of the Transaction Entry Dialog Box

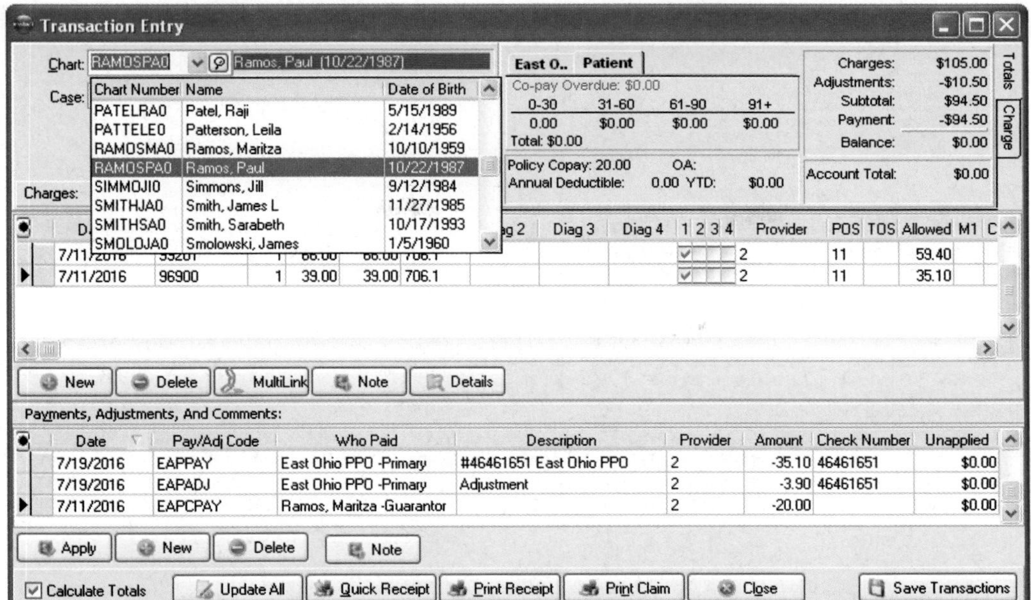

Figure 9.15 Chart Drop-down List After *RAMOSP* Is Keyed

important to know how to search for a chart number. One way is to key the first several letters of a patient's last name. As the letters are keyed, the first chart number in the list that matches is highlighted. In the example in Figure 9.15, the letters *RAMOSP* were keyed. The program highlights the first patient with a chart number beginning with those letters—in this case, Paul Ramos. If this is the correct patient, pressing Tab selects the patient and closes the drop-down list. If a different patient is desired, the up and down arrow keys are used to move up or down in the list.

Case

The Case field lists the case that relates to the current charges or payments. Recall from Chapter 5 that transactions are linked to a case. The drop-down list in the Case box displays case numbers and descriptions for the patient (see Figure 9.16). By default, the transactions for the most recent case are displayed. Transactions for other cases can be displayed by changing the selection in the Case box. Only one case can be opened at a time.

Additional Information

The remaining areas in the patient/account information section of the Transaction Entry dialog box contain information that is entered automatically by the program and cannot be edited. The dates and figures are automatically updated after a new transaction is entered and saved.

The aging, copay, and deductible section (see Figure 9.14) displays account aging information for the patient and the insurance carriers. By default, the Patient tab is displayed. The Patient tab contains the following information:

- Whether a copayment is overdue
- The outstanding balance for 0–30, 31–60, 61–90, and 91+ days, and the total amount outstanding

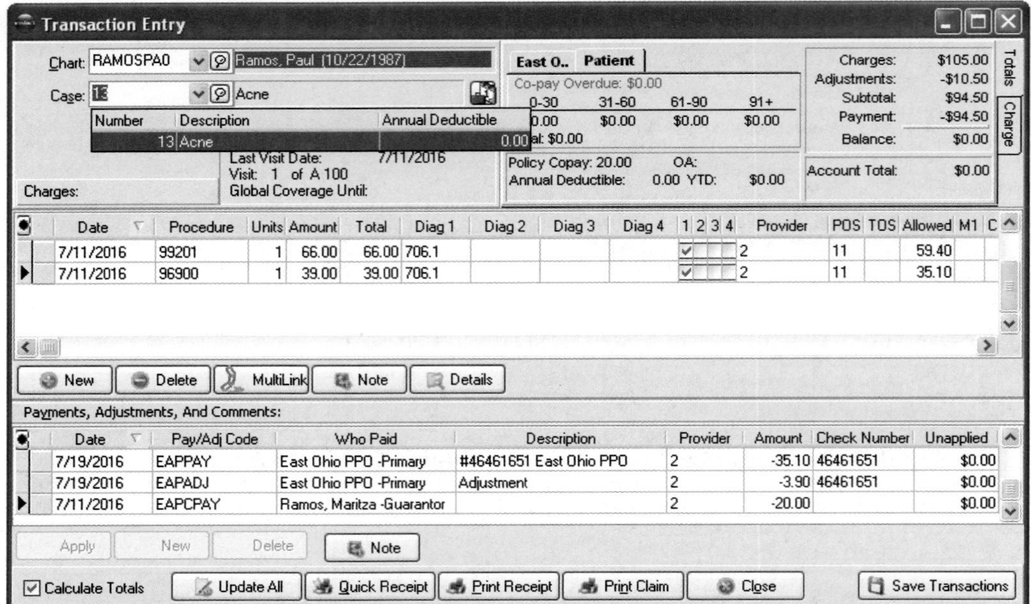

Figure 9.16 Case Drop-down List for the Patient Listed in the Chart Box

- The amount of the copayment for the patient's health plan
- The amount of the annual deductible and the amount paid toward the deductible year-to-date

The Insurance tab, which is not visible until you click the tab title (the name of the patient's insurance carrier), contains similar information, except that it displays aging information for the carrier.

Charge Transactions

Charges for procedures performed by a provider are posted in the charges section in the middle of the Transaction Entry dialog box (see Figure 9.13). The process used to post charges differs depending on whether an office uses a paper encounter form or an electronic encounter form. When a paper encounter form is used, a member of the billing staff enters each procedure charge manually; when an electronic encounter form is used, the charges are reviewed and then the procedure charges are automatically posted in the Transaction Entry dialog box.

Figure 9.17 shows a paper encounter form and an electronic encounter form for the same office visit. The red arrows show the location of the procedure and diagnosis codes on both forms.

When charges are posted in the Transaction Entry dialog box from Medisoft Clinical Patient Records (MCPR), most of the fields listed in this section are completed by the program. The fields in the Charges section of the Transaction Entry dialog box include the following:

New In an office using paper encounter forms, the process of posting charges begins with clicking the New button (see Figure 9.18). This button is not used when posting charges from MCPR unless charges not listed on the electronic encounter form have to be entered.

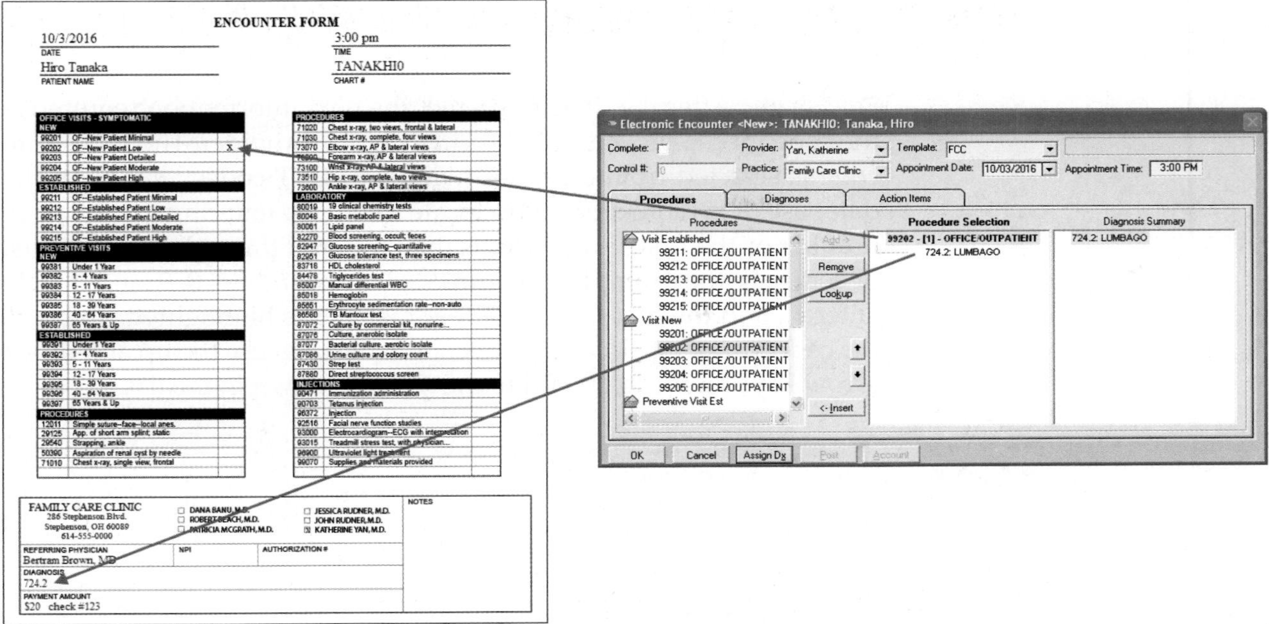

Figure 9.17 Comparison of Paper and Electronic Encounter Forms

Date	Procedure	Units	Amount	Total	Diag 1	Diag 2	Diag 3	Diag 4	1 2 3 4	Provider	POS	TOS	Allowed	M1	C
7/11/2016	99201	1	66.00	66.00	706.1				✓	2	11		59.40		
7/11/2016	96900	1	39.00	39.00	706.1				✓	2	11		35.10		

New | Delete | MultiLink | Note | Details

Figure 9.18 Charges Area in the Transaction Entry Dialog Box with the New Button Highlighted

Date When the New button is clicked, the program automatically enters the current date in the Date box (see Figure 9.19). If this is not the date on which the procedures were performed, it must be changed. To change the default date for these boxes, any of these methods can be used:

- The Set Program Date command on the File menu can be clicked.
- The Date button in the lower-right corner of the screen can be clicked. (This must be done before the New button is clicked in the Transaction Entry dialog box.)
- The information that is already in the Date box can be keyed over with the desired date.

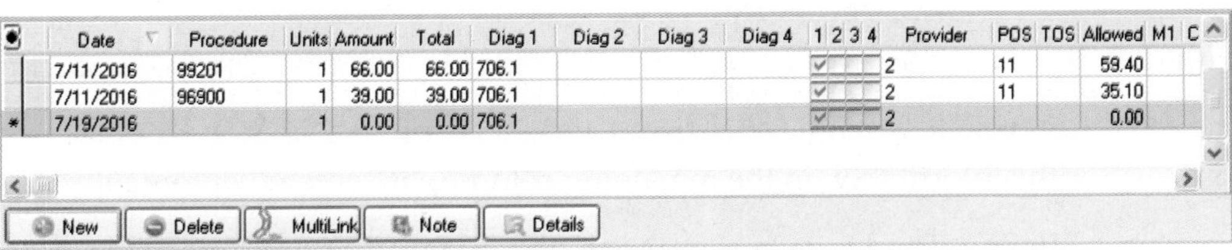

Date	Procedure	Units	Amount	Total	Diag 1	Diag 2	Diag 3	Diag 4	1 2 3 4	Provider	POS	TOS	Allowed	M1	C
7/11/2016	99201	1	66.00	66.00	706.1				✓	2	11		59.40		
7/11/2016	96900	1	39.00	39.00	706.1				✓	2	11		35.10		
7/19/2016		1	0.00	0.00	706.1				✓	2			0.00		

New | Delete | MultiLink | Note | Details

Figure 9.19 Date Displayed in the Date Column After the New Button Is Clicked (New Entry Highlighted in Yellow)

When encounters are posted from MCPR, the date is entered automatically.

Procedure After the date is entered, the next information required is the code for the procedure performed by the provider. The procedure code is selected from a drop-down list of CPT codes already in the database. It is more efficient to locate a code by entering the full code number or the first several digits than to scroll through the entire list of codes. In the example in Figure 9.20, the numbers *8, 0,* and *0* were entered, and the first CPT code that matches is highlighted. To select the code, press Tab. If a different code is desired, use the up and down arrow keys on the keyboard to move up or down in the list.

Date	Procedure	Units	Amount	Total	Diag 1	Diag 2	Diag 3	Diag 4	1 2 3 4	Provider	POS	TOS	Allowed	M1	C
7/11/2016	99201	1	66.00	66.00	706.1				✓	2	11		59.40		
7/11/2016	96900	1	39.00	39.00	706.1				✓	2	11		35.10		
7/19/2016	80048	1	0.00	0.00	706.1				✓	2			0.00		

Code 1	Description
73100	Wrist x-ray, AP and lateral views
73510	Hip x-ray, complete, two views
73600	Ankle x-ray, AP and lateral views
80048	Basic metabolic panel
80061	Lipid panel
82270	Blood screening, occult; feces
82947	Glucose screening--quantitative
82951	Glucose tolerance test, three specimens

New

Payments, Adjustme

Date				Provider	Amount	Check Number	Unapplied
7/11/2016				2	-20.00		$0.00
7/19/2016	EAPPAY	East Ohio PPO -Primary	#46461651 East Ohio PPO	2	-39.40	46461651	$0.00

Figure 9.20 Procedure Drop-down List After the Numbers *8, 0,* and *0* Are Entered

Only one procedure code can be assigned for each transaction. If multiple procedures were performed for a patient, each must be a separate transaction (unless a MultiLink code, which is discussed later in the chapter, is used).

If a CPT code for a procedure is not listed, it can be added to the database by pressing the F8 key or by clicking Procedure/Payment/Adjustment Codes on the Lists menu. This may be done without exiting the Transaction Entry dialog box.

After the code is selected and the Tab key is pressed, the program automatically enters data in the other columns (see Figure 9.21). These entries are described in the paragraphs that follow. If additional information must be added, use the Tab key to move to the box in the appropriate column.

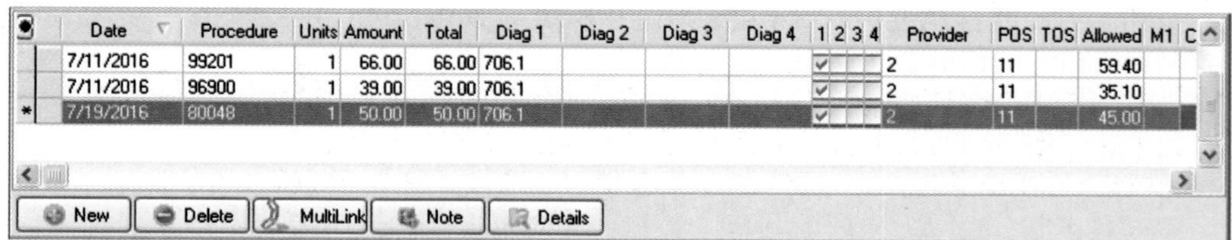

Figure 9.21 Charges Section of the Transaction Entry Dialog Box After a Procedure Code Is Selected

When encounters are posted from MCPR, the procedure codes and the information in the remaining columns are entered automatically.

Units The Units box indicates the quantity of the procedure. Normally, the number of units is one. In some cases, however, it may be more than one.

Amount The Amount box lists the charge amount for a procedure. The amount is entered automatically by the system based on the CPT code and insurance carrier. Each CPT code stored in the system has a charge amount associated with it. These amounts are determined by the fee schedule of the office.

Total To the right of the Amount box is the Total box. This field displays the total charges for the procedures performed. The amount is calculated by the system; the number in the Units box is multiplied by the number in the Amount box.

Diagnosis The Diag 1, 2, 3, and 4 boxes correspond to the information in the Diagnosis tab of the Case folder. If a patient has several different diagnoses, the diagnosis that is most relevant to the procedure is used.

1, 2, 3, 4 The 1, 2, 3, and 4 boxes to the right of the Diag 1, 2, 3, and 4 boxes indicate which diagnoses should be used for this charge. A check mark appears in each Diagnosis box for which a diagnosis was entered in the Diag 1, 2, 3, and 4 boxes.

Provider The Provider box lists the code number of a patient's assigned provider. If a patient sees a different provider for a visit, the Provider box can be changed to list that provider instead.

POS When the PM/EHR is set up for use in a practice, an option is provided to set a default POS code. In addition, POS codes can be assigned to specific procedure codes when they are set up in the Procedure/Payment/Adjustment Codes List. For purposes of this book, the default code has been set to 11 for provider's office.

TOS *TOS* stands for "type of service." Medical offices may set up a list of codes to indicate the type of service performed. For example, 1 may indicate an examination, 2 a lab test, and so on. The TOS code is specified in the Procedure/Payment/Adjustment entry for each CPT code.

Allowed This is the amount allowed by the health plan associated with this patient for this procedure. The value comes from the Allowed Amounts tab of the Procedure/Payment/Adjustment dialog box.

M1 The M1 box is for a CPT code modifier. The grid in the Transaction Entry dialog box can be changed to allow entry of up to four modifiers per line.

Co-Pay A check mark in this box indicates that the code entered in the Procedure column requires a copayment.

Buttons in the Charges Area of the Transaction Entry Dialog Box

Five buttons are provided at the bottom of the Charges area: New, Delete, MultiLink, Note, and Details. The New button, used to create a new charge entry, has just been discussed.

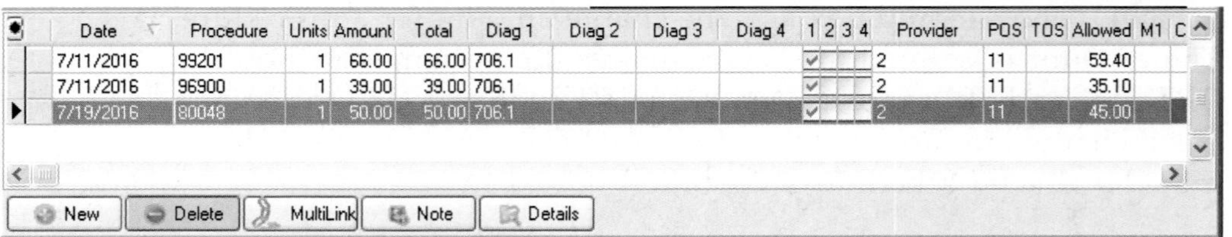

Figure 9.22 Transaction Selected for Deletion Indicated by Line Pointer at Left

Delete Button To delete a charge transaction, it is necessary to select the charge that is to be deleted. This is accomplished by clicking in any of the boxes associated with that transaction (Date, Procedure, Units, Amount, and so on). Clicking in a box selects the transaction, indicated by the black triangle pointer at the far left box on the line (see Figure 9.22).

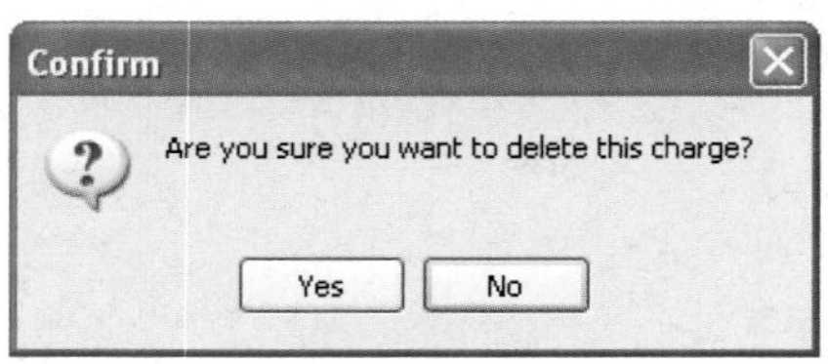

Figure 9.23 Confirm Dialog Box Displayed After Clicking the Delete Button

Once the desired transaction is selected, it is ready for deletion. Clicking the Delete button causes a confirmation message to be displayed (see Figure 9.23). To continue with the deletion, click the Yes button. To cancel the deletion, click the No button.

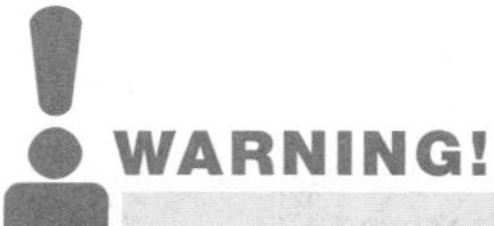

WARNING!

All transactions can be deleted from within the Transaction Entry dialog box. Caution should be exercised when using the Delete feature. Deleted data cannot be recovered.

MultiLink codes groups of procedure code entries that relate to a single activity

MultiLink Button Medisoft provides a feature that saves time when entering multiple CPT codes that are related to the same activity but that are not bundled by payers. **MultiLink codes** are groups of procedure code entries that relate to a single activity. For example, a MultiLink code could be created for the procedures related to diagnosing strep throat: 99211 OF—Established patient, minimal; 87430 Strep test; and 85025 Complete CBC w/auto diff. WBC.

Figure 9.24 MultiLink Button

Clicking the MultiLink button (see Figure 9.24) in the Transaction Entry dialog box displays the MultiLink dialog box (see Figure 9.25). After the code, such as STREPM, is selected from the drop-down list of MultiLink codes already in the database, the Create Transactions button is clicked. This causes the system to automatically enter all the procedure codes associated with the procedure in the list of transactions at the bottom of the Transaction Entry dialog box, eliminating the need to enter each CPT code separately (see Figure 9.26). The MultiLink feature saves time by reducing the number of procedure code entries, and it also reduces omission errors. When procedure codes are entered as a MultiLink, it is impossible to forget to enter a procedure, since all the codes that are in the MultiLink group are entered automatically.

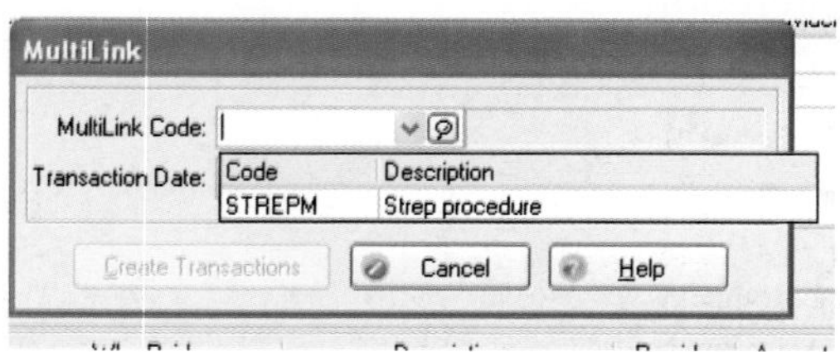

Figure 9.25 MultiLink Code Drop-down List

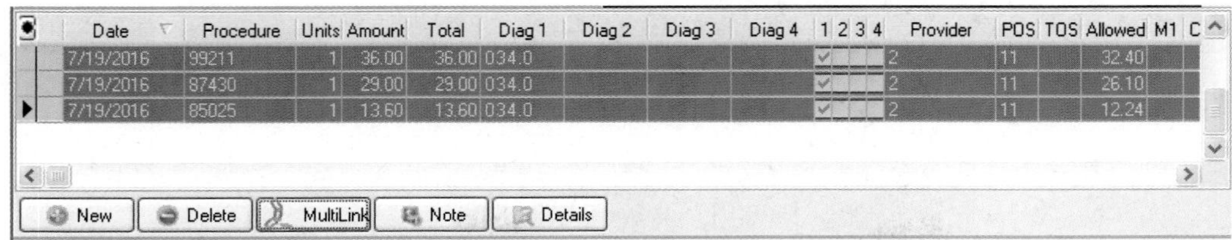

Date	Procedure	Units	Amount	Total	Diag 1	Diag 2	Diag 3	Diag 4	1 2 3 4	Provider	POS	TOS	Allowed	M1	C
7/19/2016	99211	1	36.00	36.00	034.0					2	11		32.40		
7/19/2016	87430	1	29.00	29.00	034.0					2	11		26.10		
7/19/2016	85025	1	13.60	13.60	034.0					2	11		12.24		

Figure 9.26 Charge Transactions Created with STREPM MultiLink Code

Note Button The Note button is used to enter additional information about a particular procedure. When the Note button is clicked, the Transaction Documentation dialog box is displayed (see Figure 9.27).

In the Type field, Medisoft provides a list of types of documentation in the drop-down list (see Figure 9.28). Some of the information entered here is transmitted with electronic claims.

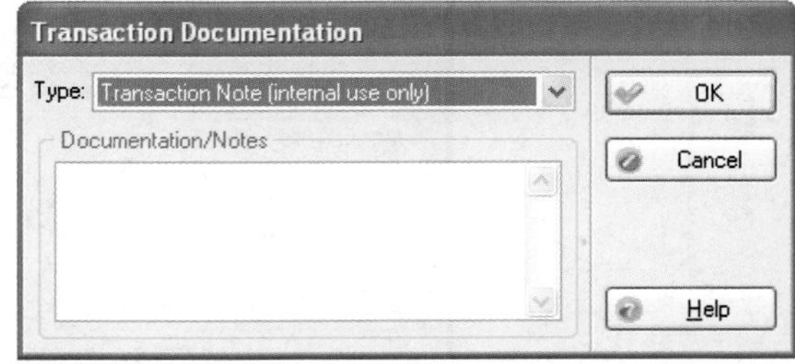

Figure 9.27 Transaction Documentation Dialog Box, Where Notes About a Transaction Are Entered

Details Button When clicked, the Details button displays a dialog box that is used to enter drug/prescription information for a charge.

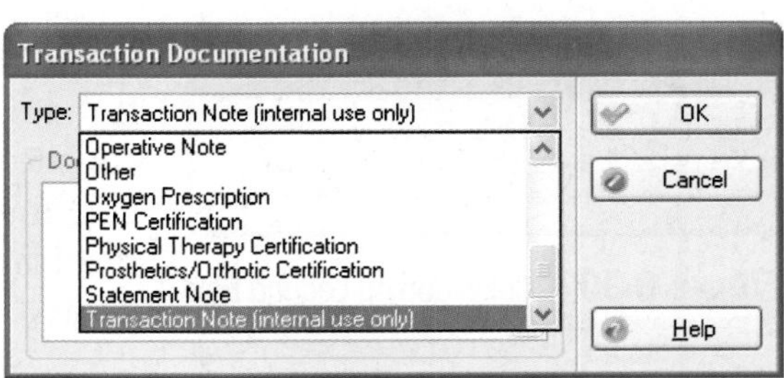

Figure 9.28 Some of the Many Types of Transaction Documentation Available in Medisoft

Color Coding in Transaction Entry

Transactions in Medisoft are color-coded, making it easy to determine the status of a charge or payment. Color codes are set up using the Program Options selection on the File menu.

In the medical practice used in this text/workbook, three color codes are applied to the status of a charge:

1. No payment: gray
2. Partially paid charge: aqua
3. Overpaid charge: yellow

Charges that have been paid in full are not colored and appear white.

To display a list of color codes used in the Transaction Entry dialog box, click the right mouse button in the white area below the list of transactions, and a shortcut menu is displayed (see Figure 9.29).

When the Show Color Legend option is selected, the Color-Coding Legend box appears on the screen (see Figure 9.30). The box lists the meaning of the color codes used in Transaction Entry—three for charges, and three for payments. The color codes used to indicate the status of a payment are discussed later in the chapter.

Figure 9.31 shows a charge entry on 7/19/2016 for procedure 99211. The line is shaded light blue to indicate that the charge has been partially paid. The other two charges are gray, indicating that no payment has been made for them.

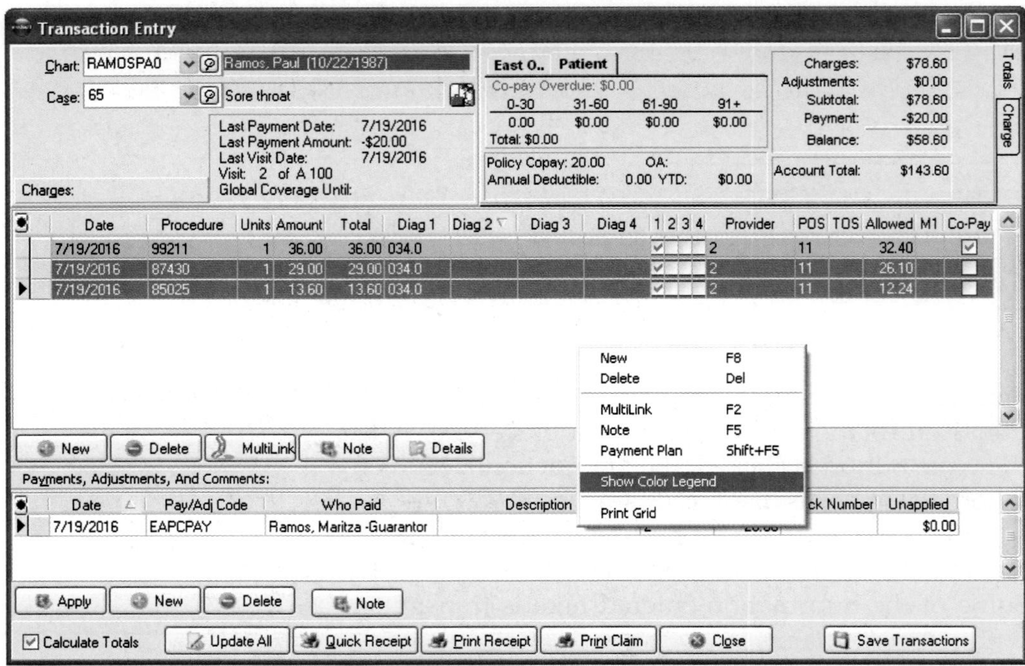

Figure 9.29 Shortcut Menu with Show Color Legend Option Highlighted

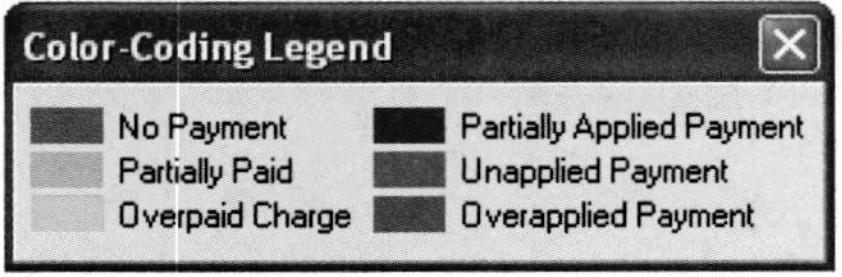

Figure 9.30 Color-Coding Legend Box

Saving Charges

If the transactions have been posted manually from a paper encounter form, they must be saved. Transactions are saved by clicking the Save Transactions button located at the bottom of the Transaction Entry dialog box (see Figure 9.31). Transactions posted from MCPR are automatically saved.

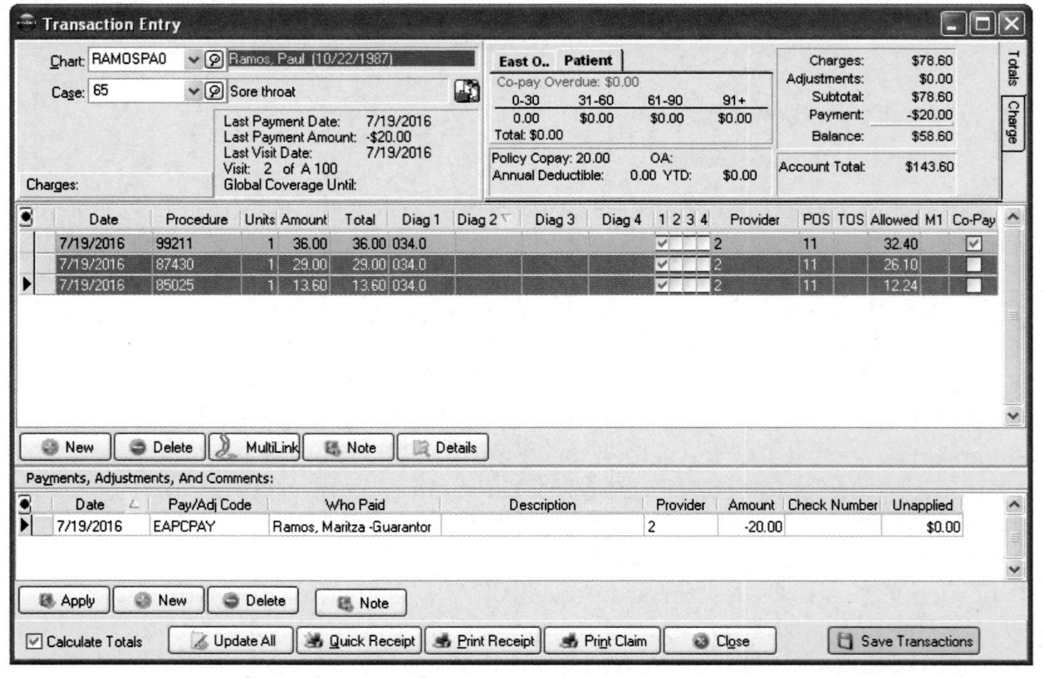

Figure 9.31 Transaction Entry Dialog Box with Save Transactions Button Highlighted

Transactions can also be saved by clicking the Update All button located in the same row of buttons. When Update All is clicked, the transactions are saved, and the program checks all fields for missing or invalid information and displays various messages, such as a warning that the date entered is in the future.

The other buttons located in this row, Quick Receipt and Print Receipt, are used to print a walkout receipt for a patient (covered later in this chapter). The Print Claim button is discussed in Chapter 10. The Close button simply closes the Transaction Entry dialog box.

Editing Transactions

The most efficient way to edit a transaction is to click in the field that needs to be changed and enter the correct information. For example, to change the procedure code, click in the Procedure box, and either key a new code or select a new code from the drop-down list. After changes are made, the data must be saved. To view the updated amounts in the patient/account information area, click the Update All button near the bottom of the Transaction Entry dialog box. Note that edits must be made before claims are sent to the insurance carrier.

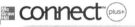

connect plus+ EXERCISE 9.3

POSTING CHARGES FROM A PAPER ENCOUNTER FORM

Using the information on Source Document 5, post the charges for John Fitzwilliams's office visit on October 3, 2016.

Date: October 3, 2016

1. Click the Activities menu. Select Enter Transactions. The Transaction Entry dialog box opens.
2. Click in the Chart field, and key ***FI.*** Notice that the chart number for John Fitzwilliams is highlighted on the drop-down list.
3. Press the Tab key. Verify that Acute gastric ulcer is the active case in the Case box. Notice that there are already charges and payments listed for this case, since this is an existing medical condition for which the patient has been treated in the past.
4. Click the New button in the Charges section of the dialog box.
5. Accept the default in the Date box (10/3/2016).
6. Click in the Procedure box, and enter ***99212*** to select the procedure code for the service checked off on the encounter form. Press Tab. Notice that the Diag 1 box and the Units box have been automatically completed. The Amount box is also automatically completed ($54.00).
7. Review the entries in the Provider (1) and POS (11) boxes. Since there are no modifiers for the procedure code, the M1 box is left blank.

(continued)

(Continued)

8. Click the New button again to enter the second procedure charge.
9. Accept the default in the Date box (10/3/2016).
10. Click in the Procedure box, and enter ***82270*** to select the procedure code for the service checked off on the encounter form. Press Tab. Review the information automatically entered.
11. Click the Save Transactions button.
12. A message appears that a $15.00 copayment is due. This will be entered in the section on copayments later in the chapter. Click the OK button.
13. The two new charges appear in the Transaction Entry dialog box.

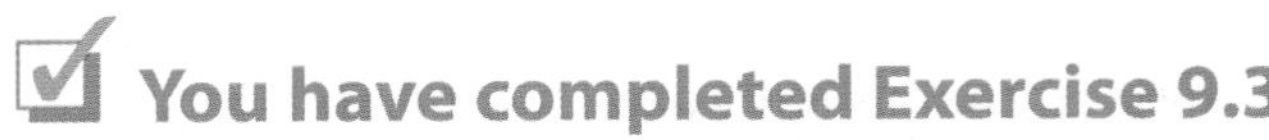

Posting Charges from an EHR

Unlike transactions on a paper encounter form, transactions from an EHR do not need to be manually posted in the Transaction Entry dialog box. After a patient visit has been documented in Medisoft Clinical Patient Records and the procedures and diagnoses have been reviewed on the electronic encounter form (EEF), the encounter data are transmitted to Medisoft Network Professional. The data are held until they are reviewed by a member of the billing staff. Once the charges have been reviewed and edited, if necessary, they are posted and automatically appear in the Transaction Entry dialog.

The Unprocessed Charges dialog box lists transactions that have been transmitted from Medisoft Clinical Patient Records, but have not yet been posted in Medisoft Network Professional (see Figure 9.32).

The Unprocessed Charges dialog box contains the following buttons:

Refresh Updates the main window with the most current data.

Edit Opens the selected transaction in the Unprocessed Transactions Edit window.

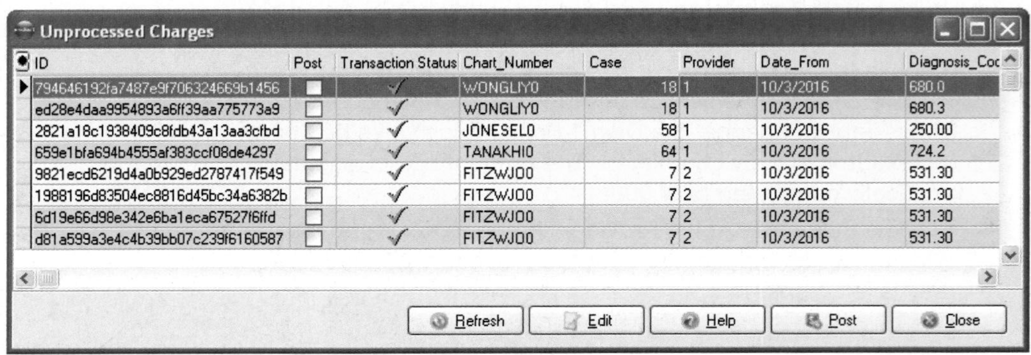

Figure 9.32 Unprocessed Charges Dialog Box

Help Accesses the Help system.

Post Posts the transaction to the patient's account.

Close Closes the window.

The columns in the dialog box correspond to information from Medisoft Clinical Patient Records. The information in all the columns must match the information in Medisoft Network Professional, or the transaction will not post correctly. For example, the patient's chart number, Social Security number, last name, and date of birth must be exact matches.

The Transaction Status column indicates whether the transaction has been validated by the program. A green check mark indicates that the transaction has been validated as ready to be posted. A yellow check mark indicates that the transaction may not post correctly due to a problem. When an attempt is made to post a transaction with a yellow check mark, a Transaction Warning dialog box is displayed (see Figure 9.33). A red X in the Transaction Status column indicates that the transaction contains an error that must be corrected before it can be posted. A transaction can be reviewed and changed by selecting it and clicking the Edit button, which opens the Unprocessed Transactions Edit dialog box.

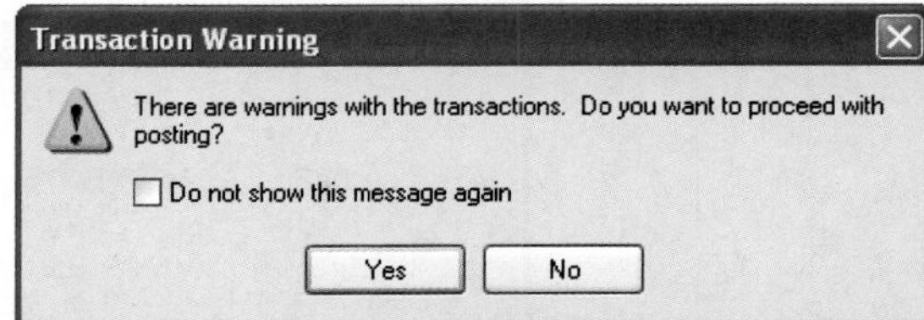

Figure 9.33 Transaction Warning Dialog Box

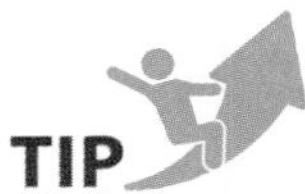

TIP

The unprocessed transaction can also be opened for editing by double clicking the entry.

The Unprocessed Transactions Edit dialog box is similar in appearance and content to the top two sections of the Transaction Entry dialog box (see Figure 9.34). Information such as the patient's chart number and case are listed, followed by transaction-specific data, including the date, procedure, units, amount, diagnosis, provider, and more.

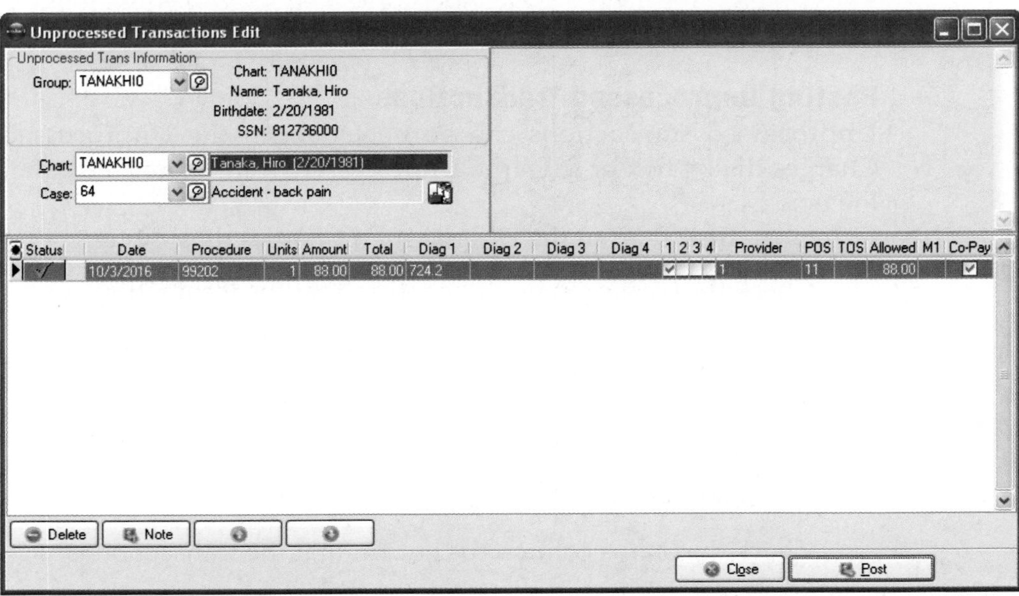

Figure 9.34 Unprocessed Transactions Edit Dialog Box

If a transaction contains errors, messages are displayed in red in the upper-right section of the dialog box. In the example in Figure 9.35, the case number and the diagnosis code do not exist in Medisoft Network Professional. Notice that the number listed in the Case field is zero. A new case can be created without leaving the Unprocessed Transactions Edit dialog box by clicking in the Case field and pressing the F8 key. The diagnosis code must be added to the database before the transactions can be posted, using the steps you learned earlier in this chapter.

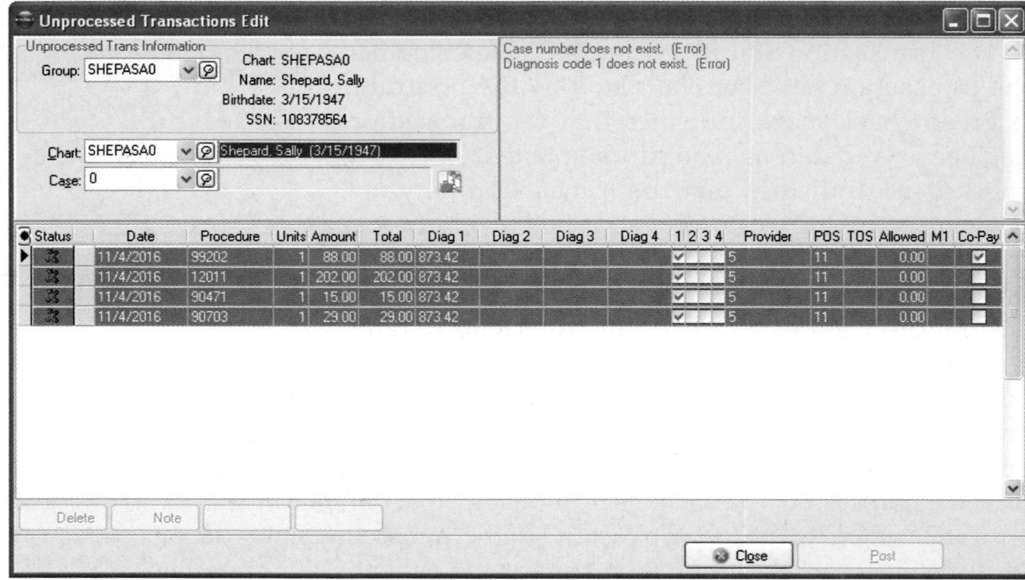

Figure 9.35 Unprocessed Transactions Edit Dialog Box with Errors

Once the errors have been corrected, the entry in the Status column changes from a red X to a green check mark, indicating that the transactions can be posted.

Posting Unprocessed Transactions

Unprocessed transactions can be posted from the Unprocessed Charges dialog box or from the Unprocessed Transactions Edit dialog box.

To post directly from the Unprocessed Charges dialog box:

1. Check the Status column to confirm that the transaction is ready to post.
2. Click the box in the Post column on the line that contains the transaction.
3. Click the Post button.

To post from the Unprocessed Transactions Edit dialog box:

1. Check the Status column to confirm that the transaction is ready to post.
2. Click the Post button.

Deleting Unprocessed Transactions

To delete an unprocessed transaction:

1. In the Unprocessed Charges dialog box, select the desired transaction and right-click the entry.
2. On the pop-up menu that appears, select Flag for Deletion. The Status column displays a trash can icon.
3. Right-click the entry, and select Delete Flagged Records on the pop-up menu.

connect plus+ EXERCISE 9.4

POSTING CHARGES FROM AN EHR, HIRO TANAKA

Review the information on Source Document 6 and the information listed in the Unprocessed Transactions Edit dialog box, and post the charges for Hiro Tanaka's office visit.

Date: October 3, 2016

1. Click the Activities menu. Click Unprocessed Transactions > Unprocessed EMR Charges. The Unprocessed Charges dialog box is displayed.
2. Click the entry for Tanaka in the list of unprocessed charges.
3. Click the Edit button to review the charges. The Unprocessed Transactions Edit dialog box opens.
4. After reviewing the charges, click the Post button. The charge disappears from the dialog box.
5. Click the Close button to close the dialog box. You are returned to the Unprocessed Charges dialog box. Notice that the charge no longer appears in the list.
6. Select Enter Transactions on the Activities menu to view the transaction you just entered.
7. Click in the Chart field, enter ***TA*** and press Enter to select Tanaka. An information box appears stating that Tanaka is allergic to penicillin. Click the OK button.
8. Tanaka's Accident—back pain case is displayed, with the charge you just posted.
9. Click the Close button to close the Transaction Entry dialog box.

You have completed Exercise 9.4

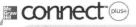

connect plus+ EXERCISE 9.5

POSTING CHARGES FROM AN EHR, JORGE BARRETT

Review the information on Source Document 7 and the information listed in the Unprocessed Transactions Edit dialog box, and post the charges for Jorge Barrett's office visit.

Date: October 21, 2016

(continued)

(Continued)

1. Click the first entry for Jorge Barrett in the list of unprocessed charges.
2. Click the Edit button to review the charges. The Unprocessed Transactions Edit dialog box opens.
3. After reviewing the charges, click the Post button. The charge disappears from the dialog box.
4. Click the Close button to close the dialog box. You are returned to the Unprocessed Charges dialog box.
5. Select Enter Transactions on the Activities menu to view the transaction you just entered.
6. Enter ***BA*** in the Chart field, and press Enter to select Barrett.
7. Barrett's hypertension case is displayed, with the charges you just posted.
8. Click the Close button to close the Transaction Entry dialog box.

You have completed Exercise 9.5

EXERCISE 9.6

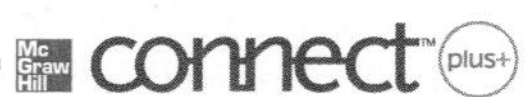

POSTING CHARGES FROM AN EHR, ELIZABETH JONES

Review the information on Source Document 8 and the information listed in the Unprocessed Transactions Edit dialog box, and post the charges from Elizabeth Jones's office visit.

Date: October 3, 2016

1. Click on the transaction for Jones in the list of unprocessed charges.
2. Click the Edit button to review the charges. The Unprocessed Transactions Edit dialog box opens.
3. After reviewing the charges, click the Post button. The charge disappears from the dialog box.
4. Click the Close button to close the dialog box. You are returned to the Unprocessed Charges dialog box.
5. Select Enter Transactions on the Activities menu to view the transaction you just entered.
6. Enter ***JO*** in the Chart field, and press Enter to select Jones.
7. Jones's diabetes case is displayed, with the charge you just posted.
8. Click the Close button to close the Transaction Entry dialog box.

You have completed Exercise 9.6

Connect Plus

EXERCISE 9.7

ADDING A MODIFIER TO A PROCEDURE BEFORE POSTING CHARGES TO AN EHR

Modifier –59 is used to indicate that two or more procedures are performed either at different anatomic sites (such as a separate lesion, site of incision, or injury) or at different patient encounters. Its use means that the physician expects to be reimbursed for both procedures, as they are separate and distinct.

The Medisoft Unprocessed Transactions Edit dialog box shows these two procedure codes for Li Y Wong:

11100 Biopsy of arm skin lesion
11641 Excision of face lesion

Since these two procedures have been done at separate anatomical sites, the addition of a –59 modifier to code 11100 is warranted to show a distinct procedural service.

Review the information on Source Document 9, add the modifier to procedure 11100, and post the charges for Li Y Wong's office visit.

Date: October 3, 2016

1. Click the first charge for Li Y Wong in the Unprocessed Charges dialog box, and then click the Edit button. The Unprocessed Transactions Edit dialog box opens.
2. Review the charges.
3. Locate the line that contains the charge for procedure 11100 click in the M1 field. Enter ***59.***
4. Click the Post button. The charge disappears from the dialog box.
5. Click the Close button to close the dialog box. You are returned to the Unprocessed Charges dialog box.
6. Select Enter Transactions on the Activities menu to view the transaction you just entered.
7. Enter ***WO*** in the Chart field. Notice that Jo Wong is selected. Click the entry for Li Y Wong.
8. Wong's boils case is displayed, with the charges you just posted, including the –59 modifier.
9. Click the Close button to close the Transaction Entry dialog box.

 **You have completed Exercise 9.7**

9.7 Posting Patient Time-of-Service Payments

In Chapter 5, you learned that upfront collections—payments collected before the patient leaves the office—are an important part of cash flow.

Types of Time-of-Service Payments

Practices routinely collect payment for the following types of charges at the time of service:

- Previous balances
- Copayments or coinsurance
- Noncovered or overlimit fees
- Charges of nonparticipating providers
- Charges for self-pay patients
- Deductibles for patients with consumer-driven health plans (CDHPs)

Depending on the practice's financial procedures, some charges may be collected at check-in before the encounter, and others may be collected during patient checkout.

Previous Balances

Practices routinely check their patient financial records and, if a balance is due, collect it at the time of service. The steps for this procedure are covered in Exercise 5.1 on page 228.

Copayments or Coinsurance

Copayments are always collected at the time of service. In some practices, they are collected before the encounter; in others, they are collected during checkout.

The amount of copayment that is due depends on the type of service and on whether the provider is in the patient's network. Copays for out-of-network providers are usually higher than for in-network providers. Specific copay amounts may be required for office visits to primary care providers or to specialists, and for lab work, radiology services such as X-rays, and surgery.

When patients receive more than one covered service in a single day, their health plan may permit multiple copayments. For example, copays for an annual physical exam and for lab tests may both be due from the patient. Review the terms of the policy to determine whether multiple copays should be collected on the same day of service.

Coinsurance

As health care costs have risen, employers have to pay more for their employees' medical benefit plans. As a result, employers are requiring employees to pay a larger share of those costs. Annual health insurance premiums are higher, deductibles are higher, and many employers have stopped requiring small fixed-amount copayments and have replaced them with coinsurance payments that are often due at the time of service.

Charges for Noncovered/Overlimit Services

Health plans require patients to pay for noncovered (excluded) services under their policies, and do not have any say about what the providers charge for the excluded services. Likewise, in managed care plans that set limits on the usage of certain covered services, patients are responsible for paying for visits beyond the allowed number. For example, if five physical therapy visits are permitted annually, the patient must pay for any additional visits. For this reason, practices usually collect these fees at the time of service.

Charges of Nonparticipating Providers

A patient who has an encounter with a provider who participates in the plan under which he or she has coverage—such as a Medicare-participating (PAR) provider—signs an assignment of benefits statement, as noted in Chapter 5. This authorizes the provider to **accept assignment** for the patient; that is, to file claims for the patient and receive payment directly from the health plan.

If the provider is a nonparticipating (nonPAR) provider, the procedure is usually different. To avoid problems collecting later on, most practices require the patient to pay in full at the time of services. If the patient does not wish to do this, the practice often requires the patient to assign benefits so that payment can be collected directly from the insurance plan by filing a claim.

accept assignment participating physician's agreement to accept allowed charge as full payment

self-pay patients patients with no medical insurance

real-time claim adjudication (RTCA) process used to contact health plans electronically to determine visit charges

Charges for Services to Self-Pay Patients

Patients who do not have insurance coverage are called **self-pay patients.** Since not all Americans have health insurance, self-pay patient office visits are a regular occurrence in most practices. Billers follow the practice's procedures for informing patients of their responsibility for paying their bills.

Deductibles for Patients with Consumer-Driven Health Plans (CDHPs)

Patients who have consumer-driven health plans must meet large deductibles before the health plans make payments. The practice is responsible for finding out whether the deductible has been met and, if not, for collecting the fee at the time of service.

Real-Time Claim Adjudication

The ideal tool for collecting at the time of service is known as **real-time claim adjudication (RTCA).** Offered by major health plans, RTCA is an Internet-based service that allows the practice to transmit the facts of the patient's visit, such as the demographics, the diagnosis and procedure codes, dates of service, and the provider's charges. The health plan transmits a response immediately (the meaning of "real time"), indicating the amount that the health plan will pay and the amount for which the patient is responsible.

The information transmitted by the health plan allows the practice to:

- Verify that the services are covered under the policy
- Learn whether the patient has met the annual deductible and, if not, collect it (if that is the policy)
- Know the patient's financial responsibility for the visit and collect it
- Provide the patient with an explanation of benefits from the health plan so that any questions the patient has about denial of coverage or payment history can be resolved immediately

Note that the RTCA does not generate a real-time payment; the payment usually follows within twenty-four hours.

Posting Payments Made at the Time of Service in Medisoft Network Professional

Patient payments made at the time of an office visit are entered in the Transaction Entry dialog box. Payments that are received electronically or by mail, such as insurance payments and mailed patient payments, are entered in the Deposit List dialog box, which is discussed in Chapter 11. The Deposit List feature is very efficient for entering large insurance payments that must be split up and applied to a number of different patients.

The first step when entering a patient payment is to select a patient's chart number and case number in the Transaction Entry dialog box. After the chart and case numbers have been selected, a payment transaction can be entered. Payments are entered in the Payments, Adjustments, And Comments section of the Transaction Entry dialog box (see Figure 9.36).

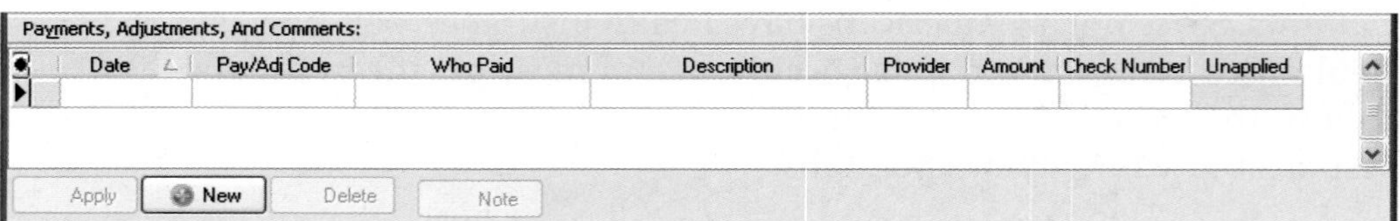

Figure 9.36 Payments, Adjustments, And Comments Area of the Transaction Entry Dialog Box

The process of creating a payment transaction begins with clicking the New button. When the New button is clicked, the program automatically enters the current date (the date that the Medisoft program date is set to) in the Date box (see Figure 9.37).

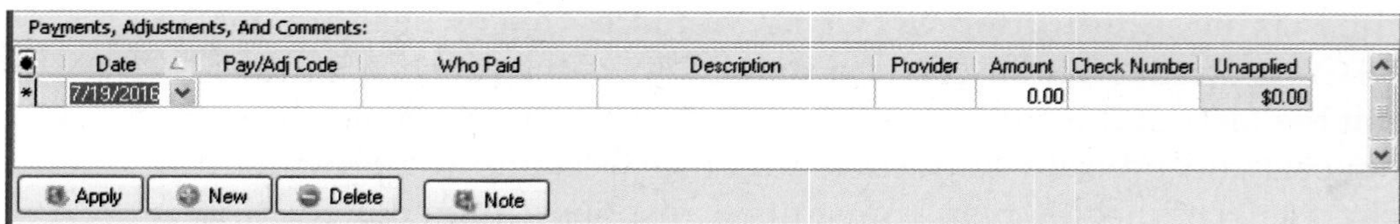

Figure 9.37 Payments, Adjustments, And Comments Area After Clicking the New Button

If this is not the date on which the payment was received, the date must be changed. To change the default date for these boxes, any of these methods can be used:

- The Set Program Date command on the File menu can be clicked.
- The Date button in the lower-right corner of the screen can be clicked. (This must be done before the New button is clicked in the Transaction Entry dialog box.)
- The date that is already in the Date box can be keyed over.

Pay/Adj Code Once the correct date is entered, pressing the Tab key moves the cursor to the Payment/Adjustment Code box. The code for a payment is selected from the drop-down list of payment codes already entered in the system (see Figure 9.38).

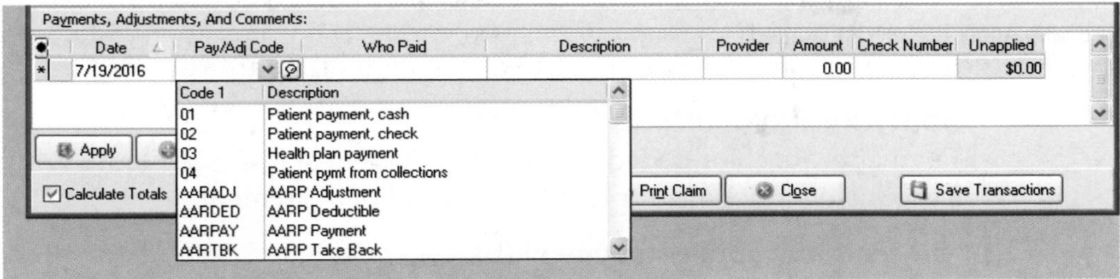

Figure 9.38 Payment/Adjustment Code Drop-down List

If a payment code is not listed, it can be added to the database by pressing the F8 key or by clicking Procedure/Payment/Adjustment Codes on the Lists menu. This may be done without exiting the Transaction Entry dialog box.

Who Paid After the code is selected and the Tab key is pressed, the program automatically completes the Who Paid box based on information stored in the database (see Figure 9.39). The Who Paid field displays a drop-down list of guarantors and carriers that are assigned in the patient case folder.

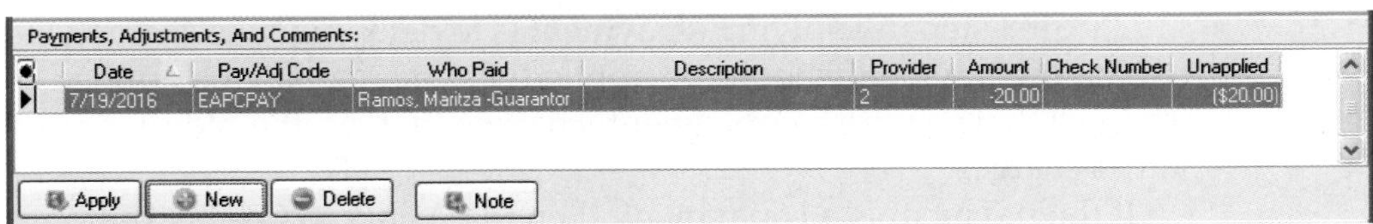

Figure 9.39 Payments, Adjustments, And Comments Area After Payment/Adjustment Code Is Entered

Description The Description field can be used to enter other information about the payment, if desired.

Provider The Provider column lists the code number of the provider.

Amount The Amount field contains the amount of payment received. If the payment is a copayment from a patient, this box is completed automatically when a payment/adjustment code is selected. Again, the program uses information stored in the database.

Check Number The Check Number field is used to record the number of the check used for payment.

Unapplied The dollar value in the Unapplied box is the amount that has not yet been applied to a charge transaction.

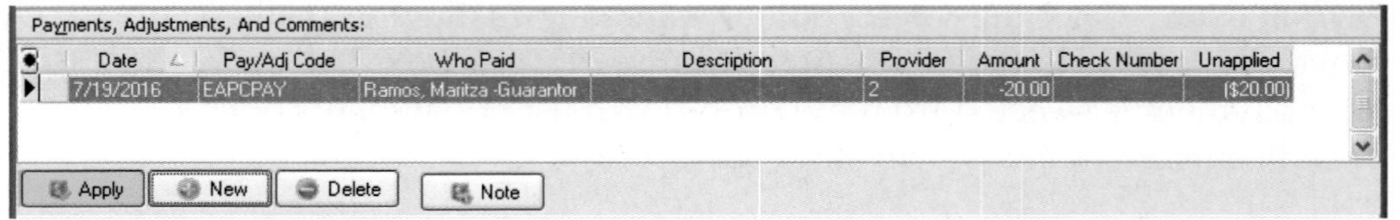

Figure 9.40 Payments, Adjustments, And Comments Area with a Color-Coded Unapplied Payment and with Apply Button Highlighted

Applying Payments to Charges

Payments are color-coded to indicate payment status (see Figure 9.40). Three color codes are applied to the status of a payment:

1. Partially applied payment (blue)
2. Unapplied payment (red)
3. Overapplied payment (pink)

Payments that have been fully applied are not colored and appear white.

Once all the necessary information is entered, it is time to apply the payment to specific charges. This is accomplished by clicking the Apply button, which causes the Apply Payment to Charges dialog box to be displayed. The Apply Payment to Charges dialog box lists information about all unpaid charges for a patient, including the date of the procedure, the document number, the procedure code, the charge, the balance, and the total amount paid (see Figure 9.41).

In the upper-right corner of the dialog box, the amount of the payment that has not yet been applied to charges is listed in the Unapplied box.

The first step in applying a payment is to determine the charge(s) to which the payment should be applied. Payments may be applied to charges that require a copayment, charges that are the oldest, or any other charges.

If the payment is a copayment, then the Apply to Co-pay button is clicked. When the Apply to Co-pay button is clicked, the program automatically applies the payment to the charge on that date that requires a copayment. Information about whether a procedure code requires a copayment is located in the General tab of the Procedure/Payment/Adjustment dialog box for that code. In the exercises in this text/workbook, copayments are required for evaluation and management codes—procedure codes that cover physicians' services performed to determine the optimum course for patient care.

If the payment should be applied to the oldest charge, the Apply to Oldest button is clicked. When the Apply to Oldest button is used, the program automatically applies the payment to the oldest charge.

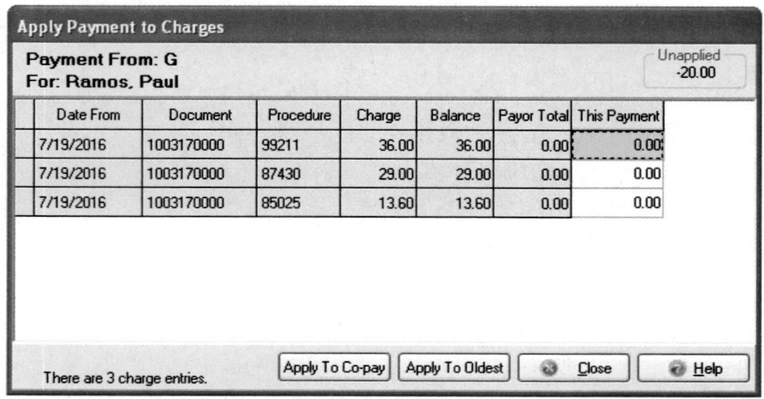

Figure 9.41 Apply Payment to Charges Dialog Box with This Payment Box Highlighted

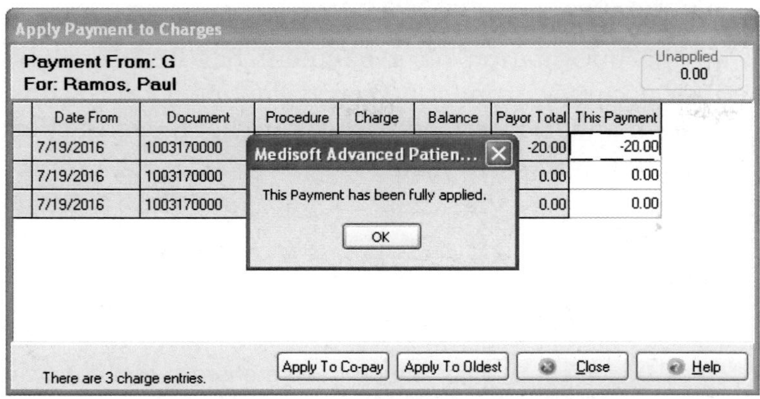

Figure 9.42 Apply Payment to Charges Dialog Box with Payment Entered

Payments may also be manually applied by clicking in the box in the This Payment column on the line that contains the charge. Clicking in the box causes a dotted rectangle to appear around the outside of the box. Enter the amount of the payment (without a decimal point), and press the Enter key. The payment is applied, and the Unapplied Amount entry is lowered by the amount of the payment.

Notice in Figure 9.42 that the payment amount has been entered in the appropriate This Payment box.

A payment can be applied to more than one charge. For example, suppose that the payment is $200.00 and that three charges have not been paid. The $200.00 payment can be applied to one, two, or all three of the charges.

Once the Apply Payment to Charges dialog box is closed, the payment appears in the Payments, Adjustments, And Comments area of the Transaction Entry dialog box (see Figure 9.43).

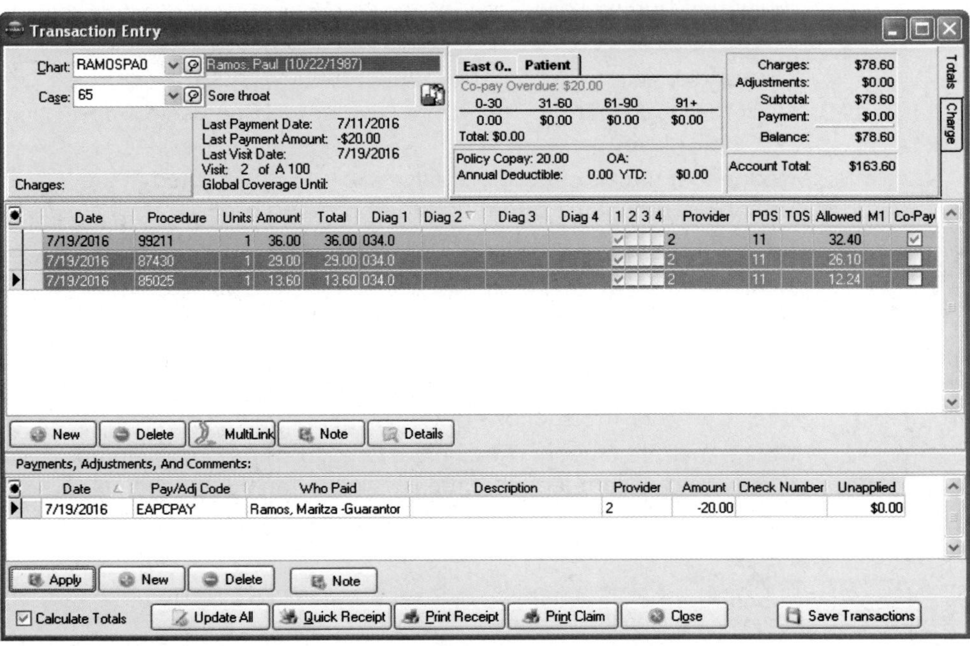

Figure 9.43 Payments, Adjustments, And Comments Area with Payment Listed and Charges Color-Coded as Partially Paid (Aqua) and No Payment (Gray)

Saving Payment Information

When all the information on a payment has been entered and checked for accuracy, it must be saved. Payment transactions are saved in the manner described earlier for charge transactions, by clicking the Save Transactions button.

EXERCISE 9.8

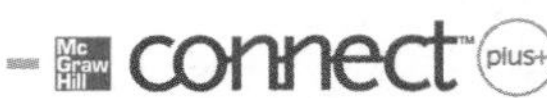

ENTERING A COPAYMENT, JOHN FITZWILLIAMS

Using Source Document 5, enter the procedure charges and copayment for John Fitzwilliams's October 3, 2016, visit.

Date: October 3, 2016

1. Click Enter Transactions on the Activities menu to open the Transaction Entry dialog box.
2. Click in the Chart box, and key ***FI*** and press Enter.
3. Verify that Acute gastric ulcer is the active case in the Case box.
4. Notice that there are already charges and payments listed for this case, since this is an existing medical condition for which the patient has been treated in the past.
5. Click the New button in the Payments, Adjustments, And Comments section of the dialog box.
6. Accept the default entry of 10/3/2016 in the Date box.
7. Click in the Pay/Adj Code box. From the drop-down list, select CHVCPAY (the code for CHAMPVA copayment), and press Tab. You will need to scroll down the list to locate the code. Notice that some of the boxes have been completed by the program.
8. Verify that Fitzwilliams, John—Guarantor is listed in the Who Paid box.
9. Notice that –15.00 has already been entered in the Amount box. Confirm that this is the correct amount of the copay by looking at Source Document 5.
10. The Unapplied Amount box should read ($15.00).
11. Click in the Check Number box, enter ***456,*** and press Tab.
12. Click the Apply button. The Apply Payment to Charges dialog box is displayed.
13. Notice that the amount of this payment (–15.00) is listed in the Unapplied box at the upper-right of the dialog box.
14. Click the Apply to Co-pay button. When the box appears that states "This payment has been fully applied," click OK.
15. Notice that –15.00 has been entered on the line for procedure code 99212, since this is the evaluation and management code for this visit.
16. Click the Close button.
17. Click the Save Transactions button.
18. Notice that the amount listed in the Unapplied Amount column is now zero. Also notice that the line listing the 99212 charge on 10/3/2016 is now aqua rather than gray, indicating that the charge has been partially paid.

You have completed Exercise 9.8

ENTERING A COPAYMENT, HIRO TANAKA

Enter the $20.00 copayment that Hiro Tanaka made while checking out. She paid with check number 123.

Date: October 3, 2016

1. Click Enter Transactions on the Activities menu.
2. In the Chart box, enter ***TA,*** and press Enter. An Information box is displayed with information about Tanaka's allergies. Click the OK button.
3. Verify that Accident—back pain is the active case in the Case box.
4. Click the New button in the Payments, Adjustments, And Comments section of the dialog box.
5. Accept the default entry of 10/3/2016 in the Date box.
6. Click in the Pay/Adj Code box. From the drop-down list, select OHCCPAY (the code for OhioCare HMO copayment), And press Tab. Notice that some of the boxes have been completed by the program.
7. Verify that Tanaka, Hiro—Guarantor is listed in the Who Paid box.
8. Notice that –20.00 has already been entered in the Amount box. Confirm that this is the correct amount of the copay by looking at Source Document 1.
9. The Unapplied Amount box should read ($20.00).
10. Click in the Check Number box, enter ***123***, and press Tab.
11. Click the Apply button. The Apply Payment to Charges dialog box is displayed.
12. Notice that the amount of this payment (–20.00) is listed in the Unapplied box at the upper-right of the dialog box.
13. Click the Apply to Co-pay button. When the box appears that states "This payment has been fully applied," click OK. The program automatically enters –20.00 in the box in the This Payment column for the 99202 procedure charge.
14. Click the Close button.
15. Click the Save Transactions button. Notice that the line listing the procedure charge has changed from gray (not paid) to aqua (partially paid), indicating that a portion of the charge has been paid.

You have completed Exercise 9.9

9.8 Creating Walkout Receipts

After a patient payment has been entered in the Transaction Entry dialog box, a walkout receipt is printed and given to the patient before he or she leaves the office. A **walkout receipt,** also known as a walkout statement, includes information on the procedures, diagnosis, charges,

walkout receipt report that lists the diagnoses, services provided, fees, and payments received and due after an encounter

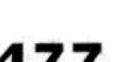

and payments for a visit. If there is a balance due, the receipt reminds the patient about the amount owed.

Receipt Options in the Transaction Entry Dialog Box

In the Transaction Entry dialog box, a walkout receipt is created via the Quick Receipt or Print Receipt buttons (see Figure 9.44). The Quick Receipt option remembers the user's preferred report format and eliminates several steps in the creation of a receipt. (*Note*: A Print Claim button also appears in the Transaction Entry dialog box; claim management is discussed in detail in Chapter 10.)

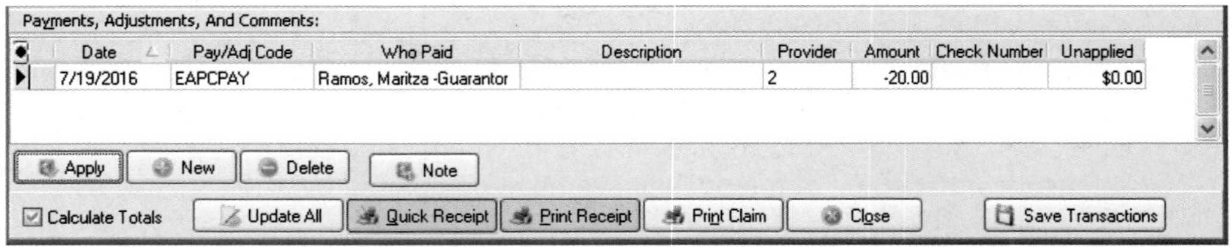

Figure 9.44 Quick Receipt and Print Receipt Buttons Highlighted in Yellow

When the Print Receipt button is clicked, the Open Report window appears with the first report highlighted, Walkout Receipt (All Transactions), as shown in Figure 9.45.

After clicking the OK button in the Open Report window, the Print Report Where? dialog box is displayed, and three options are provided (see Figure 9.46):

1. Preview the report on the screen
2. Print the report on the printer
3. Export the report to a file

Once a printing choice is made, clicking the Start button causes the Data Selection Questions window to open (see Figure 9.47). This is where the data for the receipt are selected.

Finally, when the OK button is clicked, the report is sent to its destination (on screen, to the printer, or to a file; see Figure 9.48).

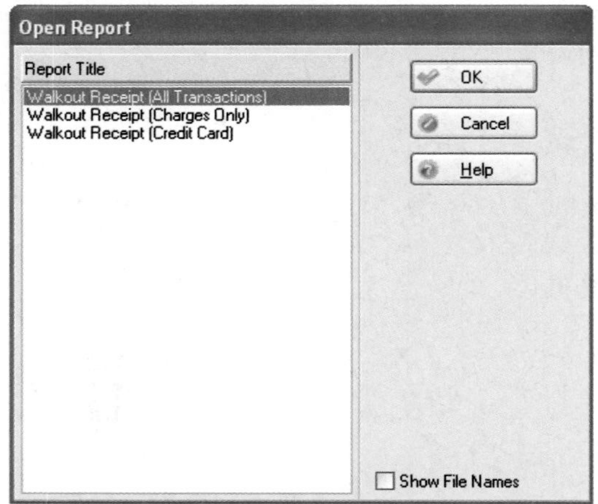

Figure 9.45 Open Report Window with Walkout Receipt (All Transactions) Selected

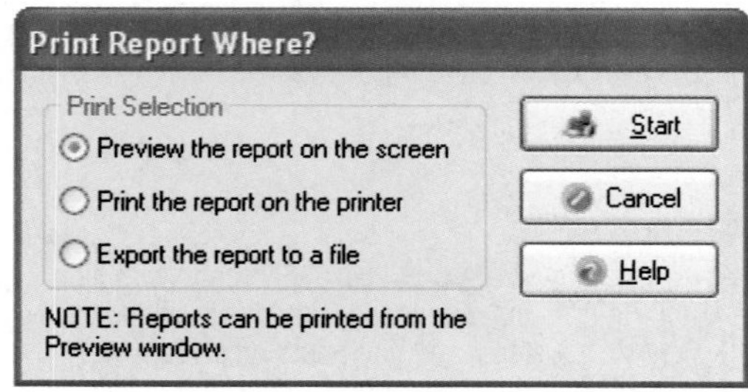

Figure 9.46 Print Report Where? Dialog Box

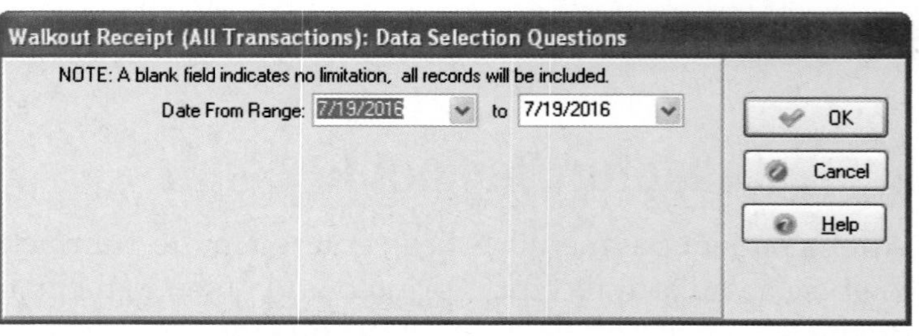

Figure 9.47 Data Selection Questions Window

Family Care Clinic
285 Stephenson Boulevard
Stephenson, OH 60089
(614)555-0000

Page: 1 7/19/2016

Patient: Paul Ramos
39 Locust Avenue
Stephenson, OH 60089

Chart #: RAMOSPA0
Case #: 65

Instructions:
Complete the patient information portion of your insurance claim form. Attach this bill, signed and dated, and all other bills pertaining to the claim. If you have a deductible policy, hold your claim forms until you have met your deductible. Mail directly to your insurance carrier.

Date	Description	Procedure	Modify	Dx 1	Dx 2	Dx 3	Dx 4	Units	Charge
7/19/2016	OF--established patient, minimal	99211		034.0				1	36.00
7/19/2016	Strep test	87430		034.0				1	29.00
7/19/2016	Complete CBC w/auto diff WBC	85025		034.0				1	13.60
7/19/2016	East Ohio PPO Copayment	EAPCPAY						1	-20.00

Provider Information
Provider Name: John Rudner MD
License: 84701
Insurance PIN:
SSN or EIN: 339-67-5000

Total Charges:	$ 78.60
Total Payments:	-$ 20.00
Total Adjustments:	$ 0.00
Total Due This Visit:	**$ 58.60**
Total Account Balance:	$ 143.60

Assign and Release: I hereby authorize payment of medical benefits to this physician for the services described above. I also authorize the release of any information necessary to process this claim.

Patient Signature: ______________________ Date: __________

Figure 9.48 Sample Walkout Receipt

connect plus+ — EXERCISE 9.10

CREATING A WALKOUT RECEIPT, JOHN FITZWILLIAMS

Open John Fitzwilliams's acute gastric ulcer case, and create a walkout receipt for his copayment of $15.00.

Date: October 3, 2016

1. Click in the Chart field. Enter ***FI*** and press Enter.
2. Verify that Acute gastric ulcer is the active case in the Case box.
3. Click the Quick Receipt button. The Print Report Where? dialog box is displayed.
4. In the Print Report Where? dialog box, accept the default selection to preview the report on the screen.
5. Click the Start button. The Preview Report window opens, displaying the walkout receipt.
6. Review the charge and payment entries listed in the top half of the receipt.

(continued)

(Continued)

7. Scroll down and review the total charges, payments, and adjustments listed in the lower-right area of the receipt.
8. Notice that a button with a printer icon is displayed at the top of the Preview Report window. In an office setting, you would click this button to send the receipt to the printer.
9. Click the Close button to exit the Preview Report window.

 **You have completed Exercise 9.10**

EXERCISE 9.11

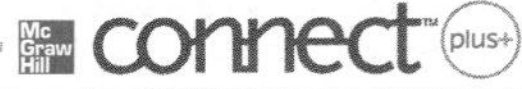

CREATING A WALKOUT RECEIPT, HIRO TANAKA

Open Hiro Tanaka's Accident—back pain case, and create a walkout receipt for her copayment of $20.00.

Date: October 3, 2016

1. Click in the Chart field, enter ***TA,*** and press Enter. An Information box is displayed with information about Tanaka's allergies. Click the OK button.
2. Verify that Accident—back pain is the active case in the Case box.
3. Click the Quick Receipt button. The Print Report Where? dialog box is displayed.
4. In the Print Report Where? dialog box, accept the default selection to preview the report on the screen.
5. Click the Start button. The Preview Report window opens, displaying the walkout receipt.
6. Review the charge and payment entries listed in the top half of the receipt.
7. Scroll down and review the total charges, payments, and adjustments listed in the lower-right area of the receipt.
8. Notice that a button with a printer icon is displayed at the top of the Preview Report window. In an office setting, you would click this button to send the receipt to the printer.
9. Click the Close button to exit the Preview Report window.

 **You have completed Exercise 9.11**

9.9 Printing Patient Education Materials

If the physician has ordered patient education materials to be given to the patient, these items are handled during checkout. For example, it may be appropriate to provide materials to help patients

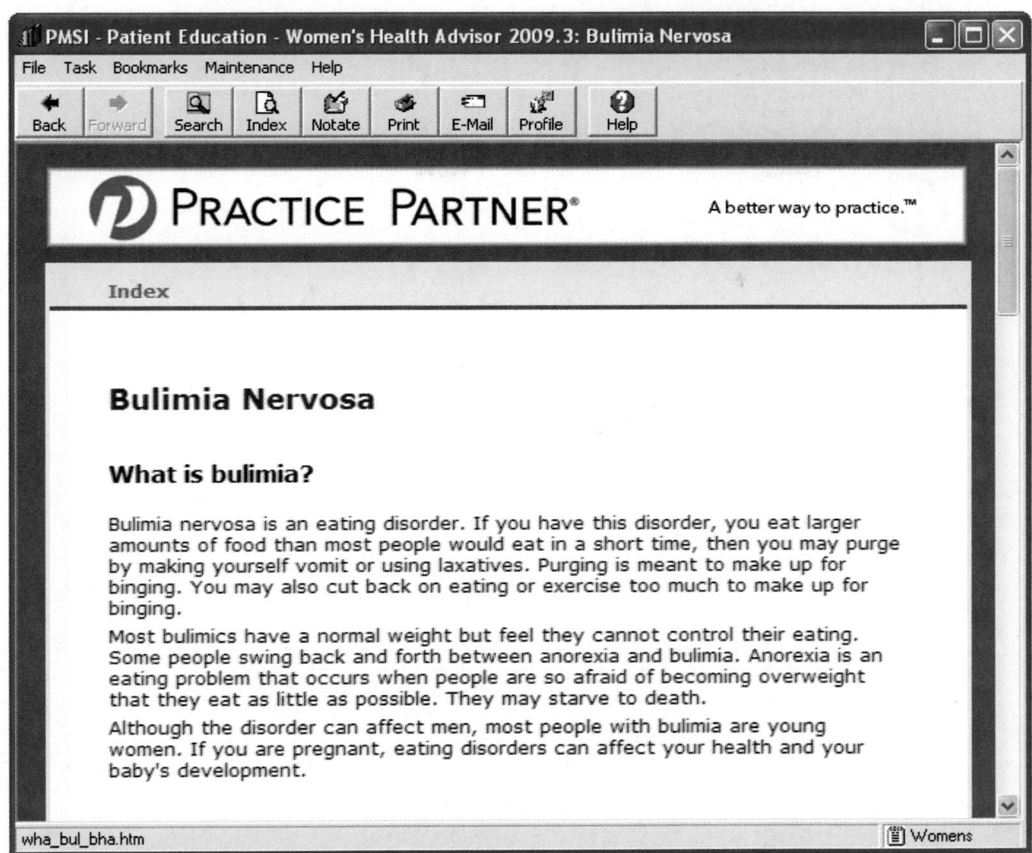

Figure 9.49 Sample Patient Education Article

better understand their diagnoses and treatments, or to provide instructions following an office procedure.

The patient education feature of MCPR provides a built-in set of patient education articles that can be printed and given to patients. The program automatically selects the appropriate education module for patients, taking into account a patient's age, sex, and diagnosis if desired. There are different sets of articles for pediatrics, adults, seniors, women, and behavioral health. The articles can either be printed or be sent by e-mail. A sample article is illustrated in Figure 9.49.

Many of the articles are available in Spanish as well as English. To select articles in Spanish, click Spanish on the main page of the education module (see Figure 9.50). Articles listed with an asterisk after the title in the English index also have Spanish-language versions.

When a patient's chart is open, the patient education articles are accessed by clicking the Pt Ed button on the toolbar. If no chart is open, the patient education articles can be accessed by clicking Patient Education on the Task menu.

The Patient Education Window

The patient education feature in MCPR opens in its own window, with its own menu and toolbar. The buttons on the toolbar, pictured

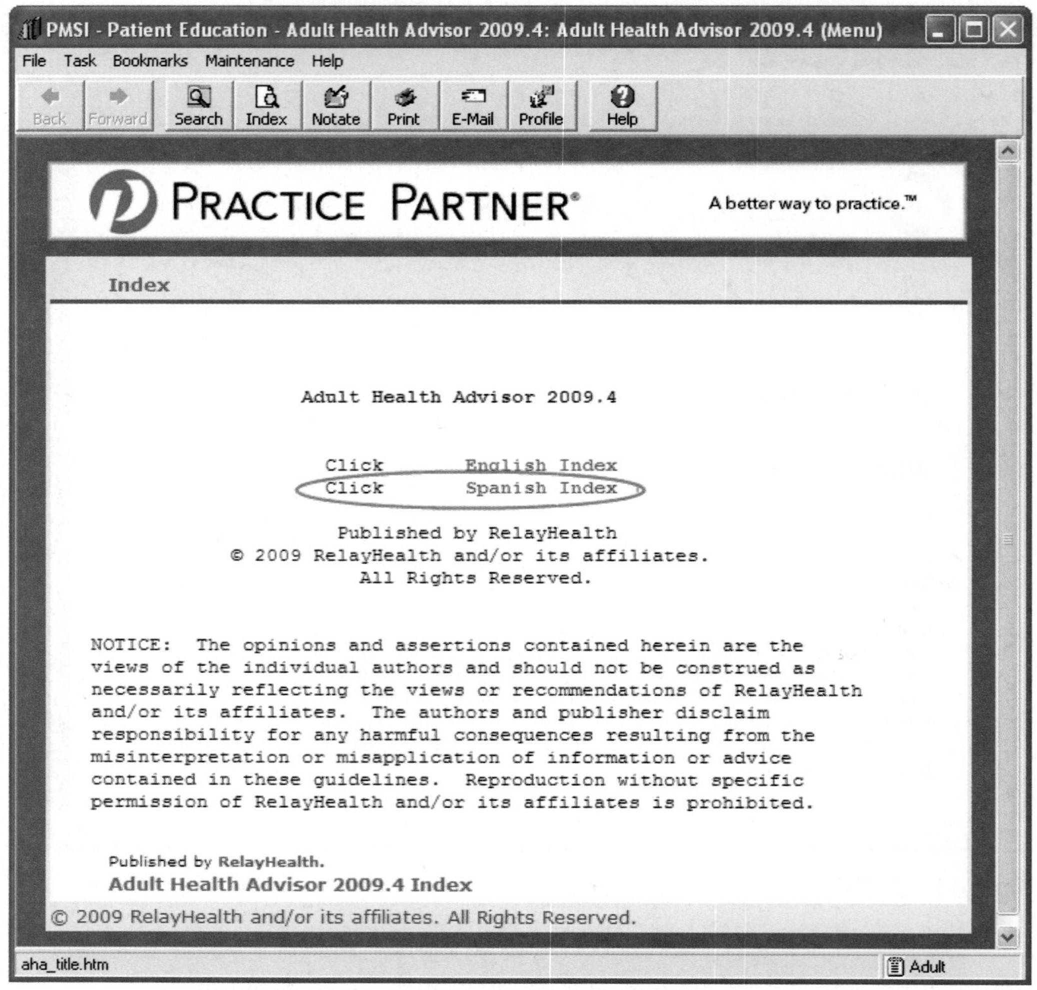

Figure 9.50 Main Page of Patient Education with Spanish Index Circled

in Figure 9.51, are used to move around in the article database:

Back, Forward Moves forward one page or back one page in the database

Search Displays the Search dialog box

Index Displays the main patient education screen, from which an English or Spanish index can be selected

Notate Attaches a note to a handout

Print Sends an article to the printer

E-Mail E-mails an article to a patient

Profile Shows and/or changes patient profile

Help Displays the education help file

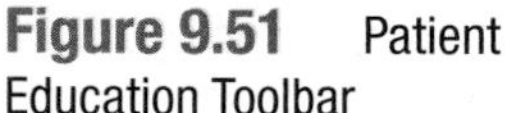

Figure 9.51 Patient Education Toolbar

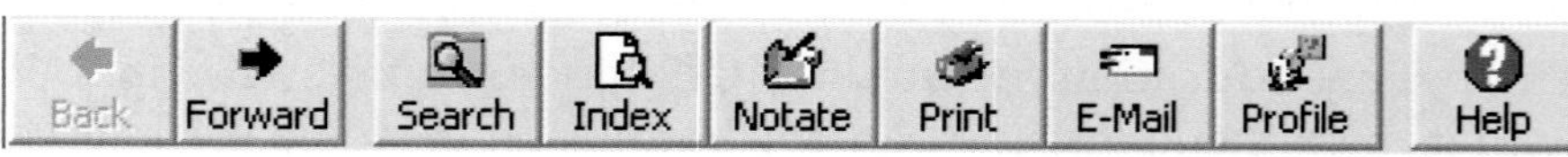

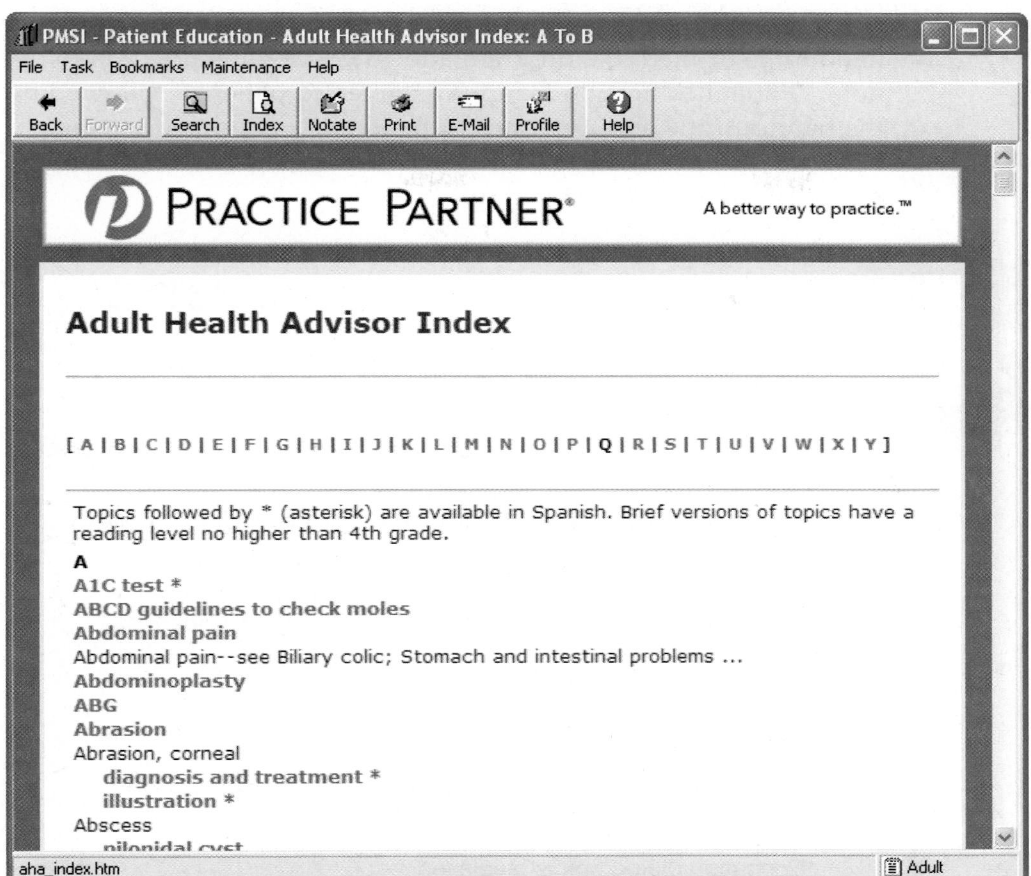

Figure 9.52 Patient Education Index Page

Using the Patient Education Index

To view the patient education index, select Index on the Task menu, click the Index button on the toolbar, or click English Index or Spanish Index on the main window. Once in the index, click on a letter from *A* through *Y* to display a list of topics for that letter (see Figure 9.52). In the list, category headings or cross-references are listed in black, and clickable articles are listed in blue. The blue type appears underlined when the mouse moves over it, just like a link on a website.

Searching for an Article

The patient education feature has a built-in search option. To view the Search dialog box, select Search on the Task menu, or click the Search button on the toolbar (see Figure 9.53).

To search for a topic:

1. In the box next to Search, type a topic or a description of the topic.
2. Click Search. The first topic that contains the description is highlighted in the topic box.
3. If the first highlighted topic is not the appropriate selection, click Search again to go to the next related topic.
4. Once you locate the desired topic, click the topic to display the handout.

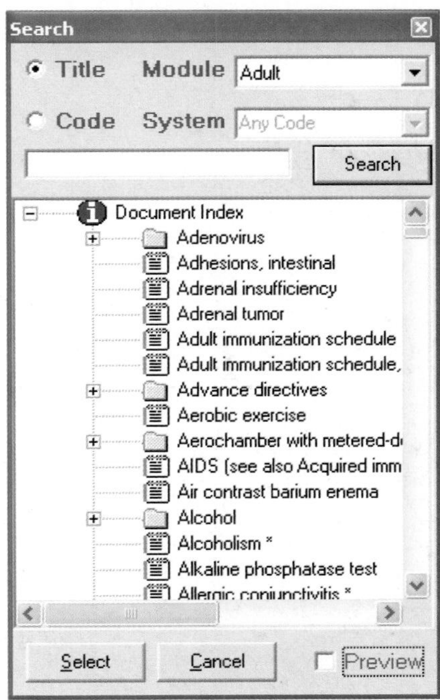

Figure 9.53 Patient Education Search Dialog Box

If the patient has a progress note created the same day that the handout is printed, the program adds the following notation to the note: "Patient Education Hand-outs given to patient," followed by the handout title and the time the handout was printed for the patient. In addition, the patient's name, ID, sex, age, and the date are printed at the top of the handout.

EXERCISE 9.12

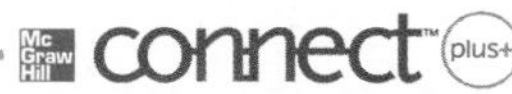

PRINTING PATIENT EDUCATION MATERIALS AT CHECKOUT

Using Source Document 3, prepare to send the two patient education articles to the printer. These will be given to the patient at checkout.

1. Click Start > All Programs > Medisoft Clinical—Client > Medisoft Clinical Client to open Medisoft Clinical Patient Records.
2. Log in as the medical assistant by entering ***MEDASST*** in the User ID field and ***master1$*** in the Password field. Click OK.
3. Click OK when the Disclaimer window appears.
4. Click the Chart button on the toolbar.
5. Enter ***BA*** in the Last Name field in the Patient Lookup dialog box.
6. Click the Lookup button.
7. With Jorge Barrett highlighted, click the OK button. Barrett's chart opens.
8. Click the Pt Ed button on the toolbar. The PMSI—Patient Education dialog box is displayed.
9. Click the Search button on the toolbar in the PMSI—Patient Education dialog box. The Search dialog box appears.
10. In the field to the left of the word Search, enter ***hypertension.***
11. Click the Search button. The section of the list that contains the entry for hypertension is displayed. Notice that the entry is a folder rather than a single article.
12. Click the plus sign to the left of the hypertension entry. A subset of entries appears. Scroll down to view all the subentries.
13. Click on the entry for essential (unknown cause).
14. Click the Select button. The article appears.
15. Review the buttons on the toolbar. Clicking the Print button sends the article to the printer. Alternatively, the E-Mail button is used to send the article to a patient via e-mail. Since you do not need to print or e-mail the article in this exercise, do not click either button.
16. To print or e-mail the second article, click the words Related topics above the article for high blood pressure. A list of related articles appears.
17. Click the entry for low-sodium diet. The low-sodium diet article appears. Again, the toolbar offers options for printing or e-mailing the article. Again, do not click either button.
18. Click the Close box at the top-right corner of the dialog box to close the PMSI—Patient Education dialog box.

 **You have completed Exercise 9.12**

chapter 9 summary

LEARNING OUTCOME	KEY CONCEPTS/EXAMPLES
9.1 List the six steps in the charge capture process. Pages 430–434	1. Access encounter data. 2. Audit coding compliance. 3. Review billing compliance. 4. Post charges. 5. Calculate, collect, and post time-of-service payments. 6. Check out patient.
9.2 Explain the purpose of auditing diagnosis and procedure code assignment. Pages 434–443	Diagnosis and procedure code assignment is audited to ensure that codes are current and correct and to ensure that the practice will receive the maximum appropriate reimbursement. The audit checks for code linkage to demonstrate medical necessity, showing that treatment was in accordance with generally accepted standards of medical practice; was clinically appropriate in terms of type, frequency, extent, site, and duration; and was not done primarily for the convenience of the patient, physician, or other health care provider.
9.3 Discuss the effect of health plans' rules on billing. Pages 443–447	Health plans' rules govern what will and will not be covered. The practice follows these rules so that the practice and the health plan have the same expectations for the payment that will be made. Not following the rules may appear to be intentional fraud and can lead to delays in processing claims and receiving payments, reduced payments. denied claims, fines and other sanctions, loss of hospital privileges, exclusion from health plans' programs, loss of the physician's license to practice medicine, and even prison sentences.
9.4 Describe the use of CPT/HCPCS modifiers to communicate billing information to health plans. Pages 447–451	A CPT/HCPCS modifier is a two-digit number that may be attached to most five-digit procedure codes. It is used to communicate special circumstances involved with a procedure, telling the health plan that the physician considers the procedure to have been altered in some way. A modifier usually affects the normal level of reimbursement for the code to which it is attached.
9.5 Discuss strategies to avoid common coding/billing errors. Pages 451–453	The following strategies can help a practice avoid common coding and billing errors: - Carefully define bundled codes and know global periods. - Use modifiers appropriately. - Follow the practice's compliance plan, especially the guidelines about physician queries.

LEARNING OUTCOME	KEY CONCEPTS/EXAMPLES
9.6 Explain the difference between posting charges from a paper encounter form and posting charges from an electronic encounter form. Pages 453–469	To post charges from a paper encounter form, the medical assistant must look for the relevant information on the form and type it into the program. By contrast, transactions from an EHR do not need to be manually posted in the Transaction Entry dialog box. After a patient visit has been documented in Medisoft Clinical Patient Records and the procedures and diagnoses have been reviewed on the electronic encounter form, the encounter data are transmitted to Medisoft Network Professional, where they are reviewed by a member of the billing staff. Once the charges have been reviewed and edited, if necessary, they are electronically posted and automatically appear in the Transaction Entry dialog.
9.7 Identify the types of payments that may be collected following a patient's visit. Pages 469–476	The following payments may be collected following a patient's visit: - Previous balances - Copayments or coinsurance - Noncovered or overlimit fees - Charges of nonparticipating providers - Charges for self-pay patients - Deductibles for patients with consumer-driven health plans
9.8 Identify the steps needed to create walkout receipts. Pages 476–480	The following steps are needed to create a walkout receipt from within the Transaction Entry dialog box: 1. In the Chart box, click the entry for the patient. 2. Select the relevant case in the Case box. 3. Click the Quick Receipt button. The Print Report Where? dialog box is displayed. 4. In the Print Report Where? dialog box, select whether to preview the report on the screen, print it, or export it to a file. 5. Click the Start button.
9.9 Describe use of a patient education feature in an electronic health record. Pages 480–484	The patient education feature in an EHR makes it possible to provide materials to help patients better understand their diagnoses and treatments, or to provide instructions following an office procedure. MCPR's patient education feature includes patient education articles in English and Spanish that can be printed and given to patients. The program automatically selects the appropriate education module for patients, taking into account their age, sex, and diagnosis if desired. There are different sets of articles for pediatrics, adults, seniors, women, and behavioral health. The articles can either be printed or be sent by e-mail.

chapter review

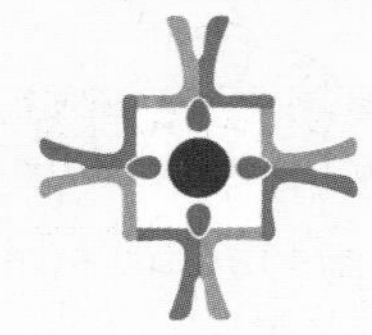

MATCHING QUESTIONS

Match the key terms with their definitions.

_____ 1. ***[LO 9.4]*** modifier
_____ 2. ***[LO 9.1]*** adjustments
_____ 3. ***[LO 9.3]*** unbundling
_____ 4. ***[LO 9.2]*** code linkage
_____ 5. ***[LO 9.1]*** charge capture
_____ 6. ***[LO 9.3]*** compliant billing
_____ 7. ***[LO 9.5]*** query
_____ 8. ***[LO 9.4]*** CCI modifier indicators
_____ 9. ***[LO 9.3]*** global period
_____ 10. ***[LO 9.3]*** bundled code

a. Billing actions that satisfy official requirements.
b. Two or more related procedure codes combined into one.
c. The process of recording billable services.
d. A number appended to a code to report particular facts.
e. Changes to a patient's account.
f. The numbers showing if the use of a modifier can bypass a CCI.
g. The days surrounding a surgical procedure when all services relating to the procedure are considered part of the surgical package.
h. A request for more information from a provider.
i. The incorrect billing practice of breaking a panel or package of services/procedures into component.
j. The clinically appropriate connection between a provided service and a patient's condition or illness.

TRUE-FALSE QUESTIONS

Decide whether each statement is true or false.

_____ 1. ***[LO 9.6]*** In Medisoft, the Unprocessed Charges window displays transactions transmitted from the EHR program that have already been posted in Medisoft.

_____ 2. ***[LO 9.7]*** Patients who do not have insurance coverage are called self-pay patients.

_____ 3. ***[LO 9.4]*** A modifier usually affects the normal level of reimbursement for the code to which it is attached.

_____ 4. ***[LO 9.9]*** In Medisoft Clinical Patient Records, some patient education handouts are available in English and in Spanish.

_____ 5. ***[LO 9.7]*** Payments are entered in two different areas of the Medisoft program: the Transaction Entry dialog box, and the Deposit List dialog box.

_____ 6. ***[LO 9.7]*** The amount of copayment that is due depends on whether the provider is in the patient's network and on the type of service.

_____ 7. ***[LO 9.3]*** Noncompliant billing refers to following these rules so that the practice and the health plan have the same expectations for the payment that will be made.

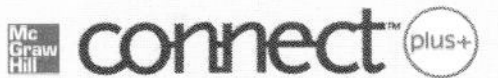

Enhance your learning at **mcgrawhillconnect.com**!
- *Practice Exercises*
- *Worksheets*
- *Activities*
- *Integrated eBook*

_____ 8. ***[LO 9.3]*** CCI edits apply to claims that bill for more than one procedure performed on the same patient, on the same date of service, by the same performing provider.

_____ 9. ***[LO 9.8]*** Walkout receipts include only information on the procedures and diagnosis for a patient visit.

_____ 10. ***[LO 9.2]*** PM/EHRs typically have a capability called claim scrubbing.

MULTIPLE-CHOICE QUESTIONS

Select the letter that best completes the statement or answers the question.

1. ***[LO 9.1]*** _________ are changes to patients' accounts.
   a. charges
   b. modifiers
   c. payments
   d. adjustments

2. ***[LO 9.1]*** _________ are the amounts a provider bills for the services performed.
   a. charges
   b. modifiers
   c. payments
   d. adjustments

3. ***[LO 9.1]*** _________ are monies received from patients and insurance carriers.
   a. charges
   b. modifiers
   c. payments
   d. adjustments

4. ***[LO 9.2]*** _________ describes the connection between a procedure code and the related diagnosis code(s).
   a. charge capture
   b. code linkage
   c. unbundling
   d. compliant billing

5. ***[LO 9.3]*** _________ is the incorrect billing practice of breaking a panel or package of services/procedures into component parts.
   a. charge capture
   b. code linkage
   c. unbundling
   d. compliant billing

6. ***[LO 9.3]*** _________ refers to following billing rules so that the practice and the health plan have the same expectations for the payment that will be made.
   a. charge capture
   b. code linkage
   c. unbundling
   d. compliant billing

7. ***[LO 9.1]*** _________ is the process of recording billable services.
   a. charge capture
   b. code linkage
   c. unbundling
   d. compliant billing

8. ***[LO 9.6]*** ________ are groups of procedure code entries that relate to a single activity.
   a. bundled codes
   b. MultiLink codes
   c. modifiers
   d. packages
9. ***[LO 9.3]*** A ________ is a group of related procedures and/or services included under a single code.
   a. bundled code
   b. MultiLink code
   c. modifier
   d. package
10. ***[LO 9.4]*** A ________ is a number appended to a code to report particular facts.
   a. bundled code
   b. MultiLink code
   c. modifier
   d. package

SHORT-ANSWER QUESTIONS

Define the following abbreviations.

1. ***[LO 9.7]*** RTCA ____________________
2. ***[LO 9.3]*** MUE ____________________
3. ***[LO 9.3]*** MEC ____________________
4. ***[LO 9.3]*** CCI ____________________
5. ***[LO 9.5]*** POS ____________________

APPLYING YOUR KNOWLEDGE

Answer the questions below in the space provided.

9.1 ***[LO 9.1]*** List the six steps in the charge capture process in order.

____

9.2 ***[LO 9.2]*** Why do you think it is important that the ICD-9-CM code set be revised twice annually?

____

9.3 ***[LO 9.2]*** How does the process of claim scrubbing help a medical practice?

____

9.4 ***[LO 9.3]*** Why is it important for medical practices to follow the practice of compliant billing?

____

chapter 10

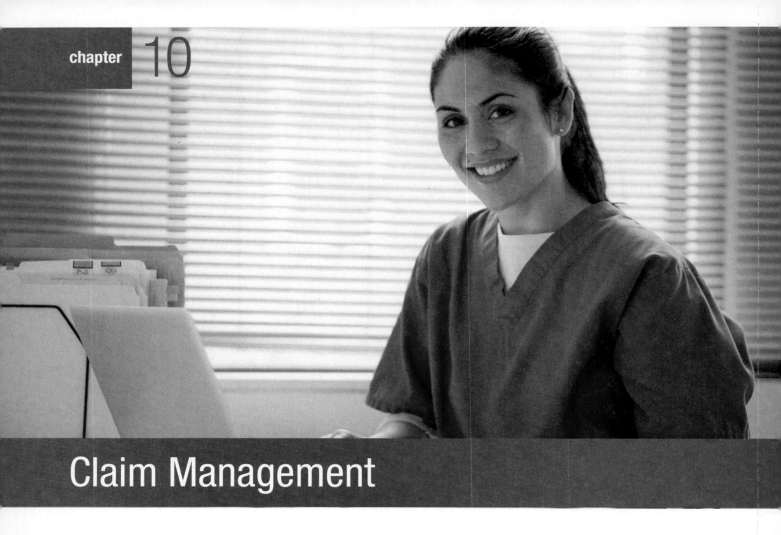

Claim Management

KEY TERMS

adjudication
aging
claim status category codes
claim status codes
claim turnaround time
CMS-1500 (08/05) claim
companion guide
crossover claim
data elements
determination
development
filter
HIPAA X12 837 Health Care Claim
HIPAA X12 276/277 Health Care Claim Status Inquiry/Response
insurance aging report
medical necessity denial
National Uniform Claim Committee (NUCC)
navigator buttons
pending
prompt payment laws
suspended
timely filing

LEARNING OUTCOMES

When you finish this chapter, you will be able to:

10.1 Briefly compare the CMS-1500 paper claim and the 837 electronic claim.

10.2 Discuss the information contained in the Claim Management dialog box.

10.3 Explain the process of creating claims.

10.4 Describe how to locate a specific claim.

10.5 Discuss the purpose of reviewing and editing claims.

10.6 Analyze the methods used to submit electronic claims.

10.7 List the steps required to submit electronic claims.

10.8 Describe how to add attachments to electronic claims.

10.9 Explain the claim determination process used by health plans.

10.10 Discuss the use of the PM/EHR to monitor claims.

"Press 2 for Claim Status Updates . . ."

"Let's just say following up on claims was a job no one particularly liked," said Chris Yakamoto, the billing specialist at the Family Care Clinic. "We'd have to call on all claims that have gone unpaid for 30 days. I spent so much time on the phone that I have the payers' recordings memorized: 'Welcome to Ohio Care's automated provider information service. For eligibility inquiries, press 1. For claim status updates, press 2.' And then the usual 'All of our agents are busy assisting other callers. Please stay on the line and the next available representative will assist you. . . .' Now claim status inquiries are sent automatically by the software. The time I used to spend on hold I now spend researching the denied and rejected claims, and I'm not so bored," Chris said.

Think about the ways in which electronic claims and electronic claim status inquiries have changed the daily routines for a billing specialist. What different skills are required to work with electronic claims? As the need for telephone follow-up lessens, what other skills are increasing in importance?

WHEN YOU FINISH THIS CHAPTER, YOU WILL ALSO BE ABLE TO USE MEDISOFT CLINICAL TO:

1. Use MNP to create Claims.
2. Locate a specific claim in MNP.
3. Review claims in MNP.
4. Transmit electronic claims in MNP.
5. Review claim edit reports in MNP.
6. Send electronic claim attachments in MNP.

SOFTWARE SKILLS

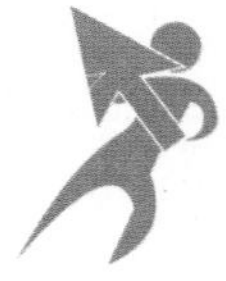

10.1 Introduction to Health Care Claims

After the charge capture process is complete, insurance claims are created for patients with insurance coverage. The insurance claim is the most important document for correct reimbursement from health plans. Claims communicate information about a patient's diagnosis, procedures, and charges to a payer. Technology makes it possible for practices to create, send, and track a large volume of claims efficiently and effectively to ensure receiving prompt payment.

The administrative team must submit clean claims with all the correct information necessary for payer processing. An error on a claim may cause the claim to be delayed or denied. Rejected claims can cost the practice twice as much as clean claims and can result in reduced cash flow. Claims that are not paid in full also have a negative effect on the practice's bottom line.

timely filing health plan's rules specifying the number of days after the date of service that the practice has to file the claim

HIPAA X12 837 Health Care Claim HIPAA standard format for electronic transmission of the claim to a health plan

CMS-1500 (08/05) claim the mandated paper insurance claim form

National Uniform Claim Committee (NUCC) organization responsible for claim content

Claims must also be submitted within the **timely filing** requirements of the particular health plan. These rules specify the number of days after the date of service that the practice has to file the claim. If it is sent later, it is not eligible for payment. For example, under the Patient Protection and Affordable Care Act (PPACA), the timely filing requirement for Medicare claims is one calendar year after the date of service.

Claim Formats

For many years, the CMS-1500 was the universal health claim accepted by most payers. The familiar red and black printed form was completed and mailed to payers. Sending paper claims has become rare with the increased use of information technology (IT) in physician practices. HIPAA/HITECH, with its emphasis on electronic transactions, has made the use of IT mandatory except in the case of very small practices and those that never send any kind of electronic health care transactions (see Chapter 2).

Today, almost all claims are sent electronically. The HIPAA standard transaction for electronic claims is the **HIPAA X12 837 Health Care Claim,** usually called the "837 claim" or the "HIPAA claim." The paper format is known as the **CMS-1500 (08/05) claim** form. Both types of insurance claims are prepared in the PM/EHR.

Claim Content

The **National Uniform Claim Committee (NUCC),** led by the American Medical Association, determines the content of both the HIPAA 837 and the CMS-1500.

CMS-1500

The concept of the health care claim is easier to understand by studying the CMS-1500, since it is a paper-based document. In this section, we provide a listing of the data elements on the CMS-1500 and the corresponding location of those data in Medisoft Network Professional (see Table 10.1). Of course, claims are not filled out by transferring information from other office documents and completing a paper form. Instead, claims are created when the PM/EHR is used to capture and organize databases of claim information. The

TABLE 10.1 **CMS-1500 Fields and Corresponding Data Locations in Medisoft Network Professional (MNP)**

Box	CMS-1500 Field Name	Data Source in MNP	Dialog Box/Tab/Field Name in MNP
Top 1	Insurance Name/Address	Insurance	***Insurance Carrier,*** Address, *Name, etc.*
Top 2	Primary, Secondary, Tertiary	Insurance	Determined by claim form selected
1	Insurance Type	Insurance	***Insurance Carrier,*** EDI/Eligibility, *Type*
1a	Insured's ID No.	Case	***Case,*** Policy 1, 2, 3, *Policy No.*
2	Patient's Name	Patient	***Patient/Guarantor,*** Name, Address, *Last Name, First Name, Middle Initial*
3	Patient's Birth Date, Sex	Patient	***Patient/Guarantor,*** Name, Address, *Birth Date, Sex*
4	Insured's Name	Case	***Case,*** Policy 1, 2, 3, *Insured*
5	Patient's Address	Patient	***Patient/Guarantor,*** Name, Address, *Street, City, State, Zip Code*
6	Patient Relation to Insured	Case	***Case,*** Policy 1, 2, 3, *Relationship to Insured*
7	Insured's Address	Patient	***Patient/Guarantor,*** Name, Address, *Street, City, State, Zip Code*
8	Patient Status	Case	***Case,*** Personal, *Marital Status, Student Status, Employment Status*
9	Other Insured's Name	Case	***Case,*** Policy 1, 2, 3, *Insured*
9a	Other Insured's Policy/Group No.	Case	***Case,*** Policy 1, 2, 3, *Policy Number, Group Number*
9b	Other Insured's Date of Birth, Sex	Patient	***Patient/Guarantor,*** Name, Address, *Birth Date, Sex*
9c	Employer/School	Patient	***Patient/Guarantor,*** Other Information, *Employer*
9d	Insurance Plan Name, Program	Insurance	***Insurance Carrier,*** Address, *Plan Name*; if empty, prints carrier name
10a	Condition Related to Employment	Case	***Case,*** Condition, *Employment Related* check box
10b	Condition Related to Auto Accident	Case	***Case,*** Condition, *Accident, Related To*
10c	Condition Related to Other Accident	Case	***Case,*** Condition, *Accident, Related To*
10d	Local Use	Case	***Case,*** Miscellaneous, *Local Use A*
11	Insured's Policy Group/FECA #	Case	***Case,*** Policy 1, *Policy Number, Group Number*
11a	Insured's Date of Birth, Sex	Patient	***Patient/Guarantor,*** Name, Address, *Birth Date, Sex*
11b	Employer/School	Patient	***Patient/Guarantor,*** Other Information, *Employer*
11c	Insurance Plan Name/Program	Insurance	***Insurance Carrier,*** Address, *Plan Name;* if empty, prints carrier name
11d	Another Health Benefit Plan?	Case	***Case,*** Policy 2, 3, *Insurance 2* or *Insurance 3*
12	Patient Signature or Authorized Signature	Patient	***Patient/Guarantor,*** Other Information, *Signature on File;* ***Insurance Carrier,*** Options and Codes, *Patient Signature on File*
13	Insured's Signature or Authorized Signature	Patient	***Patient/Guarantor,*** Other Information, *Signature on File;* ***Insurance Carrier,*** Options and Codes, *Insured Signature on File*
14	Date Current Ill/Inj/LMP	Case	***Case,*** Condition, *Injury/Illness/LMP Date*

(continued)

TABLE 10.1 *(continued)*

Box	CMS-1500 Field Name	Data Source in MNP	Dialog Box/Tab/Field Name in MNP
15	Same/Similar Date	Case	***Case,*** Condition, *Date Similar Symptoms*
16	Dates Unable to Work	Case	***Case,*** Condition, *Dates—Unable to Work*
17	Referring Provider	Case	***Case,*** Account, *Referring Provider*
17a	Referring Provider, Other Identifier, Qualifier	Referring Provider	***Referring Provider,*** Referring Provider IDs, *NPI*
17b	Referring Provider NPI	Referring Provider	***Referring Provider,*** Referring Provider IDs, *NPI*
18	Hospitalization Dates	Case	***Case,*** Condition, *Dates—Hospitalization*
19	Local Use	Case	***Case,*** Miscellaneous, *Local Use B*
20	Outside Lab? $ Charges	Case	***Case,*** Miscellaneous, *Outside Lab Work*
21	Diagnosis	Case	***Case,*** Diagnosis, Principal Diagnosis, *Default Diagnosis 1, 2, 3, 4*
22	Medicaid Resubmission	Case	***Case,*** Medicaid and Tricare, *Resubmission No., Original Reference*
23	Prior Authorization #	Case	***Case,*** Miscellaneous, *Prior Authorization Number*
24A	Dates of Service	Transaction	***Transaction Entry,*** *Date From, Date To*
24B	Place of Service	Transaction	***Transaction Entry,*** *Place of Service*
24C	EMG	Case	***Case,*** *Condition, Emergency*
24D	Procedures, Services, or Supplies	Transaction	***Transaction Entry,*** *Procedure, M1, M2, M3, M4*
24E	Diagnosis Pointer	Transaction	***Transaction Entry,*** *Diag 1, Diag 2, Diag 3, Diag 4*
24F	$ Charges	Transaction	***Transaction Entry,*** *Amount*
24G	Days or Units	Transaction	***Transaction Entry,*** *Units*
24H	EPSDT	Case	***Case,*** Medicaid and Tricare, *EPSDT*
24I	Rendering Provider, Other ID, Qualifier	Provider	***Provider,*** Provider IDs
24J	Rendering Provider ID #	Provider	***Provider,*** Provider IDs
25	Federal Tax ID	Practice	***Provider,*** Provider IDs, *Tax ID/SSN*
26	Patient's Account No.	Patient	***Patient/Guarantor,*** Name, Address, *Chart No.*
27	Accept Assignment?	Case	***Case,*** Policy 1, 2, 3, *Assignment of Benefits/Accept Assignment*
28	Total Charge	Transaction	Calculated field
29	Amount Paid	Transaction	***Transaction Entry,*** *Payment*
30	Balance Due	Transaction	Calculated field
31	Physician's Signature	Provider	***Provider,*** Address, *Signature on File;* ***Insurance Carrier,*** Address, *Signature on File*
32	Facility Address	Practice	***Facility,*** Address
32A	Facility NPI	Address	***Facility,*** Facility IDs, *NPI*
33	Billing Provider Information	Provider	***Provider,*** Address, *First Name, Middle Initial, Last Name, Street, City, State, Zip*
33A	Billing Provider NPI	Provider	***Provider:*** Provider IDs, *NPI*

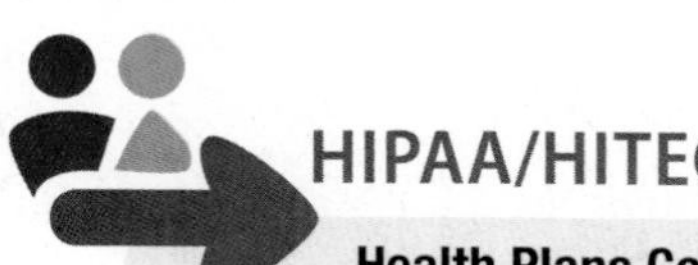

HIPAA/HITECH TIP

Health Plans Comply

Health plans cannot require providers to make changes or additions to the content of the HIPAA claim, and they cannot refuse to accept the standard transaction or to delay payment of any correctly transmitted HIPAA transaction, claims included.

program automates the formerly laborious task of creating correct claims, making it easy to update, correct, and manage the claim process.

The CMS-1500 claim has thirty-three numbered boxes representing about 150 discrete data elements. **Data elements** are the smallest units of information in a transaction. The CMS-1500 is pictured in Figure 10.1.

data element smallest unit of information in a HIPAA transaction

The HIPAA 837 Transaction

In contrast to the CMS-1500, the HIPAA 837 has a maximum of 244 segments representing about 1,054 elements. However, many of these data elements are conditional and apply to particular specialties only. Some different terms are in use with the HIPAA 837 claim, though, and a few additional information items must be relayed to the payer. For example, the HIPAA 837 uses the term *subscriber* for the insurance policyholder or guarantor, meaning the same as *insured* on the CMS-1500 claim. The HIPAA claim also requires a claim filing indicator code, which is an administrative code that identifies the type of health plan, such as Medicare Part B, Medicaid, HMO, PPO, and so on.

Examples of HIPAA claim's data elements are a patient's first name, middle name or initial, and last name. Although these are essentially the same as the data elements used to complete a CMS-1500, they are organized in a manner that is efficient for electronic transmission, rather than for use on a paper form. For example, since computers interpret blank spaces as characters, the efficient transfer of data requires removal of such spaces. As a result, the messages are not easy to read, since there is no space or line break at the end of a line.

The elements in the 837 claim are transmitted in the five major sections, or levels, of the claim:

1. Provider
2. Subscriber (guarantor/insured/policyholder) and patient (the subscriber or another person)
3. Payer
4. Claim details
5. Services

These levels are set up as a hierarchy, with the provider at the top, so that when the claim is sent electronically, data elements have to be sent only when they do not repeat previous data. For example, when the provider is sending a batch of claims, provider information is sent once for the entire batch. When the subscriber and the

1500

HEALTH INSURANCE CLAIM FORM

APPROVED BY NATIONAL UNIFORM CLAIM COMMITTEE 08/05

PICA　　　　　　PICA

CARRIER

1. MEDICARE (Medicare #) MEDICAID (Medicaid #) TRICARE CHAMPUS (Sponsor's SSN) CHAMPVA (Member ID#) GROUP HEALTH PLAN (SSN or ID) FECA BLK LUNG (SSN) OTHER (ID)

1a. INSURED'S I.D. NUMBER (For Program in Item 1)

2. PATIENT'S NAME (Last Name, First Name, Middle Initial)

3. PATIENT'S BIRTH DATE MM DD YY SEX M F

4. INSURED'S NAME (Last Name, First Name, Middle Initial)

5. PATIENT'S ADDRESS (No., Street)

6. PATIENT RELATIONSHIP TO INSURED Self Spouse Child Other

7. INSURED'S ADDRESS (No., Street)

CITY STATE

8. PATIENT STATUS Single Married Other

CITY STATE

ZIP CODE TELEPHONE (Include Area Code)

Employed Full-Time Student Part-Time Student

ZIP CODE TELEPHONE (Include Area Code)

9. OTHER INSURED'S NAME (Last Name, First Name, Middle Initial)

10. IS PATIENT'S CONDITION RELATED TO:

11. INSURED'S POLICY GROUP OR FECA NUMBER

a. OTHER INSURED'S POLICY OR GROUP NUMBER

a. EMPLOYMENT? (Current or Previous) YES NO

a. INSURED'S DATE OF BIRTH MM DD YY SEX M F

b. OTHER INSURED'S DATE OF BIRTH MM DD YY SEX M F

b. AUTO ACCIDENT? YES NO PLACE (State)

b. EMPLOYER'S NAME OR SCHOOL NAME

c. EMPLOYER'S NAME OR SCHOOL NAME

c. OTHER ACCIDENT? YES NO

c. INSURANCE PLAN NAME OR PROGRAM NAME

d. INSURANCE PLAN NAME OR PROGRAM NAME

10d. RESERVED FOR LOCAL USE

d. IS THERE ANOTHER HEALTH BENEFIT PLAN? YES NO *If yes*, return to and complete item 9 a-d.

READ BACK OF FORM BEFORE COMPLETING & SIGNING THIS FORM.

12. PATIENT'S OR AUTHORIZED PERSON'S SIGNATURE I authorize the release of any medical or other information necessary to process this claim. I also request payment of government benefits either to myself or to the party who accepts assignment below.

SIGNED DATE

13. INSURED'S OR AUTHORIZED PERSON'S SIGNATURE I authorize payment of medical benefits to the undersigned physician or supplier for services described below.

SIGNED

PATIENT AND INSURED INFORMATION

14. DATE OF CURRENT: MM DD YY ILLNESS (First symptom) OR INJURY (Accident) OR PREGNANCY(LMP)

15. IF PATIENT HAS HAD SAME OR SIMILAR ILLNESS. GIVE FIRST DATE MM DD YY

16. DATES PATIENT UNABLE TO WORK IN CURRENT OCCUPATION FROM MM DD YY TO MM DD YY

17. NAME OF REFERRING PROVIDER OR OTHER SOURCE

17a.

17b. NPI

18. HOSPITALIZATION DATES RELATED TO CURRENT SERVICES FROM MM DD YY TO MM DD YY

19. RESERVED FOR LOCAL USE

20. OUTSIDE LAB? YES NO $ CHARGES

21. DIAGNOSIS OR NATURE OF ILLNESS OR INJURY (Relate Items 1, 2, 3 or 4 to Item 24E by Line)

1. ___ . ___　　3. ___ . ___

2. ___ . ___　　4. ___ . ___

22. MEDICAID RESUBMISSION CODE ORIGINAL REF. NO.

23. PRIOR AUTHORIZATION NUMBER

	24. A. DATE(S) OF SERVICE From MM DD YY	To MM DD YY	B. PLACE OF SERVICE	C. EMG	D. PROCEDURES, SERVICES, OR SUPPLIES (Explain Unusual Circumstances) CPT/HCPCS MODIFIER	E. DIAGNOSIS POINTER	F. $ CHARGES	G. DAYS OR UNITS	H. EPSDT Family Plan	I. ID. QUAL.	J. RENDERING PROVIDER ID. #
1										NPI	
2										NPI	
3										NPI	
4										NPI	
5										NPI	
6										NPI	

25. FEDERAL TAX I.D. NUMBER SSN EIN

26. PATIENT'S ACCOUNT NO.

27. ACCEPT ASSIGNMENT? (For govt. claims, see back) YES NO

28. TOTAL CHARGE $

29. AMOUNT PAID $

30. BALANCE DUE $

31. SIGNATURE OF PHYSICIAN OR SUPPLIER INCLUDING DEGREES OR CREDENTIALS (I certify that the statements on the reverse apply to this bill and are made a part thereof.)

SIGNED DATE

32. SERVICE FACILITY LOCATION INFORMATION

a. NPI b.

33. BILLING PROVIDER INFO & PH #

a. NPI b.

PHYSICIAN OR SUPPLIER INFORMATION

NUCC Instruction Manual available at: www.nucc.org　　APPROVED OMB-0938-0999 FORM CMS-1500 (08-05)

Figure 10.1 The CMS-1500 Claim Form

patient are the same, the patient information is not needed. But if the subscriber and the patient are different people, information about both is transmitted.

Figure 10.2 shows a claim in CMS-1500 format, and Figure 10.3 shows the same claim in 837 format.

```
                                                    BLUE CROSSBLUE SHIELD
                                                    340 BOULEVARD
                                                    COLUMBUS OH 60220
P

                                               X    4965789112
MAZLOUM, ALI                 01 15 1980   X         MAZLOUM, ALI
550 CENTER ST                        X              550 CENTER ST
STEPHENSON                  OH                X     STEPHENSON                  OH
60089        614 5550894              X             60089         614 5550894
                                                    A49524
                                            X          01 15 1980     X
                                            X       STEPHENSON FOOD MART
                                            X       BLUE CROSSBLUE SHIELD
                                                           X

     SIGNATURE ON FILE                 07/01/16          SIGNATURE ON FILE

07 01 2016            INJURY

                                                           X

 924 21                         924 5
 923 9                          E821 0

07 01 16  07 01 16   11    99204            1 2 3 4   178 00 1        2456789012
07 01 16  07 01 16   11    73510                  3   124 00 1        2456789012
07 01 16  07 01 16   11    73070                2     102 00 1        2456789012
07 01 16  07 01 16   11    73090                2      99 00 1        2456789012
07 01 16  07 01 16   11    73600              1        96 00 1        2456789012
07 01 16  07 01 16   11    29540              1       121 50 1        2456789012
339675000      X      MAZLOALO      67 X                720.50               720.50
                                                            614 5550000
                                                     JOHN RUDNER MD
                                                     285 STEPHENSON BOULEVARD
SIGNATURE ON FILE                                    STEPHENSON OH
         01/01/16                                     2456789012
```

Figure 10.2 Sample Claim in CMS-1500 Format

ISA*00*   *01*CYCTRANS*ZZ*P123456*ZZ*CLAIMSCH*101108*0300*U*00401*000000001*1*P*:~
GS*HC*P123456*ECGCLAIMS*20101108*0300*1*X*004010X098A1~ST*837*0001~BHT*0019*00*11A
AAA*20101108*0300*CH~REF*87*004010X098A1~NM1*41*2*FAMILY CARE
CLINIC*****46*123456123456~PER*IC*JOHN SMITH*TE*5555555555~NM1*40*2*RELAY
HEALTH*****46*4300~HL*1*1*20*1~NM1*85*2*FAMILY CARE CLINIC*****24*033987562~N3*285
STEPHENSON BOULEVARD~N4*STEPHENSON*OH*60089~HL*1*1*22*1~SBR*P*18*A49524*BLUE
CROSS/BLUE SHIELD*****BL~NM1*IL*1*MAZLOUM*ALI****MI*4965789112~N3*550 CENTER ST.*APT
1B~N4*STEPHENSON*OH*60089~DMG*D8*19800115*M~NM1*PR*2*BLUE CROSS/BLUE
SHIELD*****PI*45678~N3*340
BOULEVARD~N4*COLUMBUS*OH*60220~CLM*67*720.5***11::1*Y*A*Y*Y*B~DTP*454*D8*20160701
~DTP*304*D8*20160701~DTP*431*D8*20160701~HI*BK:92421*BF:9239*BF:9245*BF:E8210~LX*1~SV
1*HC:99204*178*UN*1***1:2:3:4**Y~DTP*472*D8*20160701~REF*6R*600~LX*1~SV1*HC:73510*124
*UN*1***3**Y~DTP*472*D8*20160701~REF*6R*601~LX*1~SV1*HC:73070*102*UN*1***2**Y~DTP*4
72*D8*20160701~REF*6R*602~LX*1~SV1*HC:73090*99*UN*1***2**Y~DTP*472*D8*20160701~REF*
6R*603~LX*1~SV1*HC:73600*96*UN*1***1**Y~DTP*472*D8*20160701~REF*6R*604~LX*1~SV1*HC:
29540*121.5*UN*1***1**Y~DTP*472*D8*20160701~REF*6R*605~SE*9999*0001~GE*9999*1~
IEA*9999*000000001~

Figure 10.3 Sample Claim in 837 Format

HIPAA/HITECH TIP

Physician Claims: The 837P

The HIPAA transaction for electronic claims generated by physicians is called the HIPAA 837P, for professional services. The hospital version of the claim is called the 837I (institutional services), and dentists use a version called the 837D (dental services).

THINKING IT THROUGH 10.1

What are the advantages of transmitting electronic claims? Are there any potential disadvantages?

10.2 Claim Management in Medisoft Network Professional

Insurance claims are created, edited, and submitted for payment within the Claim Management area of MNP. Claims are created from transactions previously entered. After claims are created, they are either transmitted electronically or, in particular situations, printed and mailed.

The Claim Management Dialog Box

Figure 10.4 Claim Management Shortcut Button

The Claim Management dialog box is displayed by clicking Claim Management on the Activities menu or by clicking the Claim Management shortcut button on the toolbar (see Figure 10.4). The dialog box lists all claims that have already been created (see Figure 10.5). In this dialog box, existing claims can be reviewed and edited, new claims can be created, the status of existing claims can be changed, and claims can be submitted electronically or printed.

navigator buttons buttons that simplify the task of moving from one entry to another

The upper-right corner of the Claim Management dialog box contains five **navigator buttons** that simplify the task of moving from one entry to another (see Figure 10.6). The First Claim button selects

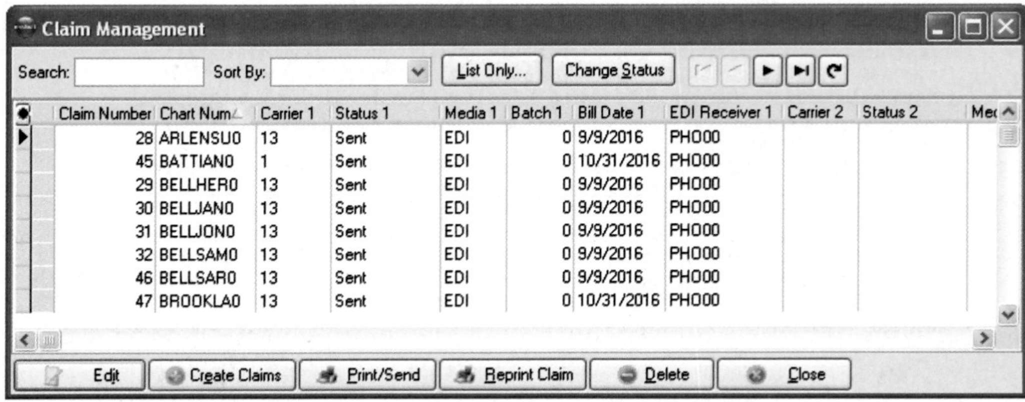

Figure 10.5 Claim Management Dialog Box

THINKING IT THROUGH 10.2

What actions can be performed in the Claim Management dialog box?

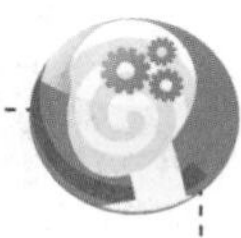

the first claim in the list and makes it active. The Previous Claim button reactivates the claim that was most recently active. The Next Claim button makes the next claim in the list active. The Last Claim button makes the last claim in the list active. The Refresh Data button is used to restore data when necessary.

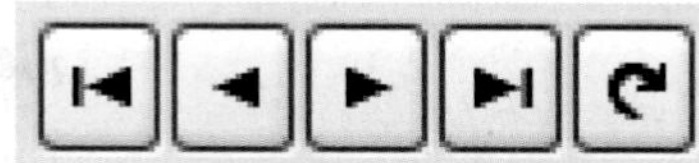

Figure 10.6 Navigator Buttons

The bottom of the Claim Management dialog box contains a number of buttons that are used for various functions (see Figure 10.5).

Edit Opens a claim for editing.

Create Claims Opens the Create Claims dialog box.

Print/Send Begins the process of sending electronic claims or printing paper claims.

Reprint Claim Reprints a claim that has already been printed.

Delete Deletes the selected claim and releases the transactions bound to the claim.

Close Closes the Claim Management dialog box.

10.3 Creating Claims

Claims are created in Medisoft Network Professional in the Create Claims dialog box. The Create Claims dialog box (see Figure 10.7) is accessed by clicking the Create Claims button in the Claim Management dialog box. This dialog box provides several filters to customize the creation of claims.

Claim Filters

A **filter** is a condition that data must meet to be selected. For example, claims can be created for services performed between the first and the fifteenth of the month. In this case, the filter is the condition that services must have been performed between the first and fifteenth of the month. Transactions that meet this criterion are included in the selection; transactions that do not fall within the date range are not included. Filters can be used to create claims for a specific patient, for a specific insurance carrier, and for transactions that exceed a certain dollar amount, among others. The following filters can be applied within the Create Claims dialog box.

filter a condition that data must meet to be selected

Transaction Dates The Transaction Dates boxes are used to specify the starting and ending dates for which claims will be created. If the boxes are left blank, transactions for all dates will be included.

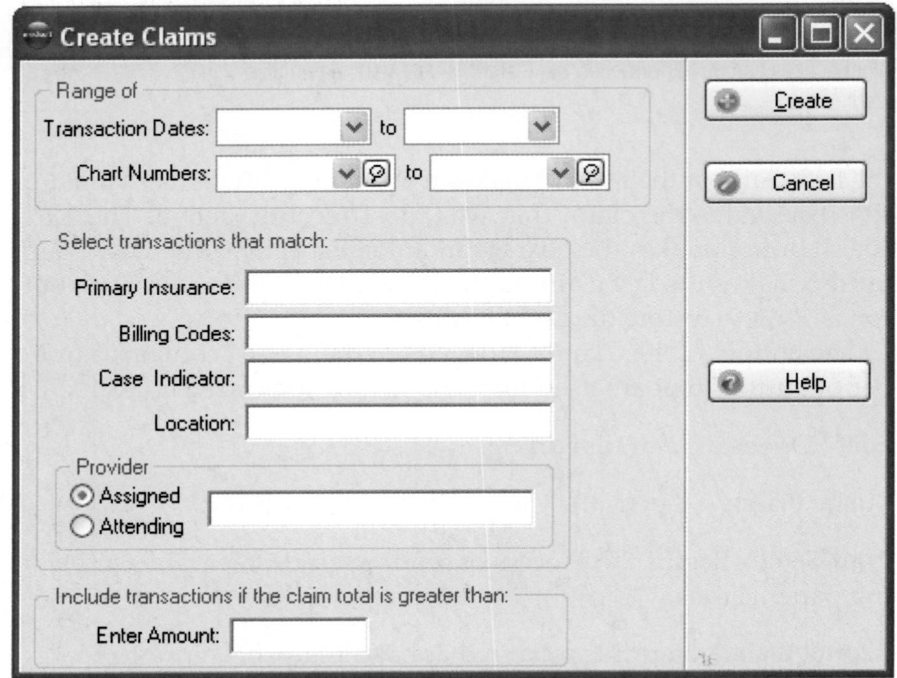

Figure 10.7 Create Claims Dialog Box

Chart Numbers The Chart Numbers boxes specify the starting and ending chart numbers for which claims will be created are entered. If the boxes are left blank, all chart numbers will be included.

Primary Insurance The carrier code for the insurance company is entered in the Primary Insurance box. If claims are being sent to a clearinghouse, more than one insurance carrier code can be entered. When more than one code is entered, commas must be placed between the codes. If claims are being sent directly to the carrier, only that carrier's code is entered.

Billing Codes The billing code is entered in the Billing Codes box. If more than one code is entered, commas must be placed between the codes.

Case Indicator If case indicators are used to classify patients (such as by type of illness for workers' compensation cases), the case indicator can be listed in the Case Indicator box. If more than one indicator is entered, commas must be placed between them.

Location Sometimes a sort is needed by location, such as all procedures done at a hospital. The location code is entered in the Location box. If more than one code is entered, commas must be placed between the codes.

Assigned The radio buttons in the Provider box indicate whether the provider is the assigned or attending provider. The assigned provider is the patient's regular physician. In the box to the right of the radio button, the provider code is entered. If more than one code is entered, commas must be placed between the codes.

Attending The attending provider is someone other than the patient's regular physician who provides treatment to the patient. In the box to the right of the radio button, the provider code is entered.

Enter Amount The dollar amount entered in this box is the minimum total amount required for a case before a claim can be created.

Any box that is not filled in will default to include all data, and all claims will be included. When all necessary information has been entered, clicking the Create button creates the claims.

connect plus+ EXERCISE 10.1

CREATING CLAIMS

Create insurance claims for patients.

Date: November 4, 2016

1. Click Start > All Programs > Medisoft > Medisoft Network Professional.
2. Click the Activities menu. Select Claim Management. The Claim Management dialog box is displayed.
3. Click the Create Claims button. The Create Claims dialog box is displayed.
4. To create claims for all transactions that have not already been placed on a claim, leave all fields in the dialog box blank.
5. Click the Create button. You are returned to the Claim Management dialog box, with the new claims added.
6. Use the scroll bars to view the claims just created.
7. Click the Close button.

You have completed Exercise 10.1

10.4 Locating Claims

At times it is necessary to select and view specific claims that have already been created. For example, claims prepared for submission to an insurance carrier can be selected and reviewed for completeness and accuracy. In addition, claims that have been rejected by insurance carriers can be selected and reviewed before resubmission.

The List Only Feature

MNP's List Only feature is used when it is necessary to list claims that match certain criteria. Filters are applied in the List

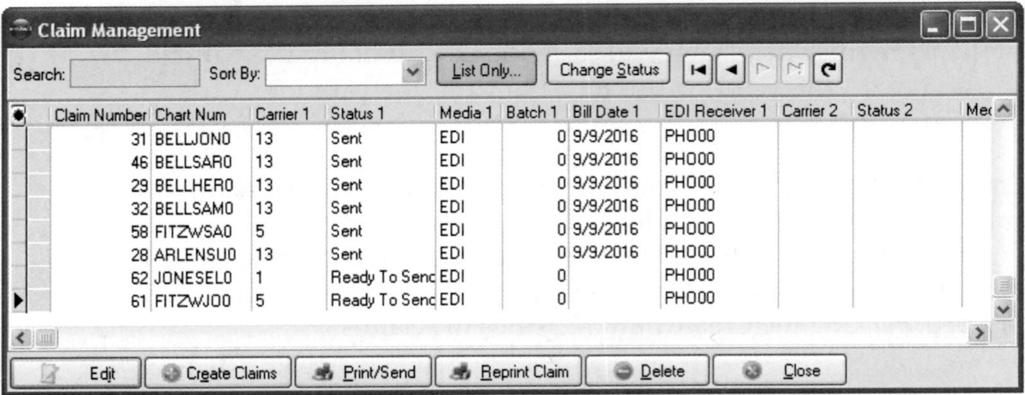

Figure 10.8 Claim Management Dialog Box with List Only… Button Highlighted in Yellow

Only Claims That Match dialog box. They can be used to view claims selectively, such as those for a specific insurance carrier and those created on a certain date. Unlike the filters in the Create Claims dialog box, those in the List Only Claims That Match dialog box do not create claims; they simply list existing claims that meet the specified criteria.

Once the filters have been applied, only the claims that match the criteria are listed at the bottom of the main Claim Management dialog box. Claims can be sorted by chart number, date created, insurance carrier, electronic claim (EDI) receiver, billing method, billing date, batch number, and claim status. Not all the boxes need to be filled in, only the ones that will be used to select the desired claims.

The List Only feature is activated by clicking the List Only… button in the Claim Management dialog box (see Figure 10.8). Clicking the button causes the List Only Claims That Match dialog box to be displayed (see Figure 10.9).

The following filters are available in the List Only Claims That Match dialog box.

Chart Number A patient's chart number is selected from the drop-down list of chart numbers.

Claim Created The date that a claim was created is entered in MMDDCCYY format.

Select Claims for Only A radio button is clicked for either all insurance carriers, primary insurance carrier only, secondary insurance carrier only, or tertiary (third) insurance carrier only. When a patient has insurance coverage with more than one carrier, the primary carrier is billed first, and then, if appropriate, the second and third carriers are billed.

Insurance Carrier An insurance carrier is selected from the drop-down list of choices.

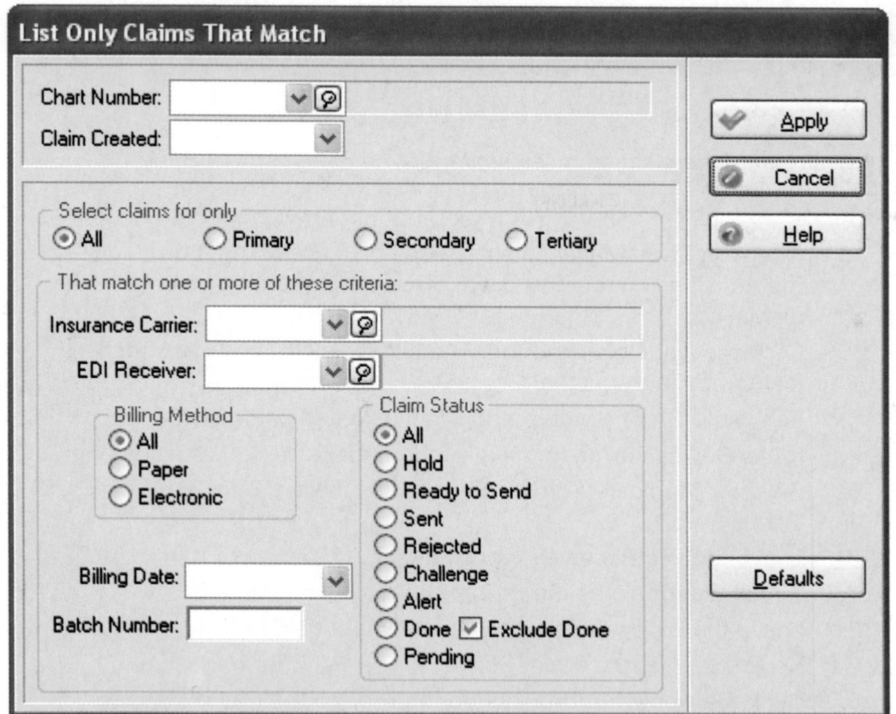

Figure 10.9 List Only Claims That Match Dialog Box

EDI Receiver An EDI receiver is selected from the choices on the drop-down list.

Billing Method In the Billing Method box, the radio button for All, Paper, or Electronic is clicked.

Billing Date The date of billing is entered in the Billing Date box.

Batch Number A batch number is entered in the Batch Number box.

Claim Status A claim status is selected from the list of radio buttons provided. If claims that have been billed and accepted (not rejected) are to be excluded from the search, the Exclude Done box is clicked. This causes a check mark to be displayed beside the option.

When the desired boxes have been filled in, clicking the Apply button applies the selected filters to the claim data. The Claim Management dialog box is displayed, listing only the claims that match the criteria selected in the List Only Claims That Match dialog box. From the Claim Management dialog box, the claims can now be edited, printed, or transmitted electronically.

To restore the Claim Management dialog box to its original settings (that is, to remove the filters selected), the List Only Claims That Match dialog box is reopened, the Defaults button is clicked, and the Apply button is clicked. All the boxes in the dialog box become blank, and the full list of claims is again displayed.

EXERCISE 10.2

connect plus+

USING THE LIST ONLY FEATURE

Find all insurance claims for Medicare that have a status of Sent.

Date: November 4, 2016

1. Open the Claim Management dialog box by selecting it on the Activities menu. The Claim Management dialog box is displayed.
2. Click the List Only... button. The List Only Claims That Match dialog box is displayed.
3. Leave the Chart Number and Claim Created fields blank.
4. In the Select Claims for Only section, make sure All is selected.
5. Select 1-Medicare from the drop-down list in the Insurance Carrier field.
6. Leave the EDI Receiver field blank.
7. Select Electronic as the Billing Method.
8. Leave the Billing Date and Batch Number fields blank.
9. Select Sent as the Claim Status.
10. Click the Apply button. You are returned to the Claim Management dialog box with only those claims that met the criteria displayed.
11. To restore the full list of claims, click the List Only... button, and then click the Defaults button.
12. Click the Apply button to return to the complete list of claims in the Claim Management dialog box.

You have completed Exercise 10.2

10.5 Reviewing Claims

An important step comes before the claims are actually transmitted—checking the claim. Most PM/EHRs provide a way for the billing specialist to review claims for accuracy. In Medisoft Network Professional, this is accomplished by using the claim edit feature, which allows claims to be reviewed and edited before they are submitted for payment. The more problems that can be spotted and solved before claims are sent to insurance carriers, the sooner the practice will receive payment.

When a claim is selected in the Claim Management dialog box, it can be edited by clicking the Edit button, or the claim itself can be double clicked. The Claim dialog box is displayed (see Figure 10.10). The top section of the Claim dialog box lists the claim number, the date the claim was created, the chart number, the patient's name, and the case number. This information cannot be edited, although the information in the five tabs can be edited.

Carrier 1 Tab

The Carrier 1 tab displays information about claims being submitted to a patient's primary insurance carrier. The following boxes are listed in the Carrier 1 tab:

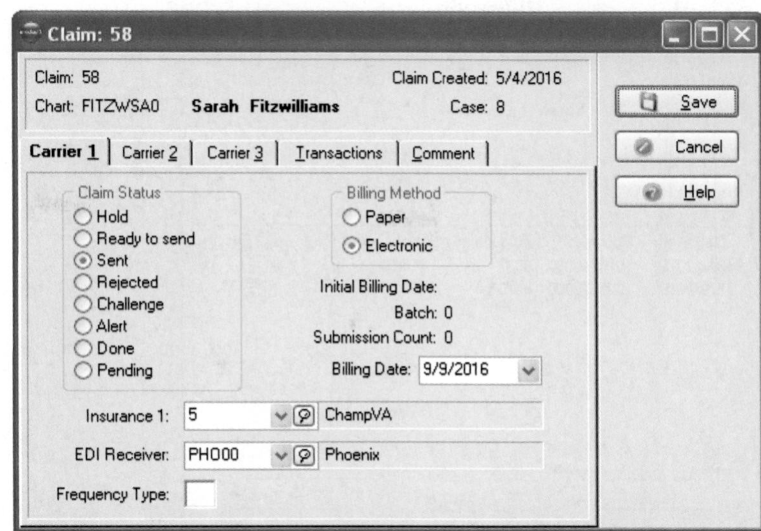

Figure 10.10 Claim Dialog Box

Claim Status The Claim Status box indicates the status of a particular claim: Hold, Ready to send, Sent, Rejected, Challenge, Alert, Done, and Pending. The radio button that reflects a claim's status should be clicked.

Billing Method The Billing Method box displays two choices: Paper and Electronic. The radio button that describes the billing method should be clicked.

Initial Billing Date If the claim was sent more than once, this box automatically displays the initial billing date.

Batch If the claim has been assigned to a batch, the batch number is displayed.

Submission Count The Submission Count area lists the number of claims submitted.

Billing Date The Billing Date box lists the most recent date the bill was sent (if the claim was submitted more than once).

Insurance 1 The Insurance 1 box lists a patient's primary insurance carrier.

EDI Receiver The EDI receiver is selected from the drop-down list.

Frequency Type This field is used with some insurance carriers when sending claims electronically. Allowed entries in this field are:

1- Original (admission through discharge claim)
6- Corrected (adjustment of prior claim)
10- Replacement (replacement of prior claim)
8- Void (voiding/cancellation of prior claim)

Carrier 2 and Carrier 3 Tabs

The Carrier 2 and Carrier 3 tabs display information about claims being submitted to a patient's secondary (Carrier 2) and tertiary (Carrier 3) insurance carriers. The boxes in these tabs are the same as the boxes in the Carrier 1 tab, with the exception of the Claim Status box and the Frequency Type box. In the Carrier 2 and Carrier 3 tabs, there is no Pending radio button in the Claim

BILLING TIP

Dropping to Paper

The phrase "dropping to paper" describes a situation in which a CMS-1500 paper claim needs to be printed and sent to a payer. Some practices, for instance, have a policy of doing this when a claim has been transmitted electronically twice but receipt of the claim is not acknowledged.

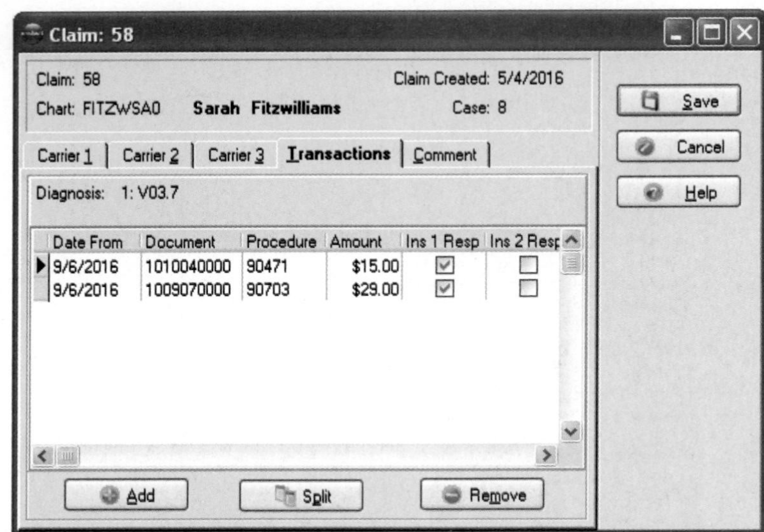

Figure 10.11 Transactions Tab

Status box, and there is no Frequency Type box. Otherwise the three tabs are the same.

Transactions Tab

The Transactions tab lists information about the transactions included in a claim. The scroll bars can be used to view all the information in the Transactions tab (see Figure 10.11).

Diagnosis The diagnosis code for the listed transactions is displayed.

Date From The Date From box lists the date on which service was provided.

Document The Document box lists the document number of a transaction.

Procedure The Procedure box displays the procedure code for a performed procedure.

Amount In the Amount box, the dollar cost of a service is displayed.

Ins 1 Resp If this box is checked, the primary insurance carrier is responsible for the claim.

Ins 2 Resp If this box is checked, the secondary insurance carrier is responsible for the claim.

Ins 3 Resp If this box is checked, the tertiary insurance carrier is responsible for the claim.

The Transactions tab also contains three buttons at the bottom of the dialog box:

Add The Add button is used to add a transaction to an existing claim.

Split The Split button removes a single transaction from an existing claim and places it on a new claim.

Remove The Remove button deletes a transaction from the claim database.

Comment Tab

The Comment tab provides a place to include specific notes or comments about the claim (see Figure 10.12). The comments are for internal use and are not transmitted or printed.

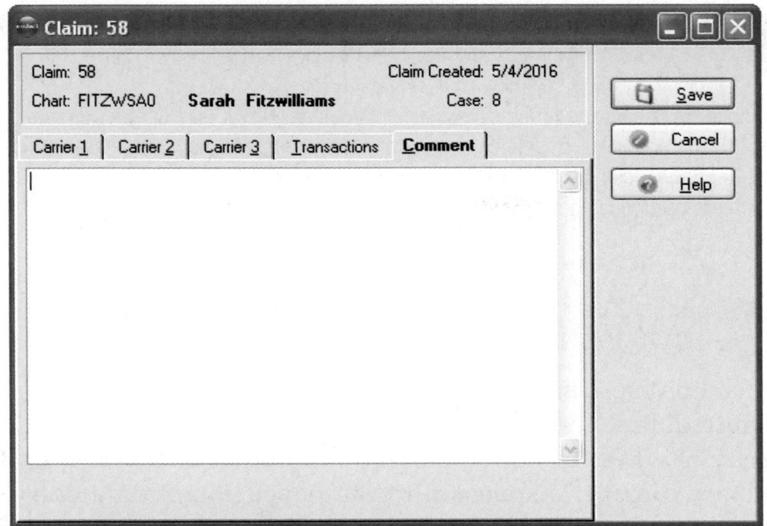

Figure 10.12 Comment Tab

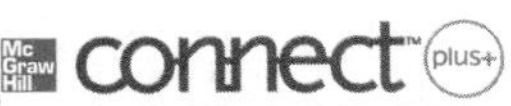

EXERCISE 10.3

REVIEWING A CLAIM

Review insurance claims for patients with East Ohio PPO as their insurance carrier.

Date: November 4, 2016

1. Click Claim Management on the Activities menu to open the Claim Management dialog box.
2. Click the List Only... button.
3. Click 13 East Ohio PPO on the drop-down list in the Insurance Carrier box.
4. Click the Apply button. You are returned to the Claim Management dialog box. Notice that only claims for patients who have East Ohio PPO as their insurance carrier are listed.
5. Click the claim for Lawana Brooks (chart number BROOKLAØ).
6. Click the Edit button to review the claim. The Claim dialog box is displayed.
7. Review the information in the Carrier 1 tab.
8. Click the Transactions tab. Review the information in the Transactions tab.
9. Click the Cancel button to exit the Claim dialog box without saving any changes. (The Cancel button does not cancel the claim; it just cancels any changes that may have been made.)
10. To restore the full list of claims in the Claim Management box, click the List Only... button, and then click the Defaults button.
11. Click the Apply button to return to the complete list of claims in the Claim Management dialog box.

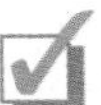 **You have completed Exercise 10.3**

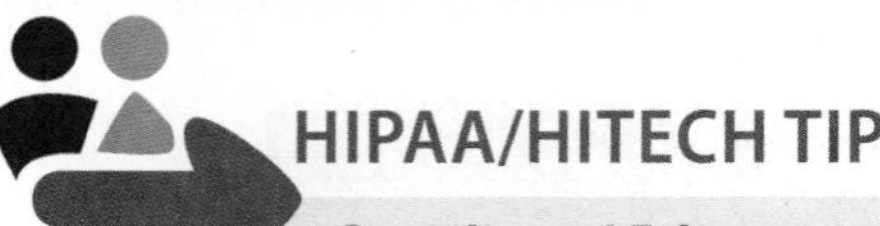

Security and Privacy

A clearinghouse is considered a business associate under HIPAA (see Chapter 2) and must follow the practice's guidelines to ensure that patients' PHI remains secure and private. Clearinghouses must receive all required data elements from providers; they cannot create or modify data content.

10.6 Methods of Claim Submission

Once claims have been created and checked, they are ready to be transmitted. Practices handle the transmission of electronic claims in a variety of ways. The three most common methods of transmitting claims are direct transmission to the payer, direct data entry, and transmission through a clearinghouse. Clearinghouses accept claim data from providers in nonstandard formats and translate them into the standard format required by the payer. A practice may choose to use a clearinghouse to transmit all claims, or it may use a combination of methods. For example, it may send claims directly to Medicare, Medicaid, and a few major commercial payers and use a clearinghouse to send claims to other payers.

Direct to the Payer

In the direct transmission approach, providers and payers exchange transactions directly without using a clearinghouse. Claims are created in the PM/EHR, and a connection is made to the payer's computer. Once connected, the claims are transmitted. In this approach, the medical practice must supply all the HIPAA data elements and follow specific EDI formatting rules. The practice may also have to purchase special software that can communicate with the payer's system.

Direct Data Entry

Direct data entry (DDE) is a method of claim transmission in which a member of the provider's billing staff manually enters claims into an application on the payer's website. Using DDE, the medical practice logs into a secure website hosted by the payer. Once connected, a staff member from the medical practice enters the claim information into an electronic form on the payer's site. Most practices that use a PM/EHR or a PM do not use DDE, since it is inefficient and susceptible to keyboarding errors.

Clearinghouse

companion guide guide published by a payer that lists its own set of claim edits and formatting conventions

Most providers send their electronic claims to a clearinghouse for a number of reasons. While all health care claims must use HIPAA transactions and code sets, each payer has its own set of claim edits and formatting conventions. These are published in what is known as a **companion guide.** Since payers publish their own

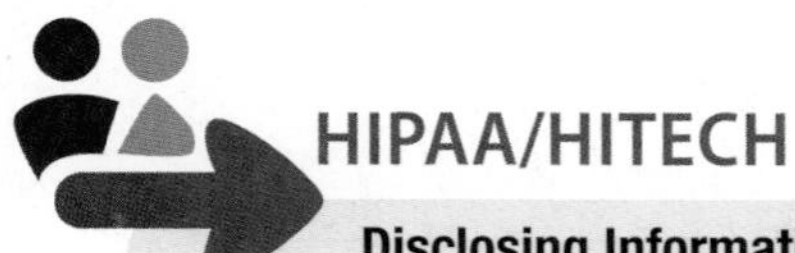

HIPAA/HITECH TIP

Disclosing Information for Payment Purposes

Under HIPAA, covered entities such as physician practices may disclose patients' PHI for payment purposes. For example, a provider may disclose a patient's name to a financial institution in order to cash a check or to a clearinghouse to initiate electronic transactions.

guides, it would be difficult for a billing specialist to know the rules of each payer. Instead, clearinghouses perform this function. In practices with a large volume of claims, it is not be practical to send electronic claims to each payer; when a clearinghouse is used, claims can be sent in one batch to one location.

At the clearinghouse, claims go through a series of edits. Then, a report indicating which claims have passed and/or failed these edits is sent to the provider. Claims that fail must be corrected and resubmitted to the clearinghouse before they can be sent to the payer.

Once the claims have cleared the clearinghouse's edits, they are sent to the payer. Rather than receive claims directly, some payers also use a clearinghouse. In these instances, the provider's clearinghouse transmits to the payer's clearinghouse. The payer's clearinghouse processes the claims before it sends them to the payer.

When the claim reaches the payer, additional editing is performed, and a status report is generated, indicating which claims were accepted and which were rejected. This report is then sent to the clearinghouse, which forwards the information to the provider. Accepted claims are sent to the payer's adjudication system for payment or denial determination. Rejected claims must be corrected and resubmitted before they can be processed.

BILLING TIP

Clearinghouses

There are many electronic claim and transaction processing firms in the health care industry. Some of the largest are RelayHealth, Emdeon, Navicure, Availity, and Gateway.

Most clearinghouses charge fees for their services. Some charge a flat fee per month regardless of the number of claims processed, while others charge on a per-claim basis.

The typical flow of a claim that is ready for transmission from a medical practice to a payer is shown in Figure 10.13.

Primary Versus Secondary and Tertiary Claims

When a patient is covered by more than one health plan, the initial claim is transmitted to the patient's primary health plan. For example, if patients are covered by Medicare and Medicaid, their claims are first submitted to Medicare and then to Medicaid. Claims billed to Medicare and then submitted to Medicaid are called **crossover claims.** The majority of Medicare carriers automatically forward crossover claims to the state Medicaid payer. Medicaid is referred to as the "payer of last resort," meaning that under federal policy all other avenues for payment must be followed first, before Medicaid will pay a claim.

crossover claim claim billed to Medicare and then submitted to Medicaid

Some insurance carriers that are secondary to Medicare are classified as complementary crossover carriers. When these carriers are involved, Medicare information about the secondary insurance carrier is already in the Medicare system.

Figure 10.13 Claim Flow Using a Clearinghouse

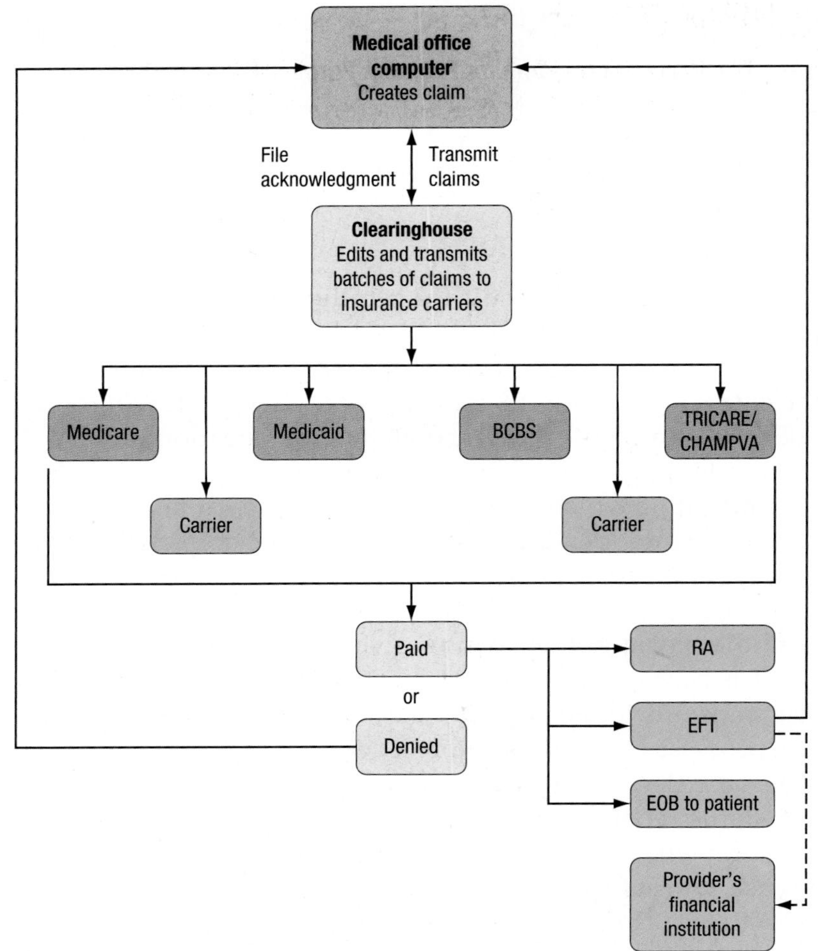

Figure 10.14 Complementary Crossover Field in the EDI/ Eligibility Tab

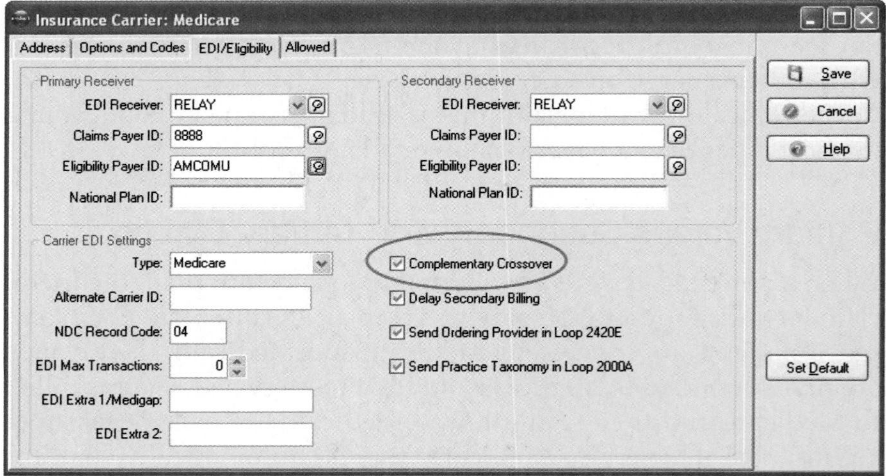

In Medisoft Network Professional, the Complementary Crossover box in the EDI/Eligibility tab of the Insurance Carrier dialog box is used to indicate a complementary claim (see Figure 10.14). When a claim is complementary, do not check the Crossover Claim box in the Policy 2 tab in the Case folder. When the Complementary Crossover box in the EDI/Eligibility tab is checked, the program does not

THINKING IT THROUGH 10.3

Why would a medical practice pay to use a clearinghouse for sending electronic claims when the practice could send claims directly to the payer for free?

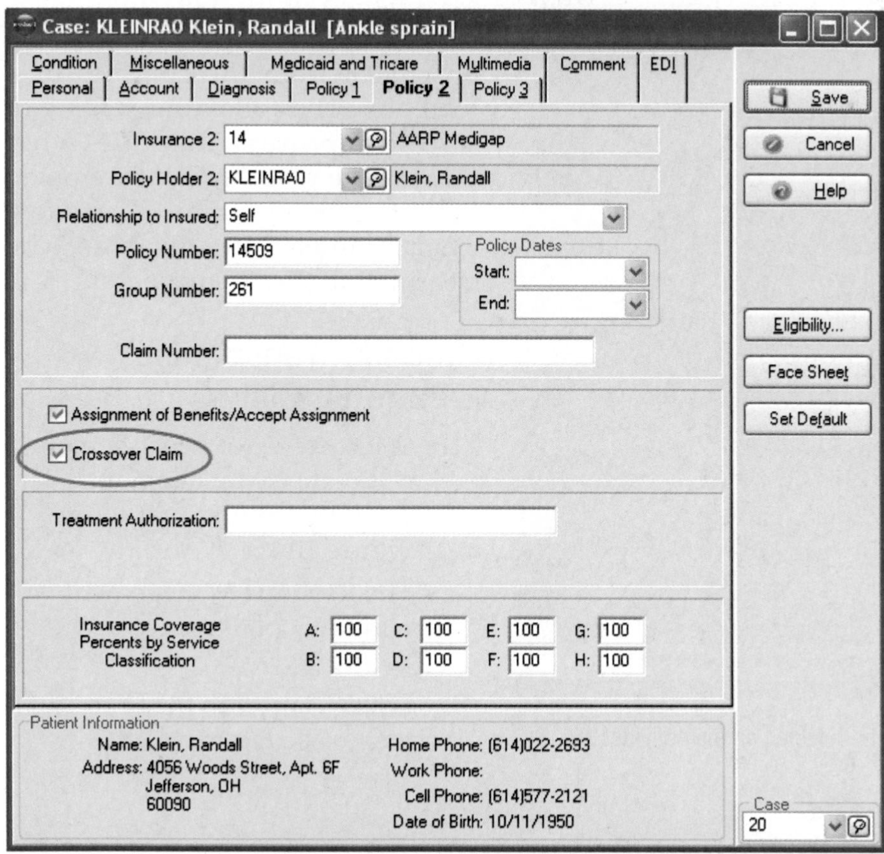

Figure 10.15 Crossover Claim Field in the Policy 2 Tab

send the secondary insurance information in the claim file but does mark the secondary claim as sent when the primary claim is sent. If the secondary claim is for a Medigap plan, do not select this box. Instead, check the Crossover Claim box in the Policy 2 tab of the Case folder (see Figure 10.15).

10.7 Submitting Claims in Medisoft Network Professional

Claims that have been created in Medisoft Network Professional (MNP) are submitted using the revenue management feature. Physician practices use Revenue Management to electronically transmit claims to clearinghouses as well as directly to payers. Before claims are sent, the program performs a number of edits, including ANSI edits, common edits, and user-defined edits. Additional edits such as CCI edits, Medicare policy edits, and global period edits require an annual subscription. The use of these edits increases the likelihood that claims will be accepted and processed by the payer in a timely manner.

The transmission of electronic claims requires that accounts be established with clearinghouses and payers, something that is not possible within the confines of a textbook. The following steps and screen captures illustrate what would take place in an office using MNP to send electronic claims to a clearinghouse. In this case, the clearinghouse is RelayHealth.

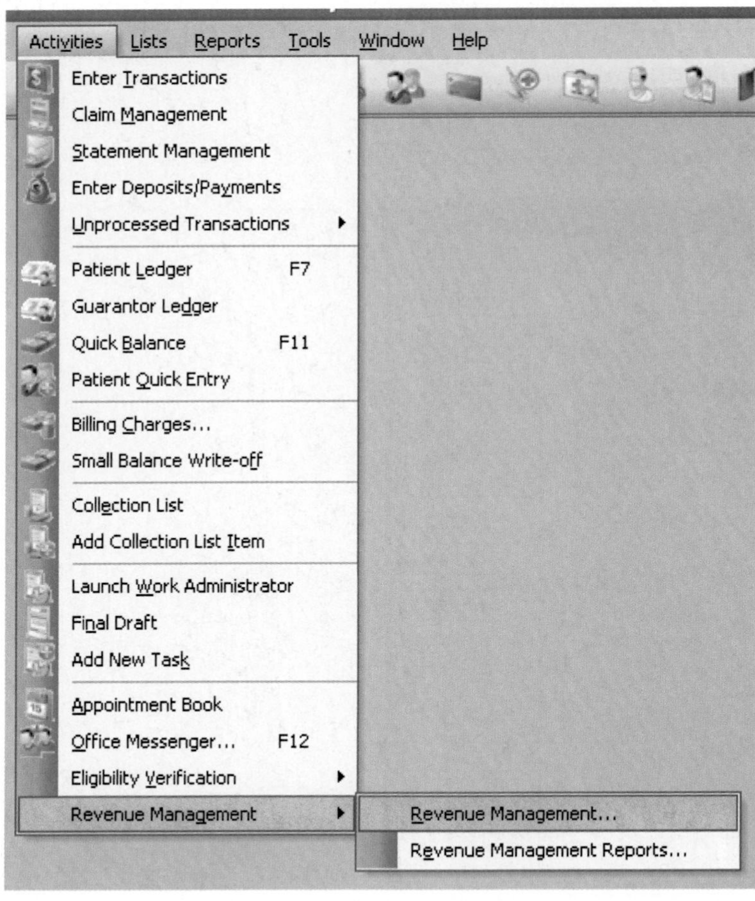

Figure 10.16 Revenue Management Selected on the Activities Menu

Steps in Transmitting Electronic Claims

1. Select Revenue Management > Revenue Management... on the Activities menu (see Figure 10.16).
2. The Revenue Management window opens (see Figure 10.17).
3. Select Claims on the Process menu (see Figure 10.18).

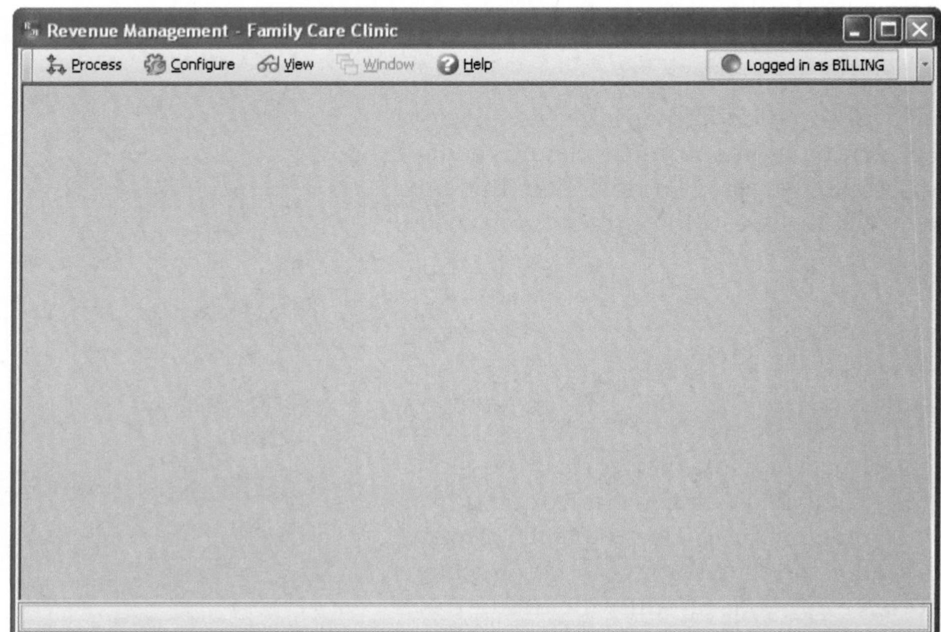

Figure 10.17 The Revenue Management Window

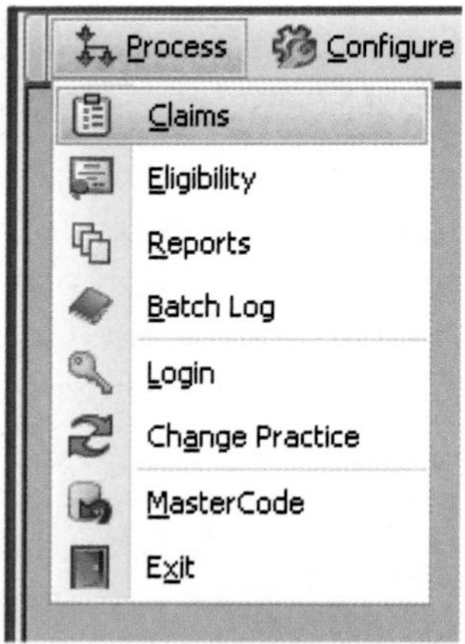

Figure 10.18 The Process Menu with Claims Selected

4. Select an EDI receiver. In this case, the receiver is RelayHealth, listed here by the code RELAY. A list of claims ready to be sent is displayed (see Figure 10.19). Notice that the entries in the Edit Status column are all "Not Checked."

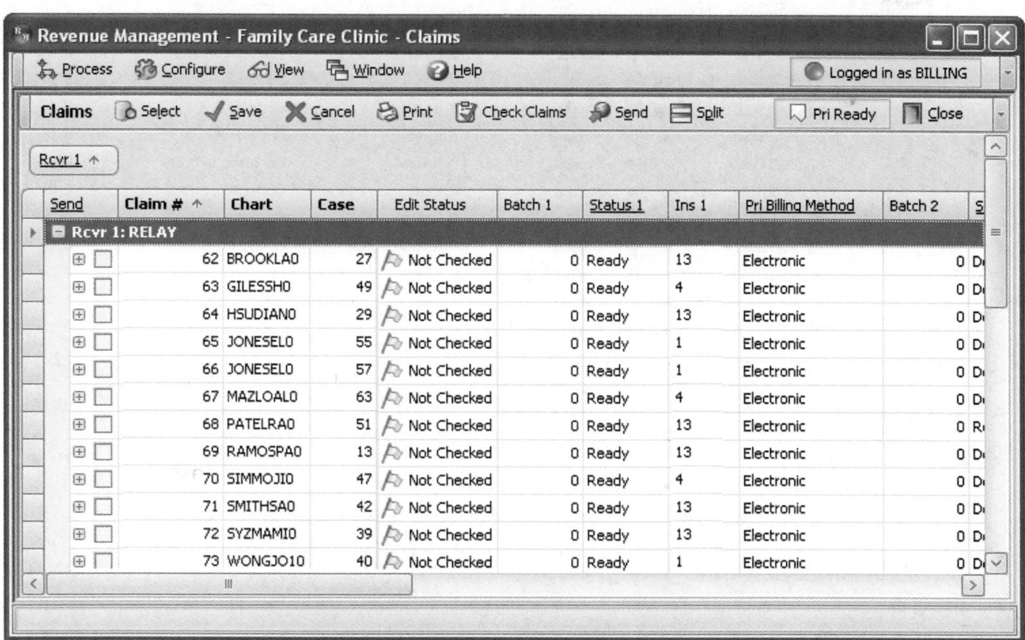

Figure 10.19 List of Claims Ready to Be Sent, by EDI Receiver

5. To perform an edit check on the claims, click Check Claims and RELAY, the EDI receiver (see Figure 10.20). The claims are checked against a number of edits, including ANSI edits, common edits, and user-defined edits.

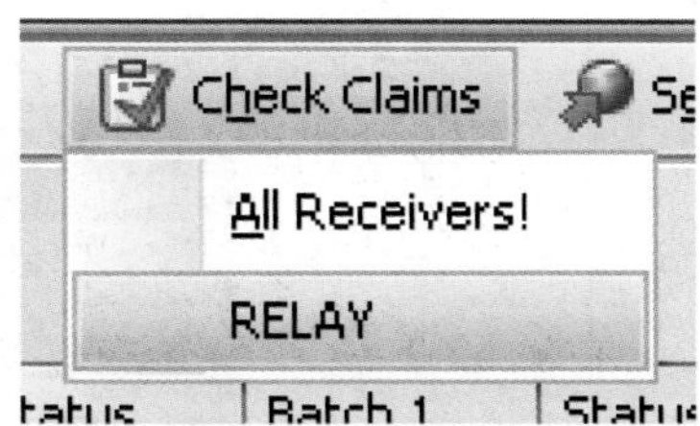

Figure 10.20 The Check Claims Menu with RELAY Selected

6. When the edit check is finished, the Edit Status column displays the status of each claim—indicated by a green, yellow, or red flag (see Figure 10.21). A green flag indicates that the claim passed the edits and is ready to send. A yellow flag indicates that there are issues with the claim—not serious enough to prevent it from being sent, but increasing the possibility that it will be rejected by the payer. A red flag indicates that the claim did not pass the first round of edits. Claims with red flags must be corrected before they can be sent. Claims can be corrected now, or an error report can be printed for later use.
7. To continue with the ready-to-send claims, select Send, select Claims, and select the EDI receiver (see Figure 10.22).
8. MNP creates a claim file and displays a preview report (see Figure 10.23).
9. If any errors are identified in the report, the claims must be edited before they can be transmitted.

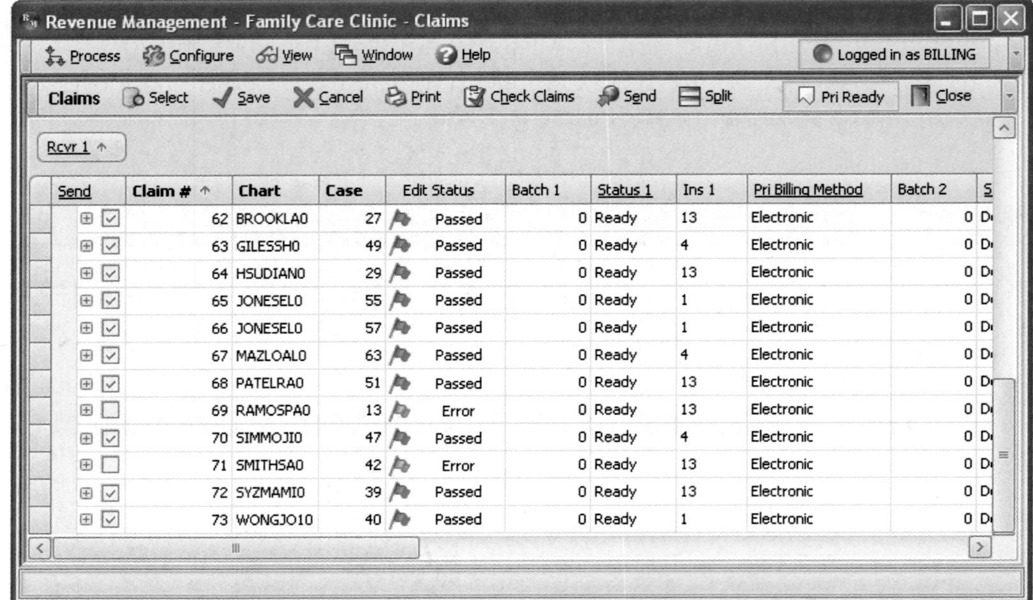

Send	Claim #	Chart	Case	Edit Status	Batch 1	Status 1	Ins 1	Pri Billing Method	Batch 2
☑	62	BROOKLA0	27	Passed	0	Ready	13	Electronic	0
☑	63	GILESSH0	49	Passed	0	Ready	4	Electronic	0
☑	64	HSUDIAN0	29	Passed	0	Ready	13	Electronic	0
☑	65	JONESEL0	55	Passed	0	Ready	1	Electronic	0
☑	66	JONESEL0	57	Passed	0	Ready	1	Electronic	0
☑	67	MAZLOAL0	63	Passed	0	Ready	4	Electronic	0
☑	68	PATELRA0	51	Passed	0	Ready	13	Electronic	0
☐	69	RAMOSPA0	13	Error	0	Ready	13	Electronic	0
☑	70	SIMMOJI0	47	Passed	0	Ready	4	Electronic	0
☐	71	SMITHSA0	42	Error	0	Ready	13	Electronic	0
☑	72	SYZMAMI0	39	Passed	0	Ready	13	Electronic	0
☑	73	WONGJO10	40	Passed	0	Ready	1	Electronic	0

Figure 10.21 List of Claims After Edits Are Performed

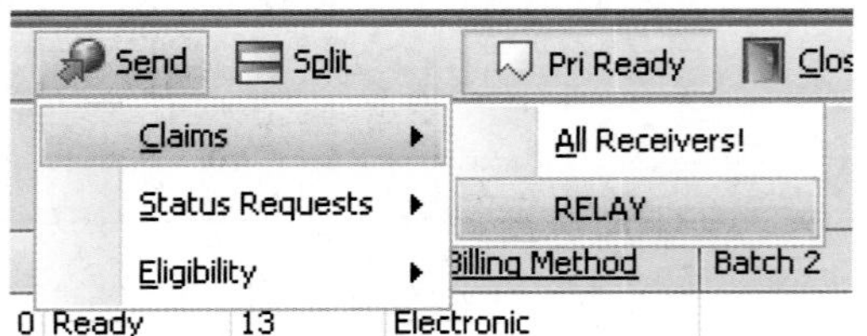

Figure 10.22 The Send Menu with Claims > RELAY Selected

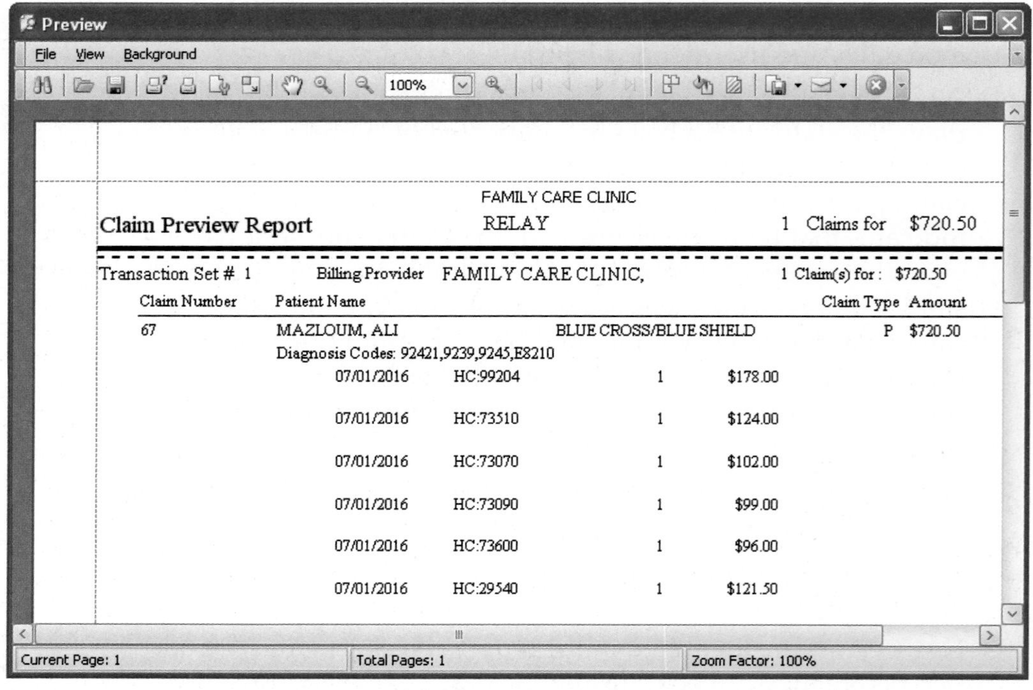

FAMILY CARE CLINIC

Claim Preview Report RELAY 1 Claims for $720.50

Transaction Set # 1 Billing Provider FAMILY CARE CLINIC, 1 Claim(s) for : $720.50

Claim Number	Patient Name				Claim Type	Amount
67	MAZLOUM, ALI	BLUE CROSS/BLUE SHIELD			P	$720.50
	Diagnosis Codes: 92421,9239,9245,E8210					
	07/01/2016	HC:99204	1	$178.00		
	07/01/2016	HC:73510	1	$124.00		
	07/01/2016	HC:73070	1	$102.00		
	07/01/2016	HC:73090	1	$99.00		
	07/01/2016	HC:73600	1	$96.00		
	07/01/2016	HC:29540	1	$121.50		

Figure 10.23 Preview Window with Claim Preview Report

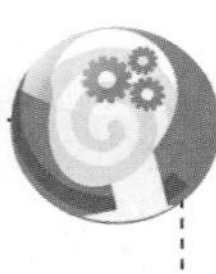

THINKING IT THROUGH 10.4

What is the purpose of using a PM/EHR that performs claim edits before a claim file is transmitted to a clearinghouse? If the clearinghouse performs edits, why is it necessary for the PM/EHR to perform edits?

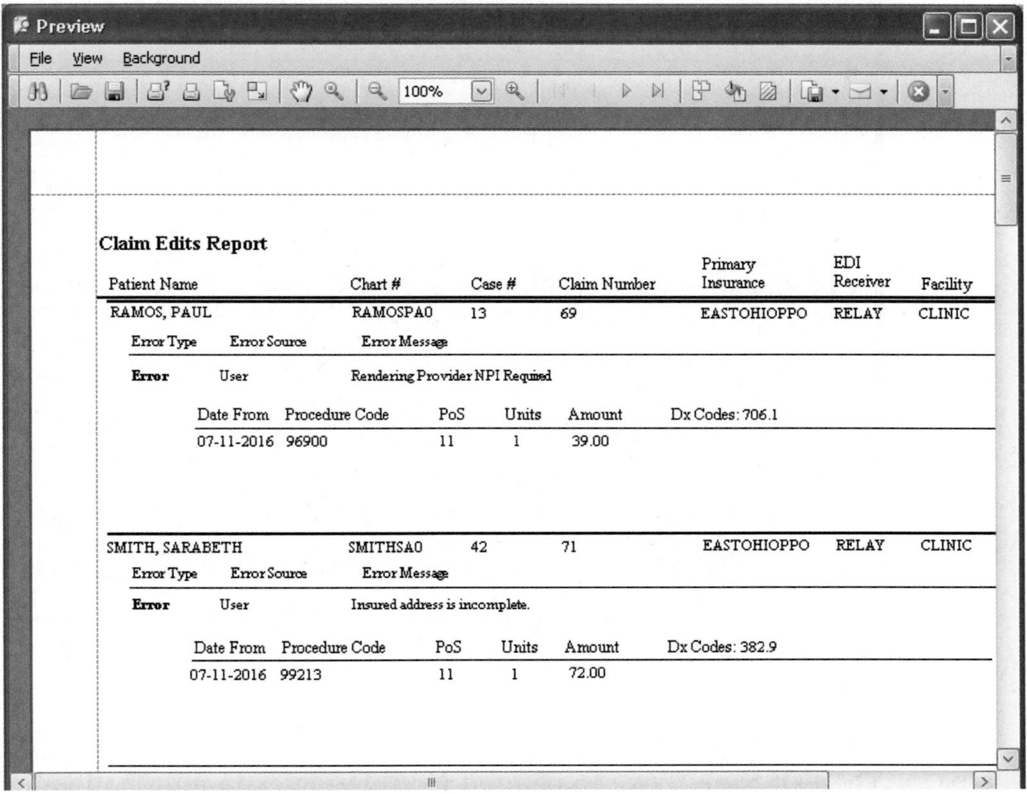

Claim Edits Report

Patient Name	Chart #	Case #	Claim Number	Primary Insurance	EDI Receiver	Facility
RAMOS, PAUL	RAMOSPA0	13	69	EASTOHIOPPO	RELAY	CLINIC

Error Type	Error Source	Error Message
Error	User	Rendering Provider NPI Required

Date From	Procedure Code	PoS	Units	Amount	Dx Codes: 706.1
07-11-2016	96900	11	1	39.00	

Patient Name	Chart #	Case #	Claim Number	Primary Insurance	EDI Receiver	Facility
SMITH, SARABETH	SMITHSA0	42	71	EASTOHIOPPO	RELAY	CLINIC

Error Type	Error Source	Error Message
Error	User	Insured address is incomplete.

Date From	Procedure Code	PoS	Units	Amount	Dx Codes: 382.9
07-11-2016	99213	11	1	72.00	

Figure 10.24 Preview Window with Claim Edits Report

10. Click the Send button to send the claim files. The files are transmitted to the clearinghouse, and the claim status is updated in MNP.

To fix the claims that did not pass the edits, review the Claim Edits Report (see Figure 10.24). This report lists the error messages associated with each claim.

10.8 Sending Electronic Claim Attachments

When a claim is sent electronically, an attachment that needs to accompany the claim, such as radiology films, must be referred to in the claim. In MNP, the EDI Report area within the Diagnosis tab of the Case dialog box is used to indicate to the payer that an attachment will accompany the claim and how the attachment will be transmitted (see Figure 10.25).

BILLING TIP

997 Functional Acknowledgment

When a payer receives a claim transmission, whether from a practice or from a clearinghouse, it sends an electronic acknowledgment of the file transmission, known as the 997 Functional Acknowledgment. This is not a standard HIPAA transaction, but it is used to report that a transaction has been received by the payer. The 997 also lists any additional errors found as a result of edits.

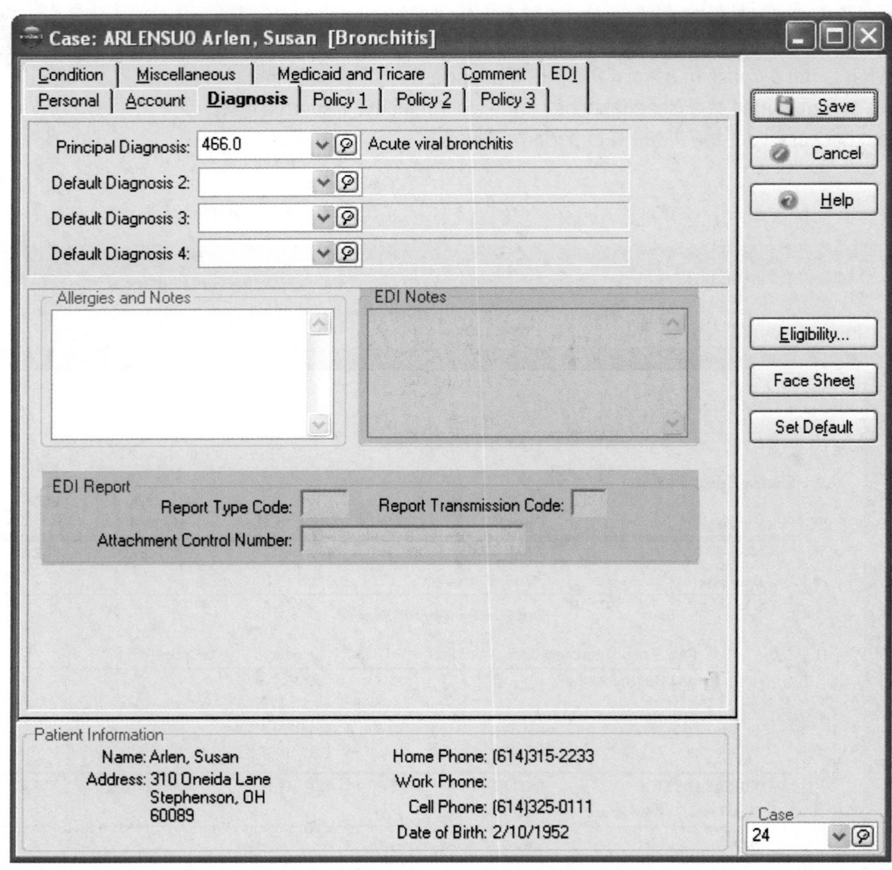

Figure 10.25 Diagnosis Tab with EDI Notes and EDI Report Fields Highlighted

EDI Notes

The EDI Notes box can be used for entering extra information for procedures and diagnoses that might be required by the patient's insurance carriers to process the electronic claim.

EDI Report

The EDI Report section contains three boxes:

1. **Report Type Code** This box is used to record the report type code—a two-digit code that indicates the type of report being attached. For example, DG is the code for a diagnostic report. Other codes include:

   107 Support data for verification

   REFERRAL To indicate a completed referral form

   AS Admission summary

   B2 Prescription

   B3 Physician order

   B4 Referral form

   CT Certification

   DA Dental models

   DG Diagnostic report

   DS Discharge summary

THINKING IT THROUGH 10.5

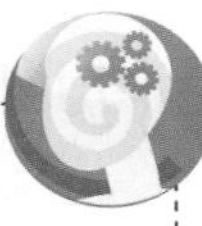

What is the purpose of the information entered in the EDI Notes and EDI Reports fields? If these fields were not completed, what might happen to a claim with an attachment?

- EB Explanation of benefits (coordination of benefits or Medicare secondary payer)
- MT Models
- NN Nursing notes
- OB Operative note
- OZ Support data for claim
- PN Physician therapy notes
- PO Prosthetics or orthotic certification
- PZ Physical therapy certification
- RB Radiology films
- RR Radiology reports
- RT Report of tests and analysis report

2. **Report Transmission Code** This box is used to record the report transmission code, a two-character code that indicates the means by which the report will be transmitted to the payer (for example, via mail, e-mail, or fax). Possible codes include:
   - AA Available on request at provider site. This means that the paperwork is not being sent with the claim at this time. Instead, it is available to the payer (or appropriate entity) at its request.
   - BM By mail.
   - EL Electronically only. Indicates that the attachment is being transmitted in a separate X12 functional group.
   - EM E-mail.
   - FX By fax.
3. **Attachment Control Number** This box contains the attachment's reference number (up to seven digits, assigned by the practice). This number is required if the transmission code is anything other than AA.

10.9 Claim Adjudication

When the health plan receives claims from the practice, it issues an electronic response to the sender showing that the transmission has been successful. Each claim then undergoes a checking process known as **adjudication,** in which the health plan follows these steps to judge how the claim should be paid:

adjudication series of steps that determine whether a claim should be paid

1. Initial processing
2. Automated review
3. Manual review
4. Determination
5. Payment

Initial Processing

Each claim's data elements are checked by the payer's front-end claims processing system. Paper claims and any paper attachments are date-stamped and entered into the payer's computer system, either by data-entry personnel or by the use of a scanning system. Initial processing might find problems such as the following:

- The patient's name, plan identification number, or place of service code is wrong.
- The diagnosis code is missing or is not valid for the date of service.
- The patient is not the correct sex for a reported gender-specific procedure code.

Claims with errors or simple mistakes are rejected, and the payer transmits instructions to the sender to fix and resubmit them. Such requests from the payer must be answered as quickly as possible by supplying the correct information and, if necessary, submitting another claim. The actual adjudication process begins when a clean claim is accepted by the payer for processing.

Automated Review

Payers' computer systems then apply edits that reflect their payment policies. For example, a Medicare claim is subject to the Correct Coding Initiative (CCI) edits (see Chapter 9). The automated review checks for the following:

1. **Patient eligibility for benefits** Is the patient eligible for the services that are billed?
2. **Time limits for filing claims** Is the claim sent within the payer's time limits for filing claims?
3. **Preauthorization and referral** Are valid preauthorization or referral numbers present as required under the payer's policies?
4. **Duplicate dates of service** Is this claim billing for a service on this date that has already been adjudicated?
5. **Noncovered services** Are the billed services covered under the patient's policy?
6. **Valid code linkages** Are the diagnosis and procedure codes properly linked for medical necessity?
7. **Bundled codes** Have surgical code bundling rules and global periods been followed?
8. **Medical review** Are the charges for services not medically necessary or over the frequency limits of the plan? The payer's medical director and other professional medical staff have a medical review program to ensure that providers give patients the most appropriate care in the most cost-effective manner. Medical review edits are based on the guidelines of the medical review program.

THINKING IT THROUGH 10.6

What effect does performing an edit to check claims before transmission to a health plan have on the speed of claim adjudication?

9. **Utilization review** Are the hospital-based health care services delivered to a member of a plan appropriate?
10. **Concurrent care** If two or more providers' work is being billed, was it medically necessary to have both treat the patient?

Manual Review

If the automated review finds problems, the claim is **suspended** and set aside for **development**—the term used by payers to indicate that more information is needed for claim processing. Such claims are sent to the medical review department, where a claim examiner reviews them. The examiner may ask the provider for clinical documentation to check:

- Where the service took place
- Whether the treatments were appropriate and a logical outcome of the facts and conditions shown in the medical record
- That the services provided were accurately reported

suspended claim status when the payer is developing the claim

development process of gathering information to adjudicate a claim

determination payer's decision about the benefits due for a claim

medical necessity denial refusal by a plan to pay for a procedure that does not meet its medical necessity criteria

Determination

For each service line on a claim, the payer makes a payment **determination**—a decision whether to (1) pay it, (2) deny it, (3) hold it for further processing, or (4) pay it at a reduced level. If the service falls within normal guidelines, it will be paid. If it is not reimbursable, the item on the claim is denied. A **medical necessity denial** may result from a lack of a clear, correct linkage between the diagnosis and procedure.

Payment

If payment is due, the payer sends it to the provider or to the provider's financial institution along with an electronic or paper document explaining the items that were paid. This remittance process is discussed in Chapter 11.

10.10 Monitoring Claim Status

Practices closely track their accounts receivable (A/R)—the money that is owed for services rendered—using the PM/EHR. The accounts receivable is made up of payments due from payers and from patients. For this reason, after claims have been accepted for processing by payers, their status is monitored.

Claim Status

Monitoring claims during adjudication requires two types of information. The first is the amount of time the payer is allowed to take to respond to the claim, and the second is how long the claim has been in process.

Timely Payment of Insurance Claims

In some instances, insurance carriers dispute claims. When a carrier contests a claim or delays payment because more information is needed, providers frequently are not given notice in a timely manner. When further documentation is requested and the physician provides the information, a health plan can further delay payment by asking for additional information or clarification. Resubmitting rejected claims is a time-consuming process, resulting in increased practice expenses and more delay in payment.

prompt payment laws state laws that mandate a time period within which clean claims must be paid; if they are not, financial penalties are levied against the payer

claim turnaround time time period in which a health plan must process a claim

aging classification of accounts receivable by length of time

insurance aging report report that lists how long a payer has taken to respond to insurance claims

Most states have enacted prompt payment laws to ensure that claims are paid in a timely manner. State **prompt payment laws** mandate a time period known as **claim turnaround time** within which clean claims must be paid, and they call for financial penalties to be levied against late payers.

If a clean claim is not paid within the allotted time frame, the payer should be notified in writing that payment has not been received according to applicable prompt payment laws. Practices should also request written explanations of all claim delays, partial payments, and denials. If satisfaction is not achieved, the applicable state or federal regulatory agency may be notified of the violation.

Aging

The other factor in claim follow-up is **aging**—how long a payer has had the claim. The PM/EHR is used to generate an **insurance aging report** that lists the claims transmitted on each day and how long they have been in process with the payer. A typical report, shown in Figure 10.26, shows claims that were sent fewer than thirty days ago, between thirty and sixty days ago, and so on. Using the report, it is easy to determine which claims require follow-up. Most practices follow up on claims that are aged less than thirty days in seven to fourteen days. Chapter 12 provides instruction on creating aging and other key practice management reports.

Primary Insurance Aging Summary

October 31, 2016

Date of Service	Procedure	- Past - 0 to 30	- Past - 31 to 60	- Past - 61 to 90	- Past - 91 to 120	- Past - 121 +	Total Balance
BCBS (04)							**614-024-9000**
Claim: 64222	Initial Billing Date: 9/23/2016		Last Billing Date: 10/14/2016				
	Insurance Totals:	$0.00	$160.00	$0.00	$0.00	$0.00	$160.00
EAST OHIO PPO (13)							**419-444-1505**
Claim: 63366	Initial Billing Date: 6/30/2016		Last Billing Date: 10/14/2016				
Claim: 63367	Initial Billing Date: 8/12/2016		Last Billing Date: 10/14/2016				
	Insurance Totals:	$0.00	$0.00	$465.00	$0.00	$655.00	$1,120.00

Figure 10.26 Primary Insurance Aging Report

HIPAA/HITECH TIP

ANSI ASC X12 5010 Format

On January 1, 2012, a new version of the standards required to submit electronic transactions will take effect. The ASC X12 Version 4010A standards, which have been in place since 2002, will be replaced by the ASC X12 Version 5010 standards. The new standards are required to accommodate ICD-10-CM, and also provide improvements to a number of electronic transactions. For the most part, the changes required will be made by PM/EHR vendors and clearinghouses, but some data changes will need to be made by the billing staff. For example, in 5010, the billing provider's address can no longer be a post office box or a lockbox.

HIPAA Health Care Claim Status Inquiry/Response

The status of a claim can also be determined at any time by sending an electronic inquiry to the payer. The **HIPAA X12 276/277 Health Care Claim Status Inquiry/Response** is the standard electronic transaction to obtain the current status of a claim during the adjudication process. The inquiry is the 276, and the response returned by the payer is the 277. Some PM/EHRs track how many days claims have been unpaid and automatically send a claim status inquiry after a certain number of days. For example, if a particular payer pays claims on the twentieth day, the program transmits a 276 for any unpaid claims aged twenty-one days.

HIPAA X12 276/277 Health Care Claim Status Inquiry/Response electronic format used to ask payers about claims

claim status category codes used to report the status group for a claim

pending claim status in which the payer is waiting for information before making a payment decision

claim status codes used to provide a detailed answer to a claim status inquiry

The HIPAA 277 transaction from the payer uses **claim status category codes** for the main types of responses:

- *A* codes are an acknowledgment that the claim has been received.
- *P* codes indicate that a claim is **pending,** that is, that the payer is waiting for information before making a payment decision.
- *F* codes indicate that a claim has been finalized.
- *R* codes indicate that a request for more information has been sent.
- *E* codes indicate that an error has occurred in transmission; usually these claims need to be resent.

These codes are further detailed by **claim status codes,** as shown in Table 10.2.

Working with Health Plans

Ensuring that claims are processed as quickly as possible requires being familiar with payers' claim-processing procedures, including:

- The timetable for submitting corrected claims, as well as for filing secondary claims (usually a period of time from the date of payment by the primary payer)

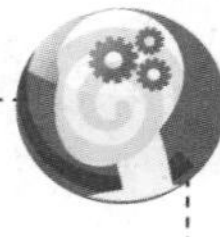

THINKING IT THROUGH 10.7

What action from the health plan would you expect if notified that a claim response is claim status code 3? Code 12?

TABLE 10.2	Selected Claim Status Codes
1	For more detailed information, see remittance advice.
2	More detailed information in letter.
3	Claim has been adjudicated and is awaiting payment cycle.
4	This is a subsequent request for information from the original request.
5	This is a final request for information.
6	Balance is due from the subscriber.
7	Claim may be reconsidered at a future date.
9	No payment will be made for this claim.
12	One or more originally submitted procedure codes have been combined.
15	One or more originally submitted procedure codes have been modified.
16	Claim/encounter has been forwarded to entity.
29	Subscriber and policy number/contract number mismatched.
30	Subscriber and subscriber ID mismatched.
31	Subscriber and policyholder name mismatched.
32	Subscriber and policy number/contract number not found.
33	Subscriber and subscriber ID not found.

- How to resubmit corrected claims that are denied for missing or incorrect data (some payers have an online or automated telephone procedure that can be used to resubmit a claim after missing information has been supplied)
- How to handle requests for additional documentation required by the payer

Requests for information should be answered as quickly as possible and should be courteous and complete.

chapter 10 summary

LEARNING OUTCOME	KEY CONCEPTS/EXAMPLES
10.1 Briefly compare the CMS-1500 paper claim and the 837 electronic claim. Pages 492–498	The CMS-1500 claim has thirty-three numbered boxes representing about 150 discrete data elements. The 837 has a maximum of 244 segments representing about 1,054 elements. Some different terms are in use with the HIPAA claim, and a few additional information items must be relayed to the payer. For example, the HIPAA 837 uses the term *subscriber* for the insurance policyholder or guarantor, rather than *insured* as on the CMS-1500 claim. The HIPAA claim also requires a claim filing indicator code, which is an administrative code used to identify the type of health plan. Although essentially the same data elements are used to complete both forms, the 837 organizes them in a manner that is efficient for electronic transmission, rather than for a paper form.
10.2 Discuss the information contained in the Claim Management dialog box. Pages 498–499	The Claim Management dialog box contains a list of all claims created, and buttons used for editing claims, creating claims, printing/sending claims, reprinting claims, and deleting claims.
10.3 Explain the process of creating claims. Pages 499–501	1. On the Activities menu, click Claim Management. The Claim Management dialog box is displayed. 2. Click the Create Claims button. 3. Add values to fields, or leave them blank to create all claims. 4. Click the Create button. The Create Claims box closes, and the new claims are listed in the Claim Management dialog box.
10.4 Describe how to locate a specific claim. Pages 501–504	The List Only feature is used to locate a claim. 1. Click the List Only... button in the Claim Management dialog box. 2. In the List Only Claims That Match dialog box, complete the fields to filter claim selection by: • Chart number • Claim created date • Carrier status • Insurance carrier • EDI receiver

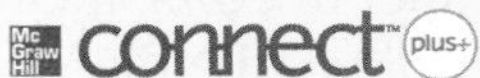

Enhance your learning at **mcgrawhillconnect.com**!
- *Practice Exercises*
- *Worksheets*
- *Activities*
- *Integrated eBook*

LEARNING OUTCOME	KEY CONCEPTS/EXAMPLES
	• Billing method • Claim status • Billing date • Batch number 3. Click Apply. The List Only Claims That Match dialog box closes, and the selected claim or claims are listed in the Claim Management dialog box.
10.5 Discuss the purpose of reviewing and editing claims. Pages 504–508	Claims are reviewed and edited to make sure they are accurate. By identifying and solving problems before claims are submitted, the practice is more likely to receive prompt payment.
10.6 Analyze the methods used to submit electronic claims. Pages 508–511	Three methods can be used to submit electronic claims: direct transmission to the payer, direct data entry, and via a clearinghouse. Each method has advantages and disadvantages. • In the direct transmission approach, the medical practice must supply all the HIPAA data elements and follow specific EDI formatting rules. The practice may also have to purchase special software that can communicate with the payer's system. • Direct data entry (DDE) is inefficient and susceptible to keyboarding errors. • Most providers send their electronic claims to a clearinghouse for a number of reasons. While all health care claims must use HIPAA transactions and code sets, each payer has its own set of claim edits and formatting conventions. It would be difficult for a billing specialist to know the rules of each payer. Practices with a large volume of claims find that it is not be practical to send electronic claims to each payer; when a clearinghouse is used, claims can be sent in one batch to one location. Also, the clearinghouse processes the claims before it sends them to the payer. Most clearinghouses charge fees for their services. Some charge a flat fee per month regardless of the number of claims processed, while others charge on a per-claim basis.
10.7 List the steps required to submit electronic claims. Pages 511–515	1. Select Revenue Management > Revenue Management... on the Activities menu. The Revenue Management main window opens. 2. Select Claims on the Process menu. 3. Select an EDI receiver. A list of claims ready to be sent is displayed. 4. To perform an edit check on the claims, click Check Claims and the name of the EDI receiver. The claims are checked against a number of edits, including ANSI edits, common edits, and user-defined edits.

LEARNING OUTCOME	KEY CONCEPTS/EXAMPLES
	5. When the edit check is finished, the Edit Status column displays the status of each claim—indicated by a green, yellow, or red flag. Claims with red flags must be corrected before they can be sent. You can view and correct the errors at this point, or you can print an error report and fix the claims at a later time. 6. To continue with the ready-to-send claims, select Send, select Claims, and select the EDI receiver. 7. Network Professional (MNP) creates a claim file and displays a preview report. 8. The preview report checks the claims for errors. If any errors are found, the claims must be edited before they can be transmitted. 9. Click the Send button to send the claim files. The files are transmitted to the clearinghouse, and the claim status is updated in MNP. 10. To fix the claims that did not pass the edits, view the Claim Edits Report, which lists the error messages associated with each claim.
10.8 Describe how to add attachments to electronic claims. Pages 515–517	Information regarding claim attachments is entered in the EDI report section of the Diagnosis tab (within the Case folder). Fields include: • Report Type Code • Report Transmission Code • Attachment Control Number
10.9 Explain the claim determination process used by health plans. Pages 517–519	Health plans follow five steps to adjudicate claims: 1. Initial processing 2. Automated review 3. Manual review 4. Determination 5. Payment
10.10 Discuss the use of the PM/EHR to monitor claims. Pages 519–522	The practice uses the PM/EHR to monitor claims by using the reports function to create an insurance aging report, which lists the claims transmitted on each day and how long they have been in process with the payer. The report makes it easy to determine which claims require follow-up. Most practices follow up on claims that are aged less than thirty days in seven to fourteen days.

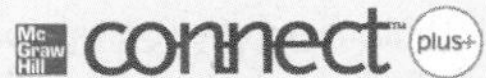

Enhance your learning at **mcgrawhillconnect.com**!

- *Practice Exercises*
- *Worksheets*
- *Activities*
- *Integrated eBook*

chapter review

MATCHING QUESTIONS

Match the key terms with their definitions.

_____ 1. ***[LO 10.10]*** claim turnaround time

_____ 2. ***[LO 10.6]*** crossover claims

_____ 3. ***[LO 10.9]*** adjudication

_____ 4. ***[LO 10.3]*** filter

_____ 5. ***[LO 10.1]*** timely filing

_____ 6. ***[LO 10.9]*** determination

_____ 7. ***[LO 10.10]*** pending

_____ 8. ***[LO 10.1]*** data elements

_____ 9. ***[LO 10.10]*** aging

_____ 10. ***[LO 10.9]*** development

a. Claim status during adjudication when the payer is waiting for information from the submitter.

b. A condition that data must meet to be selected.

c. A payer's decision about the benefits due for a claim.

d. The smallest units of information in a HIPAA transaction, such as a person's name.

e. The time period in which a health plan is obligated to process a claim.

f. The term used by payers to indicate that more information is needed for claim processing.

g. The rules that specify the number of days after the date of service that the practice has to file the claim.

h. Classification of accounts receivable by the length of time an account is due.

i. Claims that are billed to Medicare and then submitted to Medicaid.

j. The process followed by health plans to examine claims and determine benefits.

TRUE-FALSE QUESTIONS

Decide whether each statement is true or false.

_____ 1. ***[LO 10.4]*** In Medisoft Network Professional, filters are applied in the Claim Management dialog box.

_____ 2. ***[LO 10.8]*** When an attachment must accompany a claim filed electronically, specific information must be entered in the Diagnosis tab of the Case folder in Medisoft Network Professional.

_____ 3. ***[LO 10.2]*** Insurance claims are created from within the Revenue Management area of Medisoft Network Professional.

_____ 4. ***[LO 10.9]*** For each service line on a claim, the payer makes a payment adjudication—a decision whether to (1) pay it, (2) deny it, (3) hold it for further processing, or (4) pay it at a reduced level.

_____ 5. ***[LO 10.10]*** The HIPAA X12 276/277 Health Care Claim Status Inquiry/Response is the standard electronic transaction to obtain the current status of a claim during the adjudication process.

_____ 6. ***[LO 10.1]*** The HIPAA standard transaction for electronic claims is the HIPAA X12 837 Health Care Claim, usually called the HIPAA claim.

_____ 7. ***[LO 10.10]*** The HIPAA 277 transaction from the payer uses claim status category codes for the main types of responses.

_____ 8. ***[LO 10.7]*** A claim that has a yellow flag in the Edit Status column in Revenue Management must be corrected before it can be sent to a payer or clearinghouse.

_____ 9. ***[LO 10.9]*** A medical necessity denial may result from lack of a clear, correct linkage between the diagnosis and procedure.

_____ 10. ***[LO 10.6]*** Claims billed to Medicare and then submitted to Medicaid are called coordinated claims.

MULTIPLE-CHOICE QUESTIONS

Select the letter that best completes the statement or answers the question.

1. ***[LO 10.1]*** The HIPAA standard transaction for paper claims is known as the _________.
   a. HIPAA X12 837 Health Care Claim
   b. HIPAA claim
   c. CMS-1500 (08/05) Claim
   d. HIPAA X12 276/277 Health Care Claim Status Inquiry/Response

2. ***[LO 10.2]*** The upper-right corner of the Claim Management dialog box contains five _________ that simplify the task of moving from one entry to another.
   a. navigator buttons
   b. filters
   c. data elements
   d. crossover claims

3. ***[LO 10.3]*** A _________ is a condition that data must meet to be selected.
   a. transaction standard
   b. filter
   c. data element
   d. crossover claim

4. ***[LO 10.6]*** The _________ method of submitting electronic claims requires manual entry of data on the payer's website.
   a. clearinghouse
   b. direct to the payer
   c. direct data entry
   d. all of the above

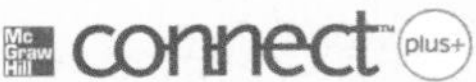
Enhance your learning at **mcgrawhillconnect.com**!
- *Practice Exercises*
- *Worksheets*
- *Activities*
- *Integrated eBook*

5. *[LO 10.5]* Medisoft Network Professional's ________ feature allows claims to be reviewed and edited before they are submitted to insurance carriers for payment.
   a. Claim Management
   b. List Only
   c. Claim Edit
   d. all of the above

6. *[LO 10.7]* To perform an edit check on claims in Revenue Management, click ________ to select the EDI receiver.
   a. Edit
   b. Edit Claims
   c. Check Claims
   d. Check

7. *[LO 10.6]* Claims billed to Medicare and then submitted to Medicaid are called ________.
   a. HIPAA claims
   b. CMS-1500 (08/05) claims
   c. crossover claims
   d. all of the above

8. *[LO 10.9]* Each claim undergoes a checking process known as ________, made up of these steps the health plan follows to judge how it should be paid.
   a. adjudication
   b. aging
   c. development
   d. pending

9. *[LO 10.9]* A ________ may result from lack of a clear, correct linkage between the diagnosis and procedure.
   a. determination
   b. medical necessity denial
   c. filter
   d. crossover claim

10. *[LO 10.10]* The ________ is the standard electronic transaction to obtain the current status of a claim during the adjudication process.
    a. HIPAA X12 837 Health Care Claim
    b. HIPAA claim
    c. CMS-1500 (08/05) Claim
    d. HIPAA X12 276/277 Health Care Claim Status Inquiry/Response

SHORT-ANSWER QUESTIONS

Define the following abbreviations.

1. ***[LO 10.1]*** NUCC ________________________________

2. ***[LO 10.1]*** HIPAA X12 276/277 ________________________

3. ***[LO 10.1]*** HIPAA X12 837 ___________________________

APPLYING YOUR KNOWLEDGE

Answer the questions below in the space provided.

10.1 ***[LO 10.1]*** Why do you think health plans have timely filing requirements?

____

____

10.2 ***[LO 10.4]*** How would you find a list of all the claims in Medisoft Network Professional from a particular day?

____

____

10.3 ***[LO 10.6]*** Why do you think Medicaid is always last to pay on claims when other insurance providers are involved?

____

____

10.4 ***[LO 10.9]*** Why do medical practices monitor the status of the claims they submit?

____

____

chapter 11

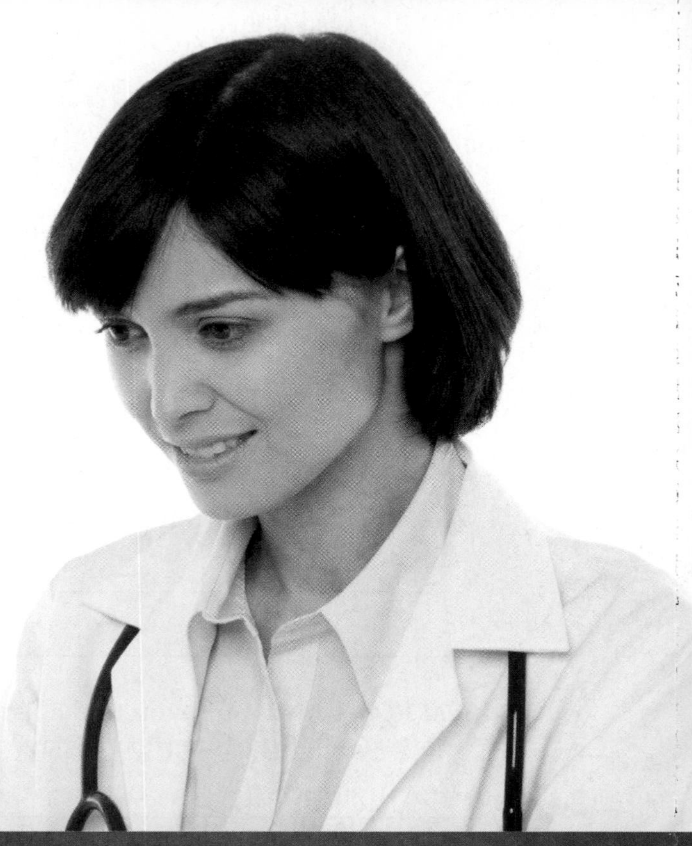

Posting Payments and Creating Statements

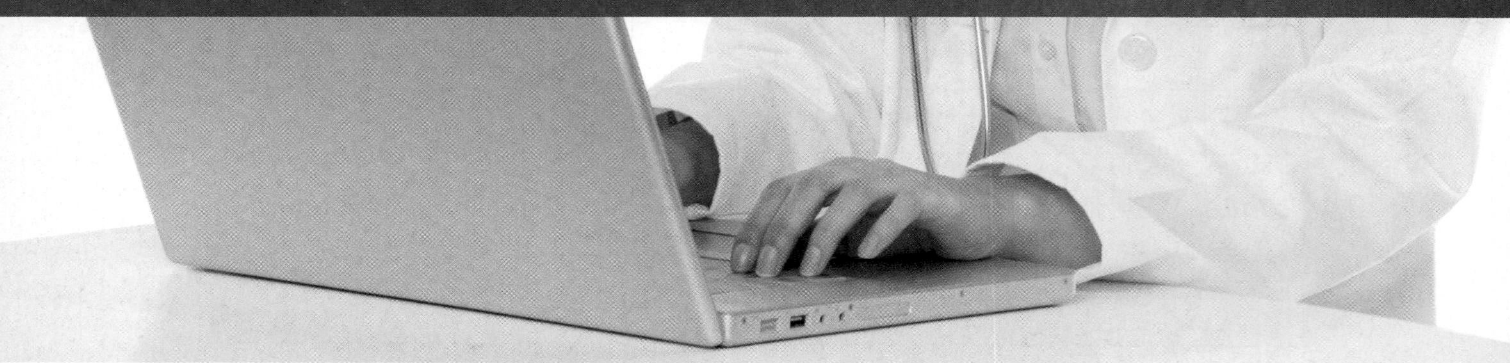

KEY TERMS

appeal
appellant
autoposting
capitation payments
claim adjustment group code (CAGC)
claim adjustment reason code (CARC)
claimant
claim control number
cycle billing
electronic funds transfer (EFT)
electronic remittance advice (ERA)
explanation of benefits (EOB)
nonsufficient funds (NSF) check
once-a-month billing
overpayment
patient statement
postpayment audit
Recovery Audit Contractor (RAC)
remainder statements
remittance advice (RA)
remittance advice remark code (RARC)
standard statements
takeback
X12 835 Electronic Remittance Advice (835)

LEARNING OUTCOMES

When you finish this chapter, you will be able to:

11.1 List the six steps for checking a remittance advice.

11.2 Describe the procedures for entering insurance payments.

11.3 Explain how to apply insurance payments to charges.

11.4 Explain how to enter capitation payments.

11.5 Discuss the purpose of appeals and postpayment audits.

11.6 Compare standard patient statements and remainder patient statements.

11.7 Explain the difference between once-a-month and cycle billing.

11.8 Explain the procedure for processing a nonsufficient funds payment.

A "Satisfied Customer"

"I'm really glad we had that ABN on file for Leila," Chris explained to Aisha over lunch. "She had given us her debit card after her last appointment so we could charge that noncovered service to it. Now a month later, she got a bill from the bank showing the payment to FCC—but she couldn't remember what it is for! I looked it up and was able to quickly explain that it was the exam she needed done before she started her new job." "Right," Aisha said, "that is why we pay good attention to that ABN policy. We need to be able to collect our fees from all our patients and also be compliant with good billing practices."

To run a successful office requires a number of related skills. In this case, the patient was really a customer calling to question a bill, and Chris was able to respond to the patient's satisfaction. Both the facts and the tone of the conversation were important in handling the situation well.

WHEN YOU FINISH THIS CHAPTER, YOU WILL ALSO BE ABLE TO USE MEDISOFT CLINICAL TO:

1. Use MNP to create a deposit from a health plan.
2. Apply an insurance payment in MNP.
3. Use MNP to enter a capitation payment.
4. Adjust a capitated account to a zero balance in MNP.
5. Use MNP to process an insurance overpayment.
6. Using MNP, create and print patient statements, and edit statement information.
7. Post a nonsufficient funds charge in MNP.

SOFTWARE SKILLS

11.1 Working with the Remittance Advice (RA)

Once a claim has been received and accepted for adjudication, the health plan determines the payment it will make for each charge. The payer then generates a remittance advice (RA) and sends it to the provider. A **remittance advice (RA)** lists patients, dates of service, charges, and the amounts paid or denied—that is, the adjustments made by the insurance carrier to the billed charges. A sample RA appears in Figure 11.1.

remittance advice (RA) document describing a payment resulting from a claim adjudication

electronic remittance advice (ERA) electronic document that lists patients, dates of service, charges, and the amounts paid or denied by the insurance carrier

X12 835 Electronic Remittance Advice (835) electronic transaction for payment explanation

claim control number unique number assigned to a claim by the sender

autoposting software feature enabling automatic entry of payments from a remittance advice

RAs cover groups of claims, not just a single claim. The claims paid on a single RA are not consecutive or logically grouped; they are usually for different patients and various dates of service. RAs list the claims that have been adjudicated within the payment cycle in different orders; they may be sorted alphanumerically by the patient account number assigned by provider, alphabetically by client name, or numerically by internal control number. A corresponding EOB sent to the patient, on the other hand, lists just the information for the recipient.

The RA may be sent in electronic format, called an **electronic remittance advice (ERA),** or in paper format. Although similar information is contained on an ERA and a paper RA, the ERA may offer additional data. The ERA that is mandated for use by HIPAA is called the **X12 835 Remittance Advice Transaction,** or simply the **835.** In addition to physicians, other health care providers receiving the 835 include hospitals, nursing homes, laboratories, and dentists.

Claim Control Number

When the practice sent a claim, the PM/EHR assigned it a **claim control number,** also known as an ID number. This number, a maximum of twenty characters, is unique to that claim. The claim control number appears on the section of the RA for that particular claim, and it is used to match the claim with the payment.

Autoposting

In practices that enable certain advanced electronic communication features of PM/EHRs, a capability called **autoposting** is used to automatically post payments listed on an ERA. This capability greatly speeds the process of handling RAs. The biller in this case performs an audit (review) function rather than a data-entry task. The program lists the posting from the ERA, and the biller accepts or overrides it.

Adjustments

An adjustment means that the payer is paying a claim or a service line differently than billed. The adjustment may be that the item is:

- Denied
- Zero pay (if accepted as billed but no payment is due)

(1) MICHAEL A. JONES, MD
414 ISLAND RD.
PAVE, OH 43068-1101

(2) PAGE: 1 OF 1
(3) DATE: 01/13/2003
(4) ID NUMBER: 010000482OH01

(5) PATIENT: SMITH (6) MARY CLAIM: 99999999999 (7) ID. NO: 0001234567 (8) PLAN CODE: P-PAR (9) MFD. REC. NO: 0555-99

(10) PROC CODE	(11) FROM DATE	(12) THRU DATE	(13) TREAT-MENT	(14) STATUS CODE	(15) AMOUNT CHRGD	(16) AMOUNT ALLWD	(17) COPAY/ DEDUCT	(18) COINS	(19) OTHER REDUCT	(20) AMOUNT APPRVD	(21) PATIENT BALANCE
99213-00	01/13/03	01/13/03	1	A	55.00	54.00	.00	5.00	.00	49.00	5.00
93000-00	01/13/03	01/13/03	1	A	40.50	39.50	.00	.00	.00	39.50	.00
81000-00	01/13/03	01/13/03	1	A	8.00	5.85	.00	.00	.00	5.85	.00
CLAIM TOTALS					103.50	94.35	.00	5.00	.00	89.35	5.00

PATIENT: ALLEN ALLAN CLAIM: 89999999999 ID. NO: 0000234567 PLAN CODE: C2000 MFD. REC. NO: 0444-88

PROC CODE	FROM DATE	THRU DATE	TREAT-MENT	STATUS CODE	AMOUNT CHRGD	AMOUNT ALLWD	COPAY/ DEDUCT	COINS	OTHER REDUCT	AMOUNT APPRVD	PATIENT BALANCE
99201-00	02/17/03	02/17/03	1	A	90.00	82.00	.00	10.00	.00	63.80	10.00
CLAIM TOTALS					90.00	82.00	.00	10.00	.00	63.80	10.00

PATIENT: JAMES JAMES CLAIM: 79999999999 ID. NO: 0001034567 PLAN CODE: STATE MFD. REC. NO:

PROC CODE	FROM DATE	THRU DATE	TREAT-MENT	STATUS CODE	AMOUNT CHRGD	AMOUNT ALLWD	COPAY/ DEDUCT	COINS	OTHER REDUCT	AMOUNT APPRVD	PATIENT BALANCE
99214-00	01/07/03	01/07/03	1	A	101.00	58.00	.00	5.00	.00	68.00	5.00
CLAIM TOTALS					101.00	68.00	.00	5.00	.00	68.00	5.00

PAYMENT SUMMARY

TOTAL AMOUNT PAID	224.35
PRIOR CREDIT BALANCE	.00
CURRENT CREDIT DEFERRED	.00
PRIOR CREDIT APPLIED	.00
NEW CREDIT BALANCE	.00
NET DISBURSED	224.35

TOTAL ALL CLAIMS

AMOUNT CHARGES	294.50
AMOUNT ALLOWED	244.35
DEDUCTIBLE	.00
COPAY/COINS	20.00
OTHER REDUCTION	.00
AMOUNT APPROVED	224.35
PATIENT BALANCE	20.00
TOTAL CREDITS	.00

CHECK INFORMATION

NUMBER	00000XXXXXX
DATE	02/27/03
AMOUNT	224.35

(22) STATUS CODES:
A - APPROVED AJ - ADJUSTMENT IP - IN PROCESS R - REJECTED V - VOID

Codes

1. Name and address of provider who rendered medical services.
2. Number of pages for the provider remittance.
3. Date the provider remittance was issued.
4. 13-digit identification number of provider who rendered medical services.
5. Name of the patient.
6. Claim number.
7. Identification number we assign to the claim.
8. Name of the member's benefit plan.
9. Number the provider's office has assigned to the patient; will be reflected only if submitted in box 26 of the red HCFA-1500 claim form.
10. Procedure code(s) describing medical services rendered.
11. Date on which medical services began.
12. Date on which medical services ended.
13. Number reflected in box 24g of the red HCFA-1500 claim form; describes the number of days or units related to the medical service.
14. The status of the claim; see box 22 for more information.
15. The amount charged by provider for performing the medical service(s).
16. The amount that we will pay.
17. The amount that has been applied to the member's deductible.
18. The amount of the copayment or the coinsurance for which the member is responsible.
19. Any plan-specific reduction for which the member may be financially responsible.
20. The amount that we will pay.
21. Any amount for which the member is financially responsible.
22. Describes the abbreviations of the status codes reflected in item 14.

Figure 11.1 Example of a Payer's Remittance Advice

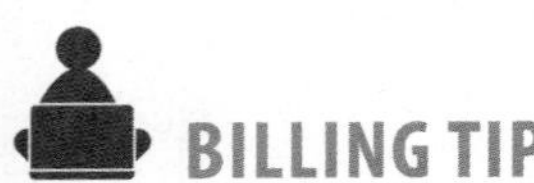

BILLING TIP

Code Updates

Claim adjustment reason codes and remark codes are updated three times each year; access www.wpc-edi.com/codes for the updated lists.

claim adjustment group code (CAGC) used on an RA/EOB to indicate the general type of reason code for an adjustment

claim adjustment reason code (CARC) used on an RA/EOB to explain why a payment does not match the amount billed

remittance advice remark code (RARC) code that explains a payer's payment decision

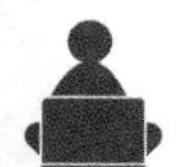

BILLING TIP

Patient Balance Billing

A group code PR with an associated reason code indicates whether a provider may bill a beneficiary for the nonpaid balance of the furnished services.

- Reduced amount paid (most likely paid according to the allowed amount)
- Less because a penalty is subtracted from the payment

To explain the determination to the provider, payers use a combination of codes: (1) a claim adjustment group code, (2) a claim adjustment reason code, and (3) a remittance advice remark code.

Claim Adjustment Group Codes

The **claim adjustment group codes,** also called group codes and abbreviated as **CAGCs,** are:

- **PR (patient responsibility)** Appears next to an amount that can be billed to the patient or insured. This group code typically applies to deductible and coinsurance or copayment adjustments.
- **CO (contractual obligations)** Appears when a contract between the payer and the provider resulted in an adjustment. This group code usually applies to allowed charges (also known as allowed amounts). CO adjustments are not billable to the patient under the contract.
- **CR (corrections and reversals)** Appears to correct a previous claim.
- **OA (other adjustments)** Used only when neither PR nor CO applies, as when another insurance is primary.
- **PI (payer-initiated reduction)** Appears when the payer thinks that the patient is not responsible for the charge, but there is no contract between the payer and the provider that states this; it might be used for medical review denials.

Claim Adjustment Reason Codes

Payers use **claim adjustment reason codes (CARCs)** to provide details about an adjustment. Examples of these codes and their meanings are provided in Table 11.1.

Remittance Advice Remark Codes

Payers may also use **remittance advice remark codes (RARCs)** for more explanation. Remark codes are maintained by CMS but can be used by all payers. Codes that start with *M* are from a Medicare code set that was in place before HIPAA but is still used, including Medicare outpatient adjudication (MOA) remark codes. Codes that begin with *N* are new. Table 11.2 shows selected remark codes.

Steps for Checking a Remittance Advice

This procedure is followed to check the remittance data:

1. Check the patient's name, claim control number, and date of service against the claim.
2. Verify that all billed CPT codes are listed.
3. Check the payment for each CPT code against the expected amount, which may be an allowed charge or a percentage of

TABLE 11.1	Selected Claim Adjustment Reason Codes
1	Deductible amount.
2	Coinsurance amount.
3	Copayment amount.
4	The procedure code is inconsistent with the modifier used, or a required modifier is missing.
5	The procedure code or bill type is inconsistent with the place of service.
6	The procedure or revenue code is inconsistent with the patient's age.
7	The procedure or revenue code is inconsistent with the patient's gender.
8	The procedure code is inconsistent with the provider type or specialty (taxonomy).
9	The diagnosis is inconsistent with the patient's age.
10	The diagnosis is inconsistent with the patient's gender.
11	The diagnosis is inconsistent with the procedure.
12	The diagnosis is inconsistent with the provider type.

TABLE 11.2	Selected Remark Codes
M11	DME, orthotics and prosthetics must be billed to the DME carrier who services the patient's Zip code.
M12	Diagnostic tests performed by a physician must indicate whether purchased services are included on the claim.
M37	Service not covered when the patient is under age 35.
M38	The patient is liable for the charges for this service as you informed the patient in writing before the service was furnished that we would not pay for it, and the patient agreed to pay.
M39	The patient is not liable for payment for this service as the advance notice of noncoverage you provided the patient did not comply with program requirements.
N14	Payment based on a contractual amount or agreement, fee schedule, or maximum allowable amount.
N15	Services for a newborn must be billed separately.
N16	Family or member out-of-pocket maximum has been met. Payment based on a higher percentage.
N210	You may appeal this decision.
N211	You may not appeal this decision.

the usual fee. Many PM/EHRs build records of the amount each payer has paid for each CPT code as these data are entered. When another RA payment for the same CPT is posted, the program highlights any discrepancy for review.

4. Analyze the payer's adjustment codes to locate all unpaid, downcoded, or denied claims for closer review.

THINKING IT THROUGH 11.1

Why is it important to double-check the data on the remittance advice?

5. Pay special attention to RAs for claims submitted with modifiers. Some payers' claim processing systems automatically ignore modifiers, and underpayment may need to be appealed.
6. Decide whether there are any items on the RA that need clarification from the payer, and follow up as necessary.

Denial Management

In most cases, insurance carriers do not fully pay the amount billed by the provider. The provider bills according to the provider's fee schedule, while the payer's rate is determined by a contract with the provider. When the RA is reviewed, the billing specialist checks to see that the amount paid is the expected amount, per the provider's contract with the payer. If a payment is not as expected, the specialist must determine the reason for the discrepancy.

Typical problems and solutions are:

- **Rejected claims** A claim that is not paid due to incorrect information must be corrected and sent to the payer according to its procedures.
- **Procedures not paid** If a procedure that should have been paid on a claim was overlooked, another claim is sent for that procedure.
- **Partially paid, denied, or downcoded claims** If the payer has denied payment, the first step is to study the adjustment codes to determine why. If a procedure is not a covered benefit or if the patient was not eligible for that benefit, typically the next step will be to bill the patient for the noncovered amount. If the claim is denied or downcoded for lack of medical necessity, a decision about the next action must be made. The options are to bill the patient, write off the amount, or challenge the determination with an appeal, as discussed later in this chapter. Some provider contracts prohibit billing the patient if an appeal or necessary documentation has not been submitted to the payer.

11.2 Entering Insurance Payments

electronic funds transfer (EFT) electronic routing of funds between banks

Many practices that receive RAs authorize the health plan to provide payment with an **electronic funds transfer (EFT)** from the health plan's bank to the provider's bank. In this case, payments are deposited directly into the provider's bank account. Otherwise, the payer sends a check to the practice, and the check is taken to the practice's bank for deposit. In either case, insurance payments must be processed so that patients' accounts are brought up to date, reflecting payments on their behalf that reduce their financial responsibility.

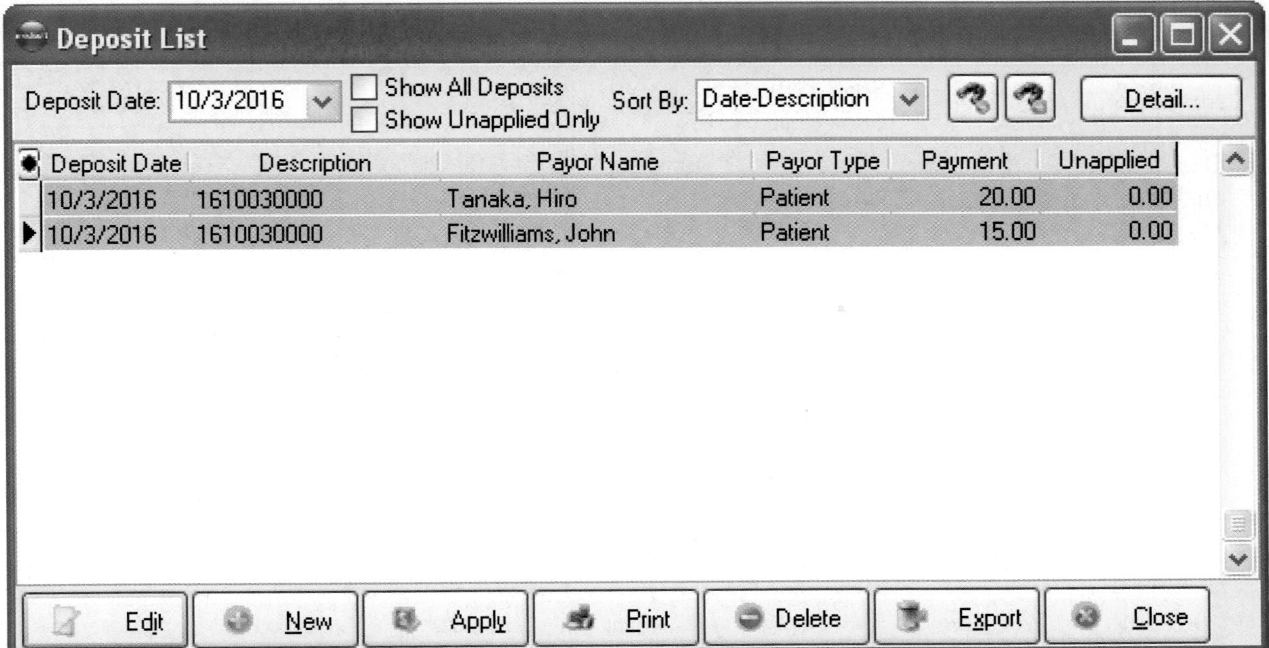

Figure 11.2 Deposit List Dialog Box

In contrast to patient payments, which are entered in the Transaction Entry dialog box, insurance payments in MNP are entered in the Deposit List dialog box (see Figure 11.2). The Deposit List dialog box is opened by selecting Enter Deposits/Payments on the Activities menu or by clicking the Enter Deposits and Apply Payments shortcut button. The Deposit/Payments area of the program is very efficient for entering large insurance payments that must be split up and applied to a number of different patients.

The Deposit List Dialog Box

The Deposit List dialog box contains the following information:

Deposit Date The program displays the current date (the Medisoft Program Date). The date can be changed by keying over the default date.

Show All Deposits If this box is checked, all payments are displayed, regardless of the date entered.

Show Unapplied Only If the Show Unapplied Only box is checked, only payments that have not been fully applied to charge transactions are displayed. If the box is not checked, all payments—both applied and unapplied—are listed.

Sort By The Sort By drop-down list offers several choices for how payment information is listed. The default is sorting payments by date and description. Payments can also be sorted by other data fields (see Figure 11.3).

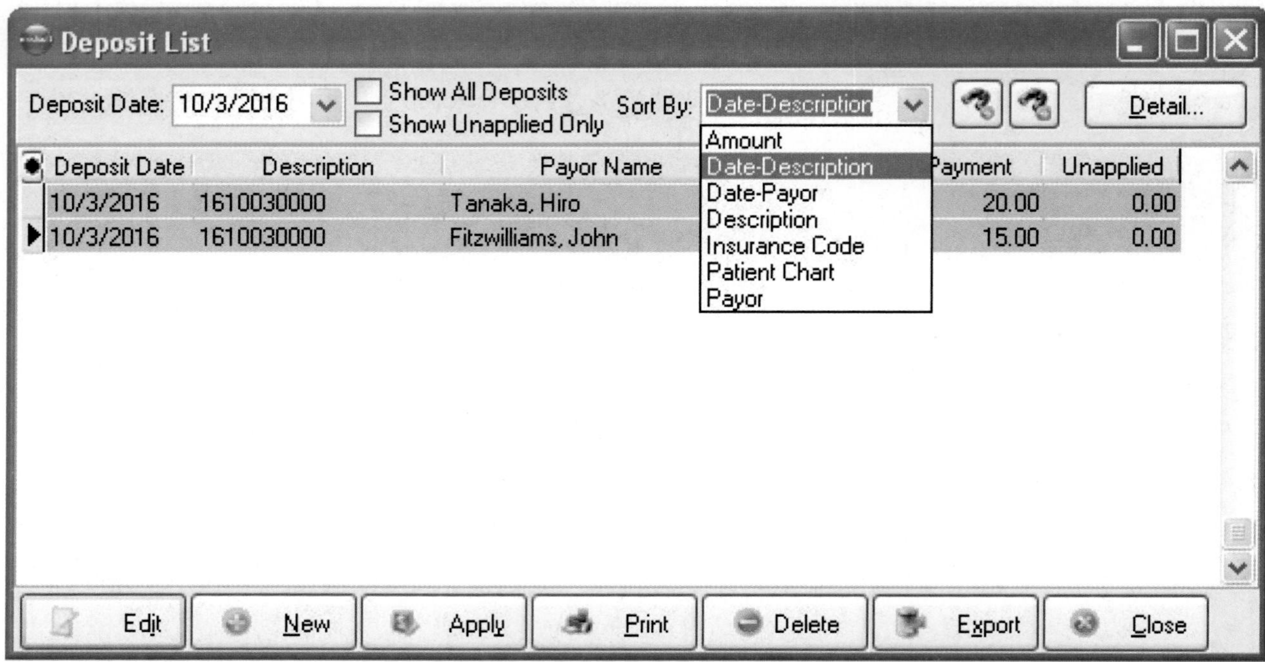

Figure 11.3 Deposit List Dialog Box with Sort By Drop-down List Displayed

Locate Buttons The Locate and Locate Next buttons, indicated by the two magnifying glass icons, are used to search for a deposit.

Detail To view a specific deposit in more detail, highlight the deposit, and click the Detail button. A dialog box opens with more information about the selected deposit (see Figure 11.4).

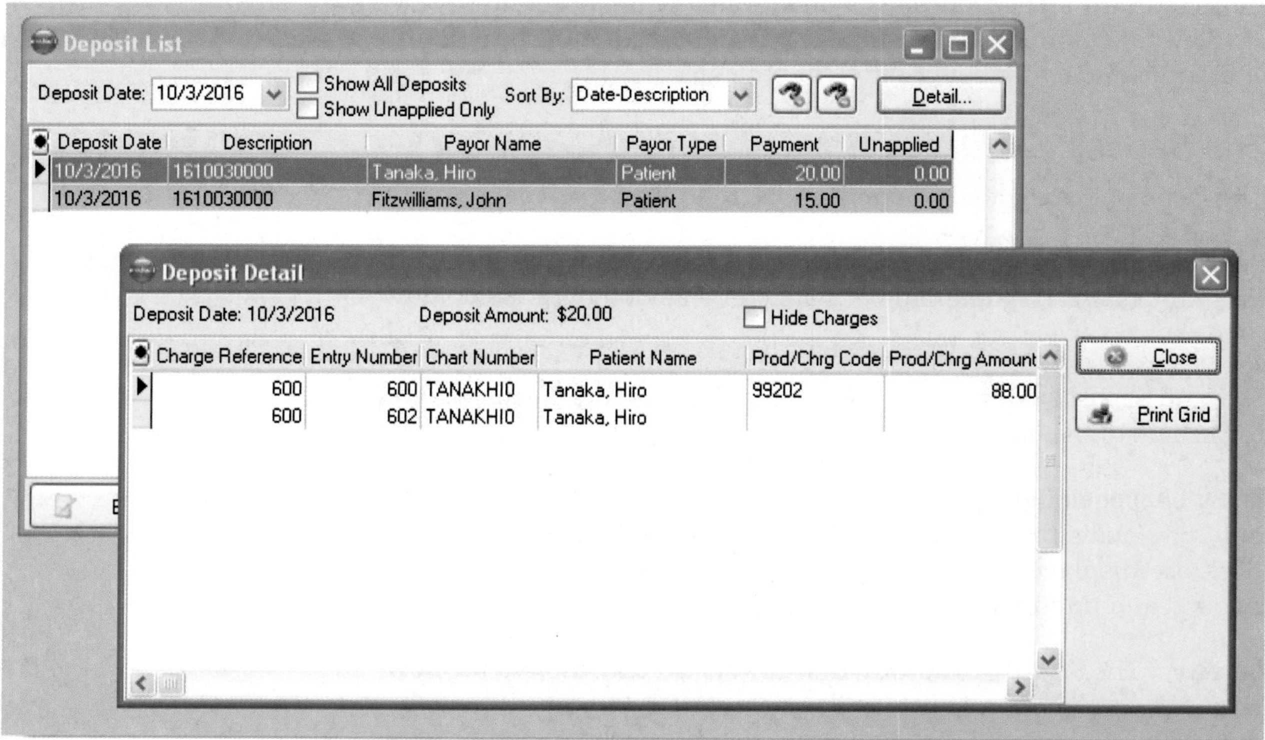

Figure 11.4 Deposit Detail Dialog Box with Deposit List Window in Background

In the middle section of the Deposit List window, information is listed for each deposit and payment, including the following:

Deposit Date Lists the date of the deposit or payment.

Description Displays whatever was entered in the Description or Check Number box in the Deposit dialog box. The Deposit dialog box is where new payments and deposits are recorded (see Figure 11.5). It is accessed by clicking the New button in the Deposit List dialog box.

Payor Name Lists the name of the insurance carrier or individual who made the payment.

Payor Type A classification column that lists whether the payment is an insurance payment, a patient payment, or a capitation payment. **Capitation payments** are made to physicians on a regular basis (such as monthly) for providing services to patients in a managed care insurance plan. (Processing capitation payments is covered in the next section of this chapter.) In traditional insurance plans, physicians are paid for the specific procedures they perform and the number of times the procedures are performed. Under a capitated plan, a flat fee is paid to the physician no matter how many times a patient receives treatment, up to the maximum number of treatments allowed per year. For example, a primary care physician with fifty patients may receive a payment of $2,500 per month for those patients, regardless of whether the physician has seen them during that month.

capitation payments payments made to physicians on a regular basis for providing services to patients in a managed care plan

Payment Lists the amount of the payment.

Unapplied Lists the amount of the deposit that has not been applied to a charge.

At the bottom of the Deposit List dialog box are buttons that perform the following actions:

Edit Opens the highlighted payment or deposit for editing.

New Opens the Deposit dialog box, where new payments and deposits are recorded.

Apply Applies payments to specific charge transactions.

Print Sends a command to print the deposit list.

Delete Deletes the highlighted transaction.

Export Exports the data in either the Quicken or QuickBooks program format.

Close Exits the Deposit List dialog box.

The Deposit Dialog Box

When the New button is clicked in the Deposit List dialog box, the Deposit dialog box appears (see Figure 11.5).

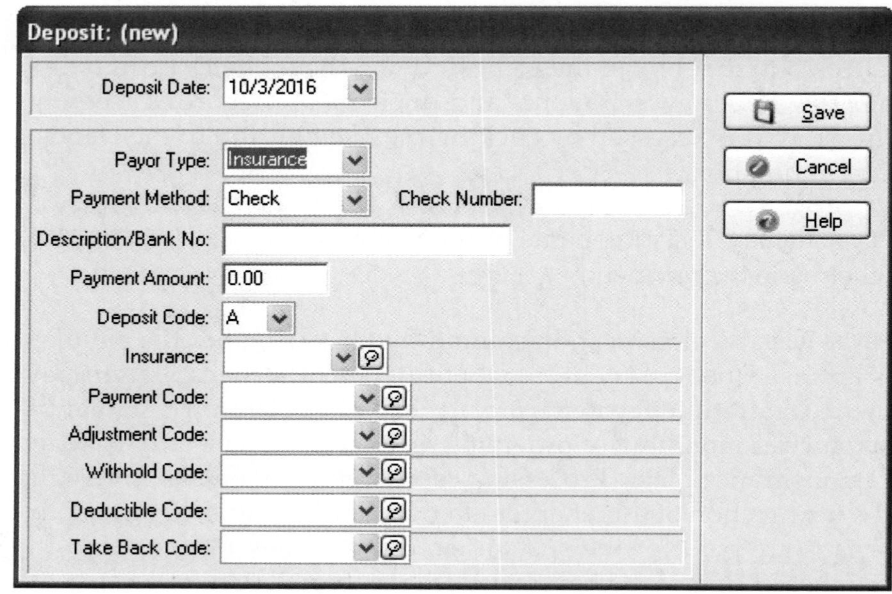

Figure 11.5 Deposit Dialog Box

The Deposit dialog box contains the following fields:

Deposit Date The program's current date is displayed by default and must be changed if it is not the date of the deposit.

Payor Type The drop-down options in this box indicate whether the payer is an insurance carrier, a capitation plan, or a patient (see Figure 11.6). Some of the boxes at the bottom of the Deposit dialog box

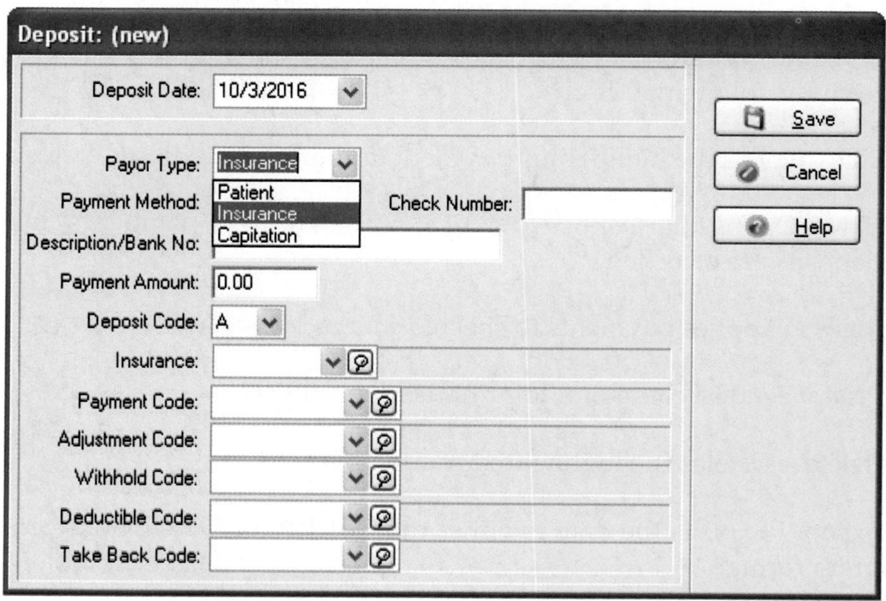

Figure 11.6 Payor Type Options in the Deposit Dialog Box

change based on the selection in this box. If Insurance is selected, the dialog box is as illustrated in Figure 11.5. If Capitation is selected, all the boxes below Insurance disappear. If Patient is chosen, the boxes listed below Deposit Code become Chart Number, Payment Code, Adjustment Code, and Copayment Code.

Payment Method This box lists whether the payment is check, cash, credit card, or electronic.

Check Number If payment is made by check, the number of the check is entered in this box.

Description/Bank No. This box can be used to enter a description of the payment, if desired.

Payment Amount The total amount of the payment is entered in this box.

Deposit Code This field can be used by practices to sort deposits according to user-defined categories.

Insurance The insurance carrier that is making the payment is selected.

Payment Code, Adjustment Code, Withhold Code, Deductible Code, and Take Back Code The appropriate codes for the insurance carrier are selected.

Once all the information has been entered and checked for accuracy, the deposit is saved by clicking the Save button (see Figure 11.7). When the deposit entry is saved, the Deposit dialog box closes, and the Deposit List dialog box reappears, with the new deposit listed (see Figure 11.8).

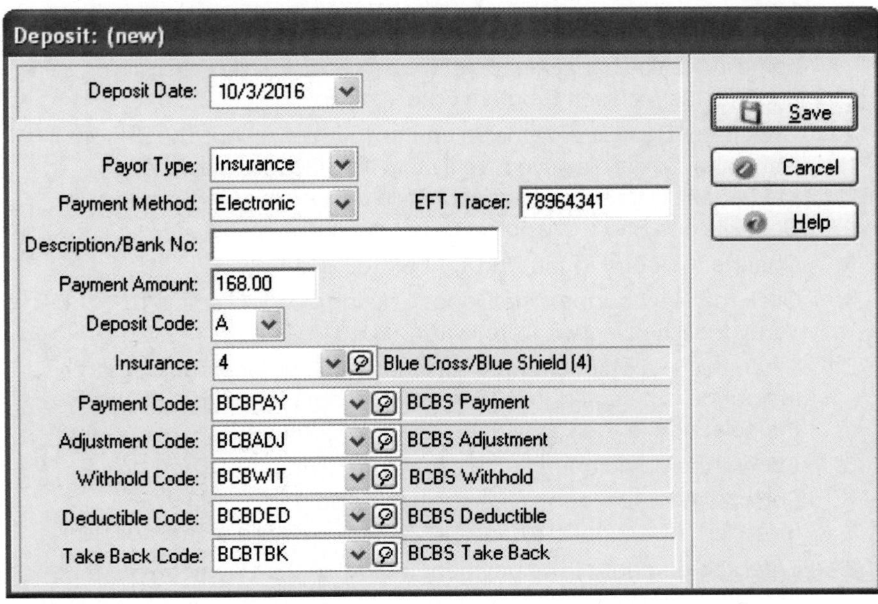

Figure 11.7 Deposit Dialog Box with Information Entered

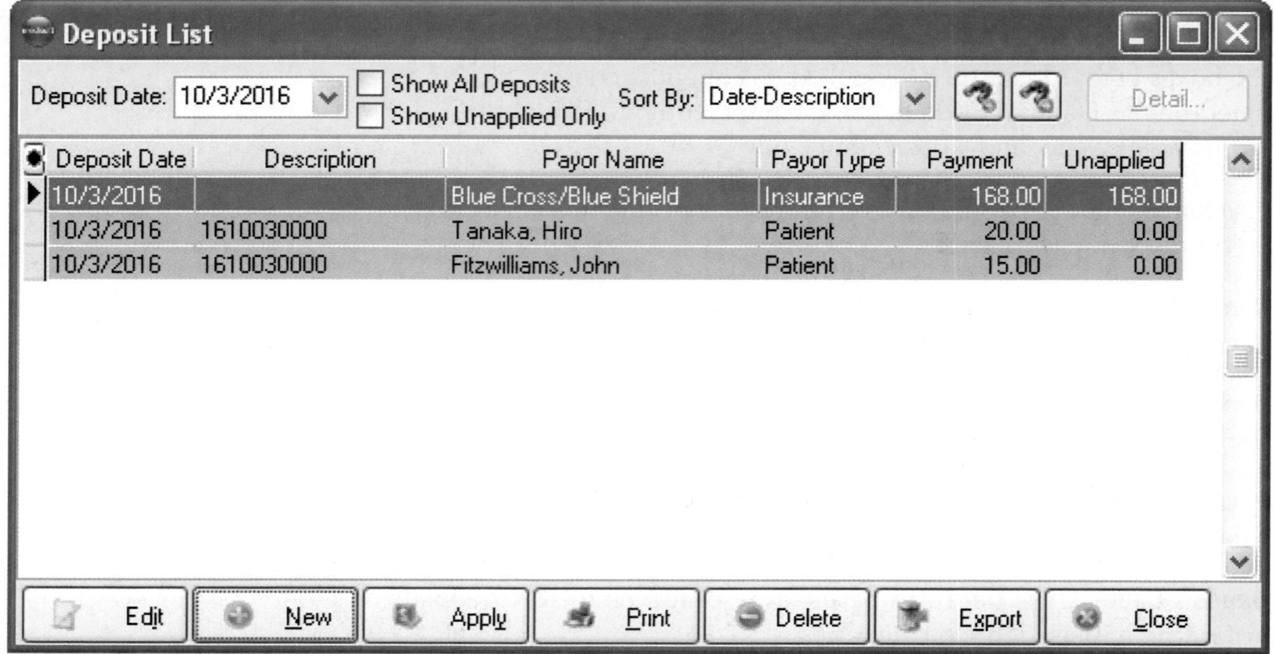

Deposit Date	Description	Payor Name	Payor Type	Payment	Unapplied
10/3/2016		Blue Cross/Blue Shield	Insurance	168.00	168.00
10/3/2016	1610030000	Tanaka, Hiro	Patient	20.00	0.00
10/3/2016	1610030000	Fitzwilliams, John	Patient	15.00	0.00

Figure 11.8 Deposit List Dialog Box with Deposit Entered

connect plus+

ENTERING A DEPOSIT: CHAMPVA

Using Source Document 10, enter the payment received from John Fitzwilliams's insurance carrier for services provided on September 6, 2016. The total amount of the remittance is $28.02. Note that John is guarantor for his daughter Sarah, so her charges and payments are included on the remittance advice.

Date: October 3, 2016

1. Verify that Medisoft Network Professional is open, that the practice name in the title bar at the top of the screen is Family Care Clinic, and that the Medisoft Program Date is set to October 3, 2016.
2. Click Enter Deposits/Payments on the Activities menu. The Deposit List dialog box is displayed. Verify that 10/3/2016 is displayed in the Deposit Date box, and that the two check boxes—Show All Deposits and Show Unapplied Only—are not checked.
3. Change the entry in the Sort By box to Date-Payor.
4. Click the New button. The Deposit dialog box is displayed. Verify that the Deposit Date is 10/3/2016.
5. Since this is a payment from an insurance carrier, confirm that Insurance is selected in the Payor Type box. If it is not, change the selection in the Payor Type box to Insurance.
6. Accept the default entry (Check) in the Payment Method box.
7. Enter ***214778924*** in the Check Number box, and press Tab twice. (The Description/Bank No. field can be left blank.)
8. Enter the amount of the payment (***28.02***) in the Payment Amount box. Press Tab.
9. Accept the default entry (A) in the Deposit Code box. Press Tab.

10. Select the insurance carrier that is making the payment (5—ChampVA) from the Insurance drop-down list. Medisoft Network Professional automatically enters the defaults for ChampVA in the code boxes.
11. Click the Save button to save the entry.
12. The Deposit List box reappears. The ChampVA insurance payment appears in the list of deposits.

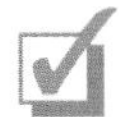 **You have completed Exercise 11.1**

11.3 Applying Insurance Payments to Charges

After a deposit has been entered, the next step is to apply the payment to the applicable transactions for each patient listed on the RA using the Apply Payment/Adjustments to Charges dialog box. To apply a deposit, the payment is highlighted in the Deposit List dialog box, and the Apply button is clicked. The Apply Payment/Adjustments to Charges dialog box opens (see Figure 11.9).

The top section of the dialog box contains information about the payer, the patient, and the amount of the payment that is unapplied.

The upper-left corner of the dialog box displays the payer's name in bold type, and the payer's name is also listed in the Ins 1 field. In Figure 11.9, the payer is Blue Cross and Blue Shield. The patient who

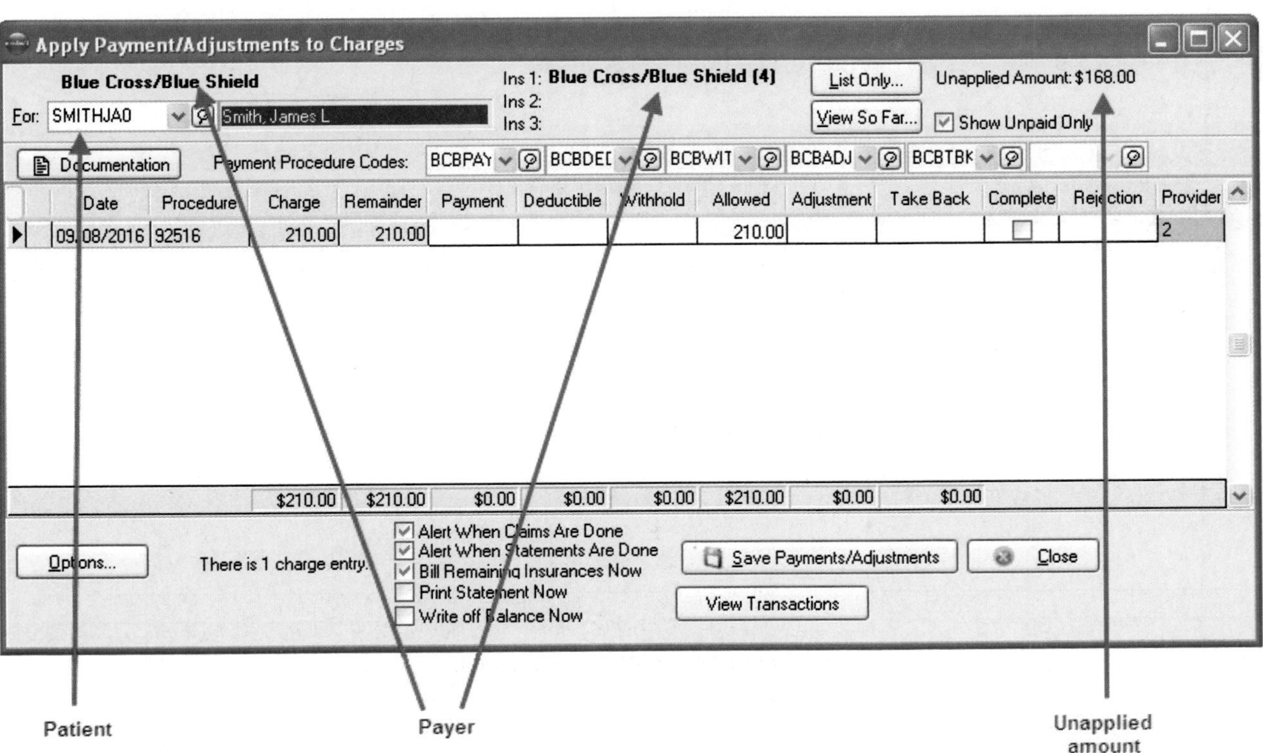

Figure 11.9 Apply Payment/Adjustments to Charges Dialog Box

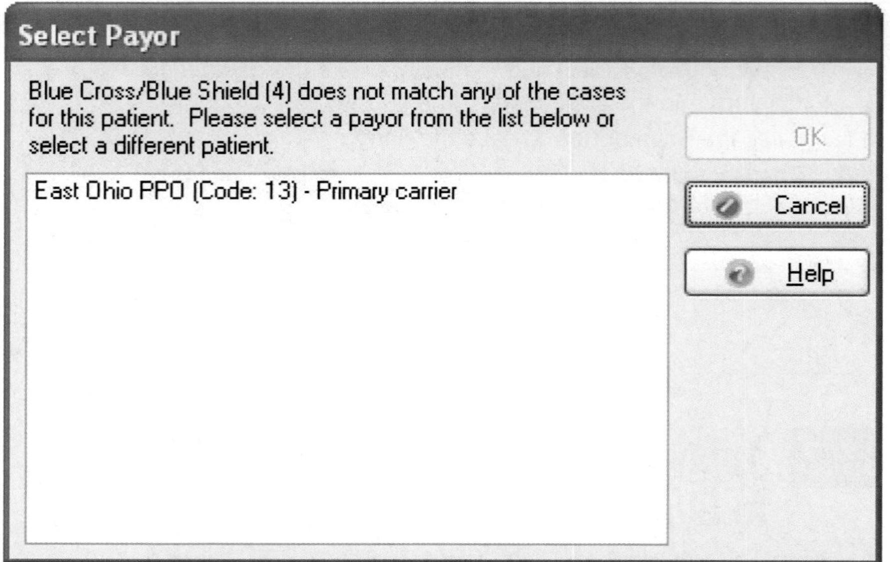

Figure 11.10 Select Payor Dialog Box

has a transaction listed on the remittance advice is selected from the drop-down list in the For box.

The upper-right area of the dialog box lists the amount of the deposit that has not yet been applied (Unapplied Amount).

Note: If a patient who does not have coverage with the insurance carrier that is making the deposit is selected, a Select Payor window opens (see Figure 11.10) with the message that the payer does not match any case for the patient. Clicking the Cancel button closes the dialog box.

The middle section of the Apply Payment/Adjustments to Charges dialog box is where payments are entered and applied (see Figure 11.11).

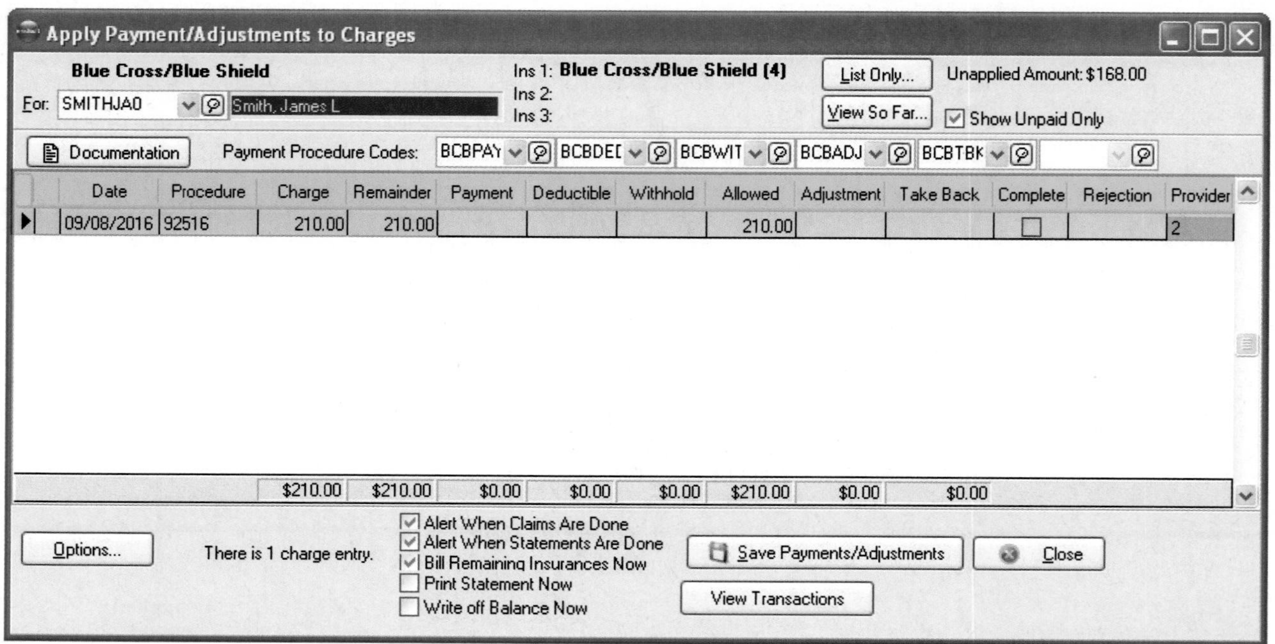

Figure 11.11 Apply Payment/Adjustments to Charges Dialog Box with Payment Entry Area Highlighted Yellow

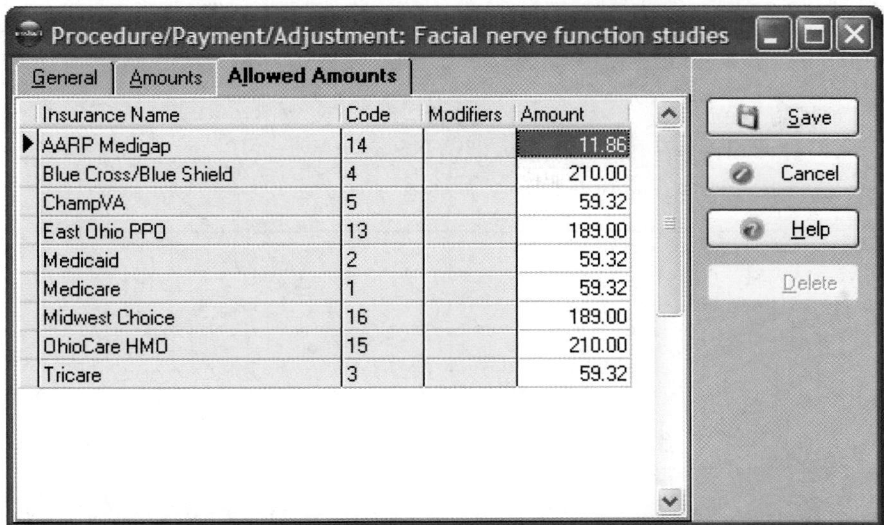

Insurance Name	Code	Modifiers	Amount
AARP Medigap	14		11.86
Blue Cross/Blue Shield	4		210.00
ChampVA	5		59.32
East Ohio PPO	13		189.00
Medicaid	2		59.32
Medicare	1		59.32
Midwest Choice	16		189.00
OhioCare HMO	15		210.00
Tricare	3		59.32

Figure 11.12 Allowed Amounts Tab in the Procedure/Payment/Adjustment Dialog Box

Date, Procedure, Charge, Remainder These fields show the date of service, procedure code, charge amount, and amount remaining for each transaction, as already entered in the database. This information cannot be edited in the dialog box.

Payment The amount of the payment for this procedure is entered. The program automatically makes this a negative sum, so it is not necessary to enter a minus sign.

Deductible If applicable, enter the amount of the deductible listed on the RA.

Withhold Some insurance companies may withhold money for multiple charges and then pay all at once. If applicable, enter the withholding amount in this field.

Allowed This is the amount allowed by the payer for this procedure. These values are located in the Allowed Amounts tab of the Procedure/Payment/Adjustment dialog box (see Figure 11.12).

Adjustment The amount entered here is the charge amount minus whatever is entered in the Allowed field. This amount is calculated by the program.

Take Back This field contains only positive adjustment amounts. It is provided when the insurance company overpays on one charge and then indicates that the overpayment should be applied as a payment for another transaction. Most times, the takeback should be applied to the same charge that had the overpayment.

Complete The program places a check in this box to indicate that the payer's responsibility is complete for this transaction.

Rejection If desired, a rejection message from the RA can be entered.

Provider This field lists the provider assigned to the transaction.

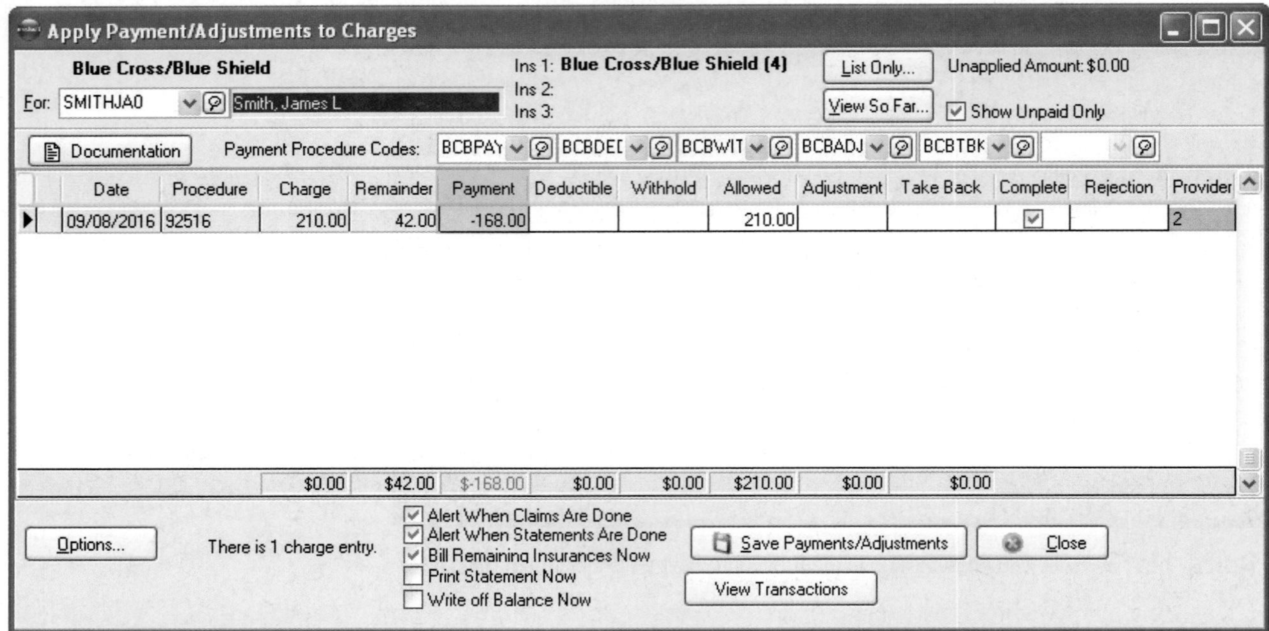

Figure 11.13 Apply Payment/Adjustments to Charges Dialog Box with Insurance Payment Entered and Highlighted

Figure 11.13 shows an Apply Payment/Adjustments to Charges dialog box with a payment entered.

The lower third of the Apply Payment/Adjustments to Charges dialog box contains several options that affect claims and statements (see Figure 11.14).

Options The Options… button is used to change the default settings for patient payment application codes.

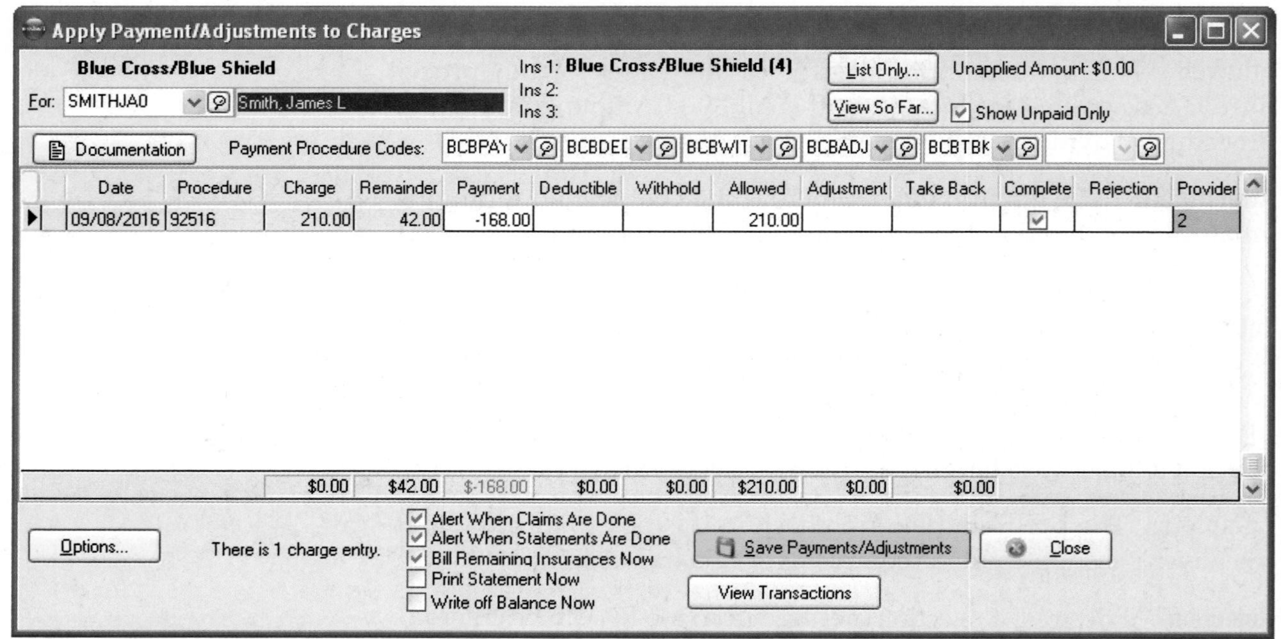

Figure 11.14 Apply Payment/Adjustments to Charges Dialog Box with Save Payments/Adjustments Button Highlighted

Alert When Claims Are Done This field determines whether a message appears as notification that a claim is done for a payer.

Alert When Statements Are Done This field determines whether a message appears as notification that a statement is done for a patient.

Bill Remaining Insurances Now If this box is checked, claims for any secondary or tertiary payer associated with the claim are created when the current insurance payment is saved.

Print Statement Now If a check mark appears in this box, the program creates a patient statement when the current insurance payment is saved.

Write Off Balance Now This field allows patient remainder balances to be written off from within this window.

Save Payments/Adjustments Clicking this button saves the payment currently being applied. Once the payment is saved, another patient can be selected in the For field, or the dialog box can be closed.

View Transactions Clicking this button opens the Transaction Entry dialog box so that the selected patient's transactions can be viewed.

connect plus+ EXERCISE 11.2

APPLYING PAYMENTS TO CHARGES: CHAMPVA

Using Source Document 10, apply the payment received from John Fitzwilliams's insurance carrier for services provided on September 6, 2016. The check includes payments for both John Fitzwilliams and his daughter Sarah.

Date: October 3, 2016

1. Verify that Medisoft Network Professional is open, that the Deposit List dialog box is displayed, and that the Medisoft Program Date is set to October 3, 2016.
2. With the ChampVA payment entry still highlighted from Exercise 11.1, click the Apply button. The Apply Payment/Adjustments to Charges dialog box appears. In the lower portion of the dialog box, make sure the first three boxes are checked and the last two (Print Statement Now and Write off Balance Now) are unchecked.
3. Key ***F*** in the For box, and press Tab to select John Fitzwilliams, since a portion of this payment is for his account. All the charge entries for John Fitzwilliams that have not been paid in full are listed. Notice that the amount listed in the Unapplied Amount box in the upper-right corner shows the full deposit amount, since nothing has been applied yet.
4. Refer to Source Document 10 to determine the first payment amount, which is for the 99211 procedure on 9/6/2016. Notice that the cursor is blinking in the Payment box for this charge. Enter ***5.68*** in the Payment box, and press Tab.

(continued)

(Continued)

5. Medisoft Network Professional automatically places a minus sign before the amount. Notice that once the payment is applied, the Complete box to the right is checked. This indicates that the transaction is complete for this payer. Also notice that the unapplied amount in the upper-right has been reduced by $5.68.
6. Press Tab seven times to move the cursor past the end of the line. As you move from column to column, the program updates the amounts in the Adjustment and Remainder boxes. The Remainder column changes to 0.00, and the amount in Adjustment column now displays −15.32.
7. Now enter the payment for procedure 84478. Enter ***8.04*** in the Payment box. Press Tab eight times to move the cursor past the end of the line. When you tab past the end of the row, the amount in the Remainder column changes to 0.00 and the amount in the Adjustment column now displays −20.96.
8. Click the Save Payments/Adjustments button to save your entry. When you click this button, an Information dialog box displays the message that the claim has been marked "done" for the primary insurance.
9. Click OK. The dialog box is cleared of the current transaction and is ready for a new transaction.
10. Now enter a payment for Sarah Fitzwilliams. Key ***F*** in the For box, and then click on her chart number in the drop-down list to display her data.
11. Notice on the RA and in the Apply Payment/Adjustments to Charges dialog box that her $15.00 copayment was applied to the charge for procedure 90471, so that the procedure now has a 0.00 remainder balance. A zero payment from the insurance plan must be entered in the Payment column. Key ***0*** in the Payment box, and press Tab eight times. The cursor moves past the end of the line and is blinking in the Payment column for the second charge.
12. Now enter the payment for procedure 90703, and press Tab eight times to update the amounts. Verify that the Remainder column for both lines now displays 0.00.
13. Click the Save Payments/Adjustments button, and then click OK. The unapplied amount in the upper-right corner now displays 0.00, showing that the full amount of the payment has been applied.
14. Click the Close button to exit the Apply Payment/Adjustments to Charges dialog box. The Deposit List box reappears, with the Unapplied column for the ChampVA deposit now displaying 0.00.
15. Without closing the Deposit List dialog box, open the Activities menu and click Enter Transactions to open the Transaction Entry dialog box.
16. Key ***F*** in the Chart box and then press Tab to display John Fitzwilliams's transaction information.
17. View the list of payments and adjustments at the bottom of the screen. In addition to the patient's $15.00 copayment on 9/6/2016, there are two payments with corresponding adjustments dated 10/3/2016. These are the payments and adjustments that were just entered in the Apply Payment/Adjustments to Charges dialog box. Payments entered in the Deposit List dialog box also appear in the Transaction Entry dialog box.

18. In the Totals tab area of the dialog box, notice that there is still a balance of $58.00 due on Fitzwilliams's account for his office visit on 10/3/2016. This amount includes two charges ($54.00 and $19.00) for procedures 99212 and 82270, totaling $73.00, minus his $15.00 copayment for the visit ($73.00 − $15.00 = $58.00).
19. Now click the Chart box and select Sarah Fitzwilliams's chart number to display her transaction information. The 10/3/2016 payment and its corresponding adjustment that you entered in the Apply Payment/Adjustments to Charges dialog box appear in the Payments, Adjustments, And Comments section, and the Account Total balance in the Totals tab area is now 0.00.
20. Close the Transaction Entry dialog box. You are back at the Deposit List dialog box.

 **You have completed Exercise 11.2**

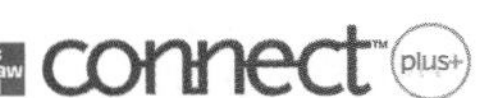

EXERCISE 11.3

ENTERING A DEPOSIT AND APPLYING PAYMENTS: EAST OHIO PPO

The medical office has just received an ERA from East Ohio PPO (see Source Document 11). The total amount of the electronic funds transfer (EFT) is $450.60. This amount includes payments for a number of patients. Enter the insurance carrier payment, and apply it to the appropriate patients. (*Note:* Source Document 11 consists of two pages.)

Date: October 3, 2016

1. Verify that the Deposit List dialog box is displayed and that the entry in the Deposit Date box is 10/3/2016.
2. Click the New button. The Deposit dialog box is displayed.
3. Accept the default setting (Insurance) in the Payor Type box.
4. Click the Payment Method box and select Electronic, since this payment was sent electronically to the practice's bank account. Notice that the Check Number box becomes an EFT Tracer box. Press Tab twice.
5. Enter the ERA ID number, ***00146972,*** in the Description/Bank No. box. Press Tab.
6. Enter ***450.60*** in the Payment Amount box. Press Tab.
7. Accept the default entry (A) in the Deposit Code box.
8. Select 13—East Ohio PPO from the drop-down list in the Insurance box. Medisoft Network Professional automatically completes the Payment, Adjustment, Withhold, Deductible, and Take Back Code boxes.
9. Click the Save button.
10. The payment entry appears in the Deposit List dialog box.
11. Now apply the payment to the specific transaction charges. With the East Ohio PPO line highlighted, click the Apply button. The Apply Payment/Adjustments to Charges dialog box appears.

(continued)

(Continued)

12. Key ***A*** in the For box, and press Tab to select Susan Arlen.
13. Locate the charge on the ERA for procedure code 99212 on 9/5/2016. Key the amount of the payment, ***28.60***, in the Payment box, and press Tab. Notice that MNP automatically checks the Complete box. Since Susan Arlen has only one insurance carrier, there is no payment forthcoming from any other carrier, and the charge is complete.
14. Press Tab seven times. As you tab past the end of the line, MNP updates the adjustment amount to −5.40 and the remainder amount to 0.00.
15. Click the Save Payments/Adjustments button.
16. Click the OK button when the Information box appears, reporting that the claim has been marked "done." The data for Susan Arlen that were visible in the Apply Payment/Adjustments to Charges dialog box are cleared, and the dialog box is ready for the next payment or adjustment. Notice also that the amount listed in the Unapplied Amount box in the upper-right corner has been reduced by the amount of the Arlen payment.
17. Now enter the payment for the next patient listed on the ERA, Herbert Bell. Key ***BE*** in the For box, and press Tab.
18. Enter the payment of ***12.40*** in the Payment box for procedure 99211 on 9/5/2016. Tab to the end of the line until the Remainder box changes to 0.00.
19. Click the Save Payments/Adjustments button, and then click the OK button.
20. Key ***BELLSAM*** in the For box, and press Tab to select Samuel Bell.
21. Enter the payment of ***28.60*** in the Payment box for procedure 99212 on 9/5/2016. Press Tab eight times.
22. Click the Save Payments/Adjustments button, and then click the OK button.
23. Continue to apply the insurance payments for Janine Bell, Jonathan Bell, and Sarina Bell using the information on Source Document 11 as follows. Key ***BELLJA*** in the For box, and press Tab to select Janine Bell.
24. Enter the first payment of ***44.80*** in the Payment box for procedure 99213 on 9/5/2016. Press Tab eight times.
25. Enter the second payment of ***111.60*** in the Payment box for the 73510 charge. Press Tab eight times. The Remainder box for both lines now reads 0.00.
26. Click the Save Payments/Adjustments button, and then click the OK button.
27. Key ***BELLJO*** in the For box, and press Tab to select Jonathan Bell.
28. Refer to Source Document 11 for the payment amount received for Jonathan Bell's 99394 procedure on 9/5/2016. Enter the amount in the Payment box, and press Tab eight times.
29. Click the Save Payments/Adjustments button, and then click the OK button.
30. Key ***BELLSAR*** in the For box, and press Tab to select Sarina Bell.
31. Refer to Source Document 11 for the payment amount received for Sarina Bell's 99213 procedure on 9/5/2016. Enter the amount in the Payment box, and press Tab eight times.

32. Click the Save Payments/Adjustments button, and then click the OK button.
33. Now that you have applied all the payments for the East Ohio PPO insurance payment, confirm that the amount in the Unapplied Amount box in the upper-right corner of the dialog box is 0.00.
34. Close the Apply Payment/Adjustments to Charges dialog box.

 **You have completed Exercise 11.3**

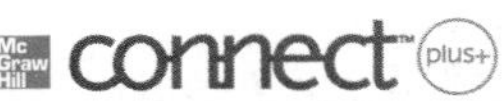

EXERCISE 11.4

ENTERING A DEPOSIT AND APPLYING PAYMENTS: BLUE CROSS AND BLUE SHIELD

The medical office has received an ERA from Blue Cross and Blue Shield (see Source Document 12). The total amount of the remittance is $310.40. This amount includes payments for a number of patients. Enter the insurance carrier payment for each patient. You will need to enter a zero payment on a charge for Sheila Giles, as one of her procedures was denied.

Date: November 3, 2016

1. Verify that the Deposit List dialog box is open and that the Medisoft Program Date has been set to November 3, 2016. Confirm that the date in the Deposit Date box is also 11/3/2016.
2. Click the New button. The Deposit dialog box is displayed.
3. Accept the default setting (Insurance) in the Payor Type box.
4. Change the entry in the Payment Method box to Electronic.
5. Enter the ERA ID number, ***001234,*** in the Description/Bank No. box. Press Tab.
6. Enter ***310.40*** in the Payment Amount box and press Tab.
7. Accept the default entry in the Deposit Code box.
8. Select 4—Blue Cross/Blue Shield in the Insurance box. Medisoft Network Professional automatically completes the code boxes.
9. Click the Save button.
10. The payment entry appears in the Deposit List dialog box.
11. Now apply the payment to the specific transaction charges. With the Blue Cross/Blue Shield line highlighted, click the Apply button. The Apply Payment/Adjustments to Charges dialog box is displayed.
12. Key ***GI*** in the For box, and press Tab to select Sheila Giles's transaction information.
13. Three charges are listed. Locate the charge for procedure code 99213 on 10/28/2016. Key the amount of the payment, ***57.60,*** in the Payment box and press Tab. Medisoft Network Professional automatically checks the Complete box, since Sheila Giles has only one insurance carrier (no payment is forthcoming from any other carrier, so the charge is complete).

(continued)

(Continued)

14. Continue pressing the Tab key until the amount listed in the Remainder column changes. Because Blue Cross/Blue Shield pays 80 percent of covered charges (80 percent of $72.00 = $57.60), and the patient is responsible for the remaining 20 percent (20 percent of $72.00 = 14.40), the Remainder column now displays $14.40.
15. Enter the payment for the next procedure listed on the ERA—71010. (*Note:* The order of procedures is different on the ERA than it is in the Apply Payment/Adjustments to Charges window. Be sure to apply the payment to the correct procedure.) Click the Payment box for the 71010 procedure, and enter the payment amount. Press Tab eight times.
16. Look again at Source Document 12. Notice that the amount paid for the final procedure, 87430, is $0.00. Read the note listed to determine why the charge was not paid. This denial of payment must be entered in MNP so that the practice billing staff will be aware that Sheila Giles is responsible for the entire amount of the charge, $29.00.
17. Click the Payment box for the 87430 procedure. Enter ***0***, and press Tab eight times. Notice that the amount listed in the Remainder column this time is the full amount of the charge, $29.00. The charge has also been marked as complete, since the insurance carrier is not responsible for the remainder amount.
18. Click the Save Payments/Adjustments button. An Information box is displayed. Click the OK button.
19. Close the Apply Payment/Adjustments to Charges dialog box; then, without closing the Deposit List dialog box, open the Transaction Entry dialog box.
20. Enter ***GI*** in the Chart box, and press Tab to display Sheila Giles's transaction data.
21. Click the Case box to display the drop-down list of cases for Sheila Giles, and then select the upper respiratory infection case.
22. In the Charges area, notice that two of the charges appear in an aqua color, which indicates that they have been partially paid. The charge that was denied by the insurance carrier—87430—is still in gray, indicating that no payment has been made.
23. Now look at the Account Total in the Totals tab area of the Transaction Entry dialog box. Sheila Giles is listed as being responsible for paying $61.60. This breaks down as follows:

Code	Charge Amount	Patient Responsible For
99213	$72.00	$14.40 (20% of charge)
71010	$91.00	$18.20 (20% of charge)
87430	$29.00	$29.00 (100% of charge)
Totals	**$192.00**	**$61.60**

24. Close the Transaction Entry dialog box.
25. Back in the Deposit List dialog box, make sure the Blue Cross/Blue Shield line is still highlighted, and click the Apply button. You are returned to the Apply Payment/Adjustments to Charges dialog box with the Unapplied Amount for the Blue Cross/Blue Shield payment displayed as $180.00.

26. Enter the payments for the second patient listed on Source Document 12, Jill Simmons. Key ***S*** in the For box and press Tab.
27. Enter the payment of ***43.20*** in the Payment box for the 99212 charge on 10/28/2016. Tab eight times. The cursor is now blinking in the Payment box for the second procedure.
28. Enter the other payment for Jill Simmons, and tab to the end of the row again until the Remainder column is updated.
29. Click the Save Payments/Adjustments button and then click the OK button. The amount listed in the Unapplied Amount box has been reduced by the amount of the Simmons payment to $96.00.
30. Now enter the payment for the last patient listed on Source Document 12, Jorge Barrett. Key ***B*** in the For box, and press Tab to select Jorge Barrett's transaction data.
31. Although two transactions are displayed in the dialog box, the first transaction is for procedure G8443, which has no charge associated with it. Click the Payment column for the second transaction, procedure 99203 on 10/21/2016.
32. Enter the payment amount listed on the RA, and then press Tab eight times.
33. Now that the entire payment has been applied, the amount listed in the Unapplied Amount box is now 0.00. Click the Save Payments/Adjustments button.
34. Close the Apply Payment/Adjustments to Charges dialog box.
35. The Deposit List dialog box reappears, and the amount in the Unapplied column for the Blue Cross/Blue Shield payment is now zero.

 **You have completed Exercise 11.4**

11.4 Entering Capitation Payments

Capitation payments are entered in the Deposit List dialog box. To indicate a capitation payment, Capitation is selected from the Payor Type drop-down list in the Deposit window (see Figure 11.15).

When a capitation payment is entered in MNP, the payment is not applied to the charges of individual patients. Under capitated plans, the health plan pays the practice a set fee to cover all the insured patients who elect to use the practice. This designated payment is made regardless of whether any of the patients visit the practice or how often they visit. However, the charges in the account of each patient who has used the practice during the month covered by the capitation payment still must be adjusted to a zero balance to indicate that the plan has met its obligation (through the capitation payment) and that the patient has also done so (by paying a copayment at the time of the office visit).

In order to adjust the patient accounts of those covered by the capitated plan, a second deposit is entered as an insurance payment with a zero amount (see Figure 11.16).

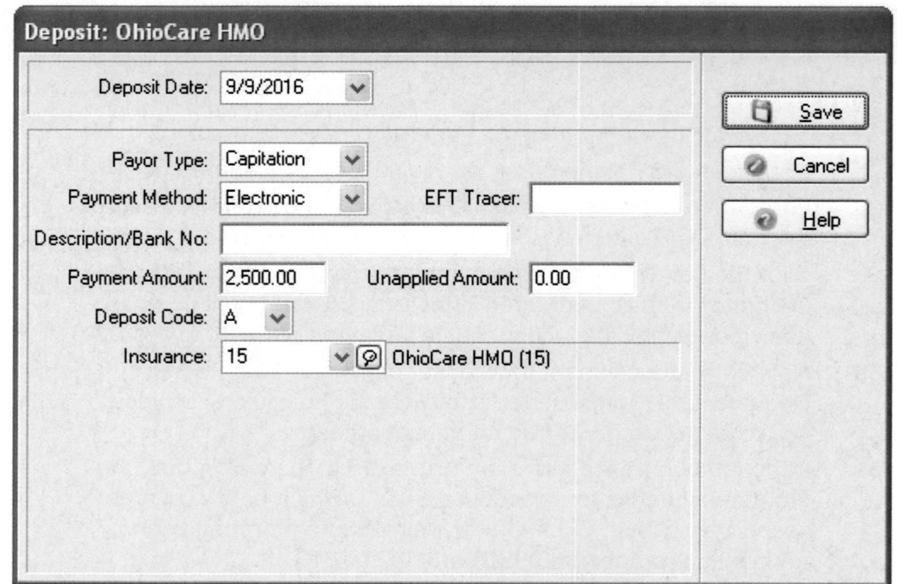

Figure 11.15 Deposit Dialog Box for a Capitation Payment

Deposit: OhioCare HMO
Deposit Date: 9/9/2016
Save
Cancel
Help
Payor Type: Insurance
Payment Method: Electronic
EFT Tracer:
Description/Bank No:
Payment Amount: 0.00
Unapplied Amount: 0.00
Deposit Code: A
Insurance: 15 OhioCare HMO (15)
Payment Code: OHCPAY OhioCare HMO Payment
Adjustment Code: OHCADJ OhioCare HMO Adjustment
Withhold Code: OHCWIT OhioCare HMO Withhold
Deductible Code: OHCDED OhioCare HMO Deductible
Take Back Code: OHCTBK OhioCare HMO Take Back

Figure 11.16 Deposit Dialog Box with a Zero Payment Amount

Once the zero amount deposit is saved, the deposit appears in the Deposit List dialog box (see Figure 11.17). The Payment column lists EOB Only, since there is no payment associated with the zero amount deposit.

The next step is to locate patients who have claims during the month covered by the capitation payment. This is accomplished using the List Only... button in the Claim Management dialog box (see Figure 11.18).

When the List Only... button is clicked, the List Only Claims That Match dialog box appears. The List Only Claims That Match

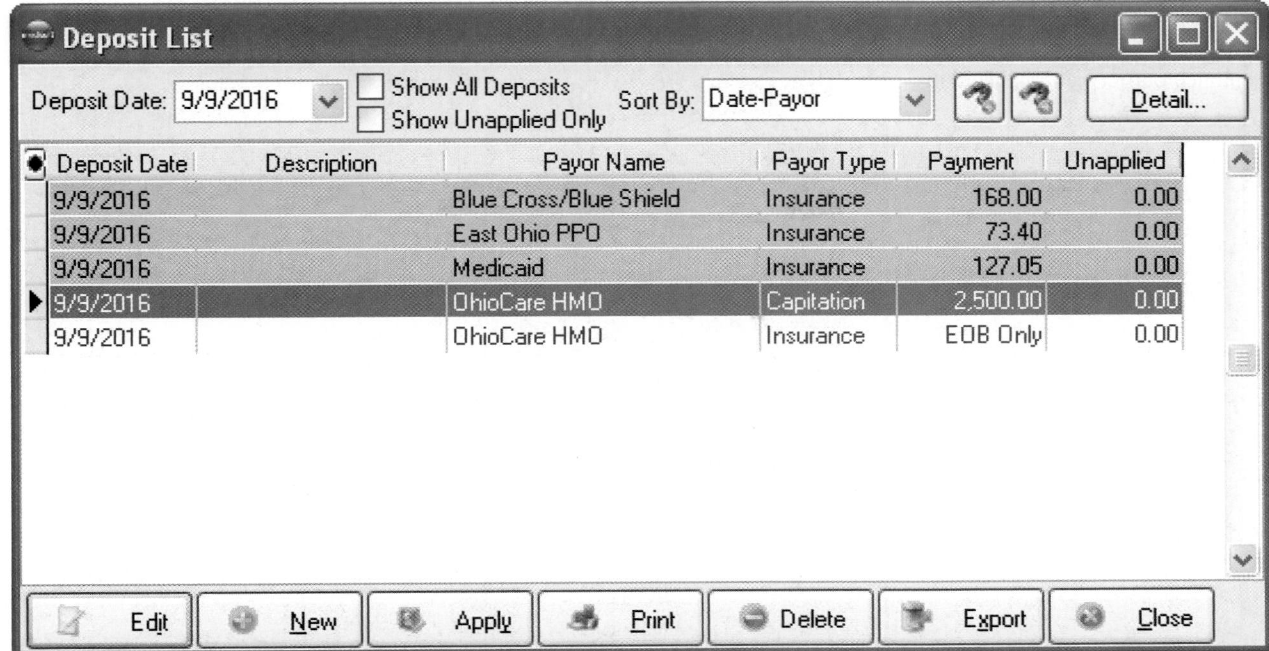

Figure 11.17 Deposit List Dialog Box with a Capitation Payment and a Zero Insurance Payment Entered

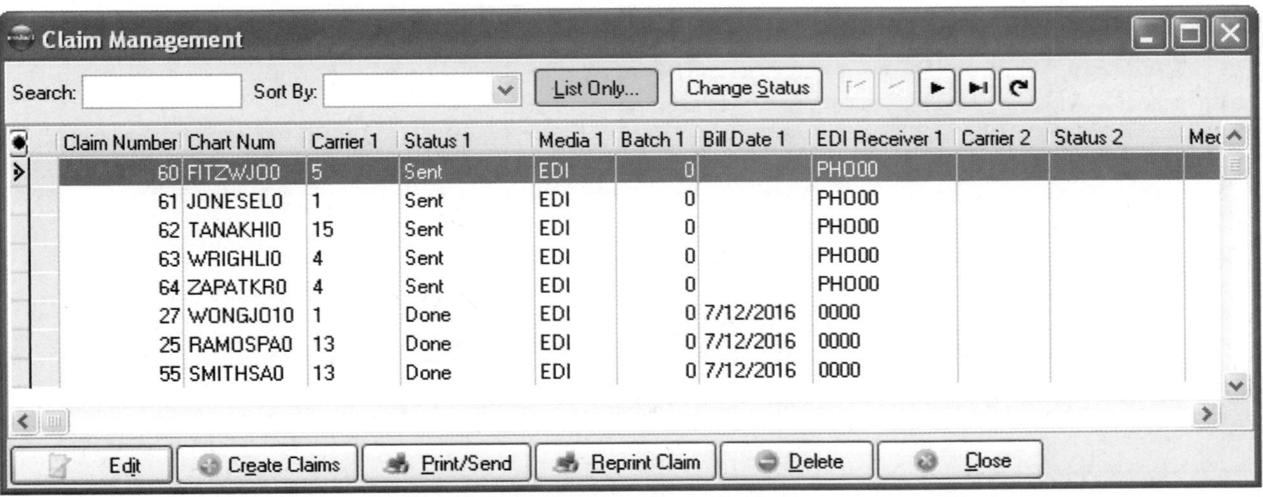

Figure 11.18 Claim Management Dialog Box with List Only... Button Highlighted

dialog box (see Figure 11.19) provides an option for searching for claims by insurance carrier. Using this option, patients with active capitated claims from a given carrier can be identified.

Once patients have been identified, the Claim Management dialog box is closed, and the Deposit List dialog box is opened. The identified patient accounts must be adjusted to a zero balance in the Apply Payment/Adjustments to Charges dialog box.

To apply the zero payment amount to these patient accounts, select the line for the deposit and click the Apply button. In the Apply Payment/Adjustments to Charges dialog box, select the chart number of each patient covered by the zero payment, and enter an adjustment equal to the outstanding balance (see Figure 11.20). In the

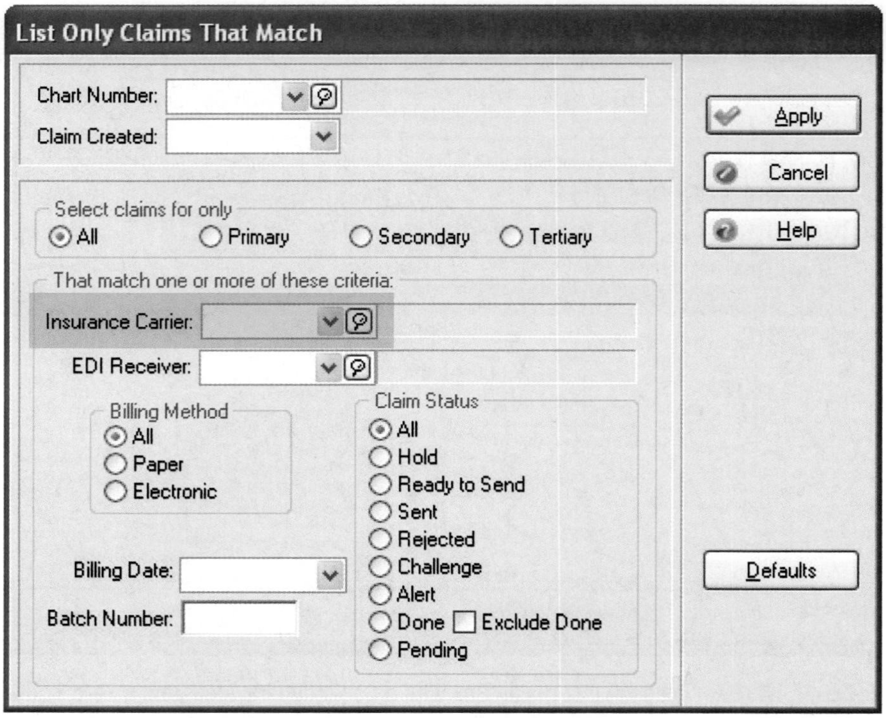

Figure 11.19 List Only Claims That Match Dialog Box with Insurance Carrier Field Highlighted

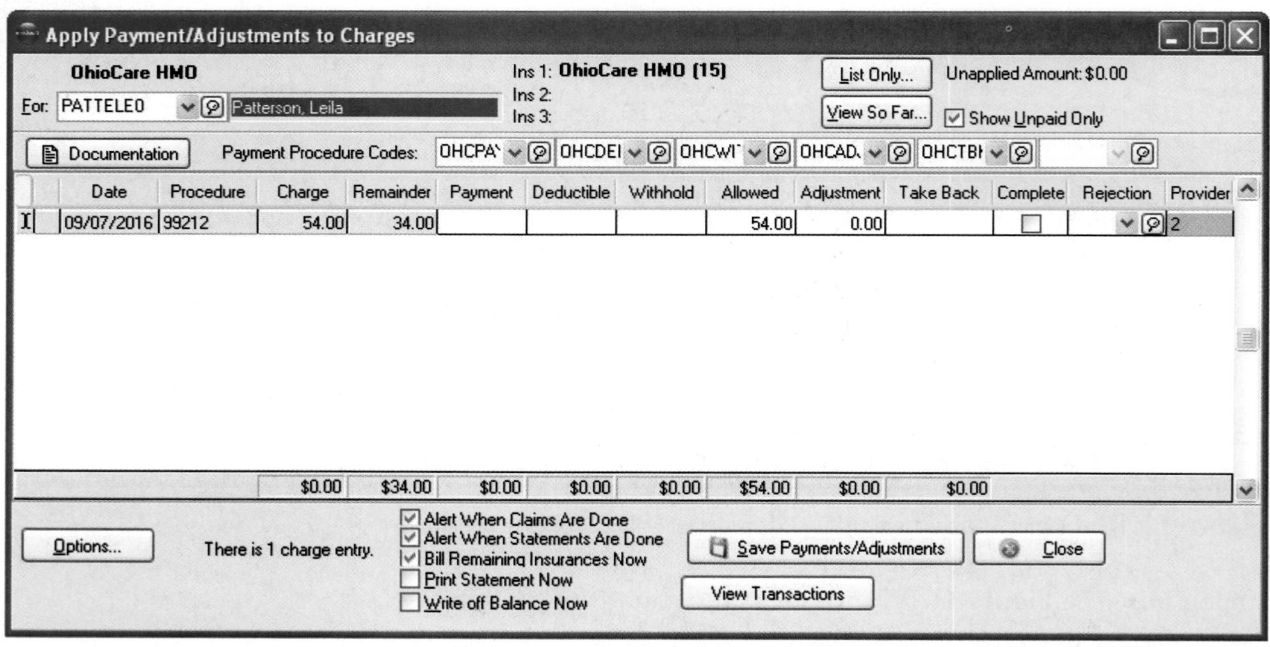

Figure 11.20 Apply Payment/Adjustments to Charges Dialog Box with Capitated Patient Account Displayed

example in Figure 11.20, the amount in the Remainder column is $34.00. This is the amount that must be entered in the Adjustment column to take the account to a zero balance. Figure 11.21 shows the dialog box after the $34.00 adjustment has been applied. Notice that the amount in the Remainder column is now zero. This procedure must be followed for each patient who has transactions during the time period covered by the capitation payment.

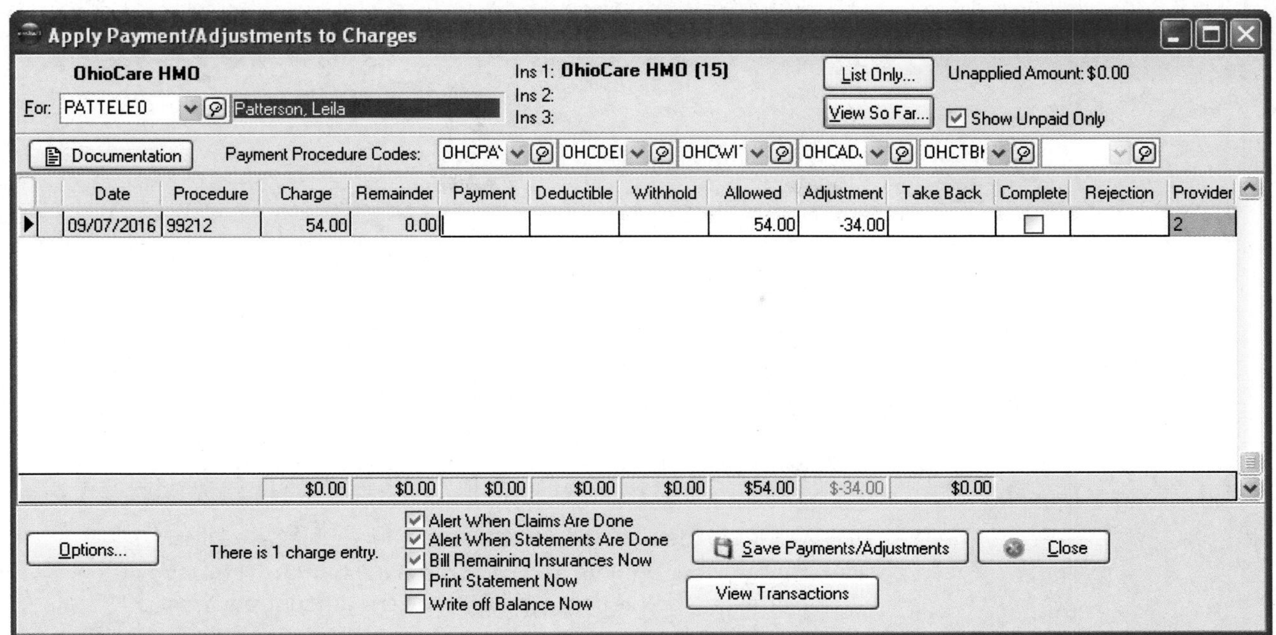

Figure 11.21 Apply Payment/Adjustments to Charges Dialog Box After the Patient Account Is Adjusted to a Zero Balance

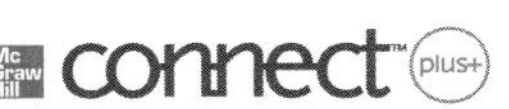

EXERCISE 11.5

ENTERING A CAPITATION PAYMENT

Using Source Document 13, enter a capitation payment from OhioCare HMO for the month of October 2016. The total amount of the electronic funds transfer is $2,500.00.

Date: November 3, 2016

1. Verify that the Deposit List dialog box is open and that the date in the Deposit Date box is 11/3/2016.
2. Click the New button. The Deposit dialog box appears.
3. Click the Payor Type box, and select Capitation.
4. Select Electronic in the Payment Method box.
5. Key ***001006003*** in the Description/Bank No. box. This is the ID number that is listed on the ERA. Press Tab.
6. Key ***2500*** in the Payment Amount box. Press Tab.
7. Accept the default entry (A) in the Deposit Code box.
8. Select 15—OhioCare HMO from the drop-down list in the Insurance box.
9. Review your entries, and click the Save button.
10. The Deposit List window reappears, displaying the payment just entered. As mentioned above, unlike other insurance payments, capitation payments are not applied to individual charges. However, amounts do need to be adjusted in the patient accounts. The next two exercises provide practice. First a zero amount payment is entered in the Deposit List dialog box. Then the zero amount payment is used to adjust the active accounts for capitated patients to a zero balance.

 **You have completed Exercise 11.5**

EXERCISE 11.6

ENTERING A ZERO AMOUNT PAYMENT

Enter a zero payment amount deposit for OhioCare HMO.

Date: November 3, 2016

1. In the Deposit List dialog box, confirm that the date in the Deposit Date box is 11/3/2016.
2. Click the New button. The Deposit dialog box is displayed.
3. In the Payor Type box, select Insurance.
4. Select Electronic in the Payment Method box.
5. Verify that 0.00 is the amount displayed in the Payment Amount box.
6. Accept the default entry (A) in the Deposit Code box.
7. Click the Insurance box, and select 15—OhioCare HMO.
8. Review your entries, and click the Save button. The Deposit List dialog box reappears with the zero amount payment displayed.

 **You have completed Exercise 11.6**

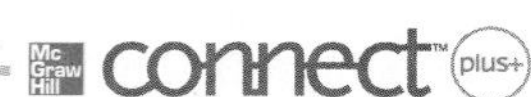

EXERCISE 11.7

ADJUSTING A CAPITATED ACCOUNT

Using the List Only Claims That Match option in Claim Management, locate the OhioCare HMO patients who visited the practice in October 2016, as these are the patients with active capitated accounts. Then, in the Apply Payment/Adjustments to Charges dialog box, enter any adjustments needed to zero out their accounts.

Date: November 3, 2016

1. Without closing the Deposit List dialog box, open the Claim Management dialog box by selecting Claim Management on the Activities menu.
2. In the Claim Management dialog box, click the List Only... button.
3. In the List Only Claims That Match dialog box, select 15—OhioCare HMO in the Insurance Carrier drop-down list. In the Claim Status options, make sure the All button is selected, and the Exclude Done box is checked to exclude claims that have already been paid.
4. Click the Apply button. The Claim Management window appears with the capitated claim listed. In this case, there is only one capitated claim. Check your screen against Figure 11.22.
5. Use the Edit button and click the Transactions tab to view the details of the claim, verifying that any transactions listed took place in October 2016. Make a note of the patient's name,

and close the Claim dialog box and the Claim Management dialog box.

6. You are returned to the Deposit List dialog box. Click the OhioCare HMO deposit that has EOB Only listed in the Payment column to select it, and then click the Apply button.
7. Key ***TA*** in the For field and press Tab to select the capitated patient, Hiro Tanaka.
8. Notice there is only one procedure on the claim. To enter the correct amount for the adjustment, identify the amount in the Remainder column.
9. Press Tab four times to move to the Adjustment column. Enter the same amount in the Adjustment column that is displayed in the Remainder column: press Backspace four times to delete the 0.00 amount, and then key ***68.00.***
10. Press Tab four times. Notice the remainder amount changes to zero.
11. Click the Save Payments/Adjustments button.
12. To verify that the account has been adjusted to a zero balance, click the View Transactions button at the bottom of the dialog box.
13. Key ***TA*** in the Chart box, press Tab, and then press OK when the two message boxes appear to display Tanaka's transaction information.
14. Notice that the adjustment has been made and the account has a zero balance. When finished viewing the data, close the Transaction Entry dialog box.
15. You are back in the Apply Payment/Adjustments to Charges dialog box. If there were other OhioCare HMO patients with capitated claims in October, you would use the For field to display their information and repeat the process for each patient's account, entering an adjustment for each transaction line that contained a remainder amount to adjust their account to a zero balance.
16. Close the Apply Payment/Adjustments to Charges dialog box.
17. Close the Deposit List dialog box.

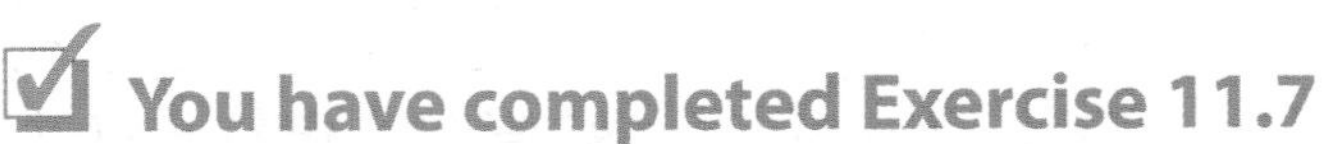

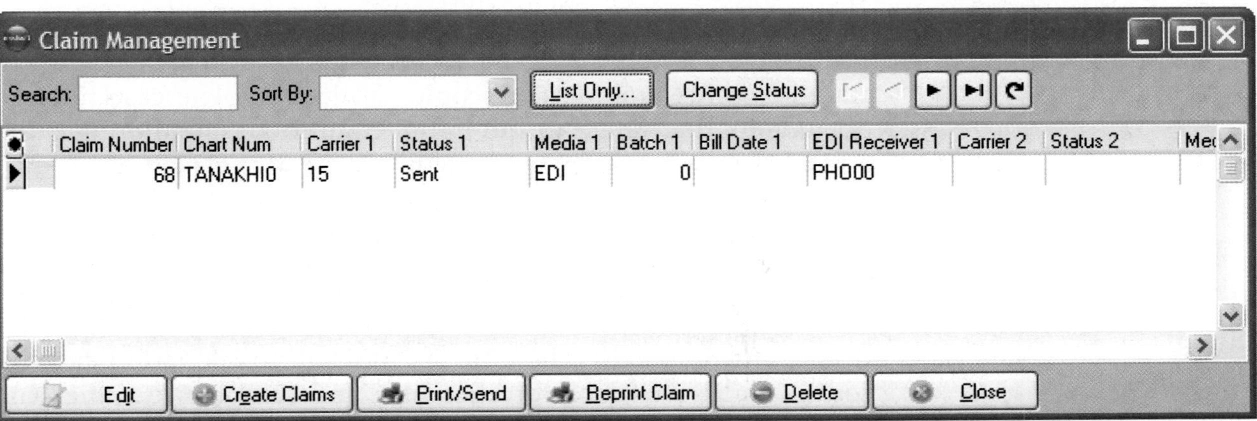

Figure 11.22 Claim Management Dialog Box with OhioCare HMO Patient Listed

11.5 Appeals, Postpayment Audits, Overpayments, and Billing of Secondary Payers

After RAs are reviewed and processed by the practice, events that may follow can alter the amount of payment. When a claim has been denied or a payment reduced by the health plan, an appeal may be filed with the payer for reconsideration, possibly reversing the nonpayment. Postpayment audits by payers may change the initial determination. Under certain conditions, refunds may be due to either the payer or the patient. Similarly, in some situations additional claims need to be created in order to generate full payments on behalf of insured patients.

The General Appeal Process

appeal request for reconsideration of a claim adjudication

claimant person or entity exercising the right to receive benefits

appellant person who appeals a claim decision

An **appeal** is a process that can be used to challenge a payer's decision to deny, reduce, or otherwise downcode a claim. A provider may begin the appeal process by asking for a review of the payer's decision. Patients, too, have the right to request appeals. The person filing the appeal is the **claimant** or the **appellant,** whether that individual is a provider or a patient.

Basic Steps

Each payer has consistent procedures for handling appeals. These procedures are based on the nature of the appeal. The practice staff reviews the appropriate procedure before starting an appeal and plans its actions according to these rules.

Appeals must be filed within a specified time after the claim determination. Most payers have an escalating structure of appeals, such as (1) a complaint, (2) an appeal, and (3) a grievance. The claimant must move through the three levels in pursuing an appeal, starting at the lowest and continuing to the highest, final level. Some payers also set a minimum amount that must be involved in an appeal process, so that a lot of time is not spent on a small dispute.

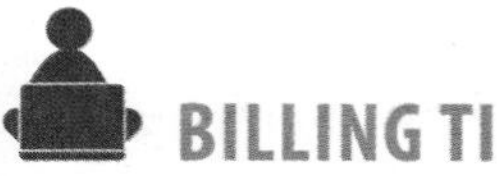

Late Claims Not Appealable
A claim that is denied because it was not filed on time is not subject to appeal.

Options After Appeal Rejection

A claimant can take another step if the payer has rejected all the appeal levels on a claim. Because they license most types of payers, state insurance commissions have the authority to review appeals that payers reject. If a claimant decides to pursue an appeal with the state insurance commission, copies of the complete case file—all documents that relate to the initial claim determination and the appeal process—are sent, along with a letter of explanation.

Postpayment Audits

As explained in Chapter 2, an audit is a systematic examination of a representative sample of documents intended to show whether particular situations exist. There are tax audits that seek underpayment, coding audits that look for upcoding, and compliance audits that seek to uncover fraudulent activities. Some audits are internal—that is, they are done in the practice by staff members or consultants to review claims and coding—and others are external, done by an outside entity such as a health plan or a government agency like the HHS Office of the Inspector General.

Health plans often conduct **postpayment audits.** Most are reviews that are used to build clinical information. Payers use audits of practices, for example, to study treatments and outcomes for patients with similar diagnoses. The patterns that are determined are used to confirm or alter best practice guidelines.

At times, however, a payer does a postpayment audit to verify the medical necessity of reported services or to uncover fraud and abuse. The audit may be based on detailed records about each provider's services that are kept by payers' medical review departments. Some payers keep records that go back for many months or years. The payer analyzes these records to assess patterns of care from individual providers and to flag outliers—those that differ from what other providers do. A postpayment audit might be conducted to check the documentation of the provider's cases or, in some cases, to check for fraudulent activities (see Chapter 2).

A good example of a postpayment audit payer program is the **Recovery Audit Contractor (RAC)** initiative of the Medicare program. The purpose of an RAC is to audit Medicare claims and determine where there are opportunities to recover incorrect payments from previously paid but noncovered services (including services that were not medically necessary), erroneous coding, and duplicate services.

RACs use a software program to analyze claims based on a practice's claim history, looking for:

- Obvious "black-and-white" coding errors (such as a well-woman exam billed for a male patient)
- Medically unnecessary treatment or wrong setting of care where information in the medical record does not support the claim
- Multiple or excessive number of units billed

Offices should respond to all RAC inquiries, since requests for information must be answered within forty-five days, or an error is declared and penalties may result.

postpayment audit review conducted after a claim is adjudicated

Recovery Audit Contractor (RAC) entity that audits Medicare claims to determine where there are opportunities to recover incorrect payments from previously paid but noncovered services, erroneous coding, and duplicate services

overpayment improper or excessive amount received by provider from payer

takeback balance that a provider owes a payer following a postpayment audit

Refunds of Overpayments

A postpayment audit may show that the health plan has overpaid a claim. From the payer's point of view, **overpayments** (also called credit balances and payer **takebacks**) are improper or excessive payments resulting from billing errors for which the provider owes refunds.

EXAMPLES

A payer may mistakenly overpay a claim.

A payer's postpayment audit may find that a claim that has been paid should be denied or downcoded because the documentation that was examined later does not support it.

A provider may collect a primary payment from Medicare when another payer is primary.

In such cases, the payer will ask for a refund (with the possible addition of interest for Medicare). If the audit shows that the claim was for a service that was not medically necessary, the provider also must refund any payment collected from the patient.

Often, the procedure is to promptly refund the overpayment. Many states require the provider to make the refund payment unless the overpayment is contested, which it may be if the provider thinks it is erroneous. A refund request may also be challenged because many practices set a time period beyond which they will not automatically issue a refund. State law may also provide for a reasonable time limit during which payers can recoup overpayments.

EXERCISE 11.8

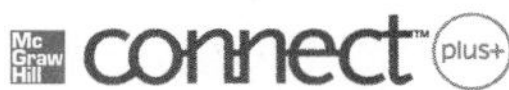

REFUNDING AN OVERPAYMENT (TAKEBACK)

ChampVA has made an overpayment on a patient's account. Using the information below, create a takeback (refund) for the overpaid amount.

Insurance Carrier: ChampVA
Date Original Payment Received: 11/11/2016
Patient Name: Gerard Verbena
Transaction Date: 10/22/2016
CPT Code: 99202
Amount Overpaid: $49.72

Date: November 29, 2016

1. Verify that Medisoft Network Professional is open and that the Medisoft Program Date is set to November 29, 2016.
2. Click Enter Deposits/Payments on the Activities menu. The Deposit List dialog box is displayed.
3. Verify that 11/29/2016 is displayed in the Deposit Date box and that the two check boxes—Show All Deposits and Show Unapplied Only—are not checked.
4. Click the New button. The Deposit dialog box appears, with the 11/29/2016 date displayed in the Deposit Date box.
5. Since this is a takeback for an insurance carrier, confirm that Insurance is selected in the Payor Type box.
6. Accept the default entry (Check) in the Payment Method box.
7. Enter the amount of the payment, ***49.72,*** in the Payment Amount box. Press Tab.
8. Accept the default entry (A) in the Deposit Code box.
9. Select the insurance carrier that is making the payment from the Insurance drop-down list. Medisoft Network Professional automatically enters the defaults for the Payment, Adjustment, Withhold, Deductible, and Take Back Code boxes.
10. Review your entries, and click the Save button.
11. The Deposit List dialog box reappears, with the ChampVA entry selected. Click the Apply button.
12. The Apply Payment/Adjustments to Charges dialog box is displayed.
13. In the For box, key ***VE*** and press Tab to select Gerard Verbena, since this takeback is for an overpayment on that account.

14. In the upper-right corner of the dialog box, if there is a check mark in the Show Unpaid Only box, click to remove it.
15. The patient's transaction information appears. Notice the amount in the Remainder column for the procedure charge listed is now −49.72, indicating the amount of the overpayment.
16. Click the Take Back column, and enter the amount to be refunded, ***49.72.*** Press Tab.
17. The amount appears in parentheses to indicate that the amount is a negative entry. Press Tab twice, until the amount in the Remainder column changes to 0.00.
18. Click the Save Payments/Adjustments button, and then click OK to save your work. The dialog box is cleared of the current transaction.
19. Click the Close button to close the Apply Payment/Adjustments to Charges dialog box.
20. Click the Close button to close the Deposit List dialog box.
21. To verify that the overpayment has been refunded to the insurance carrier, open the Transaction Entry dialog box, key ***VE,*** and press Tab to display Gerard Verbena's transaction information.
22. Notice that the Account Total in the Totals tab area of the Transaction Entry dialog box is now zero. In the Payments, Adjustments, And Comments section, the new transaction line for the takeback is displayed as an adjustment in the amount of $49.72, dated 11/29/2016. In the Pay/Adj Code column, the code CHVTBK (ChampVA Take Back) is displayed, indicating that the adjustment is a takeback from the insurance carrier.
23. Close the Transaction Entry dialog box.

 **You have completed Exercise 11.8**

Billing of Secondary Payers

If a patient has additional insurance coverage, after the primary payer's RA has been posted, the next step is to bill the second payer. The initial claim gave the primary payer information about the patient's secondary insurance policy. The secondary payer now needs to know what the primary payer paid on the claim in order to coordinate benefits. The primary claim crosses over automatically to the secondary payer in many cases—for Medicare-Medicaid and Medicare-Medigap claims as well as for others—and no additional claim is filed. For non-crossover claims, an additional claim is prepared for the secondary payer and sent with a copy of the primary payer RA.

Electronic Claims

A claim transmitted to the secondary payer with the primary RA is sent either electronically or on paper according to the payer's procedures. The secondary payer determines whether additional benefits are due under the policy's coordination of benefits (COB) provisions and sends payment with another RA to the practice (see Chapter 5).

The practice does not send a claim to the secondary payer when the primary payer handles the coordination of benefits transaction.

THINKING IT THROUGH 11.2

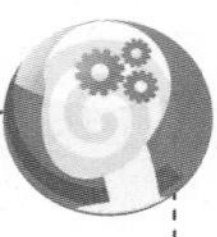

Discuss the importance of correct billing procedures to avoid problems that can arise during postpayment audits.

In this case, the primary payer electronically sends the COB transaction, which is the same HIPAA 837 that reports the primary claim, to the secondary payer. When the primary payer forwards the COB transaction, a message appears on the primary payer's RA. For example, an RA may contain the phrase "Claim Information Forwarded to," followed by the name of the secondary payer.

Paper Claims

If a paper RA is received, the procedure is to use the CMS-1500 to bill the secondary health plan that covers the beneficiary. The practice completes the claim form and sends it with the primary RA attached.

11.6 Creating Statements

patient statement list of the amount of money a patient owes, the procedures performed, and the dates the procedures were performed

explanation of benefits (EOB) document showing how the amount of a benefit was determined

A **patient statement** lists the amount of money a patient owes, organized by the amount of time the money has been owed, the procedures performed, and the dates the procedures were performed. A patient statement is created after an insurance claim has been filed and a remittance advice received.

A patient statement is sent to collect an account balance that is the patient's responsibility. This may include coinsurance charges and charges for procedures that were not covered by the insurance company. At the same time the practice receives an RA that covers a particular claim, the patient or guarantor receives a notice, called an **explanation of benefits (EOB),** that provides the same information in language appropriate for general readers. The EOB presents the charges for a date of service, the amount the insurance paid, and the amount the patient is now responsible for. By the time the practice sends a statement to an insured patient, the patient has received prior notice of what the statement will entail.

Statements are created using the Statement Management feature, which is listed on the Activities menu. Just as Claim Management provides a range of options for billing insurance carriers, Statement Management offers multiple choices for billing patients.

Statement Management Dialog Box

The Statement Management dialog box is displayed by clicking Statement Management on the Activities menu or by clicking the Statement Management shortcut button on the toolbar (see Figure 11.23). The dialog box lists all statements that have already been created (see Figure 11.24). Several actions can be performed in this dialog box: Existing statements can be reviewed and edited, new statements can be created, the status of existing statements can be changed, and statements can be printed.

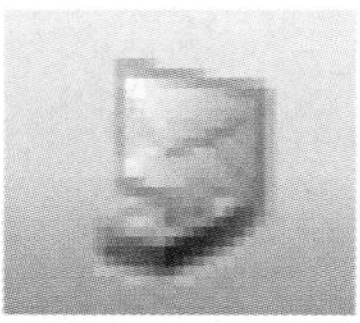

Figure 11.23 Statement Management Shortcut Button

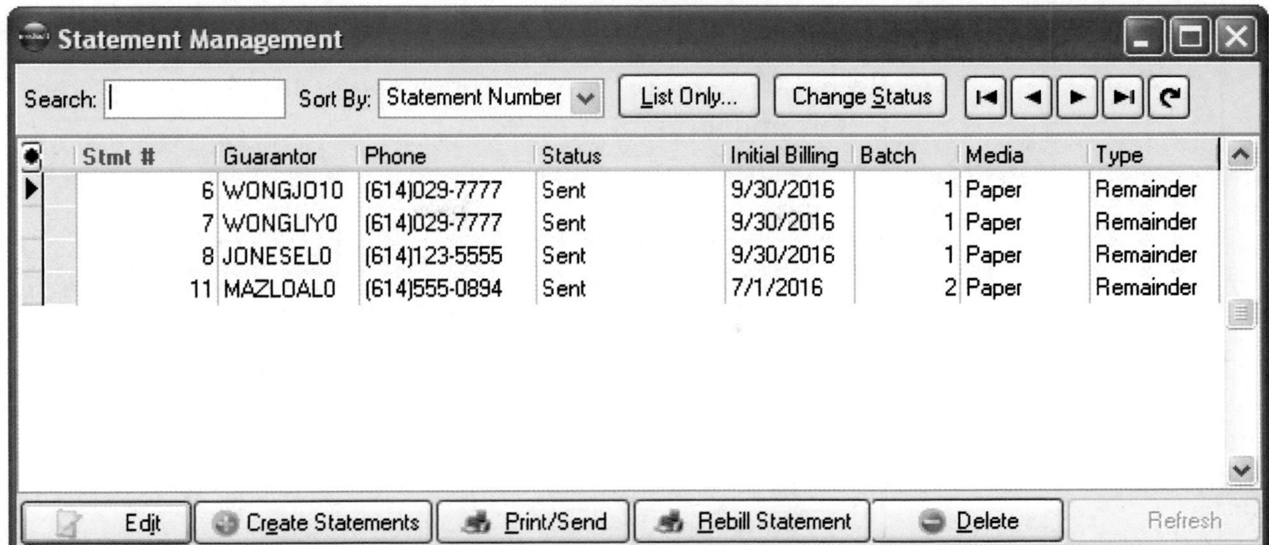

Figure 11.24 Statement Management Dialog Box

Stmt # The Stmt # column lists the statement numbers, which are generated by the program in sequential order.

Guarantor In the Statement Management dialog box, guarantors rather than patients are listed because statements are created only for the people who are financially responsible for accounts. For example, if a patient's father is the guarantor, a statement is created for the patient's father, not for the patient. In the Statement Management dialog box, the statement is listed under the father's chart number. If the man is also guarantor on his wife's account, his chart number will appear twice in the Statement Management window. When statements are printed, however, all transactions for the guarantor's child and wife are billed on one statement.

Phone The Phone column lists guarantors' phone numbers.

Status The status assigned to each statement depends on whether the statement has been billed and whether the account has a zero balance:

- **Ready to Send** Transactions that have not been billed
- **Sent** Transactions that have been billed but not fully paid
- **Done** Transactions that have been billed and fully paid

Medisoft Network Professional assigns status based on:

Initial Billing The date the statement was initially sent appears in the Initial Billing column. If a statement has been sent more than once, the most recent date is shown in the Billing Date field located in the General tab of the Statement dialog box, which is used for editing statements.

Batch The batch number assigned by MNP is displayed.

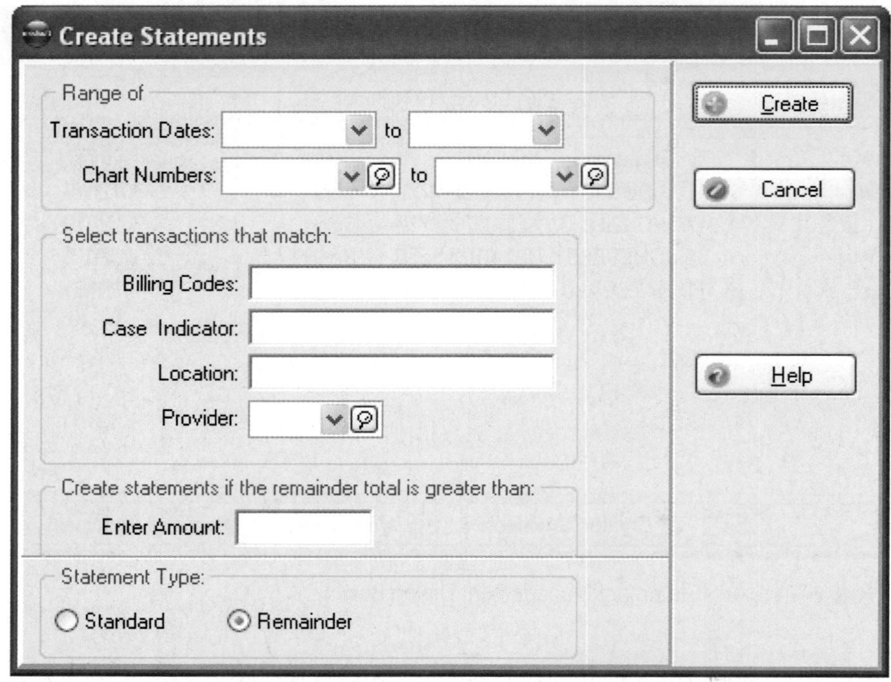

Figure 11.25 Create Statements Dialog Box

Media The format for the statement, either paper or electronic, is designated.

Type The type of statement, either Standard or Remainder, is listed.

Create Statements Dialog Box

The Create Statements dialog box is where information is entered that determines which statements are generated (see Figure 11.25).

The following filters can be applied in the Create Statements dialog box:

Transaction Dates A range of dates is entered to select transactions that occur within those dates. The dates can be entered directly by keying in the boxes, or they can be selected from the calendar that appears when the drop-down arrow is clicked. To create statements for all available transactions, leave both date boxes blank.

Chart Numbers In the Chart Numbers boxes, the starting and ending chart numbers for which statements will be created are entered. If the boxes are left blank, all chart numbers will be included.

Select Transactions That Match The options in this portion of the dialog box provide filters for creating statements for billing codes, case indicators, locations, and provider. In all instances except provider, commas must be placed between entries if more than one code is entered.

Create Statements If the Remainder Total Is Greater Than . . . Enter Amount The dollar amount entered in this box is the minimum outstanding balance required for a statement to be created. For example, if 5.00 is entered in this box, the program will not create statements for accounts with balances below $5.00. If this field is left blank, statements will be created for all accounts, regardless of the balances.

Statement Type **Standard statements** show all available charges regardless of whether the insurance has paid on the transactions. **Remainder statements** list only those charges that are not paid in full after all insurance carrier payments have been received. Once a statement type is selected, the setting remains in effect until the other type of statement is selected.

standard statements statements that show all charges regardless of whether the insurance carrier has paid on the transactions

remainder statements statements that list only charges that are not paid in full after all insurance carrier payments have been received

After all selections are complete in the Create Statements dialog box, clicking the Create button instructs the program to generate statements. (*Note:* If you click the Create button and no statements can be created, the following message appears: "No new statements were created." Click OK to close the dialog box that contains the message.)

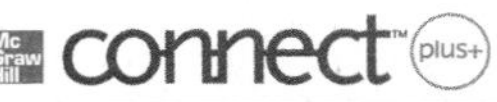

EXERCISE 11.9

CREATING STATEMENTS

Create remainder statements for all patients with chart numbers beginning with the letters *H* through *S*. *Note:* Be sure to enter *SYZMAM* instead of just *S* to select all patients whose last names begin with the letter *S*.

Date: October 28, 2016

1. Verify that Medisoft Network Professional is open and that the Medisoft Program Date is now set to October 28, 2016.
2. Select Statement Management on the Activities menu. The Statement Management dialog box appears.
3. Change the Sort By field to Statement Number.
4. Click the Create Statements button. The Create Statements dialog box is displayed.
5. Enter the chart numbers that will select all patients with last names beginning with *H* through *S* as follows. In the first Chart Number box, key ***H*** (to select the first name in the list beginning with the letter *H*) and press Tab.
6. In the second Chart Numbers box, key ***SYZMAM*** (to select Michael Syzmanski—the last name in the list beginning with the letter *S*) and press Tab.
7. Change the Statement Type field at the bottom of the dialog box from Standard to Remainder.
8. Click the Create button to generate statements.
9. A message appears stating the number of statements that have been created. In this case, one statement has been created. Click the OK button.
10. Any new statements that were created are added to the list of statements in the Statement Management dialog box, with a Ready to Send status.
11. Close the Statement Management dialog box.

You have completed Exercise 11.9

EXERCISE 11.10 connect plus+

CREATING A STATEMENT FOR A SINGLE PATIENT

Create a remainder statement for Jorge Barrett.

Date: November 30, 2016

1. Verify that the Medisoft Program Date is set to November 30, 2016.
2. Open the Statement Management dialog box.
3. Verify that the Sort By field is set to Statement Number.
4. Click the Create Statements button. The Create Statements dialog box is displayed.
5. Key ***B*** in the first Chart Numbers box, and press Tab to select Jorge Barrett's chart number. Select Jorge Barrett's chart number in the second Chart Numbers box as well.
6. Confirm that the Statement Type field at the bottom of the dialog box is set to Remainder.
7. Click the Create button to generate statements.
8. A message appears stating the number of statements that have been created. Click the OK button.
9. The new statement is added to the list of statements in the Statement Management dialog box, with a Ready to Send status.
10. Close the Statement Management dialog box.

You have completed Exercise 11.10

11.7 Editing and Printing Statements

The Edit button in the Statement Management dialog box is used to perform edits on account statements (see Figure 11.26). The three tabs in the Statement dialog box contain important information about the statement.

General Tab

The following information is located in the General tab:

Status These buttons indicate the current status of the statement.

Billing Method The statement can be either paper or electronic.

Type The Type field indicates whether the statement is standard or remainder.

Initial Billing Date The Initial Billing Date is the date the statement was first created.

Batch The batch number assigned to the statement appears.

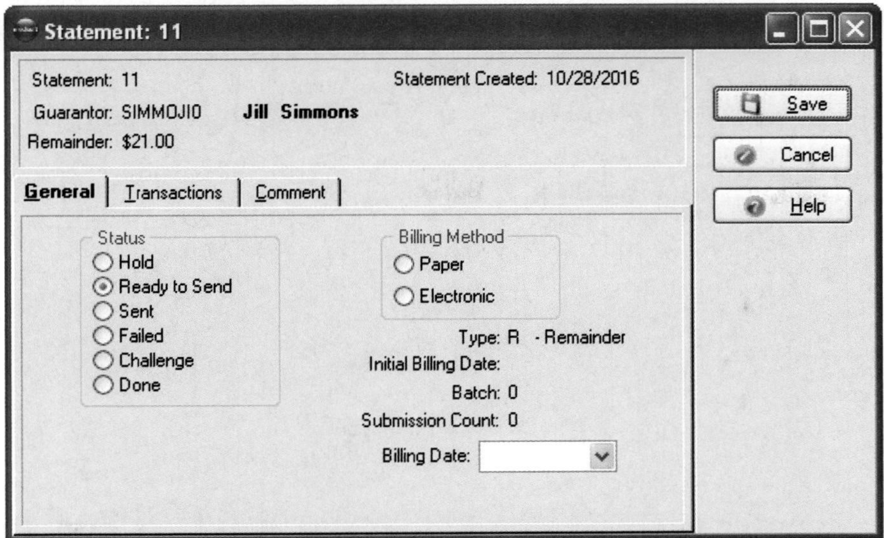

Figure 11.26 Statement Dialog Box

Submission Count This entry shows how many times a statement has been sent or printed.

Billing Date The most current billing date is displayed.

Transactions Tab

The Transactions tab lists the transactions placed on the statement (see Figure 11.27). The buttons at the bottom of the tab are used to add transactions to the statement, split transactions, or remove transactions from the statement.

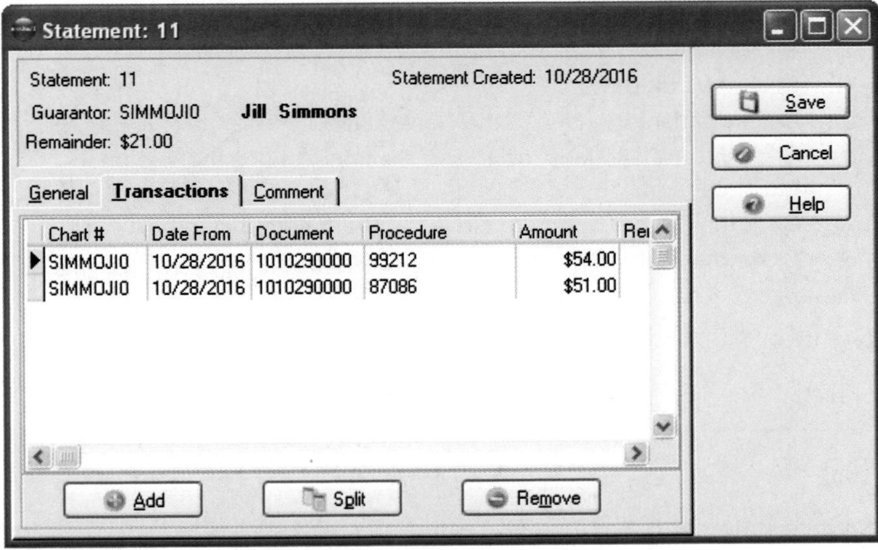

Figure 11.27 Transactions Tab

Comment Tab

The Comment tab provides a place to include notes about the statement (see Figure 11.28).

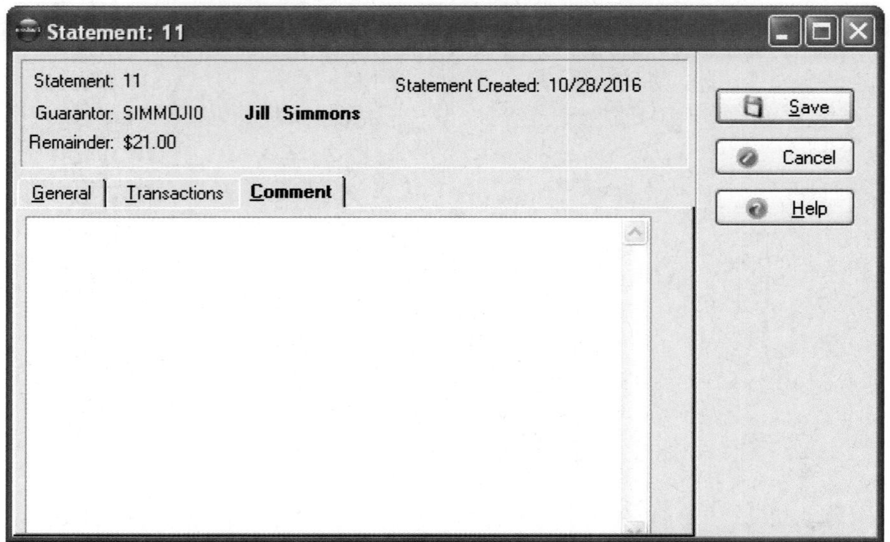

Figure 11.28 Comment Tab

EXERCISE 11.11

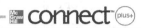

REVIEWING A STATEMENT

Review the statement created in Exercise 11.10.

Date: November 30, 2016

1. Verify that Medisoft Network Professional is open and that the Medisoft Program Date is set to 11/30/2016.
2. Select Statement Management on the Activities menu. The Statement Management dialog box appears.
3. Click the statement created for Jorge Barrett in Exercise 11.10 to highlight it.
4. Click the Edit button.
5. Review the information in the General tab.
6. Click the Transactions tab to see the transactions that are on the statement.
7. Click the Cancel button to close the Statement dialog box.
8. Close the Statement Management dialog box.

 **You have completed Exercise 11.11**

Once statements have been created, the next step is to send them to a printer or to transmit them electronically. When the Print/Send button is clicked, the Print/Send Statements dialog box is displayed (see Figure 11.29). This dialog box lists options for choosing the type of statement that will be created—Paper or Electronic. Paper statements are printed and mailed by the practice. Electronic statements are sent electronically to a processing center, which prints and mails them.

The Exclude Billed Paid Entries box designates whether transactions that have been billed and paid are left out of the statement processing.

When the Paper button is selected and the OK button clicked, the Open Report dialog box appears (see Figure 11.30).

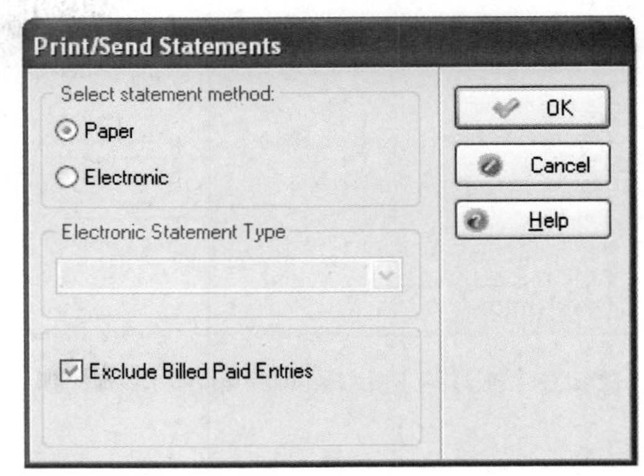

Figure 11.29 Print/Send Statements Dialog Box

Selecting a Format

The report selected in this dialog box must match the type of statement selected in the Statement Type field of the Create Statements dialog box—either Standard or Remainder. If Remainder was checked, statements will print only if one of the five Remainder Statement report formats is selected in the Open Report window:

1. Remainder Statement (0, 30, 60, 90)
2. Remainder Statement (All Payments)
3. Remainder Statement (All Pmts/Deduct)
4. Remainder Statement (Combined Payments)
5. Remainder Statement-WZ(SM)

Likewise, for Standard statements to print, one of the other patient statement report formats on the list must be chosen, such as Patient Statement (All Payments).

After selecting the report format, click the OK button to display the Print Report Where? dialog box, which asks whether to preview the

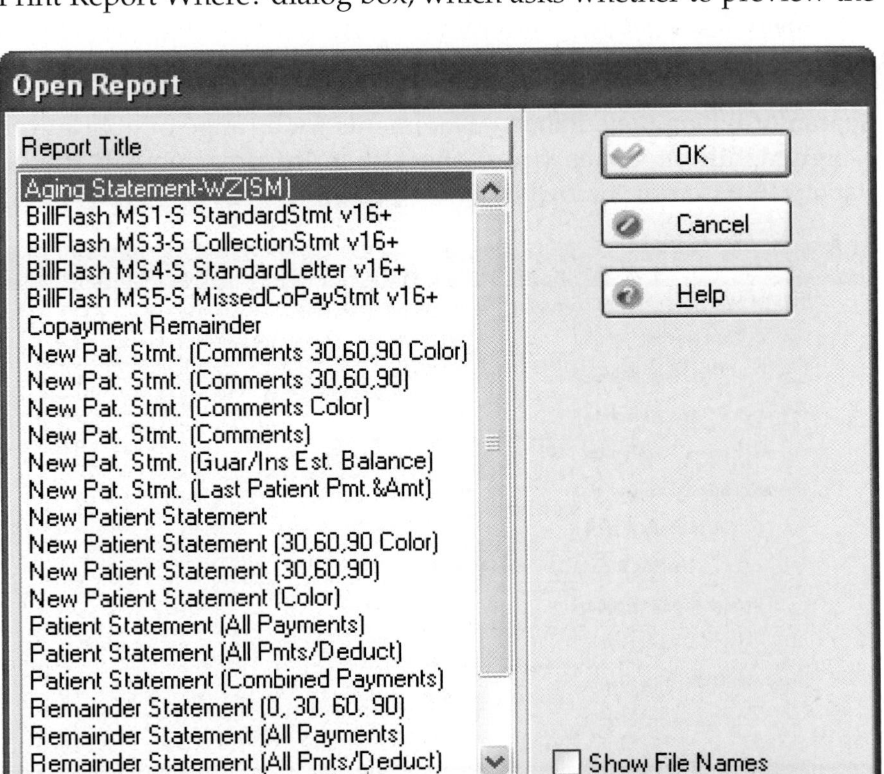

Figure 11.30 Open Report Dialog Box

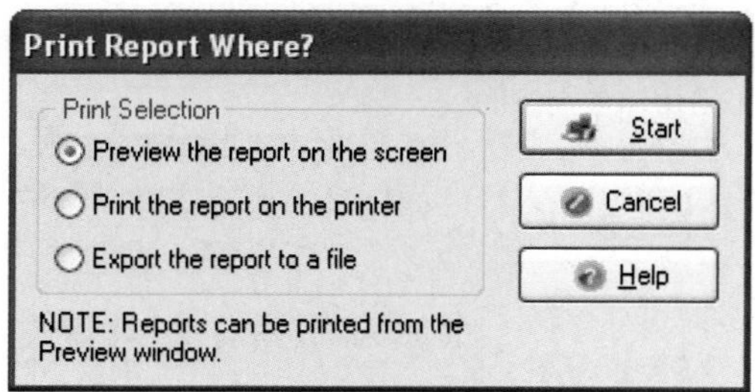
Print Report Where?
Print Selection
Preview the report on the screen
Print the report on the printer
Export the report to a file
Start
Cancel
Help
NOTE: Reports can be printed from the Preview window.

Figure 11.31 Print Report Where? Dialog Box

report on screen, send the report directly to the printer, or export the report to a file format (see Figure 11.31).

Once the Start button is clicked, the Data Selection Questions dialog box appears (see Figure 11.32).

Selecting the Filters and Printing the Statements

once-a-month billing type of billing in which statements are mailed to all patients at the same time each month

cycle billing type of billing in which statement printing and mailing is staggered throughout the month

The fields in the Data Selection Questions dialog box are used to filter statement selections. For example, to print statements for a certain group of patients, entries are made in the Chart Number Range field. In **once-a-month billing,** all statements are printed and mailed at once. Many practices use cycle billing instead. In a **cycle billing** system, patients are divided into groups, and statement printing and mailing is staggered throughout the month. For example, statements for guarantors whose last names begin with the letters *A* to *G* are mailed on the first of the month; those with last names that begin with *H* to *S* are mailed on the eighth of the month, and so on.

In addition to the Chart Number Range filter, other available filters include the following:

Date From Range Statements within a range of dates.

Insurance Carrier #1 Range Statements for a range of insurance carriers.

Statement Total Range Statements for guarantors with a balance within a specified range.

Guarantor Billing Code Range Statements for a range of guarantors assigned billing codes (from the Other Information tab in the Patient/Guarantor dialog box).

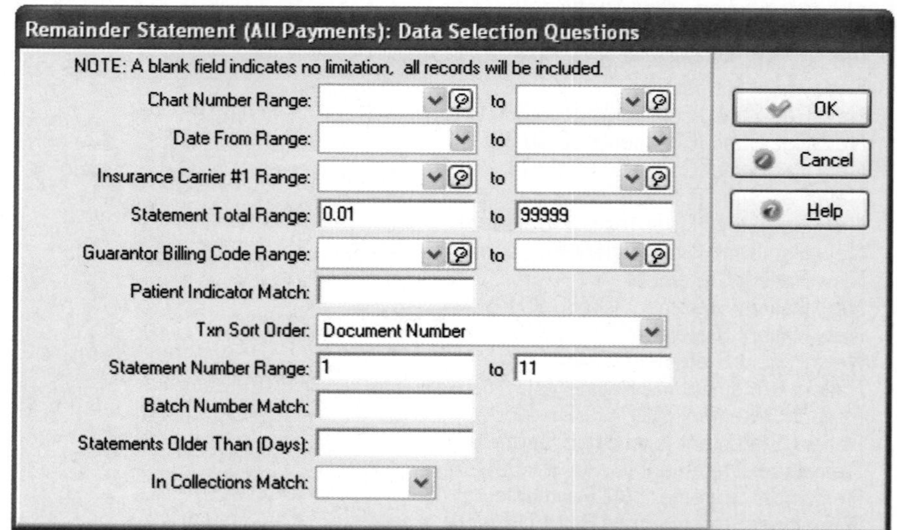
Remainder Statement (All Payments): Data Selection Questions
NOTE: A blank field indicates no limitation, all records will be included.
Chart Number Range: to
Date From Range: to
Insurance Carrier #1 Range: to
Statement Total Range: 0.01 to 99999
Guarantor Billing Code Range: to
Patient Indicator Match:
Txn Sort Order: Document Number
Statement Number Range: 1 to 11
Batch Number Match:
Statements Older Than (Days):
In Collections Match:
OK
Cancel
Help

Figure 11.32 Remainder Statement (All Payments): Data Selection Questions Dialog Box

Patient Indicator Match Statements for patients assigned a particular patient indicator (from the Other Information tab in the Patient/Guarantor dialog box).

Txn Sort Order Transactions can be listed on the statement by Date of Service (Date From), Document Number, or Entry Number.

Statement Number Range Statements for a range of statement numbers (assigned by MNP).

Batch Number Match Statements in a particular batch (assigned by MNP).

Statements Older Than (Days) Statements that are older than a specified number of days.

In Collections Match Statements for accounts that are in collections.

If no changes are made to the default entries in the Data Selection Questions dialog box, all statements that have a status of Ready to Send or Sent are included in the batch. To avoid printing statements with a Sent status, and to print only those with a Ready to Send status, a zero is entered in the Batch Number Match field. All statements that are Ready to Send have a batch number of zero. Figure 11.33 displays a sample remainder statement.

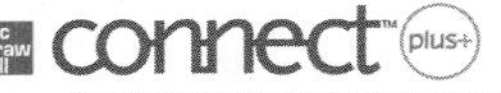

EXERCISE 11.12

PRINTING STATEMENTS

Print remainder statements for all patients with last names beginning with the letter *H* and ending with the letter *S*. *Note:* Be sure to enter *SYZMAM* instead of just *S* to select all patients whose last names begin with the letter *S*.

Date: October 28, 2016

1. Verify that Medisoft Network Professional is open and that the Medisoft Program Date is set to October 28, 2016.
2. Open the Statement Management dialog box.
3. Click the Print/Send button. The Print/Send Statements dialog box is displayed.
4. Verify that Paper is selected as the statement method and that the Exclude Billed Paid Entries box is checked. Click the OK button.
5. In the Open Report dialog box that appears, select Remainder Statement (All Payments). Click the OK button.
6. In the Print Report Where? dialog box, accept the default option to preview the report on screen. Click the Start button. The Data Selection Questions dialog box for Remainder Statements (All Payments) is displayed.
7. In the Chart Number Range boxes, enter the chart numbers that will select all patients with last names beginning with *H* through *S*.
8. In the Batch Number Match field, key ***0***, so that only statements with a Ready to Send status will be printed. Click the OK button.

(continued)

(Continued)

9. Medisoft Network Professional displays the statement to be printed in the Preview Report window.
10. To print the statement, the Print button at the top of the Preview Report window would be selected. Close the Preview window. (*Note:* In an actual office setting, if the statement is not printed, the changes that occur in the Statement Management dialog box, as described in the next step, do not occur.)
11. After a statement is printed, its status and initial billing date are updated in the Statement Management dialog box. Notice that Jill Simmons's statement now has a status of Sent and an initial billing date of 10/28/2016.
12. Close the Statement Management dialog box.

You have completed Exercise 11.12

EXERCISE 11.13

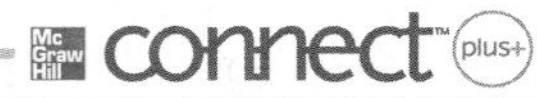

PRINTING A STATEMENT FOR A SINGLE PATIENT

Print a remainder statement for Jorge Barrett.

Date: November 30, 2016

1. Verify that the Medisoft Program Date is set to November 30, 2016.
2. Open the Statement Management dialog box.
3. Click the Print/Send button. The Print/Send Statements dialog box is displayed.
4. Verify that Paper is selected as the statement method and that the Exclude Billed Paid Entries box is checked. Click the OK button.
5. In the Open Report dialog box that appears, accept Remainder Statement (All Payments). Click the OK button.
6. In the Print Report Where? dialog box, accept the default option to preview the report on screen. Click the Start button. The Data Selection Questions dialog box for Remainder Statements (All Payments) is displayed.
7. In both Chart Number Range boxes, key ***B*** and press Tab to select Jorge Barrett.
8. In the Batch Number Match field, key ***0,*** so that only statements with a Ready to Send status will be printed. Click the OK button.
9. View the statement that is displayed.
10. To print the statement, the Print button at the top of the Preview Report window would be selected. Close the Preview window.
11. Notice that Jorge Barrett's statement now has a status of Sent and an initial billing date of 11/30/2016.
12. Close the Statement Management dialog box.

You have completed Exercise 11.13

Family Care Clinic
285 Stephenson Boulevard
Stephenson, OH 60089
(614)555-0000

Statement Date	Chart Number	Page
11/30/2016	BARREJO0	1

Make Checks Payable To:
Family Care Clinic
285 Stephenson Boulevard
Stephenson, OH 60089
(614)555-0000

Jorge Barrett
54 Juniper Court
Stephenson, OH 60089

Date of Last Payment: 11/3/2016 Amount: -96.00 Previous Balance: 0.00

Patient: Jorge Barrett Chart Number: BARREJO0 Case: Hypertension

Dates	Procedure	Charge	Paid by Primary	Paid By Guarantor	Adjustments	Remainder
10/21/16	99203	120.00	-96.00		0.00	24.00

Amount Due
24.00

Figure 11.33 Sample Remainder Statement

11.8 Nonsufficient Funds (NSF)

nonsufficient funds (NSF) check check that is not honored by the bank because the account lacks funds to cover it

When a patient makes a payment by check and does not have adequate funds in his or her checking account to cover the check, it is not honored by the bank. Such a check is referred to as a **nonsufficient funds (NSF) check.** It is also commonly called a "bounced" or a "returned" check. A bank may also not honor a check if the account has been closed. When a practice receives an NSF notice from a bank, an adjustment is made in the patient's account, since the patient now owes the practice the amount of the returned check. In addition, most practices charge a fee for a returned check. The maximum amount of the fee is governed by state laws.

In MNP, the fee for the returned check is entered in the Charges section of the Transaction Entry dialog box, and the adjustment is entered in the Payments, Adjustments, And Comments section.

EXERCISE 11.14

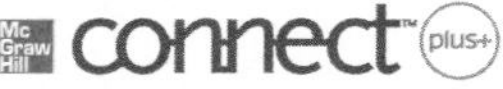

PROCESSING AN NSF CHECK

Kristin Zapata's check number 1033, in the amount of $247.50, was returned for insufficient funds. Process an NSF fee and adjustment for the returned check.

Date: October 3, 2016

1. Verify that Medisoft Network Professional is open and that the Medisoft Program Date is set to October 3, 2016.
2. Open the Transaction Entry dialog box.
3. In the Chart box, key ***Z,*** and press Tab to select Kristin Zapata's transaction information.
4. Verify that Preventive Exam is displayed in the Case box.
5. Click the New button in the Charges section of the dialog box.
6. Accept the date entry of 10/3/2016 and press Tab.
7. To enter the fee for the returned check, click the Procedure box to display the drop-down list of codes.
8. Key ***N*** and select NSFFEE (Returned check fee) from the list. Press Tab. The program automatically enters $35.00 in the Amount column.
9. Next, to enter the adjustment for the full amount of the returned check, click the New button in the Payments, Adjustments, And Comments section of the dialog box.
10. Accept the default entry of 10/3/2016 in the Date box.
11. Click the Pay/Adj Code box. Key ***N*** and select NSF (Returned check) from the drop-down list, and press Tab twice (no information is entered in the Who Paid box).
12. Enter ***Returned Check*** in the Description box, and press Tab twice to go to the Amount box.
13. Enter ***247.50*** in the Amount box, and press Tab. Notice that the amount is listed as a positive amount.

14. Enter the check number for the returned check in the Check Number field.
15. Click the Apply button. The Apply Adjustment to Charges dialog box is displayed.
16. Notice that the amount of the adjustment ($247.50) is listed in the Unapplied box in the upper-right corner of the dialog box.
17. Click the white box in the This Adjust. column in the row with the $247.50 charge on 8/28/2016. Key ***247.50,*** and press Enter.
18. Click the Close button.
19. In the Charges section of the dialog box, notice that the line for the 99385 charge that was white (fully paid) is now gray (no payment received). The line for the $35.00 fee (NSFFEE) is also gray, since it has not been paid.
20. Click the Save Transactions button to save your work.
21. Close the Transaction Entry dialog box.

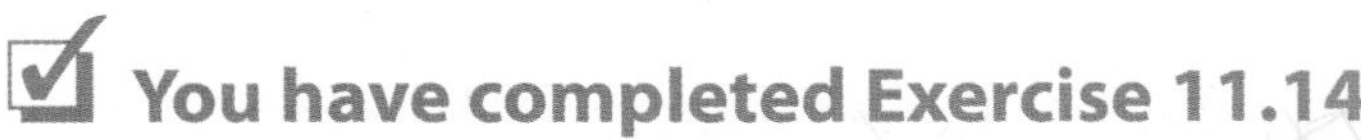
You have completed Exercise 11.14

chapter 11 summary

LEARNING OUTCOME	KEY CONCEPTS/EXAMPLES
11.1 List the six steps for checking a remittance advice. Pages 532–536	1. Check the patient's name, claim control number, and date of service against the claim. 2. Verify that all billed CPT codes are listed. 3. Check the payment for each CPT code against the expected amount. 4. Analyze the payer's adjustment codes to locate all unpaid, downcoded, or denied claims for closer review. 5. Pay special attention to RAs for claims submitted with modifiers. Some payers' claim processing systems automatically ignore modifiers, and underpayment may need to be appealed. 6. Decide whether any items on the RA need clarification from the payer, and follow up as necessary.
11.2 Describe the procedures for entering insurance payments. Pages 536–543	1. Click Enter Deposits/Payments on the Activities menu. The Deposit List dialog box is displayed. 2. Click the New button. The Deposit dialog box is displayed. 3. Select Insurance in the Payor Type box. 4. Select the appropriate entry in the Payment Method box. 5. Complete the Check Number box if entering a check or the EFT Tracer box if entering an electronic payment. 6. Enter the appropriate number in the Description/Bank No. field. 7. Enter the amount of the payment in the Payment Amount box. 8. Select the insurance carrier from the Insurance drop-down list. The program automatically completes the remaining fields. 9. Click the Save button to save the entry.
11.3 Explain how to apply insurance payments to charges. Pages 543–553	1. Click Enter Deposits/Payments on the Activities menu. The Deposit List dialog box is displayed. 2. In the list of deposits, click once on the payment that will be applied. The Apply Payment/Adjustments to Charges dialog box appears. 3. In the For box, select the first patient listed on the remittance advice. 4. Locate the first charge, enter the payment in the Payment column, and press Tab to the end of the first row. Follow the same steps for each procedure charge for that patient.

LEARNING OUTCOME	KEY CONCEPTS/EXAMPLES
	5. Click the Save Payments/Adjustments button. Click OK on the information dialog box that displays the message that the claim has been marked "done" for the primary insurance. 6. If there are additional patients for whom the payment should be applied, repeat the procedure for each patient. 7. When all payments have been applied, click the Close button.
11.4 Explain how to enter capitation payments. Pages 553–559	1. Click Enter Deposits/Payments on the Activities menu. The Deposit List dialog box is displayed. 2. Click the New button. The Deposit dialog box is displayed. 3. Select Capitation in the Payor Type box. 4. Select the appropriate entry in the Payment Method box. 5. Complete the Check Number box if entering a check or the EFT Tracer box if entering an electronic payment. 6. Enter the appropriate number in the Description/ Bank No. field. 7. Enter the amount of the payment in the Payment Amount box. 8. Select the insurance carrier from the Insurance drop-down list. 9. Click the Save button to save the entry, and close the Deposit dialog box. 10. In the Deposit List dialog box, click the New button. The Deposit dialog box appears. 11. In the Payor Type box, select Insurance. Press Tab. 12. Select Electronic in the Payment Method box. 13. Verify that 0.00 is the amount displayed in the Payment Amount box. 14. Select the insurance carrier from the Insurance drop-down list. 15. Click the Save button. The Deposit List dialog box reappears with the zero amount payment displayed. 16. Open the Claim Management dialog box by selecting Claim Management on the Activities menu. 17. Click the List Only... button.

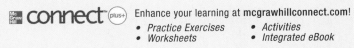

LEARNING OUTCOME	KEY CONCEPTS/EXAMPLES
	18. In the List Only Claims That Match dialog box, select the insurance carrier from the Insurance Carrier drop-down list. In the Claim Status options, make sure the All button is selected, and the Exclude Done check box is checked. 19. Click the Apply button. The Claim Management window appears with the capitated claim listed. 20. Use the Edit button and click the Transactions tab to view the details of the claim, verifying that any transactions listed took place on the dates covered by the payment. Make a note of the patient's name, and close the Claim dialog box and the Claim Management dialog box. 21. You are returned to the Deposit List dialog box. Select the deposit, and click the Apply button. 22. Select the capitated patient in the For field, and press Tab. 23. Enter the correct amount for the adjustment by identifying the amount in the Remainder column. Press Tab repeatedly, until the remainder amount changes to zero. 24. Click the Save Payments/Adjustments button. 25. Follow the same steps to identify other patients with claims covered by the capitation payment, and enter an adjustment for each transaction line that had a remainder amount. 26. Close the Apply Payment/Adjustments to Charges dialog box. 27. Close the Deposit List dialog box.
11.5 Discuss the purpose of appeals and postpayment audits. Pages 560–564	An appeal is used to challenge a payer's decision to deny, reduce, or otherwise downcode a claim. Most postpayment audits are used to build clinical information, but at times payers do postpayment audits to verify the medical necessity of reported services or to uncover fraud and abuse. The payer analyzes providers' records to assess patterns of care from individual providers and to flag those that differ from what other providers do. A postpayment audit might be conducted to check the documentation of the provider's cases or, in some cases, to check for fraudulent activities.
11.6 Compare standard patient statements and remainder patient statements. Pages 564–568	A standard patient statement shows all available charges regardless of whether the insurance has paid on the transactions. A remainder statement lists only the charges that are not paid in full after all insurance carrier payments have been received.

LEARNING OUTCOME	KEY CONCEPTS/EXAMPLES
11.7 Explain the different between once-a-month and cycle billing. Pages 568–575	In once-a-month billing, all statements are printed and mailed at once. In cycle billing, patients are divided into groups, and statement printing and mailing is staggered throughout the month. For example, statements for guarantors whose last names begin with the letters *A* to *G* are mailed on the first of the month; those with last names that begin with *H* to *S* are mailed on the eighth of the month, and so on.
11.8 Explain the procedure for processing a nonsufficient funds payment. Pages 576–577	1. Open the Transaction Entry dialog box, and select the patient in the Chart box. 2. Verify that that the appropriate case is displayed in the Case box. 3. Click the New button in the Charges section of the Transaction Entry dialog box. 4. To enter the fee for the returned check, click the Procedure box. Select NSFFEE (NSF fee for a returned check) from the drop-down list, and press Tab. The program automatically enters the amount in the Amount column. 5. To enter the adjustment for the full amount of the returned check, click the New button in the Payments, Adjustments, And Comments section of the dialog box. 6. Click in the Pay/Adj Code box. Select NSF from the drop-down list, and press Tab twice. 7. Enter ***Returned Check*** in the Description box, and press Tab twice to go to the Amount box. 8. Enter the amount in the Amount box, and press Tab. 9. Press Tab again, and enter the check number in the Check Number field. 10. Click the Apply button. The Apply Adjustment to Charges dialog box is displayed. 11. Click the white box in the This Adjust. column for the charge; enter the amount, and press Enter. 12. Click the Close button. 13. Click the Save Transactions button.

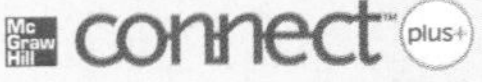

Enhance your learning at **mcgrawhillconnect.com!**

- *Practice Exercises*
- *Worksheets*
- *Activities*
- *Integrated eBook*

chapter review

MATCHING QUESTIONS

Match the key terms with their definitions.

_____ 1. ***[LO 11.2]*** capitation payments

_____ 2. ***[LO 11.7]*** cycle billing

_____ 3. ***[LO 11.1]*** electronic remittance advice (ERA)

_____ 4. ***[LO 11.8]*** nonsufficient funds (NSF) check

_____ 5. ***[LO 11.7]*** once-a-month billing

_____ 6. ***[LO 11.6]*** patient statement

_____ 7. ***[LO 11.5]*** postpayment audit

_____ 8. ***[LO 11.6]*** remainder statements

_____ 9. ***[LO 11.2]*** electronic funds transfer (EFT)

_____ 10. ***[LO 11.1]*** autoposting

a. A list of the amount of money a patient owes, organized by the amount of time the money has been owed, the procedures performed, and the dates the procedures were performed.

b. A type of billing in which patients are divided into groups and statement printing and mailing is staggered throughout the month.

c. A review conducted after a claim is adjudicated.

d. A software feature enabling automatic entry of payments from a remittance advice.

e. Payments made to physicians on a regular basis (such as monthly) for providing services to patients in a managed care insurance plan.

f. An electronic document that lists patients, dates of service, charges, and the amounts paid or denied by the insurance carrier.

g. The electronic routing of funds between banks.

h. A type of billing in which statements are mailed to all patients at the same time each month.

i. Statements that list only those charges that are not paid in full after all insurance carrier payments have been received.

j. A check that is not honored by the bank because the account lacks funds to cover it.

TRUE-FALSE QUESTIONS

Decide whether each statement is true or false.

_____ 1. ***[LO 11.5]*** An appeal is a process that can be used to challenge a payer's decision to deny, reduce, or otherwise downcode a claim.

_____ 2. ***[LO 11.2]*** Capitation payments are made to physicians on a regular basis.

_____ 3. ***[LO 11.6]*** Standard statements list only those charges that are not paid in full after all insurance carrier payments have been received.

_____ 4. ***[LO 11.4]*** Capitation payments are entered in the Claim Management dialog box.

______ 5. ***[LO 11.1]*** RAs cover groups of claims, not just a single claim.

______ 6. ***[LO 11.7]*** In cycle billing, all statements are printed and mailed at once.

______ 7. ***[LO 11.5]*** The purpose of an RAC is to audit Medicare claims and determine where there are opportunities to recover incorrect payments from previously paid but noncovered services, erroneous coding, and duplicate services.

______ 8. ***[LO 11.2]*** EFT occurs when the payer sends a check to the practice, and the check is taken to the practice's bank for deposit

______ 9. ***[LO 11.8]*** A nonsufficient funds (NSF) check is also commonly called a "bounced" or a "returned" check.

______ 10. ***[LO 11.3]*** To apply a deposit in MNP, the payment is highlighted in the Deposit List dialog box, and the Apply button is clicked.

MULTIPLE-CHOICE QUESTIONS

Select the letter that best completes the statement or answers the question.

1. ***[LO 11.1]*** The ERA that is mandated for use by HIPAA is called the X12 835 Remittance Advice Transaction or simply the ________.
   a. X12
   b. 835
   c. RAT
   d. 12

2. ***[LO 11.3]*** To apply a deposit in MNP, the payment is highlighted in the Deposit List dialog box, and the ________ button is clicked.
   a. Apply
   b. Save
   c. Edit
   d. New

3. ***[LO 11.7]*** Which of these tabs appear in the Statement dialog box?
   a. General tab
   b. Comment tab
   c. Transactions tab
   d. all of the above

4. ***[LO 11.4]*** In order to adjust the patient accounts of those covered by the capitated plan, a second deposit is entered as an insurance payment with ________.
   a. a positive amount
   b. a negative amount
   c. an equal amount
   d. a zero amount

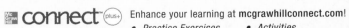

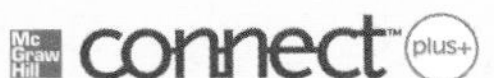

5. ***[LO 11.8]*** The maximum amount of the fee a practice can apply when it receives an NSF check is governed by ________.
   a. the practice's financial policy
   b. federal laws
   c. state laws
   d. local laws

6. ***[LO 11.1]*** Payers use ________ to provide details about an adjustment.
   a. claim adjustment group codes (CAGCs)
   b. claim adjustment reason codes (CARCs)
   c. remittance advice remark codes (RARCs)
   d. all of the above

7. ***[LO 11.2]*** What type of payments are made to physicians on a regular basis for providing services to patients in a managed care insurance plan?
   a. takeback
   b. capitation
   c. autoposting
   d. none of the above

8. ***[LO 11.6]*** A(n) ________ lists the amount of money a patient owes, organized by the amount of time the money has been owed, the procedures performed, and the dates the procedures were performed.
   a. patient statement
   b. explanation of benefits (EOB)
   c. standard statement
   d. remainder statement

9. ***[LO 11.2]*** Many practices that receive RAs authorize the health plan to provide payment with a(n) ________.
   a. remittance advice (RA)
   b. explanation of benefits (EOB)
   c. nonsufficient funds (NSF) check
   d. electronic funds transfer (EFT)

10. ***[LO 11.5]*** The person filing an appeal is the ________.
   a. claimant
   b. appellant
   c. appealer
   d. both a and b

SHORT-ANSWER QUESTIONS

Define the following abbreviations.

1. ***[LO 11.6]*** EOB ____________________
2. ***[LO 11.8]*** NSF ____________________
3. ***[LO 11.5]*** RAC ____________________
4. ***[LO 11.1]*** RA ____________________
5. ***[LO 11.1]*** RARC ____________________
6. ***[LO 11.2]*** EFT ____________________
7. ***[LO 11.1]*** ERA ____________________
8. ***[LO 11.1]*** CAGC ____________________
9. ***[LO 11.1]*** CARC ____________________

APPLYING YOUR KNOWLEDGE

Answer the questions below in the space provided.

11.1 ***[LO 11.6]*** Randall Klein calls. He would like to know whether Medicare has paid any of the charges for his September office visit. How would you look up this information in MNP?

____

____

11.2 ***[LO 11.6]*** Why do many practices send out remainder statements rather than standard statements?

____

____

11.3 ***[LO 11.4]*** What would happen if a capitated patient account was not adjusted to a zero balance?

____

____

CHAPTER 11 REVIEW CHAPTER 11 REVIEW

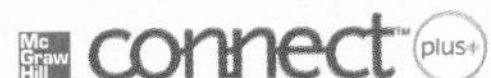

Enhance your learning at **mcgrawhillconnect.com!**

- *Practice Exercises*
- *Worksheets*
- *Activities*
- *Integrated eBook*

11.4 ***[LO 11.1]*** What is the purpose of reviewing a remittance advice before entering payments and adjustments?

____

____

11.5 ***[LO 11.1]*** If payments and adjustments listed on a remittance advice were not posted and applied to patients' accounts, what would the consequence be?

____

____

11.6 ***[LO 11.6]*** If statements were not created and mailed to patients, what would the consequence be?

____

____

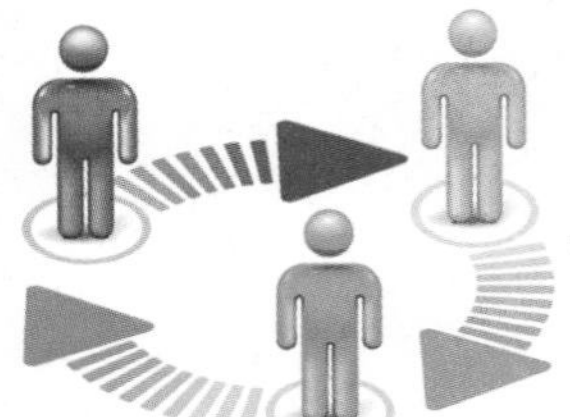

part four

Producing Reports and Following Up

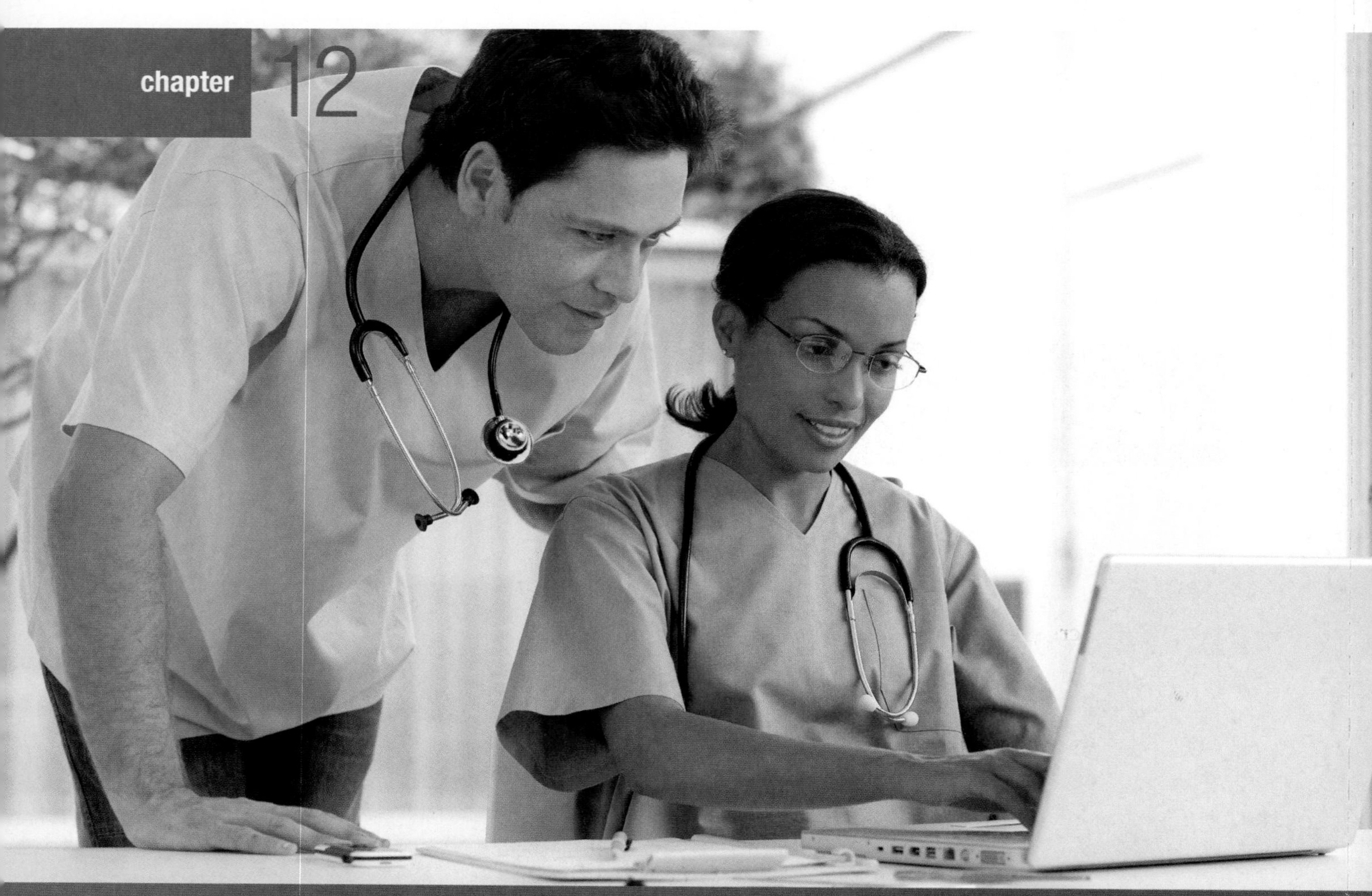

Financial and Clinical Reports

KEY TERMS

aging report
day sheet
insurance aging report
patient aging report
patient day sheet
patient ledger
patient registry
payment day sheet
performance measures
practice analysis report
procedure day sheet
production by provider report
retention
selection boxes

LEARNING OUTCOMES

When you finish this chapter, you will be able to:

12.1 List the three types of financial reports available in Medisoft Network Professional (MNP).

12.2 Describe how to select data to be included in a MNP report.

12.3 Compare patient, procedure, and payment day sheets.

12.4 Discuss the purpose of a practice analysis report.

12.5 Explain how to create a production by provider report.

12.6 List the steps for creating a patient ledger report.

12.7 Describe how to create a standard patient list report.

12.8 Describe the use of Medisoft Reports to create a report.

12.9 Explain how aging reports are used in a medical practice.

12.10 Explain how to access MNP's built-in custom reports.

12.11 Describe the process of editing reports in MNP's Report Designer.

12.12 List the reasons for using reports for tracking specific clinical data.

12.13 Discuss the regulatory obligations for the retention of patient medical records.

An Investment Pays Off

Opening the envelope with the check from the Medicare PQRI program, Aisha says, "This is a nice bonus payment—I think our new PM/EHR is paying off!"

Investments in health care informatics may take some time to "earn their keep." As you study this chapter, think about the use of reports for effective control of revenue as well as for improved heath care.

WHEN YOU FINISH THIS CHAPTER, YOU WILL ALSO BE ABLE TO USE MEDISOFT CLINICAL TO:

1. Produce patient, procedure, and payment day sheets using MNP.
2. Produce other standard reports, including a practice analysis report, a production by provider report, a patient ledger report, and a standard patient list report, using MNP.
3. Use MNP's Medisoft Reports feature to create a report.
4. Access MNP's built-in custom reports.
5. Modify a report using MNP's Report Designer.

SOFTWARE SKILLS

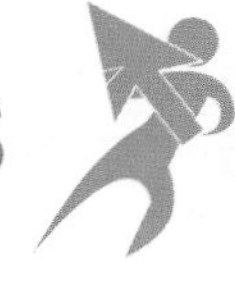

12.1 Types of Reports in Medisoft Network Professional

Reports are an important tool in managing a medical office. They provide useful information about the day-to-day operations in the practice. Providers and office managers ask for different reports at different times. Some managers want to see daily reports of each day's transactions, while others want to see reports on particular patients' accounts on a weekly or bimonthly basis.

Some reports are financial in nature and are used frequently by billing and practice management staff to monitor and control the revenue cycle. Other reports are based on clinical data and are used both for research into improved treatments and for participating in incentive programs from payers that encourage health information technology use.

Medisoft Network Professional offers several options for creating reports, all of which can be accessed via the Reports menu (see Figure 12.1). These options include:

- Standard reports
- Medisoft Reports . . .
- Design Custom Reports and Bills . . .

Standard reports include many of the basic reports used by a medical office, such as day sheets, practice analysis reports, production reports, and patient ledgers. Medisoft Reports include over a hundred reports not included in the standard reports. Finally, custom reports are created and modified using the Medisoft Report Designer program.

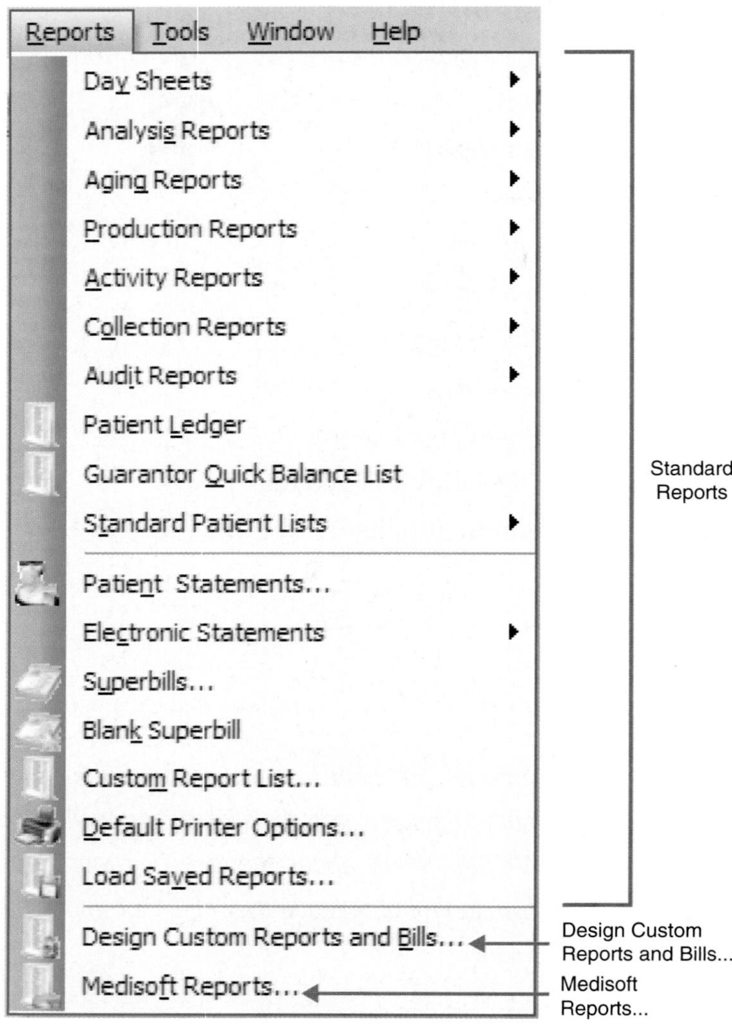

Figure 12.1 Reports Menu

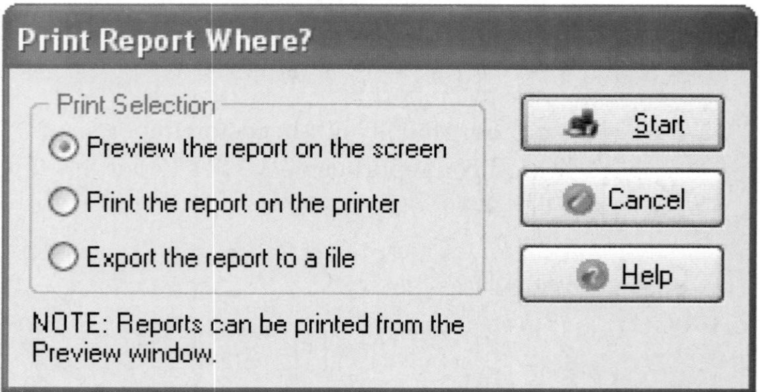

Figure 12.2 The Print Report Where? Dialog Box

Selecting Output Options

In MNP, the process of creating a report begins with selecting a report from the Reports menu. When a report is selected, a dialog box appears with the option to preview the report on the screen, send it to a printer, or export it to a file (see Figure 12.2).

Print Preview

100% 1 Close

Family Care Clinic

Patient Day Sheet

Show all data where the Date From is between 9/6/2016, 9/6/2016

Entry	Date	Document	POS	Description	Provider	Code	Amount
FITZWJO0	**Fitzwilliams, John**						
380	09/06/2016	1009070000	11		2	CHVCPAY	-15.00
471	09/06/2016	0506020000	11		2	99211	36.00
472	09/06/2016	0506020000	11		2	84478	29.00
			Patient Charges	Patient Receipts	Adjustments		Patient Balance
			$65.00	-$15.00	$0.00		$58.00
FITZWSA0	**Fitzwilliams, Sarah**						
563	09/06/2016	1010040000	11		1	90471	15.00
565	09/06/2016	1009070000	11		1	90703	29.00
566	09/06/2016	1009070000	11		1	CHVCPAY	-15.00
			Patient Charges	Patient Receipts	Adjustments		Patient Balance
			$44.00	-$15.00	$0.00		$0.00
GARDIJO0	**Gardiner, John**						
385	09/06/2016	1009070000	11		1	99211	36.00
387	09/06/2016	1009070000	11		1	OHCCPAY	-20.00
			Patient Charges	Patient Receipts	Adjustments		Patient Balance
			$36.00	-$20.00	$0.00		$0.00
KLEINRA0	**Klein, Randall**						
388	09/06/2016	1009070000	11		2	99212	54.00
389	09/06/2016	1009070000	11		2	29540	121.50
390	09/06/2016	1009070000	11		2	99070	20.00
			Patient Charges	Patient Receipts	Adjustments		Patient Balance
			$195.50	$0.00	$0.00		$0.00

Page 1 of 2

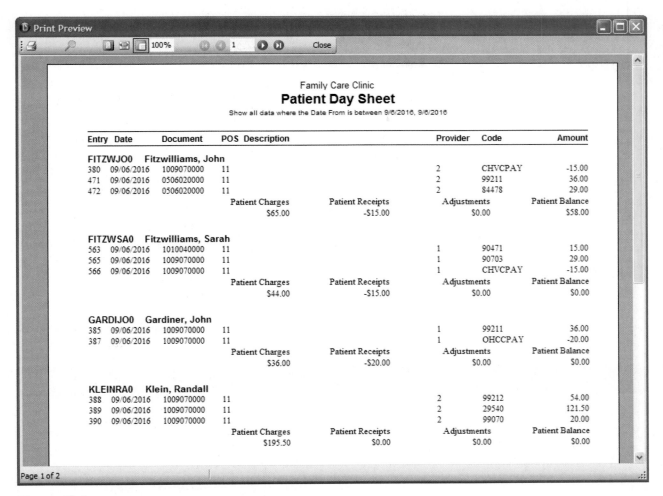

Figure 12.3 Print Preview Window

Figure 12.4 Buttons on Print Preview Toolbar

If the preview option is selected, the report will be displayed in a Print Preview window. This window, common to all reports, provides options for viewing or printing a report (see Figure 12.3). The buttons on the Print Preview toolbar control how a report is displayed on the screen and how to move from page to page within a report (see Figure 12.4).

Print The Print button is used to print the report.

Search Data The Search Data button performs a case-sensitive text search in the report displayed in the preview window.

Window Display The next three buttons are used to change the display of the report, which makes locating specific information in it easier. From left to right, the choices are whole page, page width, and percentage. A percentage can be entered in place of 100 percent for zooming in or out of the report.

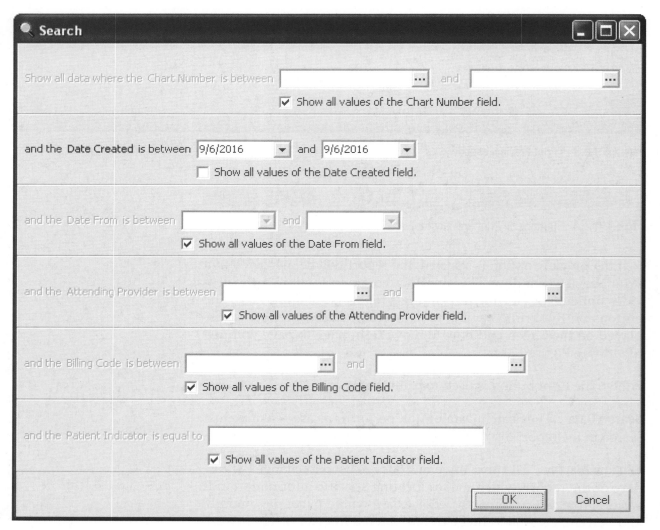

THINKING IT THROUGH 12.1

Why do you think that it is important to review reports on billing and collections on a regular basis?

Navigate Four triangle buttons, two on the left and two on the right, are used to move through pages of a multipage report. The First Page button, furthest on the left, moves to the beginning of a report. The Prior Page button moves to the page that precedes the one currently displayed. The bar between the two sets of triangle buttons indicates the number of the current page. To the right of the bar are the other two triangle buttons. The Next Page button moves to the page following the current one. The Last Page button moves to the end of a report. If a button is dimmed, it means that there are no more pages in the direction indicated by the triangle. If a button is bright blue, there is an additional page or pages in the report.

Close This command is used to close the Print Preview window.

Search

Show all data where the Chart Number is between ... and ...
☑ Show all values of the Chart Number field.

and the Date Created is between 9/6/2016 and 9/6/2016
☐ Show all values of the Date Created field.

and the Date From is between and
☑ Show all values of the Date From field.

and the Attending Provider is between ... and ...
☑ Show all values of the Attending Provider field.

and the Billing Code is between ... and ...
☑ Show all values of the Billing Code field.

and the Patient Indicator is equal to
☑ Show all values of the Patient Indicator field.

OK Cancel

Figure 12.5 Search Dialog Box for Patient Day Sheet Report

12.2 Selecting Data for a Report

Once a selection is made in the Print Report Where? dialog box and the Start button is clicked, the Search dialog box is displayed. This dialog box is used to select the range of data that will be included in the report (see Figure 12.5). While the exact contents of the Search box vary from report to report, the way selections are made does not change. Once you learn how to use the Search dialog box, you can create any report.

The Search dialog box contains a number of fields called selection boxes. Some reports have one selection box in a Search box, while others, such as the Patient Day Sheet Search box in Figures 12.5 and 12.6, have many. The **selection boxes** determine what data are included in the report.

selection boxes fields within the Search dialog box that are used to select the data that will be included in a report

Some selection boxes use a drop-down list for entering data; others use a button with three dots (see Figures 12.7a and 12.7b). This button is known as a Lookup button, since clicking it causes the Lookup dialog box to be displayed. You already know how to use a

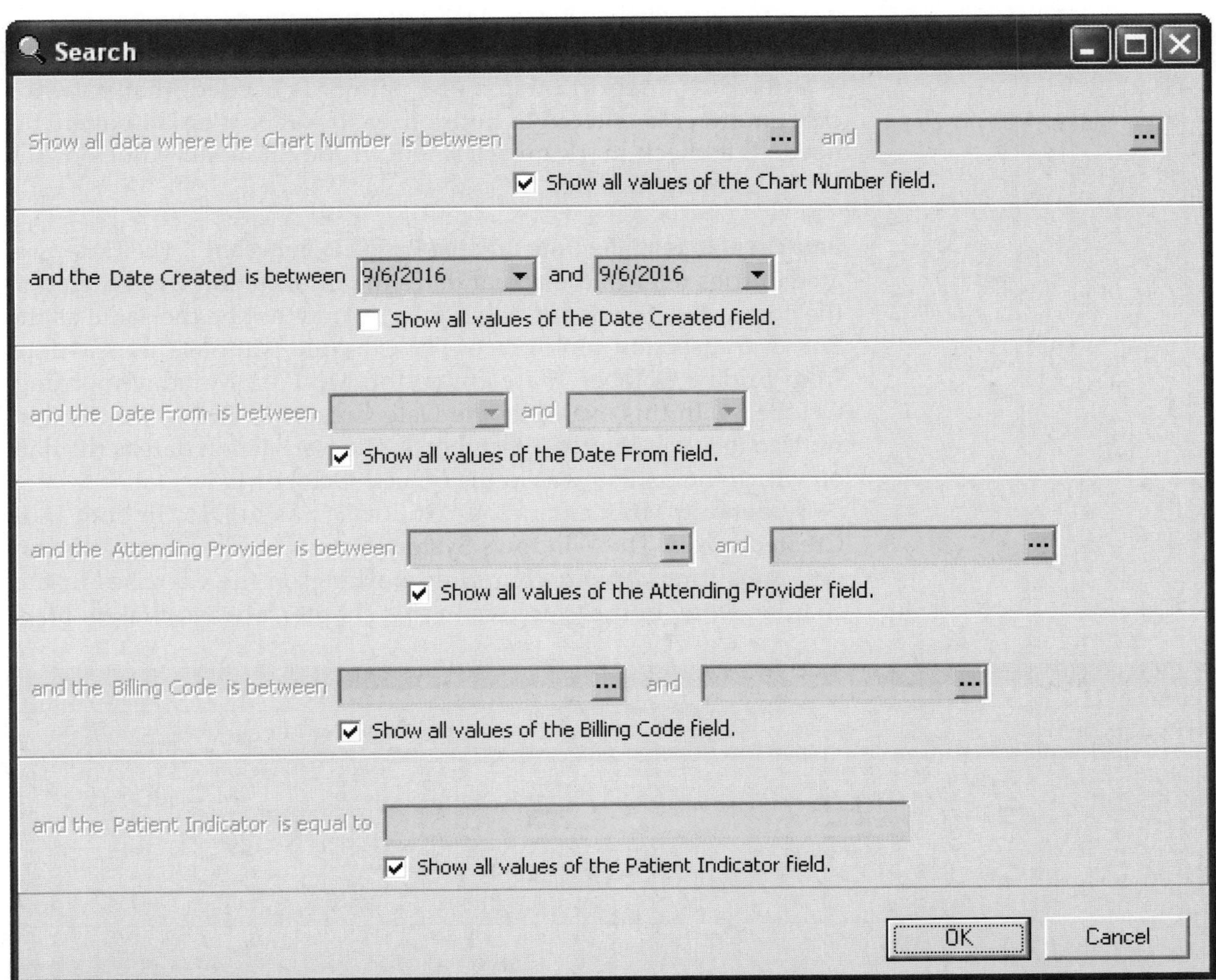

Figure 12.6 Search Dialog Box for Patient Day Sheet Report with Selection Boxes Highlighted in Yellow

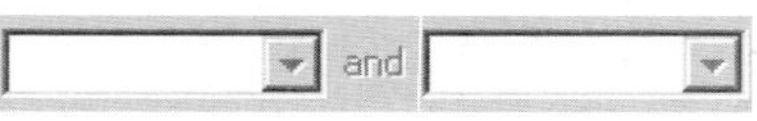

Figure 12.7a Selection Boxes with Drop-down List Buttons

drop-down list. The Lookup button is similar to a drop-down list; however, instead of displaying a limited list, when the Lookup button is clicked, a Lookup dialog box opens displaying a full list of choices from the database for that field (see Figure 12.8). When you click an item in the dialog box (for example, a chart number), that item is automatically inserted into the selection box.

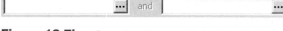

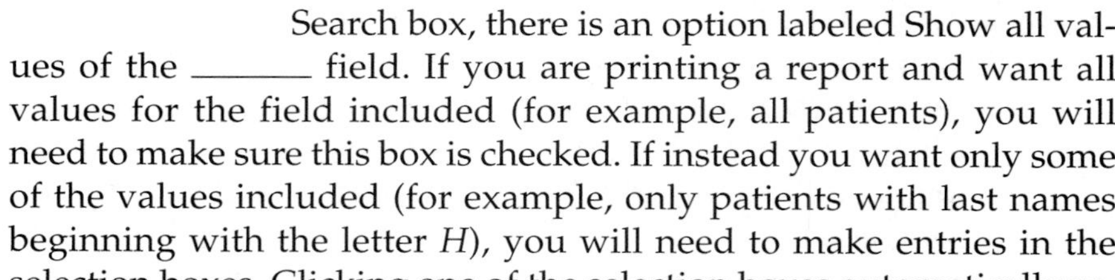

Figure 12.7b Selection Boxes with Lookup Buttons

Beneath each selection box or set of boxes in the Search box, there is an option labeled Show all values of the ______ field. If you are printing a report and want all values for the field included (for example, all patients), you will need to make sure this box is checked. If instead you want only some of the values included (for example, only patients with last names beginning with the letter *H*), you will need to make entries in the selection boxes. Clicking one of the selection boxes automatically removes the check mark from the Show all values box.

In the Patient Day Sheet Search box pictured in Figures 12.5 and 12.6, selections can be made to include some or all of the following data:

Chart Number (Show all data where the Chart Number is between) In the two Chart Number boxes, a range of chart numbers for patients is entered. If a report on just one patient is needed, that patient's chart number is entered in both boxes. If a report on all patients is needed, a check mark must remain in the Show all values of the Chart Number field box.

Date Created (and the Date Created Range is between) The Date Created entries refer to the actual dates the information was entered in the computer. The date created may or may not be the same as the date a transaction took place. For example, suppose transactions from Friday, October 1, are entered in MNP on Monday morning, October 4. In this example, the Date Created value is the date the transaction was entered—October 4. The transaction date is the date on which the patient was in the office—October 1.

By default, MNP enters the Windows System Date in both Date Created boxes. The Windows System Date is today's date—the day you are sitting at your computer working on the exercises in this chapter. *Note:* **In the exercises in this chapter, always click to place**

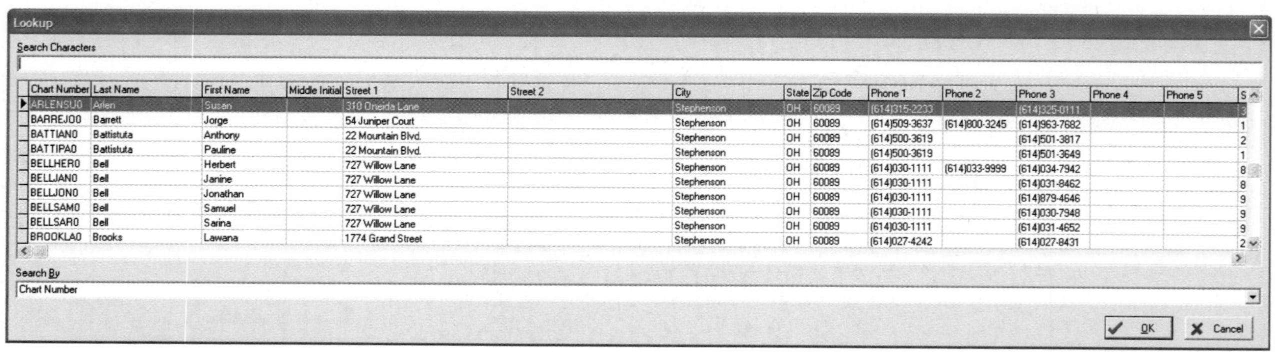

Figure 12.8 The Lookup Dialog Box That Is Displayed When the Lookup Button in the Chart Number Selection Box Is Clicked

a check mark in the Show all values of the Date Created field box. Because the exercises take place in the future (2016), if you do not show all values, the program will not find all the data it needs to create the report, and no report will be created.

Date From (and the Date From is between) The Date From entries refer to the actual dates of the transactions. If the day sheet report is for September 5, 2016, then 12/5/2016 is entered in both fields. At the beginning of each exercise, these fields must be changed to the date listed before step 1 of the exercise.

Note: There are two ways of entering dates in the Search dialog box. You can use the keyboard to enter the numbers and slashes. For example, January 1, 2016, would be keyed as 1/1/2016. The other way of entering dates is to use the pop-up calendar. The pop-up calendar is displayed when you click the down arrows at the right side of the box that contains the date (see Figure 12.9). Once this calendar is visible, clicking the month in the blue banner at the top of the calendar displays a list of the months (see Figure 12.10). Clicking any month in the

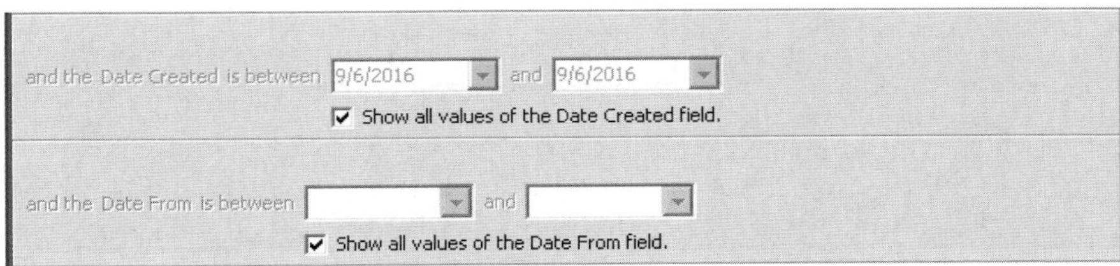

Figure 12.9 Down Arrows (Highlighted in Yellow) Used to Display the Pop-up Calendar

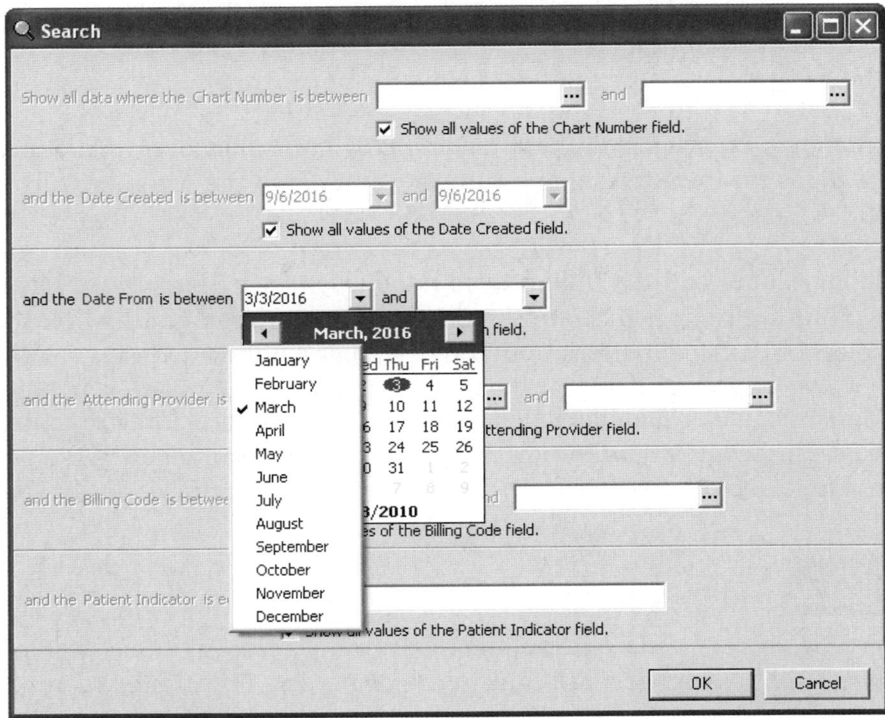

Figure 12.10 List of Months in the Pop-up Calendar

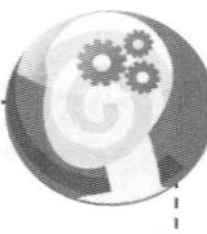

THINKING IT THROUGH 12.2

What is the advantage of learning how to use the Search dialog box?

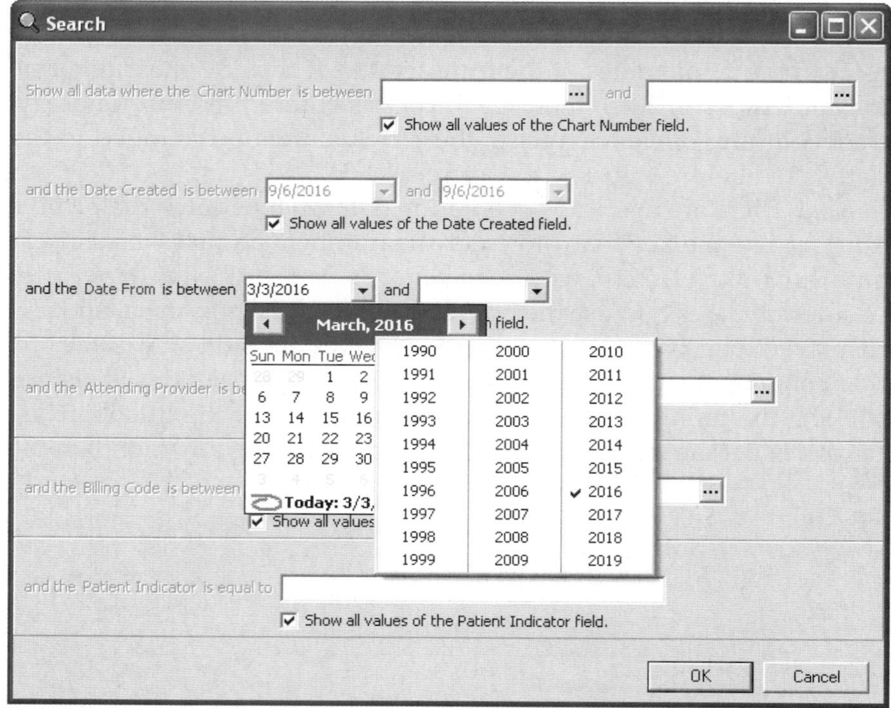

Figure 12.11 List of Years in the Pop-up Calendar

list changes the calendar to that month. Clicking the year in the blue banner displays a list of years. Clicking any year in the list changes the calendar to that year (see Figure 12.11). The day is changed by clicking the desired day in the calendar below the blue banner.

Attending Provider (and the Attending Provider is between) A range of codes for the attending providers is entered in the Attending Provider fields.

Billing Code (and the Billing Code is between) If the practice uses MNP's Billing Code feature, codes can be entered in this box to select only those patients with the designated billing codes.

Patient Indicator (and the Patient Indicator is equal to) If the practice has assigned a Patient Indicator code to each patient, an entry can be made to select only those patients who match a specific code.

12.3 Day Sheets

day sheet a report that provides information on practice activities for a twenty-four-hour period

A **day sheet** is a standard report that provides information on practice activities for a twenty-four-hour period. In MNP, there are three types of day sheet reports: patient day sheets, procedure day sheets,

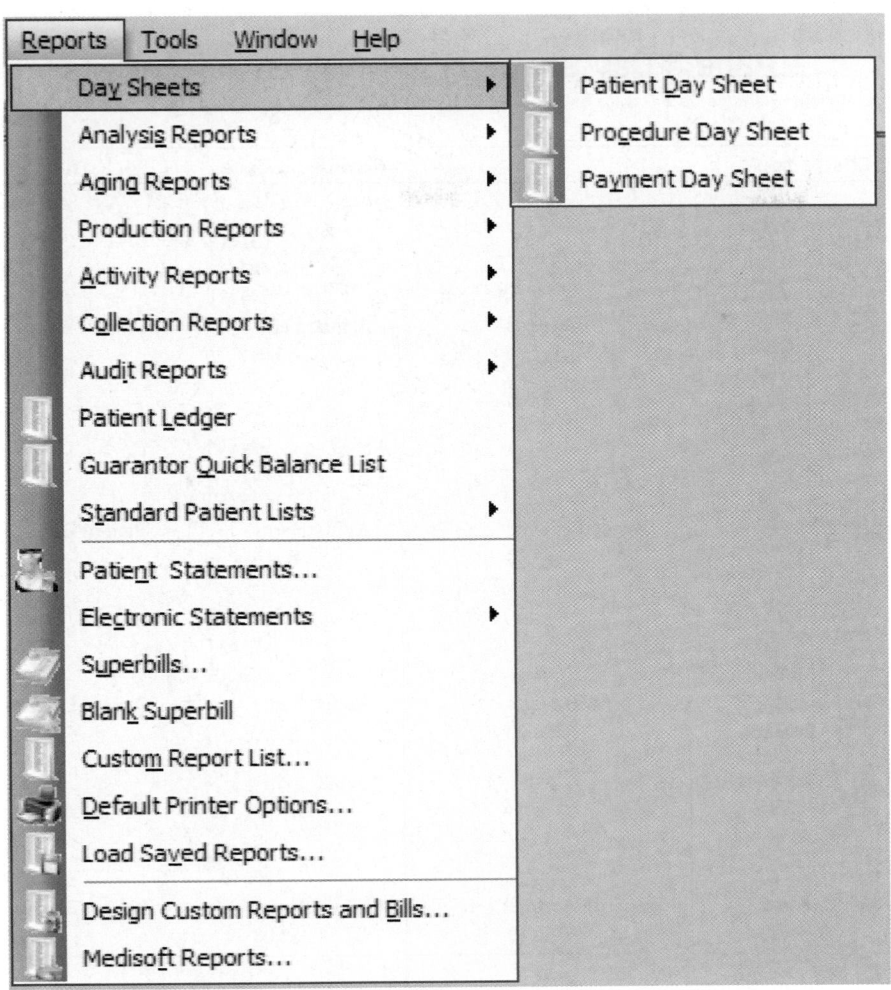

Figure 12.12 Reports Menu with Day Sheets Submenu Displayed

and payment day sheets. Options to view or print the three types of day sheets are located on the Reports menu, within the Day Sheets submenu (see Figure 12.12).

Patient Day Sheet

At the end of the day, a medical practice often prints a **patient day sheet,** which is a summary of the patient activity on that day (see Figures 12.13a and 12.13b). Medisoft Network Professional's version of this report lists the procedures for a particular day, grouped by patient, in alphabetical order by chart number. It includes:

patient day sheet a summary of patient activity on a given day

- Procedures performed for a particular patient or group of patients
- Charges, receipts, adjustments, and balances for a particular patient or group of patients
- A summary of a practice's charges, payments, and adjustments

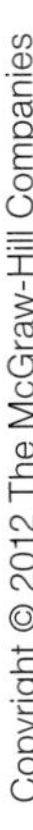

Family Care Clinic

Patient Day Sheet

Show all data where the Date From is between 9/6/2016, 9/6/2016

Entry	Date	Document	POS	Description	Provider	Code	Amount
FITZWJO0	**Fitzwilliams, John**						
380	09/06/2016	1009070000	11		2	CHVCPAY	-15.00
471	09/06/2016	0506020000	11		2	99211	36.00
472	09/06/2016	0506020000	11		2	84478	29.00
			Patient Charges	Patient Receipts	Adjustments		Patient Balance
			$65.00	-$15.00	$0.00		$58.00
FITZWSA0	**Fitzwilliams, Sarah**						
563	09/06/2016	1010040000	11		1	90471	15.00
565	09/06/2016	1009070000	11		1	90703	29.00
566	09/06/2016	1009070000	11		1	CHVCPAY	-15.00
			Patient Charges	Patient Receipts	Adjustments		Patient Balance
			$44.00	-$15.00	$0.00		$0.00
GARDIJO0	**Gardiner, John**						
385	09/06/2016	1009070000	11		1	99211	36.00
387	09/06/2016	1009070000	11		1	OHCCPAY	-20.00
			Patient Charges	Patient Receipts	Adjustments		Patient Balance
			$36.00	-$20.00	$0.00		$0.00
KLEINRA0	**Klein, Randall**						
388	09/06/2016	1009070000	11		2	99212	54.00
389	09/06/2016	1009070000	11		2	29540	121.50
390	09/06/2016	1009070000	11		2	99070	20.00
			Patient Charges	Patient Receipts	Adjustments		Patient Balance
			$195.50	$0.00	$0.00		$0.00

Figure 12.13a Page 1 of a Patient Day Sheet Report

EXERCISE 12.1

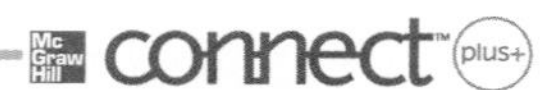

CREATING A PATIENT DAY SHEET

Create a patient day sheet report for October 3, 2016.

Date: October 3, 2016

1. Verify that Medisoft Network Professional is open, that the practice name in the title bar at the top of the screen is Family Care Clinic, and that the Medisoft Program Date is set to October 3, 2016.
2. On the Reports menu, click Day Sheets and then Patient Day Sheet. The Print Report Where? dialog box appears.
3. Accept the default selection to preview the report on the screen. Click the Start button.
4. The Search dialog box is displayed. Leave the Chart Number fields blank.
5. Under the Date Created range boxes, make sure to click the check box labeled Show all values of the Date Created field. This will clear the current Date Created range boxes to include all dates for this field.
6. Click in the first Date From box. Enter ***10/3/2016***. Click in the second Date From box, and enter the same date.
7. Leave all other fields in the Search box blank. This will select data for all patients and attending providers for October 3, 2016. Click the OK button.

Family Care Clinic

Patient Day Sheet

Show all data where the Date From is between 9/6/2016, 9/6/2016

Entry	Date	Document	POS	Description	Provider	Code	Amount
				Total # Patients	4		
				Total # Procedures	8		
				Total Procedure Charges	$340.50		
				Total Product Charges	$0.00		
				Total Inside Lab Charges	$0.00		
				Total Outside Lab Charges	$0.00		
				Total Billing Charges	$0.00		
				Total Charges	$340.50		
				Total Insurance Payments	$0.00		
				Total Cash Copayments	$0.00		
				Total Check Copayments	-$50.00		
				Total Credit Card Copayments	$0.00		
				Total Patient Cash Payments	$0.00		
				Total Patient Check Payments	$0.00		
				Total Credit Card Payments	$0.00		
				Total Receipts	-$50.00		
				Total Credit Adjustments	$0.00		
				Total Debit Adjustments	$0.00		
				Total Insurance Debit Adjustments	$0.00		
				Total Insurance Credit Adjustments	$0.00		
				Total Insurance Withholds	$0.00		
				Total Adjustments	$0.00		
				Net Effect on Accounts Receivable	$290.50		

Figure 12.13b Page 2 of a Patient Day Sheet Report

8. The patient day sheet report is displayed in the Print Preview window.
9. If necessary, use the scroll bar to view additional entries on the first page of the report.
10. Notice at the top of the Print Preview window that the triangle next to the number 1 is bright blue. This indicates that there is more than one page in the report. Click the triangle just to the right of 1 to advance to the second page of the report.
11. Follow the same procedure to view the third page of the report.
12. To print the report, you would click the Print button on the top left of the Print Preview window. It is not necessary to print the reports created in the exercises in this chapter.
13. Click the red Close box at the top right of the window or the Close button on the Print Preview toolbar to exit the Print Preview window.

 **You have completed Exercise 12.1**

Family Care Clinic

Procedure Day Sheet

Show all data where the Date From is between 9/6/2016, 9/6/2016

Entry	Date	Chart	Name	Document	POS	Debits	Credits
29540							
389	9/6/2016	KLEINRA0	Klein, Randall	1009070000	11	121.50	
		Total of 29540		Quantity: 1		$121.50	$0.00
84478							
472	9/6/2016	FITZWJO0	Fitzwilliams, John	0506020000	11	29.00	
		Total of 84478		Quantity: 1		$29.00	$0.00
90471							
563	9/6/2016	FITZWSA0	Fitzwilliams, Sarah	1010040000	11	15.00	
		Total of 90471		Quantity: 1		$15.00	$0.00
90703							
565	9/6/2016	FITZWSA0	Fitzwilliams, Sarah	1009070000	11	29.00	
		Total of 90703		Quantity: 1		$29.00	$0.00
99070							
390	9/6/2016	KLEINRA0	Klein, Randall	1009070000	11	20.00	
		Total of 99070		Quantity: 1		$20.00	$0.00
99211							
471	9/6/2016	FITZWJO0	Fitzwilliams, John	0506020000	11	36.00	
385	9/6/2016	GARDIJO0	Gardiner, John	1009070000	11	36.00	
		Total of 99211		Quantity: 2		$72.00	$0.00
99212							
388	9/6/2016	KLEINRA0	Klein, Randall	1009070000	11	54.00	
		Total of 99212		Quantity: 1		$54.00	$0.00
CHVCPAY							
380	9/6/2016	FITZWJO0	Fitzwilliams, John	1009070000	11		-15.00
566	9/6/2016	FITZWSA0	Fitzwilliams, Sarah	1009070000	11		-15.00
		Total of CHVCPAY		Quantity: 2		$0.00	-$30.00
OHCCPAY							
387	9/6/2016	GARDIJO0	Gardiner, John	1009070000	11		-20.00
		Total of OHCCPAY		Quantity: 1		$0.00	-$20.00
					Total of Codes:	$340.50	-$50.00
					Balance:	$290.50	

Figure 12.14 Procedure Day Sheet

Procedure Day Sheet

procedure day sheet a report that lists all the procedures performed on a particular day, in numerical order

A **procedure day sheet** lists all procedures performed on a particular day and gives the dates, patients, document numbers, places of service, debits, and credits relating to them (see Figure 12.14). Procedures are listed in numerical order. Procedure day sheets are printed by clicking Day Sheets and then Procedure Day Sheet on the Reports menu. The same Search dialog box used for a patient day sheet is displayed, except that a range of procedure codes rather than patients can be selected. A procedure day sheet will be

THINKING IT THROUGH 12.3

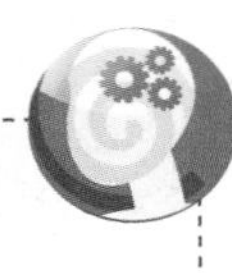

How do patient day sheets, procedure day sheets, and payment day sheets differ?

Family Care Clinic

Payment Day Sheet

Show all data where the Date From is between 9/6/2016, 9/6/2016

Entry	Date	Document	Description	Chart	Code	Amount
1	**Yan, Katherine**					
566	9/6/2016	1009070000		FITZWSA0	CHVCPAY	-15.00
387	9/6/2016	1009070000		GARDIJO0	OHCCPAY	-20.00
			Count: 2		Provider Total	-$35.00
2	**Rudner, John**					
380	9/6/2016	1009070000		FITZWJO0	CHVCPAY	-15.00
			Count: 1		Provider Total	-$15.00
			Report Totals			
			Total # Payments			3
			Total Payments			-50.00

Figure 12.15 Payment Day Sheet

generated only for data that meet the selection criteria. If any box is left blank, all values are included in the report. The report can be previewed on the screen, printed, or exported to a file.

Payment Day Sheet

A **payment day sheet** lists all payments received on a particular day, organized by provider (see Figure 12.15). It is printed by clicking Day Sheets and then Payment Day Sheet on the Reports menu. The same Search dialog box is displayed, but with fewer data fields.

A payment day sheet will be generated only for data that meet the selection criteria. If any box is left blank, all values for that box are included in the report. Again, the report can be previewed on the screen, printed, or exported to a file.

payment day sheet a report that lists all payments received on a particular day, organized by provider

12.4 Analysis Reports

Medisoft Network Professional includes a number of standard reports that provide information about practice finances. These reports are known as analysis reports. The Analysis Reports submenu is shown in Figure 12.16. The following paragraphs provide a description of each report. Not all reports can be created in student exercises because data have not been sent to insurance carriers and patients.

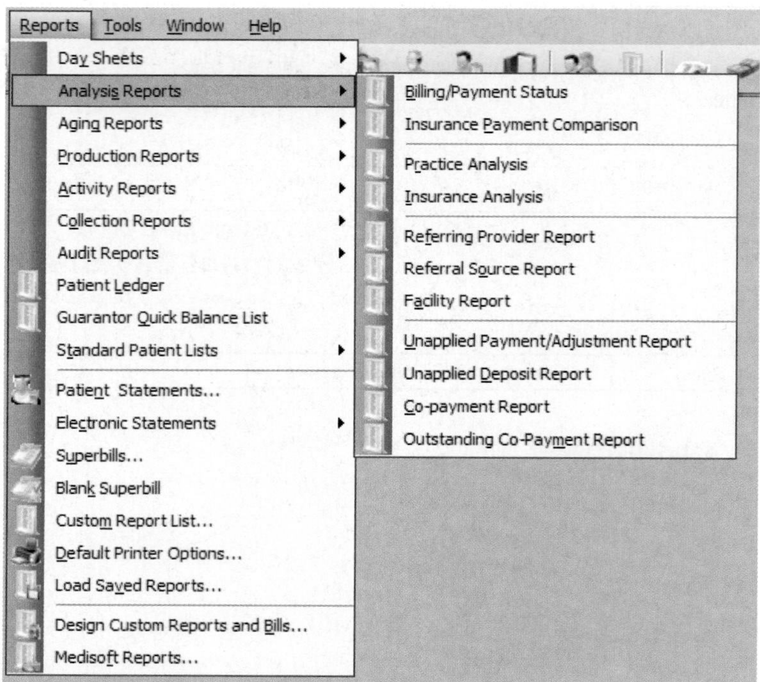

Figure 12.16 The Analysis Reports Submenu

Billing/Payment Status Report

The billing/payment status report lists the status of all transactions that have responsible insurance carriers, showing who has paid and who has not been billed (see Figure 12.17). The report is in a column format sorted first by chart number and then by case. Every chart number listed shows a patient balance and any unapplied payments or unapplied adjustments. An asterisk (*) next to a number indicates that the payer has made a complete payment for that transaction. Information in this report can be used by a practice to determine whether billing charges can be applied to a patient account.

Insurance Payment Comparison

The insurance payment comparison report isolates a procedure code and shows the payments applied to it from up to five insurance carriers. It is used to determine the average amount different carriers are paying for a given procedure or a range of procedures. In the Insurance Carrier #1 box, the Lookup button is used to select an insurance carrier code. Additional codes are selected using the Add to List button. For each procedure code, the report shows the procedure code and description, the standard charge, the average payment of each insurance carrier selected for the report, and the total current charges for the procedure.

Practice Analysis Report

practice analysis report a report that analyzes the revenue of a practice for a specified period of time

Medisoft Network Professional's **practice analysis report** analyzes the revenue of a practice for a specified period of time, usually a

Family Care Clinic

Billing/Payment Status Report

Show all data where the Patient Reference Balance is between 0.01,999999999999.99
Show all data where the Date From is between 10/1/2016, 10/31/2016

Date	Document	Procedure	Amount	Policy 1	Policy 2	Policy 3	Guarantor	Adjustments	Balance
BARREJO0	**Jorge Barrett (614)509-3637**								
Case 67	1: Blue Cross/Blue Shield			(614)024-9000					
	2:								
	3:								
10/21/2016	1610210000	99203	120.00	-96.00*	0.00*	0.00*	11/30/2016	0.00	24.00
								SubTotal:	24.00
								Unapplied Payments and Adjustments:	96.00
								Case Balance:	120.00
								Patient Reference Balance:	24.00
BATTIAN0	**Anthony Battistuta (614)500-3619**								
Case 25	1: Medicare			(215)599-0000					
	2:								
	3:								
10/27/2016	1009280000	82947	25.00	10/31/2016	0.00*	0.00*	Not Billed	0.00	25.00
10/27/2016	1009280000	99212	54.00	10/31/2016	0.00*	0.00*	Not Billed	0.00	54.00
								SubTotal:	79.00
								Unapplied Payments and Adjustments:	0.00
								Case Balance:	79.00
								Patient Reference Balance:	79.00
BROOKLA0	**Lawana Brooks (614)027-4242**								
Case 27	1: East Ohio PPO			(419)444-1505					
	2:								
	3:								
10/28/2016	1010290000	73600	96.00	10/31/2016	0.00*	0.00*	Not Billed	0.00	96.00
10/28/2016	1010290000	99212	54.00	10/31/2016	0.00*	0.00*	-20.00	0.00	34.00
								SubTotal:	130.00
								Unapplied Payments and Adjustments:	0.00
								Case Balance:	130.00
								Patient Reference Balance:	130.00
FITZWJO0	**John Fitzwilliams (614)002-1111**								
Case 7	1: ChampVA			(614)024-7000					
	2:								
	3:								
10/3/2016	1006230000	82270	19.00	Not Billed	0.00*	0.00*	Not Billed	0.00	19.00
10/3/2016	1006230000	99212	54.00	Not Billed	0.00*	0.00*	-15.00	0.00	39.00
								SubTotal:	58.00
								Unapplied Payments and Adjustments:	-50.00
								Case Balance:	8.00
								Patient Reference Balance:	58.00

Figure 12.17 Sample First Page of Billing/Payment Status Report

month or a year (see Figures 12.18a and 12.18b). The report can be used to generate medical practice financial statements. It can also be used for profit analysis. The summary at the end of the report breaks down the information into total charges, total payments and copayments, and total adjustments.

Family Care Clinic

Practice Analysis

Show all data where the Date From is between 9/1/2016, 9/30/2016

Code	Description	Amount	Units	Average	Cost	Net
02	Patient payment, check	-299.50	2	-149.75	0.00	-299.50
29540	Strapping, ankle	121.50	1	121.50	0.00	121.50
50390	Aspiration of renal cyst by needle	551.00	1	551.00	0.00	551.00
73510	Hip x-ray, complete, two views	124.00	1	124.00	0.00	124.00
84478	Triglycerides test	29.00	1	29.00	0.00	29.00
90471	Immunization administration	15.00	1	15.00	0.00	15.00
90703	Tetanus injection	29.00	1	29.00	0.00	29.00
92516	Facial nerve function studies	210.00	1	210.00	0.00	210.00
93000	Electrocardiogram--ECG with interpr	84.00	1	84.00	0.00	84.00
99070	Supplies and materials provided	20.00	1	20.00	0.00	20.00
99201	OF--new patient, minimal	66.00	1	66.00	0.00	66.00
99211	OF--established patient, minimal	144.00	4	36.00	0.00	144.00
99212	OF--established patient, low	324.00	6	54.00	0.00	324.00
99213	OF--established patient, detailed	216.00	3	72.00	0.00	216.00
99214	OF--established patient, moderate	105.00	1	105.00	0.00	105.00
99394	Preventive est., 12-17 years	222.00	1	222.00	0.00	222.00
AARPAY	AARP Payment	-19.57	3	-6.52	0.00	-19.57
BCBDED	BCBS Deductible	0.00	1	0.00	0.00	0.00
BCBPAY	BCBS Payment	-168.00	2	-84.00	0.00	-168.00
CHVCPAY	ChampVA Copayment	-30.00	2	-15.00	0.00	-30.00
EAPADJ	East Ohio PPO Adjustment	-12.60	2	-6.30	0.00	-12.60
EAPCPAY	East Ohio PPO Copayment	-160.00	8	-20.00	0.00	-160.00
EAPPAY	East Ohio PPO Payment	-73.40	2	-36.70	0.00	-73.40
MCDADJ	Medicaid Adjustment	-479.95	2	-239.97	0.00	-479.95
MCDCPAY	Medicaid Copayment	-10.00	1	-10.00	0.00	-10.00
MCDPAY	Medicaid Payment	-127.05	2	-63.52	0.00	-127.05
MEDADJ	Medicare Adjustment	-212.73	6	-35.46	0.00	-212.73
MEDPAY	Medicare Payment	-209.42	7	-29.92	0.00	-209.42
OHCADJ	OhioCare HMO Adjustment	-50.00	2	-25.00	0.00	-50.00
OHCCPAY	OhioCare HMO Copayment	-40.00	2	-20.00	0.00	-40.00

Figure 12.18a Page 1 of Practice Analysis Report

EXERCISE 12.2

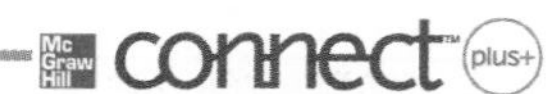

CREATING A PRACTICE ANALYSIS REPORT

Creating a practice analysis report for October 2016.

Date: October 31, 2016

1. Verify that Medisoft Network Professional is open and that the Medisoft Program Date is set to October 31, 2016.
2. On the Reports menu, click Analysis Reports and then Practice Analysis. The Print Report Where? dialog box appears.
3. Accept the default selection to preview the report on the screen. Click the Start button.
4. The Search dialog box is displayed. Leave the Code 1 fields blank.
5. Make sure the box to show all values for the Date Created field is checked.
6. Enter ***10/1/2016*** in the first Date From box, press Tab, and enter ***10/31/2016*** in the second. This will select data for the month of October 2016.
7. Click the OK button. The practice analysis report is displayed in the Print Preview window.

Family Care Clinic

Practice Analysis

Show all data where the Date From is between 9/1/2016, 9/30/2016

Code	Description	Amount	Units	Average	Cost	Net
		Total Procedure Charges				$2,260.50
		Total Global Surgical Procedures				$0.00
		Total Product Charges				$0.00
		Total Inside Lab Charges				$0.00
		Total Outside Lab Charges				$0.00
		Total Billing Charges				$0.00
		Total Insurance Payments				-$597.44
		Total Cash Copayments				$0.00
		Total Check Copayments				-$240.00
		Total Credit Card Copayments				$0.00
		Total Patient Cash Payments				$0.00
		Total Patient Check Payments				-$299.50
		Total Credit Card Payments				$0.00
		Total Debit Adjustments				$0.00
		Total Credit Adjustments				$0.00
		Total Insurance Debit Adjustments				$0.00
		Total Insurance Credit Adjustments				-$755.28
		Total Insurance Withholds				$0.00
		Net Effect on Accounts Receivable				$368.28
		Practice Totals				
		Total # Procedures				60
		Total Charges				$4,977.50
		Total Payments				-$2,558.64
		Total Adjustments				-$755.86
		Accounts Receivable				$1,712.72

Figure 12.18b Page 2 of Practice Analysis Report

8. Notice at the top of the Print Preview window that the triangle next to the number 1 is bright blue, indicating that there is more than one page in the report. Click the triangle just to the right of 1 to advance to the second page of the report.
9. Review the second page of the report. Notice that both triangle buttons to the right of the number 1 at the top of the Print Preview window are now dimmed. This indicates that you are viewing the last page of the report.
10. Click the red Close box at the top right of the window or the Close button on the Print Preview toolbar to exit the Print Preview window.

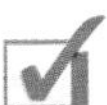 **You have completed Exercise 12.2**

Insurance Analysis

The insurance analysis report tracks charges, insurance payments received during a specified period, and copayments applied to accounts that include those procedures. It is usually printed at the end of the month. The amount listed as the outstanding balance displays the total charges, subtracting the full amount of the charge if the insurance payment was made.

Referring Provider Report

The referring provider report enables a practice to determine the origins of revenue derived from providers who have referred patients to the practice. The report lists the percentage of total income that was generated by referring providers.

Referral Source Report

The referral source report tracks the source of referrals that are not from other medical offices or providers, such as referrals from established patients.

Facility Report

The facility report tracks the revenue coming in from patients who are treated at different facilities. For the facility report to work properly, facilities must be set up using the Facilities option on the Lists menu. Then the appropriate facility must be entered in the Account tab for each patient's case. The filters include a case facility range and a date from range.

Unapplied Payment/Adjustment Report

The unapplied payment/adjustment report lists payments or adjustments that have not been fully applied. Information about the payment or adjustment includes the case, document number, posting date, code, code description, transaction amount, and unapplied amount.

Unapplied Deposit Report

The unapplied deposit report lists deposits that have unapplied amounts. The report includes the date, code, payer name, payer type, deposit amount, and unapplied amount.

Co-Payment Report

This report lists patients who have copayment transactions. It shows the amount paid, how much was applied, and how much, if any, was left unapplied.

Outstanding Co-Payment Report

This report shows patients who have outstanding copayment transactions. The report shows the copayment amount expected, the actual amount paid, and the amount due.

THINKING IT THROUGH 12.4

What is the importance of the referring provider report?

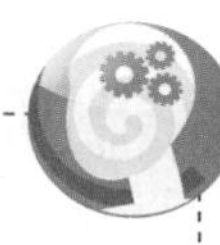

12.5 Production Reports

Production reports are standard reports that provide incoming revenue information for various aspects of the practice. Figure 12.19 shows the Production Reports submenu on the Medisoft Reports menu. There are three regular production reports and three summary production reports.

Production by Provider Report

The **production by provider report** lists incoming revenue information for each provider in the practice (see Figure 12.20). Charges are listed chronologically by date of service and include the chart number, procedure code, charge amount, and allowed amount. For each charge listed, the report shows the expected payments and adjustments—from the insurance carriers and the guarantor—and the actual payments and adjustments that were applied to the charge. The report displays information for one provider or a range of providers. Each provider's data are printed on a separate page.

production by provider report a report that lists incoming revenue information for each provider in the practice

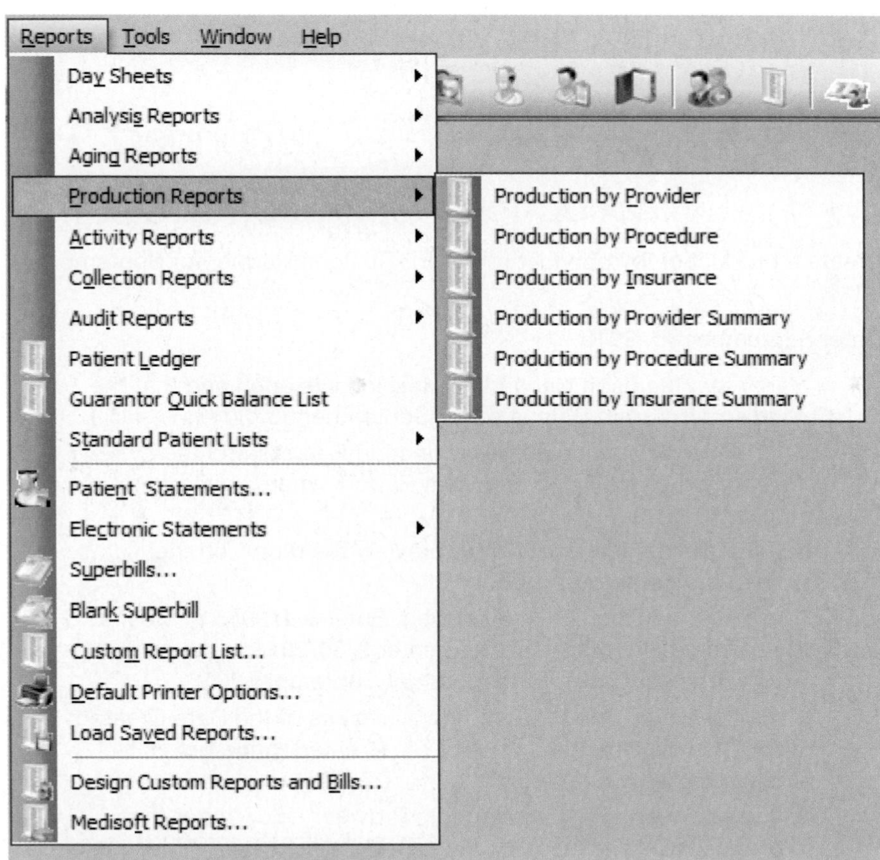

Figure 12.19 The Production Reports Submenu

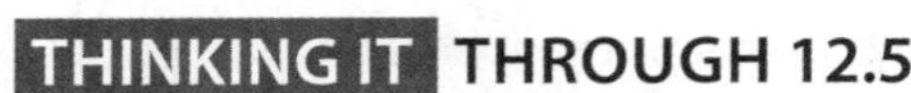

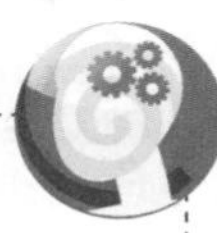

THINKING IT THROUGH 12.5

What do production reports allow the practice to predict?

Family Care Clinic

Production by Provider

Show all data where the Date From is between 9/1/2016, 9/30/2016

Provider: 1 - Yan, Katherine

				Primary Insurance				Secondary Insurance		Tertiary Insurance		Guarantor	
	Procedure Code	Charge Amount	Allowed Amount	Expected Payment	Actual Payment	Expected Adjustment	Actual Adjustment	Expected Payment	Actual Payment	Expected Payment	Actual Payment	Expected Payment	Actual Payment
Date of Service: 9/6/2016													
FITZWSA0	90703	29.00	14.30	0.00	-14.30	-14.70	-14.70	0.00	0.00	0.00	0.00	-14.30	0.00
FITZWSA0	90471	15.00	15.00	0.00	0.00	0.00	0.00	0.00	0.00	0.00	0.00	-15.00	-15.00
GARDIJO0	99211	36.00	36.00	0.00	0.00	0.00	-16.00	0.00	0.00	0.00	0.00	-36.00	-20.00
	Totals:	80.00	65.30	0.00	-14.30	-14.70	-30.70	0.00	0.00	0.00	0.00	-65.30	-35.00
Date of Service: 9/7/2016													
RAMOSMA0	99213	72.00	64.80	0.00	-44.80	-7.20	-7.20	0.00	0.00	0.00	0.00	-64.80	-20.00
	Totals:	72.00	64.80	0.00	-44.80	-7.20	-7.20	0.00	0.00	0.00	0.00	-64.80	-20.00
Date of Service: 9/9/2016													
WONGJO10	99212	54.00	37.36	0.00	-29.89	-16.64	-16.64	0.00	0.00	0.00	0.00	-37.36	0.00
WONGLIY0	99211	36.00	20.68	0.00	-16.54	-15.32	-15.32	0.00	0.00	0.00	0.00	-20.68	0.00
	Totals:	90.00	58.04	0.00	-46.43	-31.96	-31.96	0.00	0.00	0.00	0.00	-58.04	0.00
Date of Service: 9/20/2016													
JONESEL0	93000	84.00	25.72	0.00	-20.58	-58.28	-58.28	0.00	0.00	0.00	0.00	-25.72	0.00
JONESEL0	99214	105.00	80.15	0.00	-64.12	-24.85	-24.85	0.00	0.00	0.00	0.00	-80.15	0.00
	Totals:	189.00	105.87	0.00	-84.70	-83.13	-83.13	0.00	0.00	0.00	0.00	-105.87	0.00
Provider Totals:		431.00	294.01	0.00	-190.23	-136.99	-152.99	0.00	0.00	0.00	0.00	-294.01	-55.00

Figure 12.20 Production by Provider Report

EXERCISE 12.3

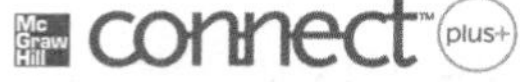

CREATING A PRODUCTION BY PROVIDER REPORT

Create a production by provider report for Dr. John Rudner for September 2016.

Date: September 30, 2016

1. Verify that Medisoft Network Professional is open and that the Medisoft Program Date is set to September 30, 2016.
2. On the Reports menu, click Production Reports and then Production by Provider. The Print Report Where? dialog box appears.
3. Accept the default selection to preview the report on the screen. Click the Start button.
4. The Search dialog box is displayed. Enter ***9/1/2016*** in the first Date From field, press Tab, and enter **9/30/2016** in the second. This will select data for the month of September 2016.
5. Click the check box for the Show all values of the Date Created field. This will clear the current Date Created range boxes to include all dates for this field.
6. In the selection area for Attending Provider field, rather than select all values of the Attending Provider field, you will use the Lookup button to select a single attending provider. Click in the Show all values of the Attending Provider field box to remove

the check mark. Then click the Lookup button that is located to the right of the first Attending Provider selection box.

7. The Lookup dialog box appears with a list of providers. Click the line with Dr. John Rudner's information to select it, and then click the OK button at the lower-right corner of the dialog box.
8. The provider code for Dr. John Rudner—2—is displayed in the first Attending Provider field. Press Tab to move to the second Attending Provider field and key **2** to select the same provider. This will select production data for Dr. Rudner only.
9. Leave all other fields in the Search box blank. Click the OK button.
10. The production by provider report is displayed in the Print Preview window.
11. Notice that the triangle buttons on either side of the number 1 at the top of the Print Preview window are dimmed. This indicates that the report has only one page, since it is for only one provider.
12. After viewing the report, click the Close button on the Print Preview toolbar to exit the Print Preview window.

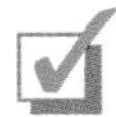 **You have completed Exercise 12.3**

Production by Procedure Report

The production by procedure report lists incoming revenue information for each procedure code in the practice's database. For each charge listed in the report, the expected payments and adjustments from the primary insurance carrier are shown side by side with the actual payments and adjustments that were applied to the charge. Data for each code are displayed on a separate page.

Production by Insurance Report

The production by insurance report lists incoming revenue information for each insurance carrier in the practice's database. As with the other two production reports, the Production by Insurance report compares expected payments and adjustments with actual payments and adjustments. Each insurance carrier's data are listed on a separate page.

Production Summary Reports

The three summary reports that follow in the Production Reports submenu—Production Summary by Provider, Production Summary by Procedure, and Production Summary by Insurance—are based on the same information as the Production by Provider, Production by Procedure, and Production by Insurance reports, respectively. As seen in the Production by Provider report in Figure 12.20, regular production reports contain many details. The summary reports display only a summary of those details.

12.6 Patient Ledger Reports

patient ledger a report that lists the financial activity in each patient's account

A **patient ledger** lists the transaction details of a patient's account, including charges, payments, and adjustments (see Figures 12-21a and 12-21b). Like day sheets, analysis reports, and production

Family Care Clinic

Patient Account Ledger

As of October 31, 2016

Show all data where the Date From is between 1/1/1980, 10/31/2016

Entry	Date	POS	Description	Procedure	Document	Provider	Amount
ARLENSU0	**Susan Arlen**			(614)315-2233			
	Last Payment: -28.60		On: 10/3/2016				
359	09/05/2016	11		99212	1009060000	5	54.00
361	09/05/2016	11		EAPCPAY	1009060000	5	-20.00
643	10/03/2016		East Ohio PPO	EAPPAY	1009060000	5	-28.60
644	10/03/2016		Adjustment	EAPADJ	1009060000	5	-5.40
						Patient Total:	0.00
BARREJO0	**Jorge Barrett**			(614)509-3637			
	Last Payment: -96.00		On: 11/3/2016				
634	10/21/2016	11		G8443	1610210000	4	0.00
635	10/21/2016	11		99203	1610210000	4	120.00
						Patient Total:	120.00
BATTIAN0	**Anthony Battistuta**			(614)500-3619			
	Last Payment: 0.00		On:				
425	10/27/2016	11		99212	1009280000	4	54.00
426	10/27/2016	11		82947	1009280000	4	25.00
						Patient Total:	79.00
BELLHER0	**Herbert Bell**			(614)030-1111			
	Last Payment: -12.40		On: 10/3/2016				
364	09/05/2016	11		EAPCPAY	1009060000	2	-20.00
362	09/05/2016	11		99211	1009060000	2	36.00
645	10/03/2016		East Ohio PPO	EAPPAY	1009060000	2	-12.40
646	10/03/2016		Adjustment	EAPADJ	1009060000	2	-3.60
						Patient Total:	0.00
BELLJAN0	**Janine Bell**			(614)030-1111			
	Last Payment: -156.40		On: 10/3/2016				
368	09/05/2016	11		EAPCPAY	1009060000	3	-20.00
365	09/05/2016	11		99213	1009060000	3	72.00
366	09/05/2016	11		73510	1009060000	3	124.00
649	10/03/2016		East Ohio PPO	EAPPAY	1009060000	3	-44.80
650	10/03/2016		Adjustment	EAPADJ	1009060000	3	-7.20
651	10/03/2016		East Ohio PPO	EAPPAY	1009060000	3	-111.60
652	10/03/2016		Adjustment	EAPADJ	1009060000	3	-12.40
						Patient Total:	0.00
BELLJON0	**Jonathan Bell**			(614)030-1111			
	Last Payment: -179.80		On: 10/3/2016				
371	09/05/2016	11		EAPCPAY	1009060000	3	-20.00
369	09/05/2016	11		99394	1009060000	3	222.00
653	10/03/2016		East Ohio PPO	EAPPAY	1009060000	3	-179.80
654	10/03/2016		Adjustment	EAPADJ	1009060000	3	-22.20
						Patient Total:	0.00

Figure 12.21a First Page of Patient Account Ledger Report

Family Care Clinic
Patient Account Ledger
As of October 31, 2016
Show all data where the Date From is between 1/1/1980, 10/31/2016

Entry	Date	POS	Description	Procedure	Document	Provider	Amount
ZAPATKRO	**Kristin Zapata**			(614)033-0044			
		Last Payment: -247.50	On: 9/21/2016				
580	08/28/2016	11		99385	0803270000	1	247.50
583	09/10/2016		Carrier 1 Deductible -$247.50	BCBDED	0803270000	1	0.00
582	09/20/2016		#456789 Blue Cross/Blue Shield	BCBPAY	0803270000	1	0.00
584	09/21/2016	11		02	0807010000	1	-247.50
665	10/03/2016	11		NSFFEE	1610030000	1	35.00
666	10/03/2016	11	Returned Check	NSF	1610030000	1	247.50
					Patient Total:		282.50
					Ledger Total:		$2,154.12

Figure 12.21b Last Page of Patient Account Ledger Report

reports, the patient ledger report is one of the standard reports in MNP. The information it provides is especially useful when there is a question about a patient's account.

The patient account ledger report is created by clicking Patient Ledger on the Reports menu. The Print Report Where? dialog box is displayed. After the preview, print, or export selection is made, the Search dialog box is displayed, as it is with the other reports. It provides options to select by chart numbers, patient reference balances, dates, attending providers, billing codes, and patient indicators. A patient account ledger is generated only for data that meet the selection criteria.

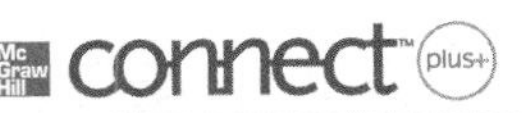

EXERCISE 12.4

CREATING A PATIENT ACCOUNT LEDGER

Create a patient account ledger for October 2016 for patients whose last names begin with the letters *R* through *Z*.

Date: October 31, 2016

1. Verify that Medisoft Network Professional is open and that the Medisoft Program Date is set to October 31, 2016.
2. On the Reports menu, click Patient Ledger. The Print Report Where? dialog box is displayed.
3. Accept the default selection to preview the report on the screen. Click the Start button.
4. The Search dialog box is displayed. In the selection area for Chart Number, rather than select all values of the Chart Number field, you will use the Lookup button to select a range of chart numbers. Click in the Show all values of the Chart Number field box to remove the check mark. Then click the Lookup button that is located to the right of the first Chart Number selection box.

(continued)

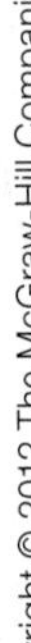

(Continued)

5. In the Search Characters field in the Lookup dialog box, key ***R***. Notice that the program moves to RAMOSMA0, the first chart number that begins with the letter *R*. Click the OK button at the lower-right corner of the dialog box to accept the chart number selection.
6. The Lookup box disappears, and you are returned to the Search dialog box. Notice that the chart number for the patient you selected in the Lookup box is now in the first Chart Number selection field.
7. Click the Lookup button in the second Chart Number selection field. The Lookup box appears. Key ***Z*** in the Search Characters box. The chart for Kristin Zapata is selected. Click the OK button to accept the selection.
8. The chart number for the second patient you selected is now in the second Chart Number selection field.
9. Now you need to enter the dates. Click the first Date From field, and enter ***10/1/2016***.
10. Click the second Date From field, and enter ***10/31/2016***. Click the OK button.
11. The report is displayed in the Print Preview window. Notice in the Print Preview toolbar at the top of the screen that the triangle buttons on either side of the number 1 are dimmed, indicating that the report has only one page. Scroll to the end of the page to see the ledger total.
12. After reviewing the report, click the appropriate button to exit the Print Preview window.

You have completed Exercise 12.4

12.7 Standard Patient Lists

Medisoft Network Professional includes several convenient reports for identifying patients by diagnosis or insurance carrier. These reports are accessed via the Standard Patient Lists submenu on the Reports menu (see Figure 12.22).

The Patient by Diagnosis report lists diagnosis code, chart number, patient name, age, attending provider, facility, and date of last visit. The Patient by Insurance Carrier report lists patients sorted by provider or facility, and then by their insurance carrier.

EXERCISE 12.5

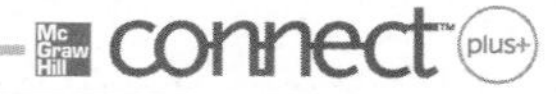

CREATING A PATIENT BY INSURANCE CARRIER LIST

Create a Patient by Insurance Carrier list for all patients in the practice.

Date: October 31, 2016

1. Verify that Medisoft Network Professional is open and that the Medisoft Program Date is still set to October 31, 2016.

2. On the Reports menu, click Standard Patient Lists, and then Patient by Insurance Carrier. The Print Report Where? dialog box is displayed.
3. Accept the default selection to preview the report on the screen. Click the Start button.
4. Accept the Show all values of the Code field entry in the Search box. Click the OK button.
5. The report, called Patient Census by Carrier (Primary), is displayed in the Print Preview window.
6. Let your cursor hover over the second triangle button to the right of the number 1 on the toolbar until the name of the button (Last Page) is displayed. Click the Last Page button to view the last page of the report.
7. Then click the first triangle button on the toolbar (the First Page button) to return to the first page of the report.
8. When finished viewing the report, exit the Print Preview window.

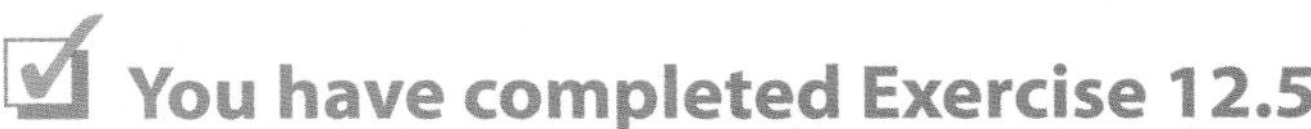

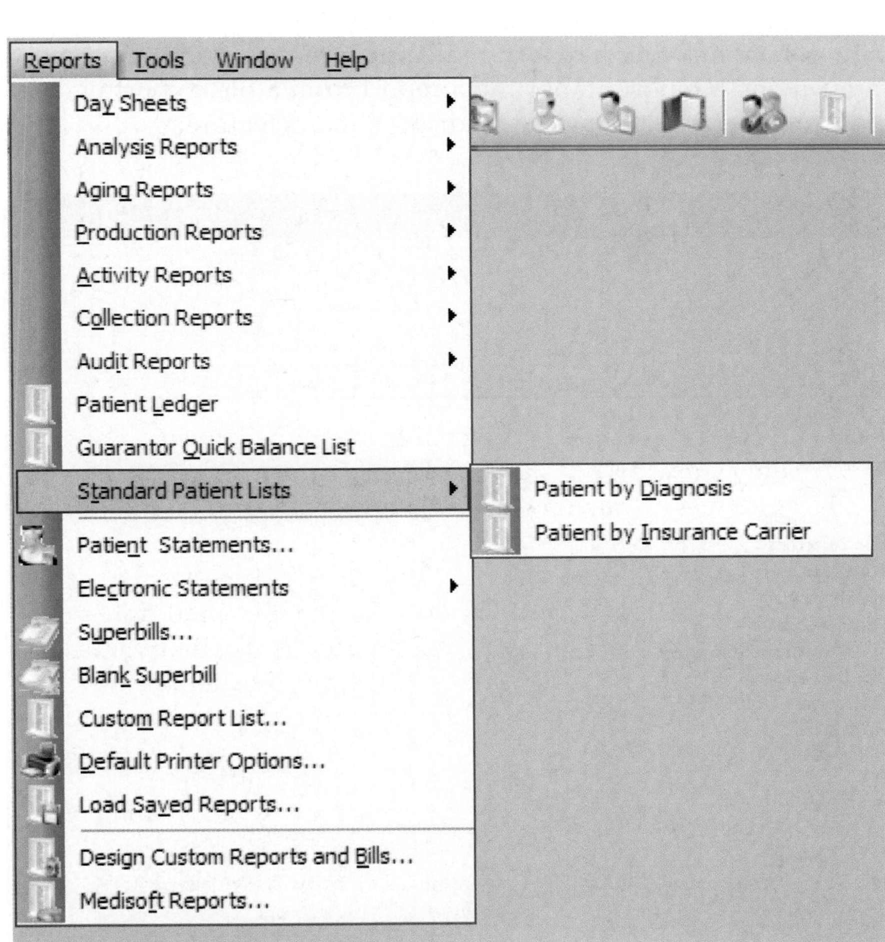

Figure 12.22 Reports Menu with Standard Patient Lists Submenu Displayed

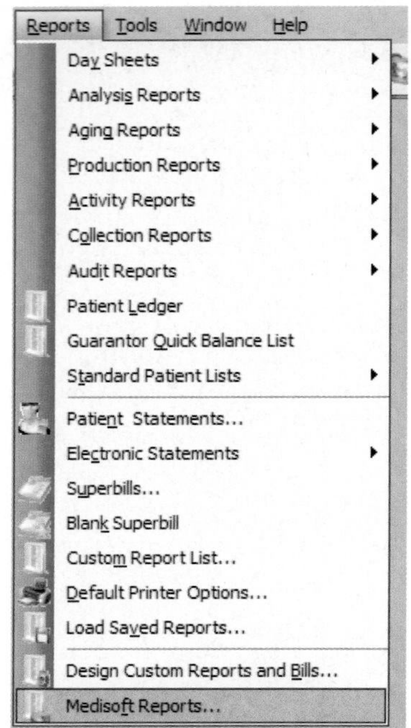

Figure 12.23 The Medisoft Reports Option on the Reports Menu

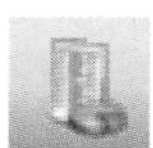

Figure 12.24 The Medisoft Reports Shortcut Button

12.8 Navigating in Medisoft Reports

The Medisoft Reports feature is new in Version 16. It does not replace existing reports, but instead provides access to over a hundred reports. To start the Medisoft Reports feature, select Medisoft Reports on the Reports menu (see Figure 12.23), or click the shortcut button on the toolbar (see Figure 12.24).

The Medisoft Reports application window features its own main window that contains menu items and a toolbar with shortcut buttons (see Figure 12.25).

The window is divided into two sections: an All Folders area and a Contents of All Folders area. The All Folders section displays the reports directory and the subfolders in the directory. The Contents of All Folders section lists the individual reports included in the folder that is selected in the All Folders list. In Figure 12.26, the Aging Power Pack folder is selected in All Folders, and the reports within the Aging Power Pack folder are listed in Contents of All Folders.

Above the All Folders and Contents of All Folders area, the Medisoft Reports window has its own menu bar, toolbar, and search area.

The Medisoft Reports Menus

The Medisoft Reports menus include File, View, and Help. The File menu, displayed in Figure 12.27, contains commands for creating a new folder, deleting a report, renaming a report, printing a report, previewing a report, importing a report from a file, exporting a report to a file, and closing the Medisoft Reports feature.

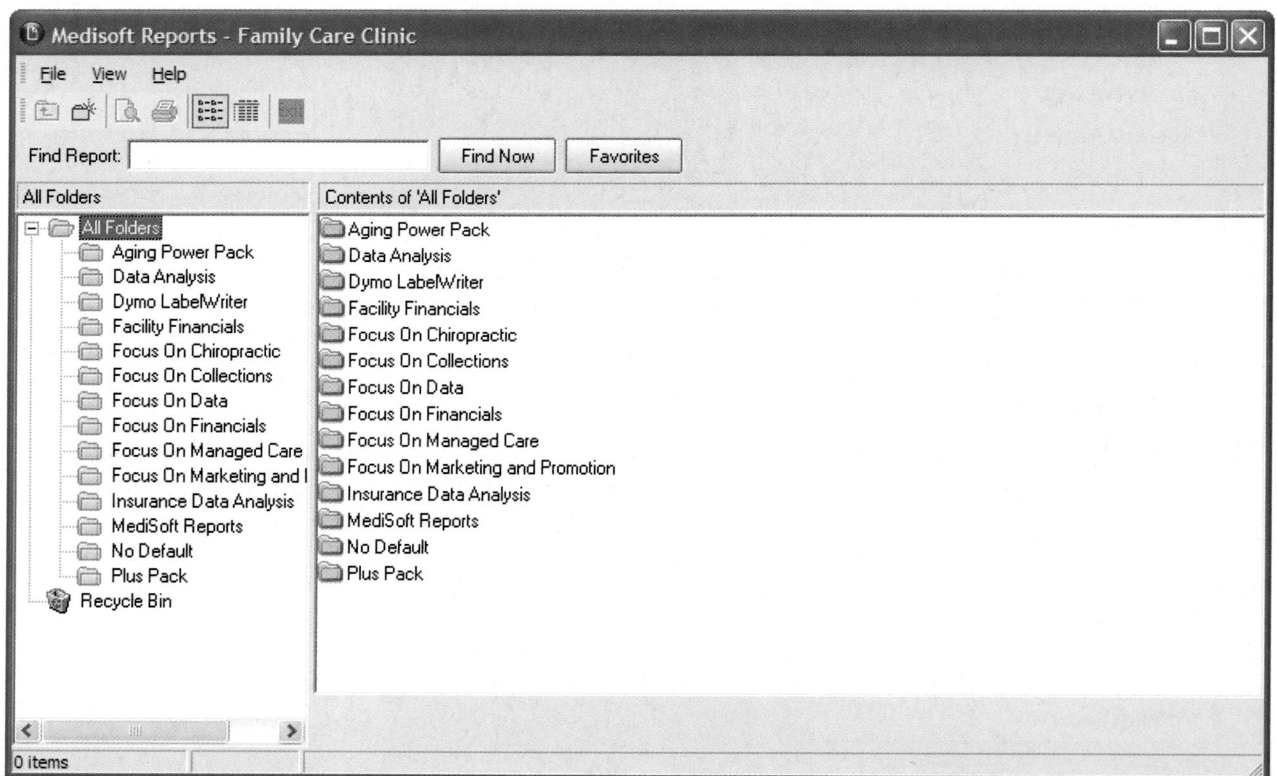

Figure 12.25 The Medisoft Reports Window

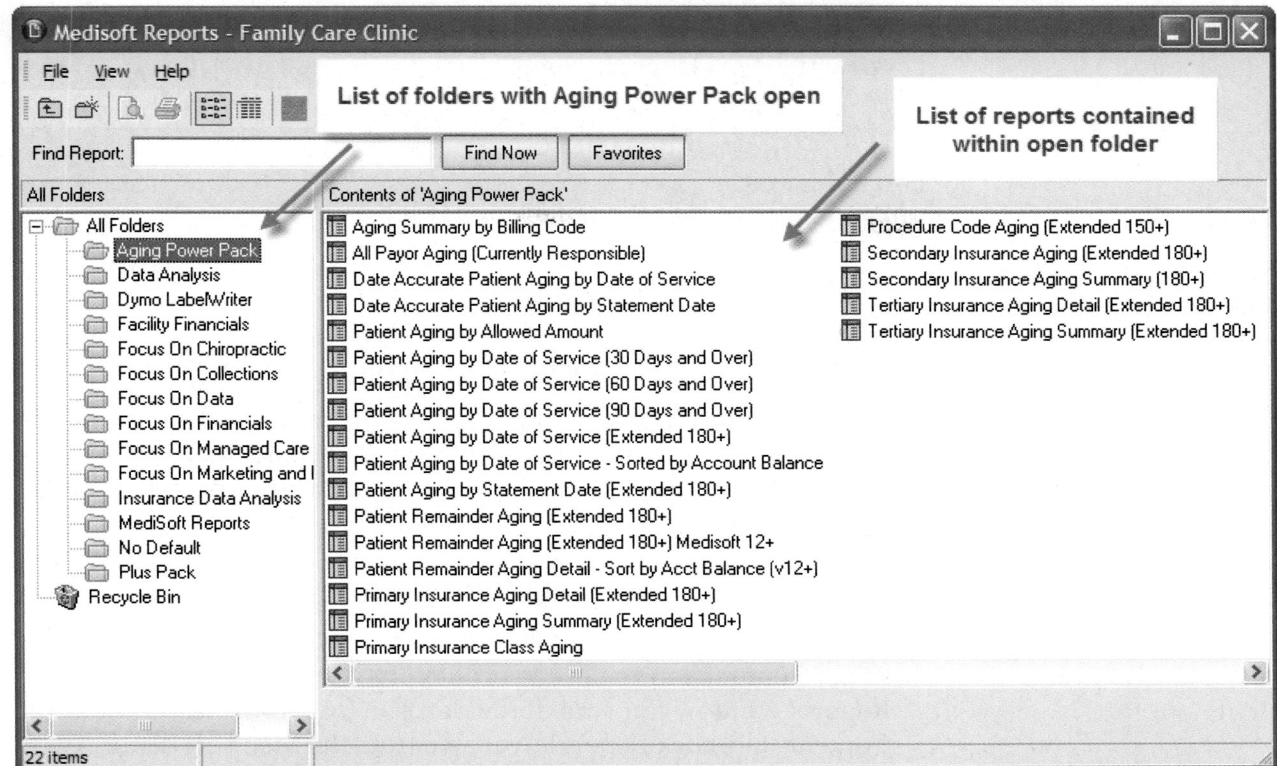

Figure 12.26 The Medisoft Reports Window with the Aging Power Pack Folder Selected

Commands on the View menu include options for displaying the toolbar and status bar, and whether to display the Contents of All Folders list of reports in List view or in Detail view (see Figure 12.28).

The Help menu contains entries for viewing help contents, navigating to Medisoft's website, viewing Medisoft Reports file location and path, and displaying the version of Medisoft Reports you are using. The Help menu is pictured in Figure 12.29.

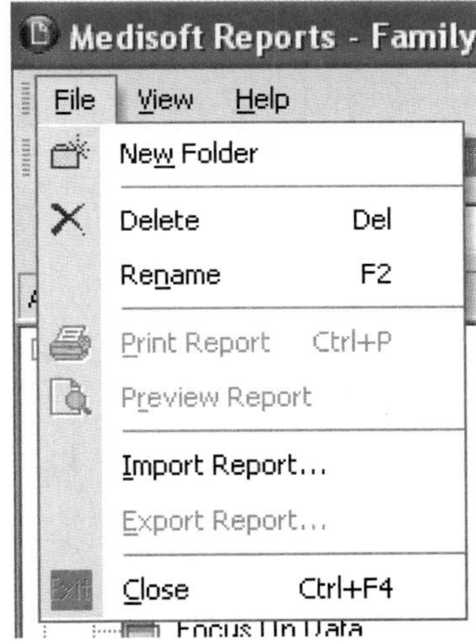

Figure 12.27 The Medisoft Reports File Menu

The Medisoft Reports Toolbar

Below the menu bar is a toolbar featuring shortcut buttons (see Figure 12.30). From left to right, these buttons are used for:

- Moving up a folder level
- Creating a new folder
- Previewing a report
- Printing a report

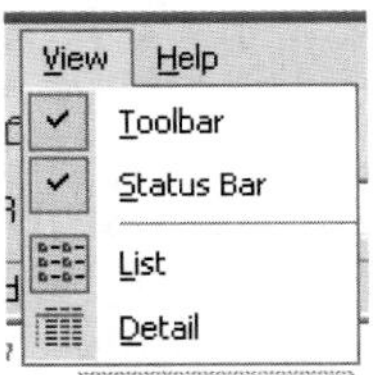

Figure 12.28 The Medisoft Reports View Menu

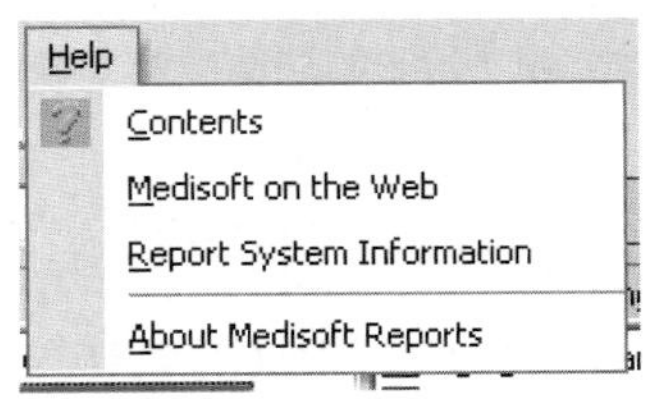

Figure 12.29 The Medisoft Reports Help Menu

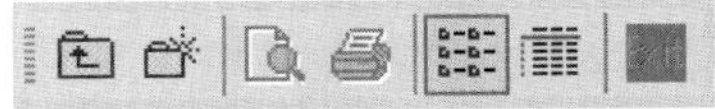

Figure 12.30 The Medisoft Reports Toolbar

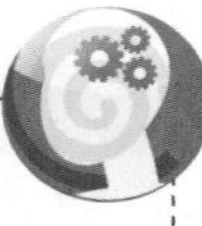

THINKING IT THROUGH 12.6

Some of the reports listed on the Reports menu can also be created using the Medisoft Reports feature. What advantages does the Reports menu offer? What advantages does the Medisoft Reports feature offer?

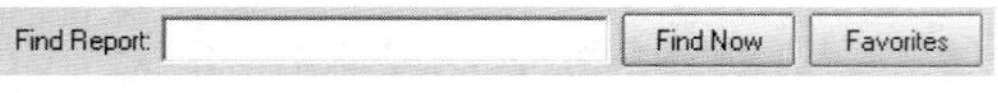

Figure 12.31 The Medisoft Reports Find Report Box

- Displaying reports in a list
- Displaying report details
- Exiting the application

The Medisoft Reports Find Box

Below the toolbar are the Find Report box and the Find Now button, which are used for searching for specific reports, and the Favorites button, which displays reports marked as favorites (see Figure 12.31).

The Medisoft Reports Help Feature

To view descriptions of all the reports available in Medisoft Reports, select Contents on the Medisoft Reports Help menu. The Medisoft Reports window appears. In the left side of the window, under the Contents tab, click Reports Available from the Medisoft Reports window (see Figure 12.32). Scroll down the window for a full listing of the reports and their descriptions.

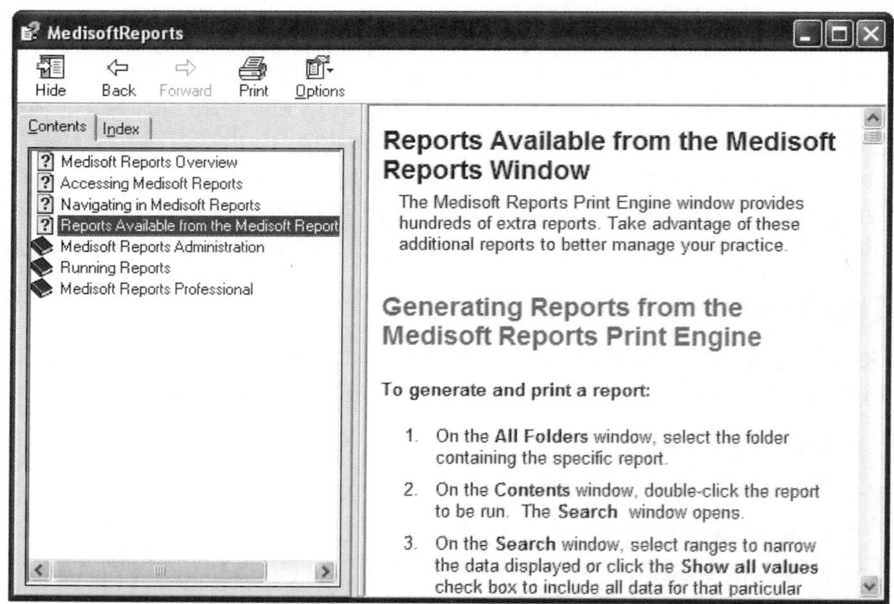

Figure 12.32 Contents of the Medisoft Reports Help File with Reports Available from the Medisoft Reports Window Selected

12.9 Aging Reports

aging report a report that lists the amount of money owed to the practice, organized by the amount of time the money has been owed

Aging reports are of particular importance to medical billing specialists. An **aging report** lists the amount of money owed to the practice, organized by the amount of time the money has been owed. Medical practices use aging reports to determine which accounts require follow-up to collect past-due balances. A **patient aging report** lists a patient's balance by age, date and amount of the last payment, and telephone number.

patient aging report a report that lists a patient's balance by age, date and amount of the last payment, and telephone number

insurance aging report a report that lists how long a payer has taken to respond to insurance claims

An **insurance aging report** shows how long a payer has taken to respond to each claim. This information is used to compare the response time with the terms of the practice's contract with the payer. For example, a practice may discover that a payer is routinely responding to claims ten days later than the claim turnaround time specified in the contract. In that case, the practice manager might review the situation with the payer's customer service manager and ask the payer to adhere to its guidelines.

Standard aging reports are contained on the Reports menu under the Aging Reports submenu. Additional aging reports are also contained in the Medisoft Reports feature. Refer back to Figure 12.26 to see the list of aging reports available in the Aging Power Pack folder of the Medisoft Reports feature. The exercise that follows provides practice in creating an aging report using the Medisoft Reports feature.

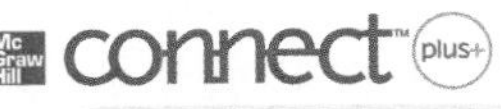

EXERCISE 12.6

CREATING A PATIENT AGING REPORT

Create a patient aging report for the period ending September 30, 2016, using the Medisoft Reports feature.

Date: September 30, 2016

1. Verify that Medisoft Network Professional is open and that the Medisoft Program Date is set to September 30, 2016.
2. On the Reports menu, click Medisoft Reports. The Medisoft Reports window is displayed.
3. In the All Folders list on the left side of the window, double click the Aging Power Pack folder to display its contents. The contents are listed in the area of the window to the right of the All Folders column.
4. Locate the Date Accurate Patient Aging by Date of Service report, and double click it. A Search box appears.
5. In the Charges/Payments/Adj box, enter ***9/30/2016***, if it is not already displayed. Then click OK.
6. The patient aging by date of service report is displayed in the Print Preview window. After viewing the report, click the Close button to close the window.
7. You are returned to the Medisoft Reports window.
8. Select Close on the File menu, or click the red Close box, to close the Medisoft Reports window and return to the main MNP window.

 **You have completed Exercise 12.6**

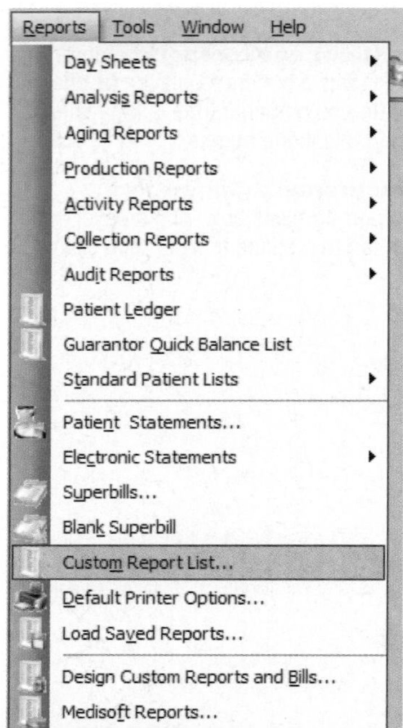

Figure 12.33 Custom Report List Option on the Reports Menu

12.10 Custom Reports

In addition to its standard reports on the Reports menu and the reports in the Medisoft Report feature, MNP has a number of built-in custom reports, including:

- Lists of addresses, billing codes, EDI receivers, patients, patient recalls, procedure codes, providers, and referring providers
- The CMS-1500 and Medicare CMS-1500 forms in a variety of printer formats
- Patient statements and walkout receipts
- Superbills (encounter forms)

The built-in custom reports, which were created in MNP using the Report Designer, are accessed via the Custom Report List option on the Reports menu (see Figure 12.33). When Custom Report List is clicked on the Reports menu, the Open Report dialog box is displayed (see Figure 12.34). When a new custom report is created, it is added to the list of custom reports displayed on the screen.

Listed under the heading Show Report Style, the Open Report dialog box contains eleven radio buttons that are used to control the list of reports displayed in the dialog box. When the All radio button is clicked, all types of custom reports are listed in the dialog box. When one of the other radio buttons is clicked, only reports of that style are listed. For example, if the Insurance Form radio button is clicked, only reports that are insurance forms are listed.

To print a custom report, highlight the title of the report by clicking it, and then click the OK button. The same options that are available with standard reports for previewing the report on the screen, sending it directly to the printer, or exporting it to a file are available with reports created through the Custom Report List option.

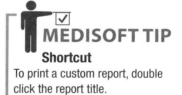

Shortcut

To print a custom report, double click the report title.

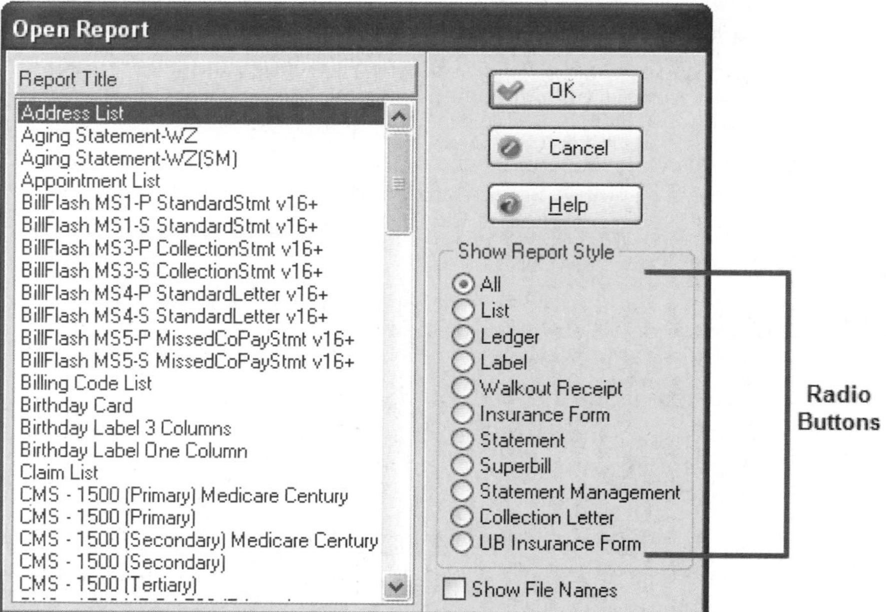

Figure 12.34 Open Report Dialog Box

EXERCISE 12.7

CREATING A LIST OF PATIENTS

Create a list of all patients.

Date: October 31, 2016

1. Verify that Medisoft Network Professional is open and that the Medisoft Program Date is set to October 31, 2016.
2. On the Reports menu, click Custom Report List.
3. In the Show Report Style panel on the right side of the dialog box, click the List radio button. Only list reports are displayed in the Open Report dialog box.
4. Select the Patient List report, and click the OK button.
5. Accept the option to preview the report on the screen. Click the Start button.
6. The Data Selection Questions dialog box appears. (*Note:* The Data Selection Questions dialog box that appears when creating custom reports serves the same purpose as the Search dialog box when creating standard reports.)
7. Leave the Chart Number Range boxes blank to select all patients. Click the OK button.
8. The patient list for the Family Care Clinic is displayed in the Preview Report window.
9. The buttons that appear in the preview window for custom reports are slightly different from those that appear for standard reports. Notice that the toolbar lists the number of pages in the report. In this case, you are viewing page 1 of 1.
10. The first three buttons on the toolbar are used to control the size of the report in the Preview Report window. Click the middle button, labeled "Zoom to 100%."
11. The report is now displayed at 100 percent. The other two buttons are labeled "Zoom to fit full page," and "Zoom to width of page." (When viewing standard reports, an actual percentage can be keyed in a percentage box on the toolbar.)
12. After viewing the report, exit the Preview Report window.

 **You have completed Exercise 12.7**

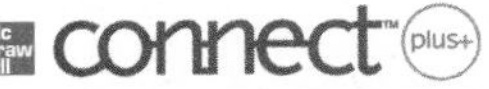

EXERCISE 12.8

CREATING A LIST OF PROCEDURE CODES

Create a list of all procedure codes in the database.

Date: October 31, 2016

1. On the Reports menu, click Custom Report List.
2. In the Show Report Style panel of the dialog box, click the List radio button.

(continued)

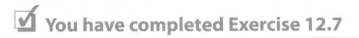

(Continued)

3. Select Procedure Code List. Click the OK button.
4. Accept the option to preview the report on the screen. Click the Start button.
5. In the Data Selection Questions dialog box, leave the Code 1 Range boxes blank to select all procedure codes. Click the OK button.
6. The procedure code list for Family Care Clinic is displayed in the Preview Report window.
7. Click the middle zoom button to display the report at 100 percent.
8. Use the triangle button to view page 2 and page 3.
9. When finished viewing the report, exit the Preview Report window.

You have completed Exercise 12.8

12.11 Using Report Designer

Medisoft Network Professional comes with a built-in program, called the Medisoft Report Designer, that allows users to modify existing reports or create new reports to add to the custom report list. The

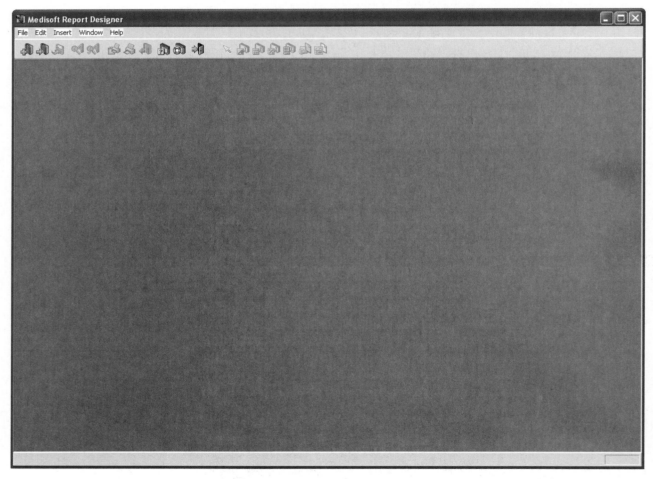

Figure 12.35 The Medisoft Report Designer Window

program provides maximum flexibility and control over data in the report and over how the data are displayed. Formatting styles include list, ledger, statement, and insurance. A report can be created from scratch, or an existing report can be used as a starting point. Although the details of how to create new custom reports with the Report Designer are beyond the coverage of this text/workbook, Exercise 12.9 offers practice using the Report Designer to modify an existing report.

The Report Designer is accessed by clicking Design Custom Reports and Bills on the Reports menu. This action displays the Medisoft Report Designer window (see Figure 12.35).

connect plus+

EXERCISE 12.9

MODIFYING A REPORT

Using the Medisoft Report Designer, modify the Patient List report so that a work telephone number replaces a home telephone number in the report.

Date: October 31, 2016

1. Verify that Medisoft Network Professional is open and that the Medisoft Program Date is set to October 31, 2016.
2. On the Reports menu, click Design Custom Reports and Bills. The Report Designer window is displayed.
3. Click Open Report on the File menu. The Open Report dialog box is displayed. Click the List radio button to display list reports only.
4. Double click Patient List in the list. The Patient List report is displayed in the Medisoft Report Designer window.
5. Double click Phone, which appears on the right between the two horizontal black lines near the top of the report, to select it.
6. Then, double click Phone again to edit it. The Text Properties dialog box is displayed. Change the entry in the Text box to "Work Phone" as follows. Click inside the Text box to activate it. Position the cursor in front of the word "Phone," and key ***Work***, so that the Text box reads "Work Phone."
7. In the Size panel of the Text Properties dialog box, be sure that the Auto Size button is checked, so the program will automatically resize the text box to accommodate the longer title.
8. Click the OK button. Work Phone is displayed in the band where Phone used to be.
9. In the green band below the band in which Work Phone appears, click the Phone 1 box to select it. Then double click the Phone 1 box again to edit its contents. The Data Field Properties dialog box is displayed.
10. The current data box, Print Patient.Phone 1, is active in the Data Field and Expressions box. Click the Edit button to change this box. The Select Data Field dialog box is displayed.
11. In the Fields column, scroll down, highlight Work Phone, and click OK. The Data Field and Expressions box now lists Print Patient. Work Phone.
12. In the Size panel, be sure the Auto Size box is checked, and click the OK button. Work Phone is displayed where Phone 1 used to be.

(continued)

(Continued)

13. On the Report Designer File menu, click Preview Report to save the file as a new report and see how the report will look when printed. The Save Report As... dialog box is displayed.
14. Press the Backspace key on your keyboard to delete the current report title (Untitled), and then key ***Patient List--Work.*** Click the OK button. The Data Selection Questions dialog box is displayed.
15. Leave the Chart Number Range boxes blank to select all patients for the report.
16. Click the OK button.
17. The Preview Report dialog box is displayed, showing the report. Notice that the last column displays a work phone number, rather than a home phone number.
18. Exit the Preview Report window.
19. Click Close on the Report Designer File menu, or click the Close button in the upper-right corner of the dialog box, to close the report file.
20. Click Exit on the Report Designer File menu, or click the Exit button on the toolbar, to leave Medisoft Report Designer.
21. You are returned to the main Medisoft Network Professional window. Select Custom Report List on the Reports menu.
22. Click the List radio button. Confirm that Patient List—Work appears in the list of custom reports.
23. Click Cancel to close the Open Report dialog box.

 **You have completed Exercise 12.9**

12.12 Preparing Clinical Reports

PM/EHRs have the potential to substantially improve the delivery of health care. For this reason, the federal government and private payers have established a number of financial incentives to guide PM/EHR implementation. For example, the CMS program called Physician Quality Reporting Initiative (PQRI), as explained in Chapter 1, gives bonuses to physicians who report to the Medicare program about their use of recognized ongoing performance measurements that underpin treatment plans for certain conditions. Likewise, more than half of commercial plans have some type of pay-for-performance programs.

Similarly, as summarized in Table 1.2, the HITECH Act requires providers to show that they are going to change the way they practice by using health information technology to improve outcomes and quality and by using EHRs in ways that accomplish the following basic goals:

- Improving quality, safety, and efficiency, while reducing disparities in the care patients receive
- Engaging patients and families in their health care

- Improving care coordination
- Ensuring adequate privacy and security protections for personal health information
- Improving population and public health

Medisoft Network Professional's reports can be used to capture the required items for performance measure reporting and for meaningful use. Using the PM/EHR saves countless hours of time and energy by automating the process of sorting through hundreds of records, searching for specific results, and generating lists and reminders for follow-up.

Performance Measure Reporting

Performance measure reporting is based on tracking the quality of care by coding certain services and test results that support nationally established **performance measures.** These performance measures are based on objective evidence of their contribution to quality patient care. Each practice's results can be compared to national standards and to the results of other practices. Common areas include the management of diabetes, cardiovascular disease, cancer screening, immunizations, infectious disease, mental health, substance abuse, and obesity. Procedure coding is based on CPT codes in the Category II section and on G codes from the PQRI section of the HCPCS code set. The Category II and G codes are supplemental tracking codes that describe clinical components that may be typically included in evaluation and management (E/M) or clinical services. Unlike regular CPT codes, no fees are associated with the Category II and G codes. Instead, under programs such as PQRI and similar private payer plans, financial payments can be earned if these services are provided for enough patients in the affected groupings—if, for example, tobacco use is assessed for all adult patients.

performance measures processes, experience, and/or outcomes of patient care, observations, or treatment that relate to one or more quality aims for health care, such as effective, safe, efficient, patient-centered, equitable, and timely care

patient registry method of reporting clinical data to payers using an online service rather than claims-based reporting

Types of Performance Measures

The types of performance measures include:

- Therapeutic interventions like medication for HBP and physical therapy for specific injuries
- Preventive interventions like mammography for breast cancer and immunizations
- Other interventions such as tobacco cessation counseling or dietary counseling to decrease risk factors associated with obesity and CAD

Reporting Methods

Practices that participate in PQRI may either report their Category II codes directly to CMS using a claims-based system that is often handled by a clearinghouse or use a **patient registry.** Patient registries are databases that collect clinical data on all the practice's patients who have specific conditions, such as diabetes or asthma, or that keep track of specific tests, such as mammograms. A registry acts as an online service that coordinates storing and reporting performance

THINKING IT THROUGH 12.7

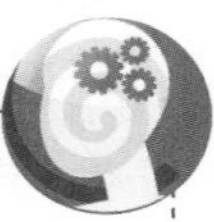

Each year, Medicare releases a new list of performance measures. As the staff member in charge of incentive programs, how would you research this year's PQRI information?

measurement data. The practice can enter the patient data as part of routine clinical activities like documentation using the PM/EHR.

Demonstrating Meaningful Use

Medisoft Network Professional's reports can also be used to analyze and report on meaningful use criteria. The initial payments of the CMS-run Medicare and Medicaid program bonuses began in May 2011. Providers are required to demonstrate meaningful use for at least ninety consecutive days to get a year's payment.

EXAMPLE

Effective screening for cervical cancer with a Pap test depends on good follow-up care in the event of abnormal test results. The EHR can establish a tracking system to ensure that the primary care physician is aware of the abnormal results, that patients' follow-up appointments are scheduled, and that patients appear for these appointments.

12.13 Record Retention

retention preservation of information on patients' medical conditions for continuity of care

Patients' medical records and financial records are retained according to the practice's policy. The practice manager or providers set the **retention** policy after reviewing the state and federal regulations that apply.

The practice's policy about keeping records is summarized in a retention schedule, a list of the items from a record that are retained and for how long they are retained. The retention schedule usually also covers the method for retention. For example, a policy might state that all established patients' records are retained in the practice's network for three years, and then copied onto removable media and sent to another storage location for another four years.

The retention schedule protects both the provider and the patient. Continuity of care is the first concern: the record must be available for anyone who is caring for the patient, within or outside of the practice. Also, records must be kept in case of a legal proceeding, For example, the provider might be asked to justify the level and nature of treatment when a claim is investigated or challenged, requiring access to documentation.

Although state guidelines cover medical information about patients, most do not specifically cover financial records. Financial records are generally saved according to federal business records

THINKING IT THROUGH 12.8

In your opinion, how will the transition to electronic health records affect record retention?

BILLING TIP

Retention Advice

The American Health Information Management Association (AHIMA) publishes guidelines called "Practice Briefs" on many topics, including retention of health information and of health care business records.

HIPAA/HITECH TIP

Disposal of Electronic Protected Health Information

The HIPAA Security Rule requires covered entities to implement policies and procedures to address the final disposition of ePHI and/or the hardware or electronic media on which it is stored. The practice must have procedures for reasonably ensuring that ePHI cannot be recovered from a device or medium such as a hard disk, floppy disk, CD, Zip disk, tape, or cartridge.

retention requirements. Under HIPAA, covered entities must keep records of HIPAA compliance for six years. For example, patients have the right to request an accounting of the disclosures that have been made of their protected health information. In general, the storage method chosen and the means of destroying the records when the retention period ends must strictly adhere to the same confidentiality requirements as patient medical records.

chapter 12 summary

LEARNING OUTCOME	KEY CONCEPTS/EXAMPLES
12.1 List the three types of reports available in Medisoft Network Professional (MNP). Pages 590–592	1. Standard reports 2. Medisoft Reports 3. Custom reports
12.2 Describe how to select data to be included in a MNP report. Pages 593–596	Data for a report are selected in the Search dialog box. The Search dialog box contains one or more selection boxes. Entering data in the selection boxes causes the data in the report to be limited to the data selected. If all data are to be included, the Show all values of the ______ field is selected.
12.3 Compare patient, procedure, and payment day sheets. Pages 596–601	A patient day sheet lists patient transactions for a day, organized alphabetically by chart number. A procedure day sheet lists patient transactions by procedure code, and is sorted numerically, then alphabetically (for codes that begin with letters). A payment day sheet lists patient transactions by provider, ordered numerically by the code assigned to the provider in MNP.
12.4 Discuss the purpose of a practice analysis report. Pages 601–607	A practice analysis report analyzes the revenue of a practice for a specified period of time, usually a month or a year. The report can be used to generate medical practice financial statements and can also be used for profit analysis.
12.5 Explain how to create a production by provider report. Pages 607–609	1. On the Reports menu, click Production Reports. Select Production by Provider. The Print Report Where? dialog box appears. 2. Accept the default option to preview the report. Click the Start button. 3. The Search dialog box is displayed. Make the necessary entries in the following selection boxes: Date From Date Created Attending Provider 4. Click the OK button. The report opens in the Print Preview window. 5. Click the Close button to exit the Print Preview window.

LEARNING OUTCOME	KEY CONCEPTS/EXAMPLES
12.6 List the steps for creating a patient ledger report. Pages 610–612	1. On the Reports menu, click Patient Ledger. The Print Report Where? dialog box appears. 2. Accept the default option to preview the report. Click the Start button. 3. The Search dialog box is displayed. Make the necessary entries in the following selection boxes: Chart Number Patient Reference Balance Date From Attending Provider Billing Code Patient Indicator 4. Click the OK button. The report opens in the Print Preview window. 5. Click the Close button to exit the Print Preview window.
12.7 Describe how to create a standard patient list report. Pages 612–613	1. On the Reports menu, click Standard Patient Lists. Select Patient by Diagnosis or Patient by Insurance Carrier from the submenu. The Print Report Where? dialog box appears. 2. Accept the default option to preview the report. Click the Start button. 3. The Search dialog box is displayed. For a Patient by Diagnosis report, make the necessary entries in the Diagnosis Code 1 selection box. For a Patient by Insurance Carrier report, make the necessary entry in the Code selection box. 4. Click the OK button. The report opens in the Print Preview window. 5. Click the Close button to exit the Print Preview window.

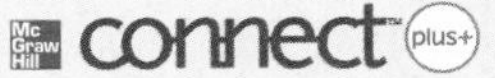

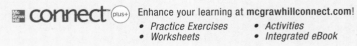

Enhance your learning at **mcgrawhillconnect.com**!

- *Practice Exercises*
- *Worksheets*
- *Activities*
- *Integrated eBook*

LEARNING OUTCOME	KEY CONCEPTS/EXAMPLES
12.8 Describe the use of Medisoft Reports to create a report. Pages 614–616	1. Select Medisoft Reports on the Reports menu. The Medisoft Reports window opens. 2. Locate the folder in the All Folders column that contains the report you want to create. 3. Double click the folder to see its contents. 4. In the list of reports that appears in the window to the right of the All Folders list, locate the report. 5. Double click the report. After several seconds, the Search dialog box appears. 6. Make the necessary entries in the selection boxes, and then click the OK button. 7. The report appears in the Print Preview window. 8. To send the report to the printer, click the Print button.
12.9 Explain how aging reports are used in a medical practice. Pages 616–617	Medical practices use aging reports to determine which accounts require follow-up to collect past-due balances. Aging reports list the amount of money owed to the practice, sorted by the amount of time the money has been owed.
12.10 Explain how to access MNP's built-in custom reports. Pages 618–620	1. Click Custom Report List on the Reports menu. The Open Report dialog box appears. 2. Select the desired report from the list of reports, and click the OK button. 3. Select the option to preview or print the report, and then click the Start button. 4. Make the necessary entries in the Data Selection Questions dialog box and click OK. 5. The report appears in the Print Preview window or is sent to the printer.

LEARNING OUTCOME	KEY CONCEPTS/EXAMPLES
12.11 Describe the process of editing reports in MNP's Report Designer. Pages 620–622	On the Reports menu, click Design Custom Reports and Bills. The Medisoft Report Designer window is displayed. Click Open Report on the File menu. Click to select a report in the list, and click the OK button, or double click the report title. When the report opens in Report Designer, double click the entry you want to change in order to select it, and double click it a second time to edit it. Enter the new wording in the appropriate text box, making sure the Auto Size button is checked, so the program will automatically resize the text box to accommodate the title. Click the OK button. Next, double click the box to select it, and double click it again to edit its contents. In the Data Field Properties dialog box, click the Edit button. In the Select Data Field dialog box, scroll to the new field, highlight it, and click OK. Make sure the Auto Size box is checked, and click the OK button. On the Report Designer File menu, click Preview Report to save the file as a new report. In the Save Report As… dialog box, key in the new title and click the OK button.
12.12 List the reasons for using reports for tracking specific clinical data. Pages 622–624	The Medisoft Clinical PM/EHR collects needed information related to clinical improvement and incentive payments and makes reporting it easier. This information can include the use of recognized ongoing performance measures that underpin treatment plans and the use of health information technology to improve outcomes and quality of care. PM/EHR facilitates the search for specific conditions and results and generates follow-up reminders. The information is entered during the regular documentation stage and is furnished electronically, saving considerable time over paper-based collection and reporting.
12.13 Discuss the regulatory obligations for the retention of patient medical records. Pages 624–625	State and federal regulations determine which records need to be retained and for how long they must be retained. The practice manager or providers set a retention policy after reviewing these regulations. Continuity of care is the first concern: the record must be available for anyone who is caring for the patient, within or outside of the practice. Also, records must be kept in case of a legal proceeding.

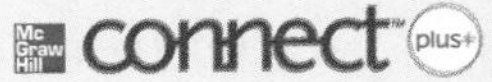

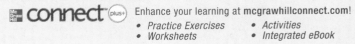

Enhance your learning at **mcgrawhillconnect.com**!

- *Practice Exercises*
- *Worksheets*
- *Activities*
- *Integrated eBook*

chapter review

MATCHING QUESTIONS

Match the key terms with their definitions.

_____ 1. ***[LO 12.9]*** aging report

_____ 2. ***[LO 12.3]*** day sheet

_____ 3. ***[LO 12.9]*** insurance aging report

_____ 4. ***[LO 12.12]*** performance measures

_____ 5. ***[LO 12.3]*** patient day sheet

_____ 6. ***[LO 12.6]*** patient ledger

_____ 7. ***[LO 12.3]*** payment day sheet

_____ 8. ***[LO 12.4]*** practice analysis report

_____ 9. ***[LO 12.3]*** procedure day sheet

_____ 10. ***[LO 12.5]*** production by provider report

a. A summary of the patient activity on a given day.

b. A report that lists incoming revenue information for each provider in the practice.

c. A report that lists the amount of money owed the practice, organized by the length of time the money has been owed.

d. A report that provides information on practice activities for a twenty-four-hour period.

e. A report that lists the financial activity in each patient's account, including charges, payments, and adjustments.

f. Processes, experience, and/or outcomes of patient care, observations, or treatment that relate to one or more quality aims for health care, such as effective, safe, efficient, patient-centered, equitable, and timely care.

g. A report that lists payments received on a given day, organized by provider.

h. A report that analyzes the revenue of a practice for a specified period of time, usually a month or a year.

i. A report that lists the procedures performed on a given day, listed in numerical order.

j. A report that lists how long a payer has taken to respond to insurance claims.

TRUE-FALSE QUESTIONS

Decide whether each statement is true or false.

_____ 1. ***[LO 12.3]*** A day sheet is a standard report that provides information on practice activities for the week.

_____ 2. ***[LO 12.11]*** The Medisoft Report Designer allows users to modify existing reports or create new reports to add to the custom report list.

_____ 3. ***[LO 12.6]*** An insurance analysis report lists the transaction details of a patient's account, including charges, payments, and adjustments.

_____ 4. ***[LO 12.9]*** A patient aging report shows how long a payer has taken to respond to each claim.

_____ 5. ***[LO 12.10]*** When a new custom report is created in MNP, it is added to the list of custom reports displayed on the screen.

_____ 6. ***[LO 12.8]*** The new Medisoft Reports feature in Version 16 replaces existing reports.

_____ 7. ***[LO 12.13]*** Retention schedules usually also cover the method for retention.

_____ 8. ***[LO 12.12]*** Patient registries are databases that collect clinical data on all the practice's patients who have specific conditions, or that keep track of specific tests.

_____ 9. ***[LO 12.7]*** In MNP, the Patient by Insurance Carrier report lists patients sorted by their insurance carrier and then by their provider or facility.

_____ 10. ***[LO 12.4]*** Medisoft Network Professional's practice analysis report analyzes the revenue of a practice for a specified period of time.

MULTIPLE-CHOICE QUESTIONS

Select the letter that best completes the statement or answers the question.

1. ***[LO 12.4]*** Medisoft Network Professional's ________ analyzes the revenue of a practice for a specified period of time, usually a month or a year.
   a. insurance aging report
   b. practice analysis report
   c. day sheet
   d. aging report
2. ***[LO 12.9]*** A(n) ________ shows how long a payer has taken to respond to each claim.
   a. aging report
   b. insurance aging report
   c. patient aging report
   d. all of the above
3. ***[LO 12.1]*** Which of the following options does MNP offer for creating reports?
   a. Medisoft reports
   b. Standard reports
   c. Design Custom Reports and Bills
   d. all of the above
4. ***[LO 12.9]*** A(n) ________ lists a patient's balance by age, date and amount of the last payment, and telephone number.
   a. aging report
   b. insurance aging report
   c. patient aging report
   d. all of the above

5. ***[LO 12.6]*** A(n) ________ lists the transaction details of a patient's account, including charges, payments, and adjustments.
   a. patient ledger
   b. day sheet
   c. aging report
   d. retention schedule

6. ***[LO 12.2]*** In MNP, the ________ determine what data are included in the report.
   a. day sheets
   b. retention schedules
   c. patient ledgers
   d. selection boxes

7. ***[LO 12.3]*** Which of the following is a summary of the patient activity on that day?
   a. patient day sheet
   b. procedure day sheet
   c. payment day sheet
   d. day sheet

8. ***[LO 12.5]*** Which of the following reports lists incoming revenue information for each procedure code in the practice's database?
   a. production by provider report
   b. production by procedure report
   c. production by insurance report
   d. production report

9. ***[LO 12.3]*** Which of the following lists all payments received on a particular day, organized by provider?
   a. patient day sheet
   b. procedure day sheet
   c. payment day sheet
   d. day sheet

10. ***[LO 12.10]*** The built-in custom reports in MNP include ________.
    a. walkout receipts
    b. superbills
    c. patient statements
    d. all of the above

SHORT-ANSWER QUESTION

Define the following abbreviation.

1. ***[LO 12.12]*** PQRI ____________________

APPLYING YOUR KNOWLEDGE

Answer the questions below in the space provided.

12.1 ***[LO 12.3]*** One of the providers in a practice asks for a report of yesterday's transactions. How would this report be created?

____

____

12.2 ***[LO 12.6]*** A patient is unsure whether she mailed a check last month to pay an outstanding balance on her account. What standard report would you use to help answer her question?

____

____

12.3 ***[LO 12.3]*** If the office manager asked you for a list of procedure codes representing services performed on a particular day, what report would you create?

____

____

12.4 ***[LO 12.9]*** What would the consequences be if a medical practice did not produce patient aging reports on a regular basis?

____

____

chapter 13

KEY TERMS

bankruptcy
collection agency
collection list
collection tracer report
Equal Credit Opportunity Act (ECOA)
Fair Debt Collection Practices Act of 1977 (FDCPA)
means test
patient refund
payment plan
small-balance account
Telephone Consumer Protection Act of 1991
tickler
Truth in Lending Act
uncollectible account
write-off

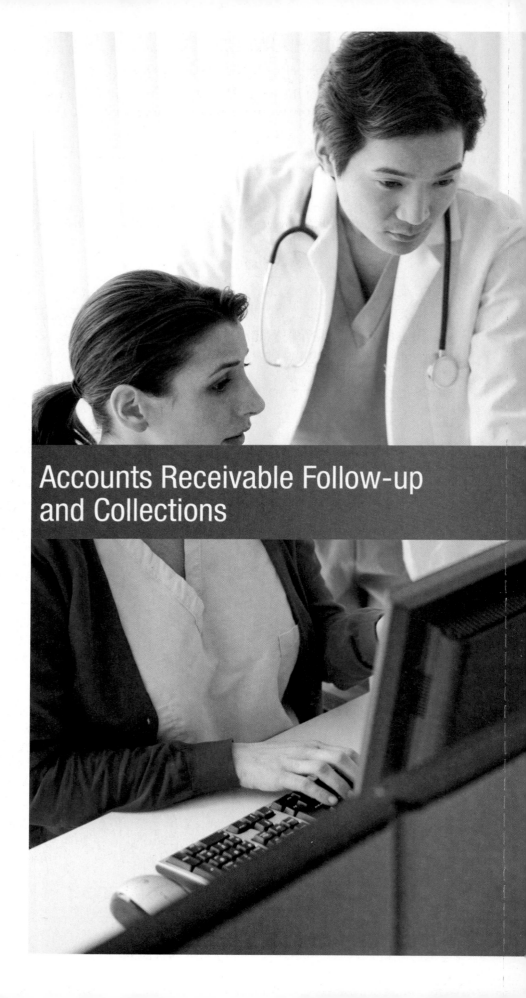

Accounts Receivable Follow-up and Collections

LEARNING OUTCOMES

When you finish this chapter, you will be able to:

13.1 Explain why it is important to collect overdue balances from patients.

13.2 Describe the way in which financial policies help establish payment expectations.

13.3 Describe the procedures followed to identify overdue accounts.

13.4 Identify the major federal laws that govern the collection process.

13.5 Explain how letters are used in collecting overdue payments.

13.6 Explain payment plans.

13.7 Discuss the use of collection agencies to pursue patients who have not paid overdue bills.

13.8 Describe the procedures for clearing uncollectible balances and small balances from patients' accounts receivable.

Tackling Problems

Chris looked over the patient aging report and noted, "Calling people to follow up on their overdue bills may be the hardest part of this job. I'm glad I know our practice's guidelines on how to have these conversations in a courteous way and how to set up payment plans that work for our patients."

Even difficult parts of the job are easier to handle when you know the right way to tackle them. As you study this chapter, think about the issue of collecting needed revenues for the practice in light of the various financial situations people are in. How would you like to be treated, if you were the patient in this case?

WHEN YOU FINISH THIS CHAPTER, YOU WILL ALSO BE ABLE TO USE MEDISOFT CLINICAL TO:

1. Analyze a patient aging report.
2. Create a tickler for an account using MNP.
3. Create a collections letter using MNP.
4. Using MNP, produce a collection tracer report.
5. Using MNP, assign a payment plan to an account.
6. Using MNP, post a payment from a collection agency.
7. Write off an uncollectible account using MNP.
8. Write off small-balance accounts using MNP.
9. Issue a patient refund using MNP.

SOFTWARE SKILLS

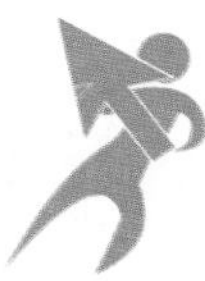

13.1 The Importance of Collections from Patients

Receiving full payment for services is a critical factor in determining the financial success of a medical practice. The average patient is now responsible for paying nearly 35 percent of medical bills, according to the Centers for Medicare and Medicaid Services (CMS). Sums that are not collected must be subtracted from income, reducing working capital, meaning that the practice might have to borrow funds and pay interest on those amounts just to pay bills. Practices collect payments from insurance carriers, as explained in Chapter 11, and from patients, as covered here.

Patients' payments are collected both at the time of service (TOS) and, for insured patients, after claim adjudication by payers. At TOS, practices routinely collect copayments and overdue balances, and may also collect either partial or full payment for visits. The majority of payments, however, are collected from patients after the payer's remittance advice and payment are transmitted to the office and a statement is mailed to the patient indicating the balance due. The collection process begins with sending these statements to patients promptly. It continues until the bill is collected or the amount due is determined to be uncollectible.

While most patients pay their bills on time, every practice has some patients who do not. Patients' reasons for not paying include:

- Lack of insurance
- Lack of financial resources
- Significant medical costs
- Consumer-directed health plans with high out-of-pocket costs
- Lack of understanding that payment is their responsibility

Members of the billing staff may be asked to work with patients and representatives of health plans to follow up on overdue accounts and unpaid claims. The goal of the follow-up is to resolve problems and collect payments.

13.2 The Financial Policy and Payment Expectations

The patient collection process begins with a clear financial policy and effective communications with patients about their financial responsibilities. When patients understand the charges and the practice's financial policy in advance, collecting payments is not usually problematic. As a result, as detailed in Chapter 5 and reviewed here, it is important to have a written financial policy that spells out patients' responsibilities.

The financial policy of a medical practice explains how the practice handles financial matters. When new patients register, they should be

THINKING IT THROUGH 13.1

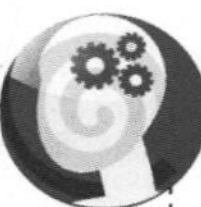

After receiving a statement in the mail, a patient calls the practice and asks to speak to the billing department. The patient believes that she has been overcharged. In your opinion, what first steps should the biller take to respond to the call? What tone should the biller use?

THINKING IT THROUGH 13.2

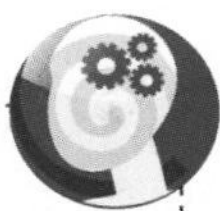

Based on the financial policy shown in Figure 13.1:

- Who is responsible for charges?
- What fee is charged if a copay is not paid at TOS?

given copies of the financial policy along with the practice's HIPAA privacy policies and patient registration material. The policy should tell patients how the practice handles:

- Collecting copayments and past-due balances
- Setting up financial arrangements for unpaid balances
- Providing charity care or using a sliding scale for patients with low incomes
- Collecting payments for services not covered by insurance
- Collecting prepayment for services
- Accepting cash, checks, money orders, and credit and debit cards

If the practice's printed or displayed payment policy covers adding finance charges on late accounts, it is acceptable to do so. The amount of the finance charge must comply with federal and state law.

Figure 13.1 shows a sample financial policy of a medical practice.

13.3 Collection Procedures

Despite the practice's efforts to communicate the financial policy to all patients, some individuals still do not pay in full and on time. Nonpayment of patient statements initiates the collection process, which involves identifying the overdue accounts and organizing them for effective follow-up.

Working with Patient Aging Reports

The medical office tracks overdue bills by reviewing the patient aging report. Like the insurance aging report, it is analyzed to determine which patients are overdue on their bills and to group them into categories for efficient collection efforts (see Figure 13.2). The patient aging report includes the patient's chart number, name, aging amounts, and total balance. The aging period begins on the date

Financial Policy of
Any Medical Practice
Any Town, USA

Thank you for choosing Any Medical Practice for your health care needs. The following information is being provided to assist you in understanding our financial policies and to address the questions most frequently asked by our patients.

Account Responsibility

You are responsible for all charges incurred on your account. It is also your responsibility to make sure all information on your account is current and accurate. Incorrect information can cause payment delays, which may result in late fees being applied to your account. Many people are under the impression that it is up to the physician and staff to make sure that all charges are paid or covered by insurance. This is not the case. Please remember that the insurance contract is between you and the insurance company, not the physician. It is your responsibility to know what your contract covers and pays and to communicate this to physicians and staff. Therefore, you are responsible for charges incurred regardless of insurance coverage.

Insurance Billing

If you have medical insurance, we will be happy to bill your insurance carrier for you. As a courtesy we will also bill the carrier of any secondary insurance coverage that you may have. Any Medical Practice contracts with many insurance companies, but due to the fact that these companies have many different plans available, it is impossible for us to know if your specific plan is included. You will need to check with your insurance company in advance. Please remember that your insurance may not cover or pay all charges incurred. Any unpaid balance after insurance is your responsibility.

Copays

All copays are due at time of service. A $5.00 billing fee is assessed if your copay is not paid at time of service. This fee will not be waived. It is your responsibility to know whether your insurance requires you to pay a copay.

No Insurance

If you have no insurance, payment in full is expected at time of service, unless payment arrangements have been made prior to your visit.

Late Fees

All patient balances are to be paid in full within 60 days. This refers to balances after your insurance has paid. If you are unable to pay your balance in full within 60 days, please contact the business office to set up a payment plan. A late fee of $20.00 per month will be assessed on patient balances over 60 days.

Cash Only

If your account has been turned over to collection, it will also be changed to a cash-only account. This means that all services will need to be paid in full at time of service. A letter will be sent to inform you if your account has been changed to a cash-only basis.

Dishonored Checks

A $25.00 service charge will be assessed on all dishonored checks.

Payment Methods

Any Medical Practice accepts cash, personal checks, and the following credit cards: Visa, MasterCard, American Express, and Discover. Payments can be made at any reception area. For your convenience, an ATM machine is located in the lobby of the building.

Figure 13.1 A Sample Medical Practice Financial Policy

Patient Aging by Date of Service

Family Care Clinic

Show all data where the Charges/Payments/Adj is on or before 9/30/2016

Chart	Name	0-30	31-60	61-90	91-120	121+	Total
FITZWJO0	Fitzwilliams, John	50.00					50.00
JONESEL0	Jones, Elizabeth	21.17	7.47				28.64
MAZLOAL0	Mazloum, Ali				720.50		720.50
SMITHJA0	Smith, James	-10.00					-10.00
WONGJO10	Wong, Jo	7.47		7.47			14.94
Report Totals:		68.64	7.47	7.47	720.50	0.00	804.08

Figure 13.2 Example of a Patient Aging Report

of the bill. The report is divided into the following categories based on each statement's beginning date:

- Current or up-to-date: 30 days
- Past due: 31–60 days
- Past due: 61–90 days
- Past due: 91+ days

Each practice sets its own procedures for the collection process. Large bills have priority over smaller ones. Usually, an automatic reminder notice and a second statement are mailed when a bill has not been paid thirty days after it was issued. Some practices phone a patient with a thirty-day overdue account. If the bill is not then paid, a series of collection letters is generated at intervals, each more stringent in its tone and more direct in its approach.

Table 13.1 provides an example of one practice's collection timeline; different approaches are used in other practices. Some practices send all accounts that are past thirty days to an outside agency.

TABLE 13.1 Patient Collection Timeline

Amount Past Due	Action
30 days	Bill patient
45 days	Call patient regarding bill
60 days	Letter 1
75 days	Letter 2 and call
80 days	Letter 3
90 days	Turn over to collections

connect plus+

EXERCISE 13.1

IDENTIFYING OVERDUE ACCOUNTS

Review the patient aging report displayed in Figure 13.2. Using the information contained in the report, locate the patient account that is 61–90 days overdue. List the chart number, patient name, past-due amounts, and account balance below. You will use this information in Exercise 13.2 to create a tickler item for the practice's collection list.

Chart Number	Name	Current 0–30	Past 31–60	Past 61–90	Past 91+	Total

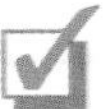

You have completed Exercise 13.1

collection list tool for tracking activities that need to be completed as part of the collection process

tickler reminder to follow up on an account

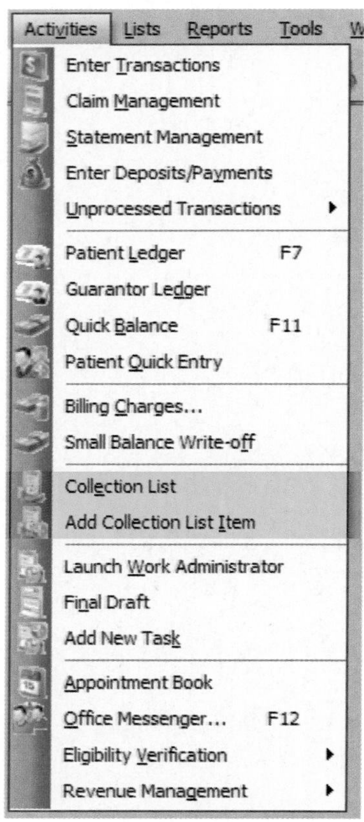

Figure 13.3 Collection List Options on the Activities Menu

Adding an Account to the Collection List

Once overdue accounts have been identified, the next step is to add collection items to a collection list. The **collection list** is designed to track activities that need to be completed as part of the collection process. Ticklers or collection reminders are displayed as collection list items. A **tickler** is a reminder to follow up on an account that is entered on the collection list.

In MNP, the selections for the Collection List feature are located on the Activities menu (see Figure 13.3).

Using the Collection List Window

The Collection List dialog box displays ticklers that have already been entered into the database (see Figure 13.4). The information displayed in the dialog box depends on the dates entered in the Date boxes in the top-left corner of the window. For example, if 9/30/2016 is entered in both boxes, only ticklers marked for follow-up on September 30, 2016, will be listed.

Options for controlling what appears in the Collection List window are at the top of the dialog box and include the following:

Date Items can be displayed for the current date, for a range of dates, or for all dates. By default, the current date (the Windows System Date) is used as the range of dates, and only those tickler items that are due on that date are displayed. To see all ticklers regardless of the date, click the Show All Ticklers box.

Show All Ticklers A check in this box results in the listing of all tickler items.

Show Deleted Only A check in this box displays only ticklers that have been deleted.

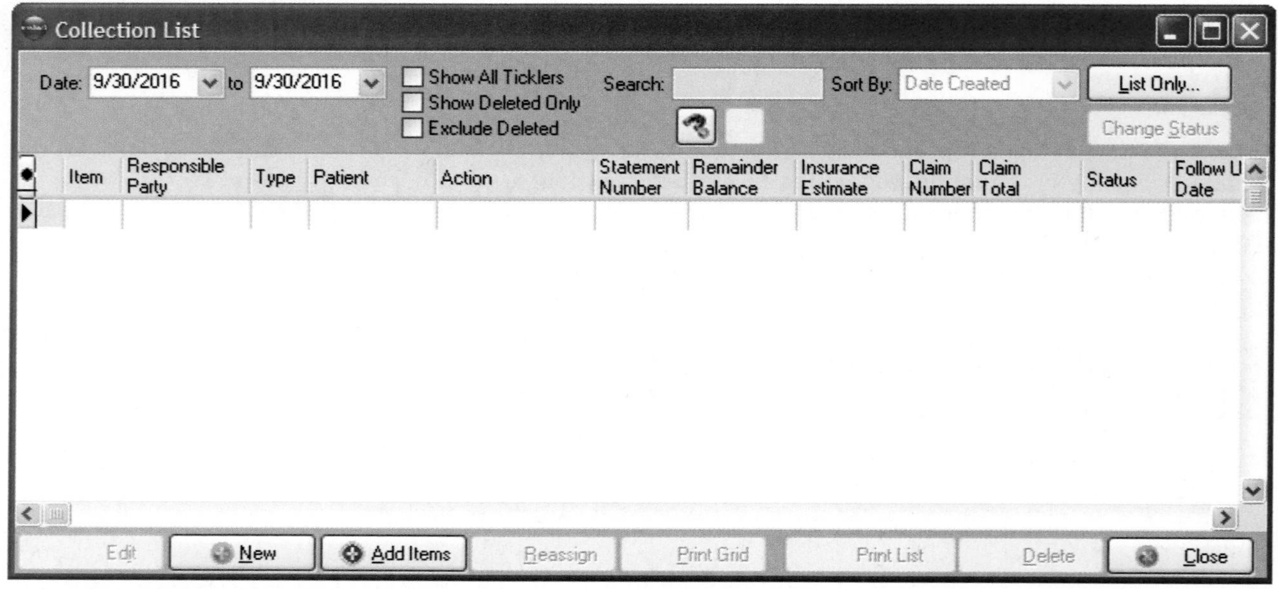

Figure 13.4 Collection List Dialog Box

Exclude Deleted A check in this box indicates that deleted ticklers are not displayed.

The Collection List dialog box contains the following information about each tickler item:

Item This unique number identifying a tickler item is assigned automatically by the program.

Responsible Party This field contains the chart number (patient/guarantor) or insurance code (insurance carrier) that identifies the responsible party for this item. By clicking the plus sign (+) that appears to the left of an entry, the field can be expanded to view more information about the responsible party. *Note:* The plus sign is visible only when a tickler has been entered.

When the responsible party is an insurance carrier, the following additional information appears (see Figure 13.5):

- Code
- Name
- Contact
- Phone
- City
- State
- Zip Code
- Group Number
- Policy Number

When the responsible party is a patient/guarantor, the following additional information is displayed (see Figure 13.6):

- Chart Number
- Name

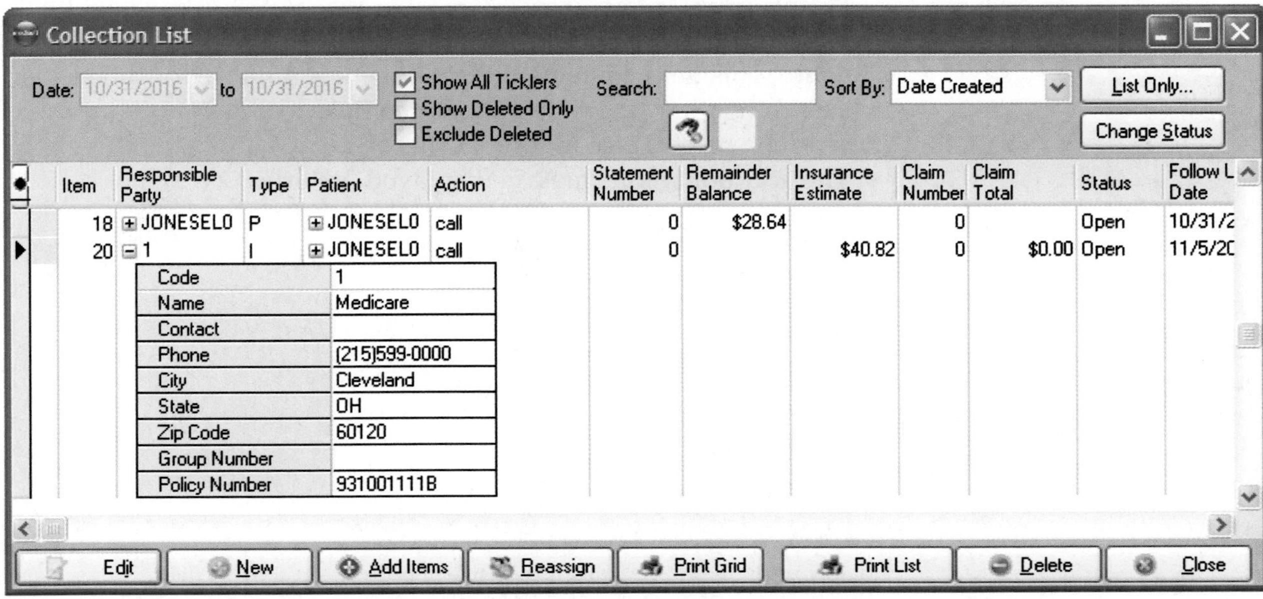

Figure 13.5 Additional Information Displayed When the Responsible Party Is an Insurance Carrier

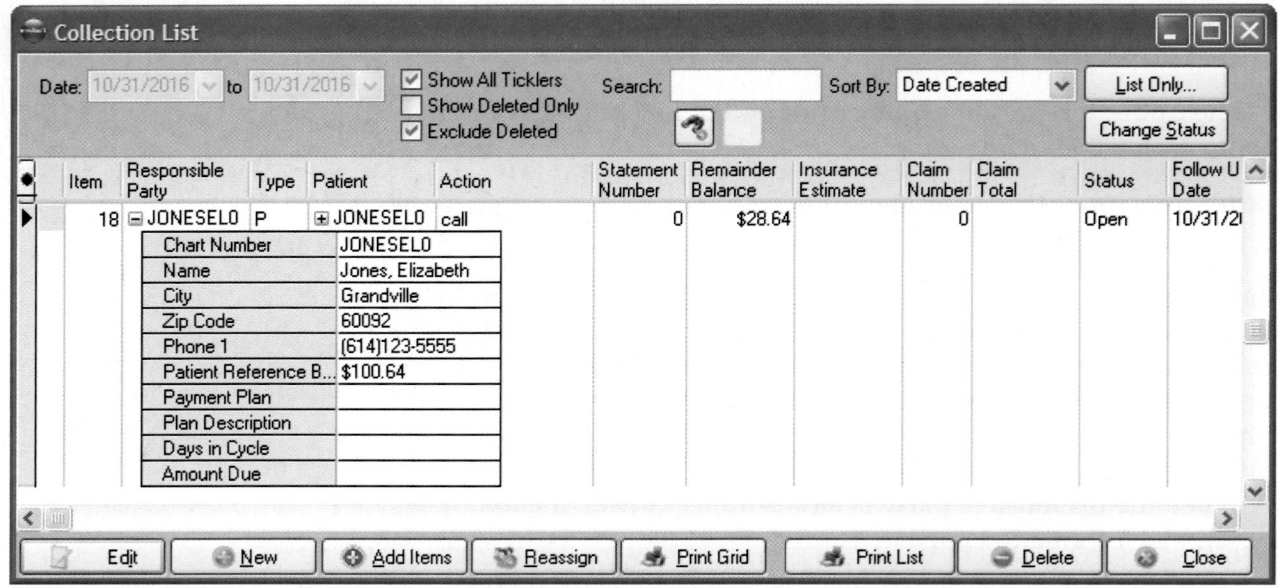

Figure 13.6 Additional Information Displayed When the Responsible Party Is a Patient/Guarantor

- City
- Zip Code
- Phone 1
- Patient Reference Balance
- Payment Plan
- Plan Description
- Days in Cycle
- Amount Due

Type The type is either a *P* for Patient or an *I* for Insurance. If the type is *P*, the responsible party is a patient. If the type is *I*, the responsible party is the insurance carrier.

Patient This field contains the patient chart number for this tickler. Clicking the plus sign (+) expands the field to show more information on the patient (see Figure 13.7).

The additional information displayed includes:

- Chart Number
- Last Name
- First Name
- Middle Initial
- Phone 1
- Zip Code
- Date of Birth
- Sex
- Patient Reference Balance
- Social Security Number

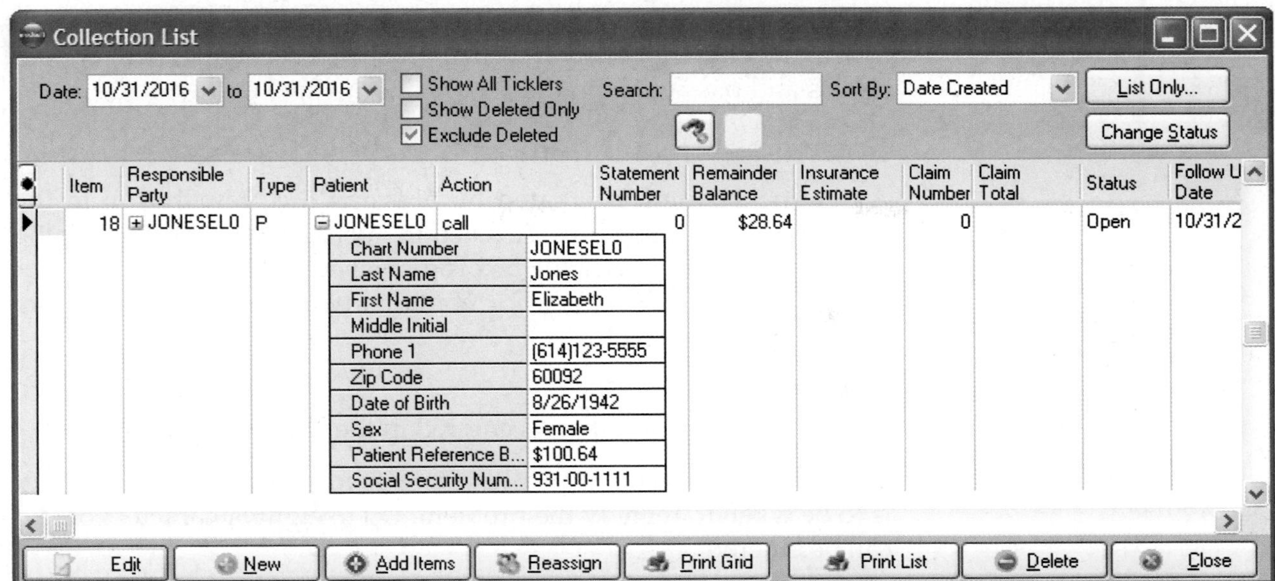

Figure 13.7 Additional Information Available in the Patient Field of the Collection List Dialog Box

Other information in the Collection List dialog box includes the following:

Action This field lists the action required. To see all of the text entered for this field, double click in the field. This opens a window showing the complete text entry.

Statement Number If the tickler is for a patient, the statement number is listed.

Remainder Balance If the responsible type is Patient, the balance reported is the patient's balance as listed in Transaction Entry. If the responsible type is Insurance, the balance reported is an estimated balance for the patient's specified carrier. This is the balance at the time the tickler is created. This balance does not refresh when payments are made to the patient's account. To manually update the amounts, the tickler must be edited and saved again.

Insurance Estimate This field displays an estimate of the amount of payment expected from the insurance carrier.

Claim Number If the tickler is for an insurance carrier, the claim number is listed in this column.

Claim Total If the tickler is for an insurance carrier, the total amount of charges on the claim is listed here.

Status The entries in the field are Open, Resolved, and Deleted.

Follow Up Date This is the date the tickler will appear on the collection list.

Date Resolved This is the date that the status of the item was changed to Resolved. Resolution is determined by the user.

User ID The User ID identifies the user who is responsible for following up on the item. In an actual practice, users are assigned login names and passwords in the Security Setup area of the program.

Entering a Tickler Item

A new tickler item is created by pressing the New button in the Collection List dialog box. This action opens the Tickler Item dialog box. The Tickler Item dialog box is displayed in Figure 13.8.

The Tickler Item dialog box contains two tabs for information: Tickler and Office Notes.

Tickler Tab

The following information is entered in the Tickler tab:

Action Required The Action Required field specifies the action that is to be taken to remedy the problem. Up to eighty characters of text can be entered.

Responsible Party Type The button selected in this field indicates whether the patient or the insurance carrier is responsible for the account balance. This entry also controls the contents of the drop-down lists for the Responsible Party field below.

Chart Number The patient's chart number is selected from the list.

Guarantor The Guarantor field lists the account guarantor chart number for this tickler item.

Responsible Party If the responsible party type is Patient, a chart number is selected from the drop-down list. If the responsible party type is Insurance, the code for an insurance carrier is selected.

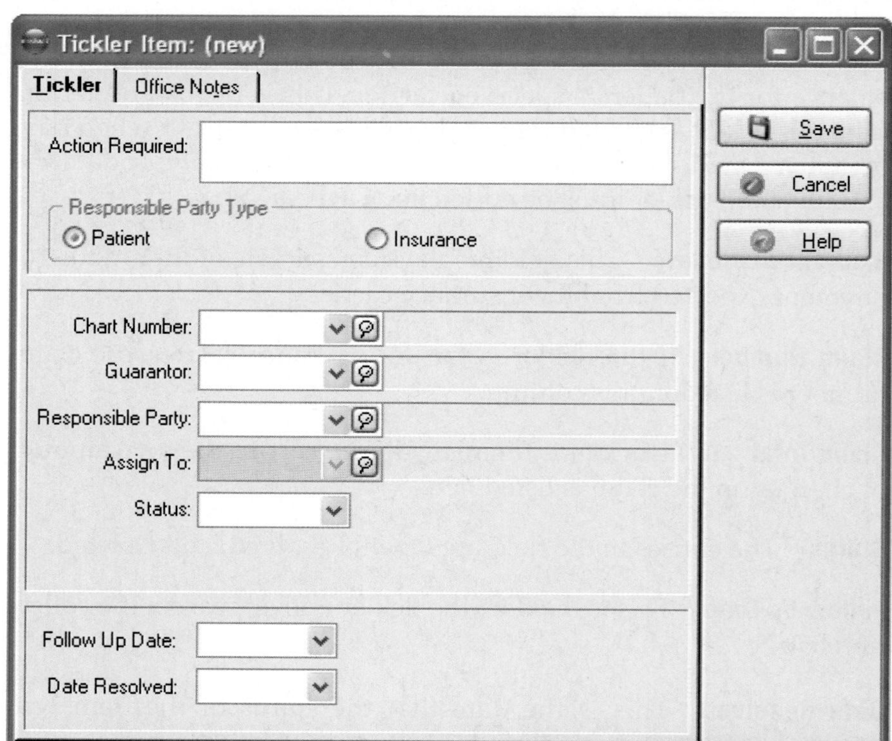

Figure 13.8 Tickler Item Dialog Box

Assign To The Assign To box lists the name of the individual responsible for following up on the tickler item. These names are set up by selecting Security Setup on the File menu. *Note:* This feature is not demonstrated in this text/workbook, so the field is grayed out, and an entry cannot be made.

Status The status of the tickler item is chosen from a drop-down list. The options are Open, Resolved, or Deleted.

Follow Up Date This is the date the tickler will appear on the collection list if the Date range in the Collection List window is used. By default, MNP enters the current date—the Windows System Date—in this field.

Date Resolved This field lists the date on which the status of the item was changed to Resolved. When the status is set to Resolved, the Date Resolved is set to the current date. Again, this is determined by the Windows System Date.

Office Notes Tab

The Office Notes tab consists of several buttons and a large area in which to enter notes. Notes that relate to the collection process of the selected tickler are entered in the large box.

When the right mouse button is clicked within the typing area, a shortcut menu is displayed (see Figure 13.9). Using this menu, notes can be edited, formatted, and printed from within the Office Notes tab.

Once a new tickler has been saved, the program automatically assigns a unique identifier code to the item.

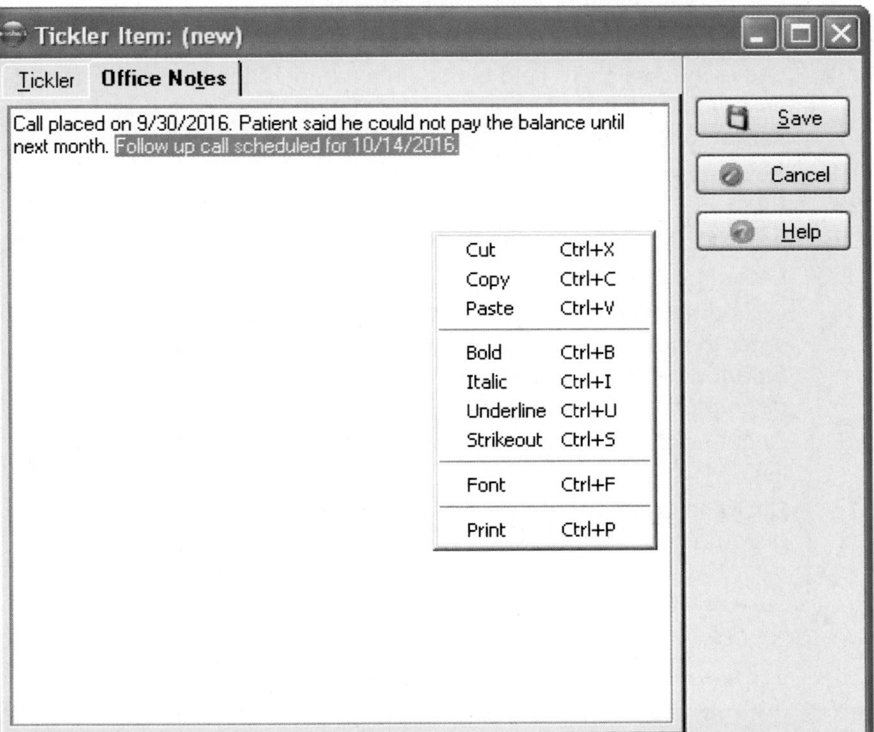

Figure 13.9 Office Notes Tab of the Tickler Item Dialog Box with Shortcut Menu Displayed

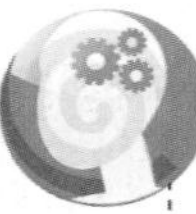

THINKING IT THROUGH 13.3

In MNP, a patient account is entered into collections by creating a tickler. One of the fields on the Tickler tab lists the guarantor. Based on what you learned here and in Chapter 5, why is it necessary to list the guarantor in the Tickler tab?

EXERCISE 13.2

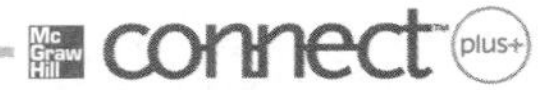

CREATING A TICKLER

Using the information in Exercise 13.1, create a tickler item for the patient whose account is 61–90 days overdue.

Date: September 30, 2016

1. Verify that Medisoft Network Professional is open, that the practice name in the title bar at the top of the screen is Family Care Clinic, and that the Medisoft Program Date is set to September 30, 2016.
2. Select Collection List on the Activities menu.
3. The Collection List dialog box is displayed. Confirm that the entry in both Date fields is 9/30/2016.
4. Click the New button to display the Tickler Item dialog box.
5. In the Action Required box, enter ***Telephone call about overdue balance. See notes.***
6. Make sure that Patient is selected as the Responsible Party Type.
7. Select the patient's chart number in the Chart Number field.
8. Select the guarantor in the Guarantor field.
9. Complete the Responsible Party field.
10. Leave the Assign To field blank. (In a real practice setting, this field would contain the name of the staff member who was assigned to follow up on this collection list item.)
11. Set the Status of the item to Open.
12. Verify that the entry in the Follow Up Date box is today's date, 9/30/2016.
13. Leave the Date Resolved field blank.
14. Click the Office Notes tab at the top of the dialog box, and enter the following text: ***Patient said she could not pay the balance on the account until her Social Security check was deposited early next week.***
15. Click the Save button. The item is added to the collection list.
16. Click the Close button to close the Collection List dialog box.

 **You have completed Exercise 13.2**

THINKING IT THROUGH 13.4

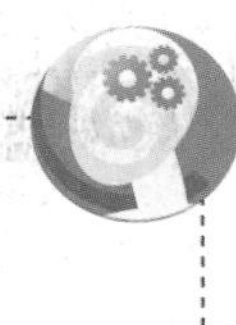

You are a biller for Family Care Clinic and are asked to call Jennifer Argada about the $38 payment that is overdue for the preschool visit of her child, Jimmy. The amount is overdue thirty days. When you call, you get the answering machine. Write a script for the phone message you would leave in this situation.

WARNING!

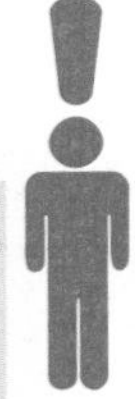

When an account is added to the collection list, the current balance for the tickler is determined. Once recorded in the tickler, it is not updated when new transactions are entered in the program.

For patient-responsible ticklers, the balance is the balance shown in the Transaction Entry window. It could also include insurance balances. For insurance-responsible ticklers, the balance is the estimated amount due from the assigned insurance carrier.

13.4 Laws Governing Patient Collections

Collections from patients are classified as consumer collections and are regulated by federal and state laws. The Federal Trade Commission enforces the **Fair Debt Collection Practices Act of 1977 (FDCPA)** and the **Telephone Consumer Protection Act of 1991** that regulate third-party collections to ensure fair and ethical treatment of debtors. The following guidelines are part of federal regulations and are also best practices in medical offices:

Fair Debt Collection Practices Act of 1977 (FDCPA) federal law regulating collection practices

Telephone Consumer Protection Act of 1991 federal law regulating collection practices

- Contact patients only once daily, and leave no more than three messages per week.
- Do not call a patient before 8 A.M. or after 9 P.M.
- Do not threaten the patient or use profane language.
- Identify the caller, the practice, and the purpose of the call; do not mislead the patient.
- Do not discuss the patient's debt with another person (called a third party).
- Do not leave a message on an answering machine that indicates the call is about a debt or send e-mail stating that the topic is debt.
- If a patient requests that all phone calls cease and desist, do not call the patient again, and contact the patient via mail.
- If a patient desires calls to be made to an attorney, do not contact the patient again, unless the attorney says to or the attorney cannot be reached.

13.5 Collection Letters

The practice's collection procedures set up the series of contacts in writing that patients will receive when they have overdue balances.

Collection Letter Series

For most patients, the collection letter is their first notice that their bill is past due. (Some practices send a second statement if the first is not paid before starting a series of letter.) Collection letters are generally brief and to the point while preserving a professional and courteous tone. They remind the patient of the practice's payment options and their responsibility to pay the debt. Practices decide what types of letters should be sent to accounts in the various past-due stages. Accounts that are further past due will receive more aggressive letters. For example, Figure 13.10a–c shows the progression in the tone of these letters.

Figure 13.10a–c Samples of Collection Letters

Date:
Patient:
Acct. #:
Balance Due: $

Dear

Your insurance company has paid its portion of your bill. You are now responsible for the remaining balance. Full payment is due, or you must contact this office within 10 days to make suitable payment arrangements. As an added payment option, you may pay by credit card, using the payment form below.

Sincerely,

<Employee signature>
<Employee name and title>

(a) First Letter

Date:
Patient:
Acct. #:
Balance Due: $

Dear

This is a reminder that your account is overdue. If there are any problems we should know about, please telephone or stop in at the office. A statement is attached showing your past account activity.

Your prompt payment is requested.

Sincerely,

<Employee signature>
<Employee name and title>

(b) Second Letter

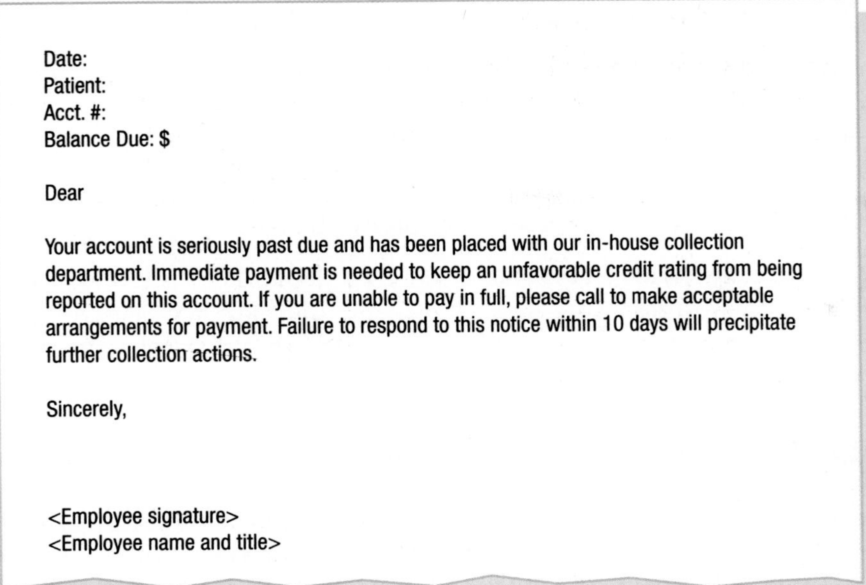

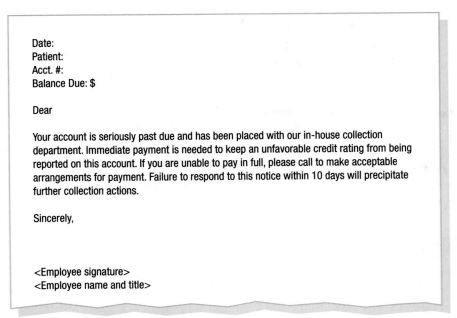

Date:
Patient:
Acct. #:
Balance Due: $

Dear

Your account is seriously past due and has been placed with our in-house collection department. Immediate payment is needed to keep an unfavorable credit rating from being reported on this account. If you are unable to pay in full, please call to make acceptable arrangements for payment. Failure to respond to this notice within 10 days will precipitate further collection actions.

Sincerely,

<Employee signature>
<Employee name and title>

(c) Third Letter

Figure 13.10a–c (*continued*)

TIP
Collection letters must comply with all debt-collection statutes—federal, state, and local.

Creating Collection Letters

A number of actions must be taken within MNP before collection letters can be sent. A patient-responsible tickler item for the patient's account must be entered in the collection list. Also, a collection letter report must be created. This report is generated when the Patient Collection Letters option is selected on the Collection Reports submenu of the Reports menu (see Figure 13.11). The collection letter

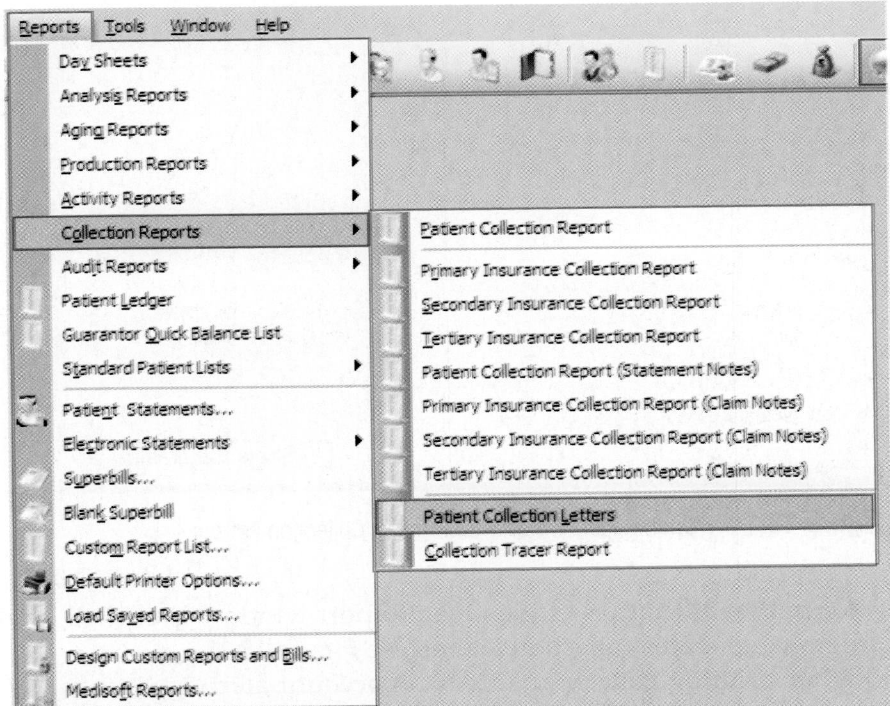

Figure 13.11 Patient Collection Letters Selected on the Collection Reports Submenu

Family Care Clinic

Collection Letter Report

10/31/2016

User ID:

Item	Status	Responsible Party	Patient Chart	Date Created	Date Resolved	Follow Up Date	Balance	# Days Old
19	Open	Kristin Zapata	ZAPATKR0	10/31/2016		10/31/2016	$247.50	0
18	Open	Elizabeth Jones	JONESEL0	10/31/2016		10/31/2016	$28.64	0

Figure 13.12 Collection Letter Report

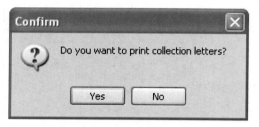

Figure 13.13 Confirm Dialog Box

report lists patients with overdue accounts to whom statements have been mailed (see Figure 13.12).

After the patient collection report is printed (or the Preview window is closed), the program displays a Confirm window that asks whether to print collection letters (see Figure 13.13).

If the Yes button is clicked, an Open Report dialog box appears (see Figure 13.14).

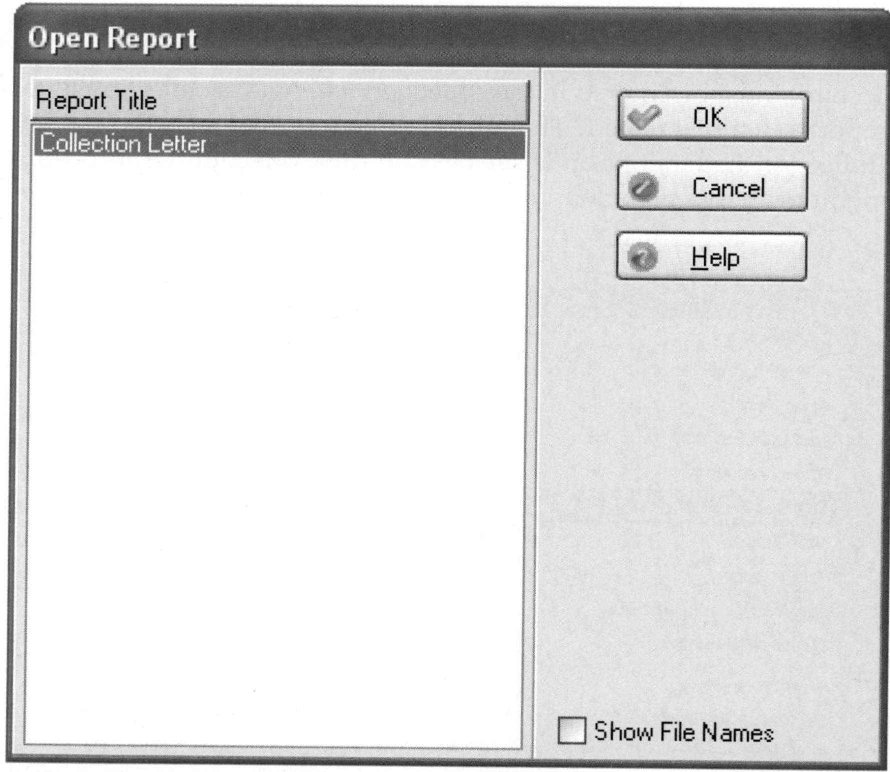

Figure 13.14 Open Report Window for Printing Collection Letters

Once the OK button in the Open Report window is clicked, the program generates collection letters (see Figure 13.15).

After printing collection letters, an account alert appears in the Transaction Entry, Quick Ledger, and Appointment Entry windows

Family Care Clinic
285 Stephenson Boulevard
Stephenson, OH 60089
(614)555-0000

Kristin Zapata
109 East Milan Avenue
Stephenson, OH 60089

10/31/2016
Patient Account: Zapata, Kristin

Dear Kristin Zapata

Our records indicate that your account with us is overdue. The total unpaid amount is *$ 282.50

If you have already forwarded your payment, please disregard this letter; otherwise, please forward your payment immediately.

Please contact us at (614)555-0000 if you have any questions or concerns about your account.

Sincerely,

Katherine Yan

ZAPATKR0

*Balance does not reflect any outstanding insurance payments

Figure 13.15 Patient Collection Letter

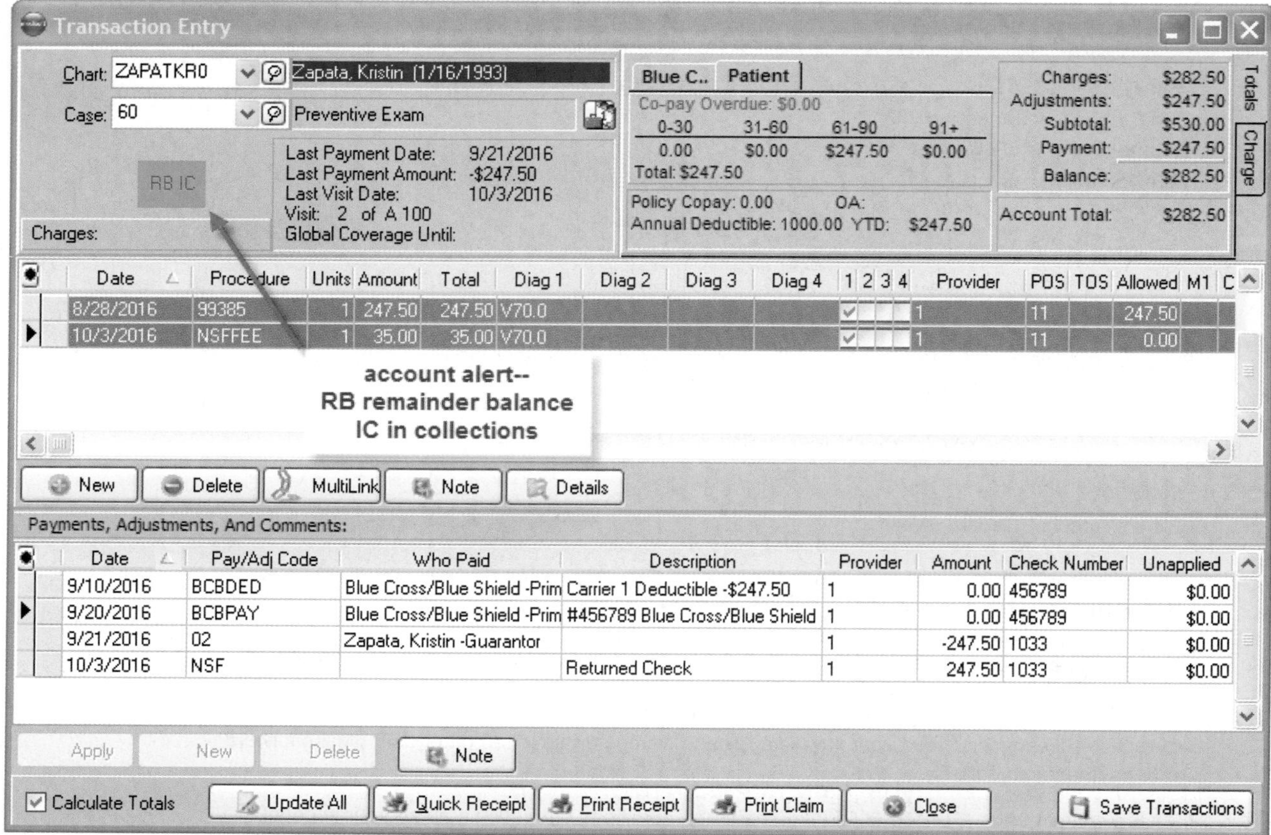

Figure 13.16 Transaction Entry Dialog Box with Account Alert Message Displayed

and remains until the patient no longer has an open tickler in the collection list. There are three account alert abbreviations:

1. RB: The patient has a remainder balance greater than the amount specified in the General tab in the Program Options window.
2. DP: The patient is delinquent on his or her payment plan.
3. IC: The patient account is in collections. (For this message to appear, a collection letter must have been printed.)

A sample account alert in the Transaction Entry window is displayed in Figure 13.16.

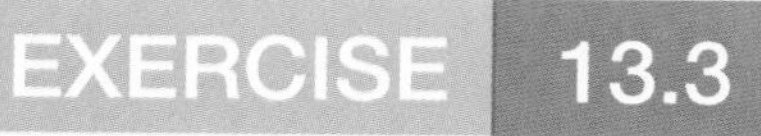

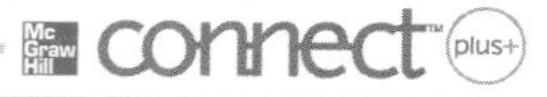

CREATING A COLLECTION LETTER

Create a collection letter for the patient you added to the collection list in Exercise 13.2.

Date: September 30, 2016

1. Verify that Medisoft Network Professional is open and that the Medisoft Program Date is set to September 30, 2016.
2. On the Reports menu, select Collection Reports and then Patient Collection Letters. The Print Report Where? dialog box appears. Accept the default entry to preview the report on the

screen, and click the Start button. The Data Selection Questions dialog box appears.

3. Leave the Responsible Party Range and the Patient Range boxes blank. Enter ***9/30/2016*** in both Follow Up Date Range boxes.
4. Leave the other boxes as they are, except for the check boxes at the bottom of the dialog box. Click the first two check boxes—Exclude items that follow Payment Plan and Generate Collection Letters. When you click the second check box, the third check box—Add to Collection Tracer—is automatically checked. All three check boxes are now checked.
5. Click the OK button. The collection letter report with Jo Wong's information appears.
6. Click the Close button to exit the Preview window.
7. A Confirm dialog box is displayed, asking if collection letters should be printed. Click the Yes button.
8. The Open Report window appears, with the Collection Letter option selected. Click OK.
9. The Print Report Where? dialog box appears. Accept the default entry to preview the report on the screen, and click the Start button.
10. The collection letter for Jo Wong is displayed in the Preview window. To print the report, you would click the print button on the toolbar. For the purposes of this text, assume the report has been printed. Click the Close button to exit the Preview window. (*Note*: In an actual office setting, if the letter is not printed, the account alert message feature illustrated in the next step will not work.)
11. Open the Transaction Entry dialog box, and select Jo Wong in the Chart field. Notice that the letters *RB IC* appear in red in the upper-left section of the window. This is an account alert message, indicating that the account has a remainder balance and is in collections. Close the Transaction Entry dialog box.

 **You have completed Exercise 13.3**

Creating a Collection Tracer Report

A **collection tracer report** is used to keep track of collection letters that were sent. The report lists the tickler item number, the responsible party, the chart number, the account balance (as of the date the tickler was created), the date the collection letter was sent, and the reasons the account is in collections (see Figure 13.17).

collection tracer report tool for keeping track of collection letters that were sent

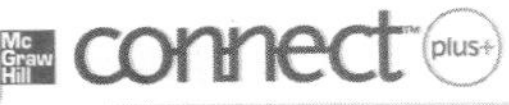

EXERCISE 13.4

CREATING A COLLECTION TRACER REPORT

Create a collection tracer report.

Date: September 30, 2016

1. Verify that Medisoft Network Professional is open and that the Medisoft Program Date is still set to September 30, 2016.

(continued)

(Continued)

2. On the Reports menu, select Collection Reports and then Collection Tracer Report.
3. In the Print Report Where? dialog box, click the Start button to preview the report on the screen.
4. In the Data Selection Questions dialog box, select Jo Wong in both Responsible Party Range boxes.
5. Leave the Date Letter Sent Range boxes blank to include all dates.
6. Click the OK button.
7. The report appears in the Preview window. When you are finished viewing the report, close the Preview window.

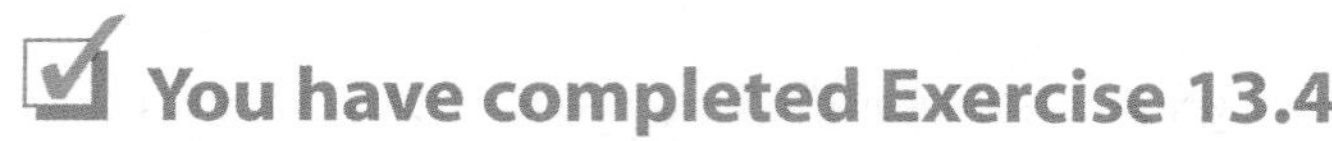
You have completed Exercise 13.4

Family Care Clinic

Collection Tracer Report

10/31/2016

Item #	Responsible Party	Patient Chart	Balance	Date Letter Sent	Reasons
Elizabeth Jones					
2	Elizabeth Jones	JONESEL0	28.64	10/31/2016	The outstanding balance is greater than 0.01.
					Total Letters Sent: 1
Kristin Zapata					
3	Kristin Zapata	ZAPATKR0	247.50	10/31/2016	The outstanding balance is greater than 0.01.
					Total Letters Sent: 1

Figure 13.17 Collection Tracer Report

payment plan agreement between a patient and a practice in which the patient agrees to make regular monthly payments over a specified period of time

Equal Credit Opportunity Act (ECOA) law that prohibits credit discrimination on the basis of race, color, religion, national origin, sex, marital status, or age, or because a person receives public assistance

13.6 Payment Plans

For large bills or special situations, some practices may offer payment plans to patients. A **payment plan** is an agreement between a patient and a practice in which the patient agrees to make regular monthly payments over a specified period of time.

Equal Credit Opportunity Act

The Federal Trade Commission (FTC) enforces the **Equal Credit Opportunity Act (ECOA),** which prohibits credit discrimination on

THINKING IT THROUGH 13.5

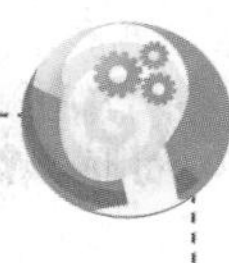

In the collection tracer report in Figure 13.17, which patient has the greater balance? How much is the patient's balance?

the basis of race, color, religion, national origin, sex, marital status, age, or because a person receives public assistance. If the practice decides not to extend credit to a particular patient while extending it to others, under the ECOA the patient has a right to know why. Factors like income, expenses, debts, and credit history are among the considerations lenders use to determine creditworthiness. The practice must be specific in answering such questions.

Financial Agreements

If no finance charges are applied to unpaid balances, this type of arrangement is between the practice and the patient, and no additional legal regulations apply. If, however, the practice adds finance charges or late fees and the payments are to be made in more than four installments, the arrangement is subject to the **Truth in Lending Act,** which is part of the Consumer Credit Protection Act. In this case, the practice notifies the patient in writing about the total amount, the finance charges (stated as a percentage), the amount of each payment and when it is due, and the date the last payment is due. The agreement must be signed by the patient.

Truth in Lending Act part of the federal Consumer Credit Protection Act that regulates collection practices related to finance charges and late fees

For example, the following schedule might be followed:

$50 balance or less: Entire balance due the first month

$51–$500 balance: $50 minimum monthly payment

$501–$1,000 balance: $100 minimum monthly payment

$1,001–$2,500 balance: $200 minimum monthly payment

Over $2,500 balance: 10 percent of the balance due each month

Collection specialists work out payment plans using patient information such as the amount of the bill, the patient's payday, the amount of disposable income the patient has, and any other contributing factors.

Assigning a Payment Plan to a Patient's Account

Most practices have a number of different plans. These plans vary depending on:

- The day of the month the payment is due (for example, 10th, 20th, 30th)
- How often the payment occurs (for example, every 30 days)
- The amount of the payment (for example, $20, $40)

If a payment plan is assigned and the patient follows the plan (that is, pays the required amount by the required date), the patient will not be sent collection letters. However, if the plan is not followed, letters will be sent.

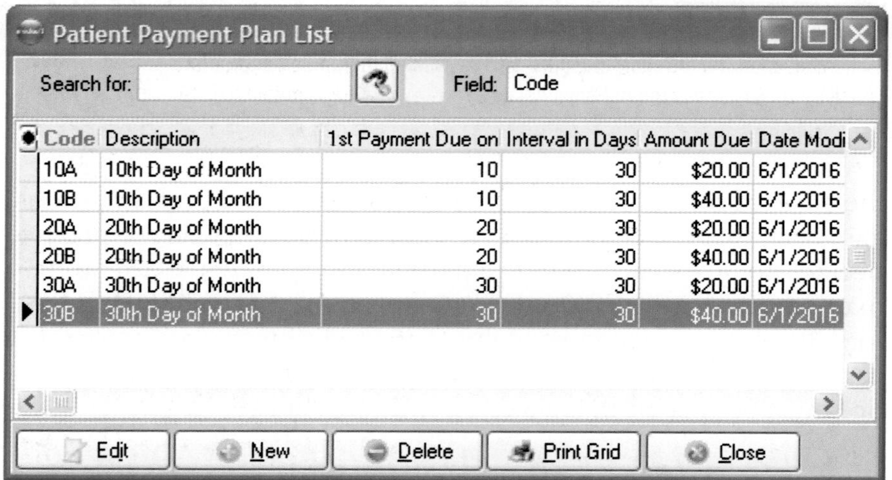

Figure 13.18 Patient Payment Plan List Dialog Box

In MNP, payment plans are set up in the Patient Payment Plan List dialog box, which is accessed via the Lists menu. Figure 13.18 shows the payment plans already set up for the Family Care Clinic.

Once set up, payment plans are assigned to patient accounts in the Payment Plan tab of the Patient/Guarantor dialog box (see Figure 13.19).

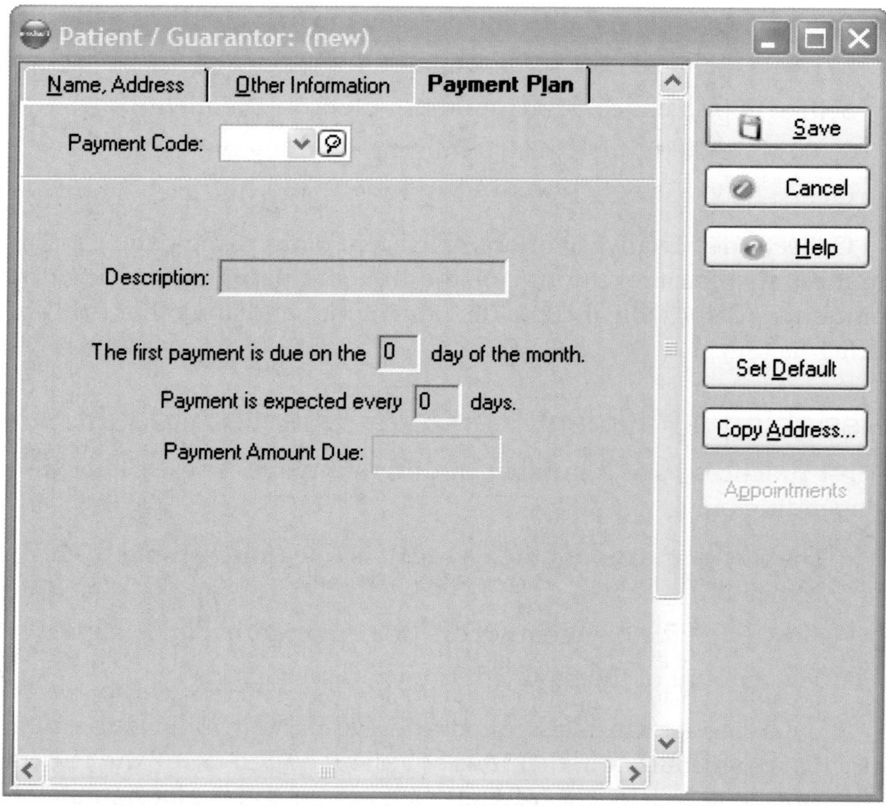

Figure 13.19 Payment Plan Tab

THINKING IT THROUGH 13.6

A patient owes the physician $2,400 for a surgical procedure. Based on the payment schedule shown in this section of the chapter, what monthly payment is the biller likely to set up?

Selecting a plan in the Payment Code field assigns a specific payment amount, due date, and schedule of payments. Once the Payment Code is entered, the program automatically completes the rest of the fields.

Mc Graw Hill connect plus+

EXERCISE 13.5

ASSIGNING A PAYMENT PLAN

Assign a payment plan to an overdue patient account.

Date: October 31, 2016

1. Verify that Medisoft Network Professional is open and that the Medisoft Program Date is set to October 31, 2016.
2. Select Patients/Guarantors and Cases on the Lists menu.
3. Key ***Z*** in the Search for box to locate Kristin Zapata's record, and click the Edit Patient button.
4. The Patient/Guarantor dialog box appears. Click the Payment Plan tab.
5. Click the triangle button in the Payment Code field to display the list of payment plan codes currently in the database. From the list, select code 20A.
6. When you select code 20A, information is displayed in the bottom panel of the dialog box. Verify that 20A is the plan that requires a $20.00 payment, every 30 days, on the 20th day of the month.
7. Click the Save button to save the new payment plan assigned to Kristin Zapata.
8. You are returned to the Patient List dialog box. Click the Close button to close the Patient List dialog box.

You have completed Exercise 13.5

13.7 Collection Agencies

Office staff members encounter a number of problems in their collections work. For example, a patient may have moved without leaving a forwarding address. After a number of collection attempts that do not produce results, some practices use collection agencies to pursue large unpaid bills. A **collection agency** is an outside firm hired to collect on delinquent accounts. The agency that is selected should have a reputation for fair and ethical handling of collections.

collection agency outside firm hired to collect on delinquent accounts

THINKING IT THROUGH 13.7

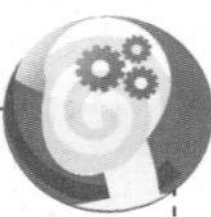

Under HIPAA and HITECH, collection agencies are considered business associates of the practice. Based on the information in Chapter 2, are business associates required to comply with the HIPAA Privacy and Security Rules?

When a patient's account is referred to an agency for collection, the office staff members no longer contact the patient or send statements. If a payment is received from a patient while the account is with the agency, the agency is notified. Collection agencies are often paid on the basis of the amount of money they collect. For example, an agency may keep 30 percent of the amount it collects.

When a payment is received from a collection agency, it must be posted to the patient's account. The agency provides a statement that shows which patients' accounts have paid and the amounts of the payments.

EXERCISE 13.6

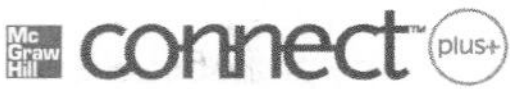

POSTING A PAYMENT FROM A COLLECTION AGENCY

The practice has received a payment from a collection agency for Ali Mazloum's account, which has an overdue balance of $720.50. Per the Family Care Clinic's financial policy, the account was assigned to the agency once it was more than ninety days past due. The statement included with the payment indicates that the agency collected 50 percent of the amount owed, or $360.25, as payment in full. The agency then subtracted its fee of 25 percent ($90.06), leaving a payment of $270.19 to the provider. Post this amount to the patient's account in MNP.

Amount owed:	$720.50
Amount collected:	$360.25
Fees:	$90.06
Net paid to provider:	$270.19

Date: October 31, 2016

1. Verify that Medisoft Network Professional is open and that the Medisoft Program Date is set to October 31, 2016.
2. On the Activities menu, click Enter Transactions. The Transaction Entry dialog box is displayed.
3. Key ***M*** in the Chart box, and press Tab to select Ali Mazloum.
4. Verify that Accidental fall is active in the Case box.
5. In the Payments, Adjustments, And Comments section of the dialog box, click the New button.
6. Verify that the entry in the Date box is 10/31/2016.
7. Click the Pay/Adj Code box twice to display the list of codes. Select the payment code 04—Collections payment, and press Tab.
8. Verify that Mazloum, Ali—Guarantor is listed in the Who Paid box.
9. Enter ***Collections payment*** in the Description field, and press Tab twice.

10. Enter the amount of the payment, ***270.19***, in the Amount box, and press Tab.
11. The Unapplied box at the end of the transaction line should read ($270.19).
12. Click the Apply button. The Apply Payment to Charges dialog box is displayed.
13. In the first line of charges, the amount owed is $178.00. Since the payment is for more than $178.00, you will enter $178.00 toward this charge and the remaining amount to the other charges. Enter ***178.00*** in the This Payment box for the first charge, and press Enter.
14. Check the amount that is listed in the upper-right corner of the dialog box to see the amount of the payment that is still unapplied (–92.19). Enter the remaining unapplied amount to the charge on the second line, and press Enter.
15. Click the Close button.
16. Back in the Transaction Entry dialog box, click the Save Transactions button to save the entry for the collections payment.
17. Notice that the previous account total, $720.50, has been reduced by the amount of the collections payment, $270.19, and is now $450.31. Close the Transaction Entry dialog box.

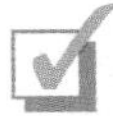 **You have completed Exercise 13.6**

13.8 Write-offs and Refunds

When all collection attempts have been exhausted and the cost of continuing to pursue the debt is higher than the total amount owed, the collection process is ended. Medical practices have policies on how to handle bills they do not expect to collect. Usually, the amount owed is called an **uncollectible account** or a bad debt.

uncollectible account account that does not respond to collection efforts and is written off the practice's expected accounts receivable

means test process of fairly determining a patient's ability to pay

Types of Uncollectible Accounts

The most common reason an account becomes uncollectible is that a patient cannot pay the bill. Under federal and state laws there are **means tests** that help a practice decide whether patients are indigent (categorized as poor). Patients complete a form that is used to evaluate their ability to pay. A combination of factors, such as their income level (verified by recent federal tax returns) compared to the federal poverty level, their other expenses, and the practice's policies, are used to determine what percentage of the bill will be declared uncollectible.

Other reasons for uncollectible accounts include the following:

- A patient cannot be located.
- A patient has died. Large unpaid balances of deceased patients may be pursued, either by filing an estate claim or by working in a considerate manner with the deceased patient's family members.

bankruptcy declaration that a person is unable to pay his or her debts

write-off balance that has been removed from a patient's account

- A patient has filed for **bankruptcy.** Debtors may choose to file for bankruptcy when they determine that they will not be able to repay the money they owe. When a patient files for bankruptcy, the practice, which is considered to be an unsecured creditor, must file a claim in order to join the group of creditors that may receive some compensation for unpaid bills. Claims must be filed by the date specified by the bankruptcy court, or the right to any money from the bankruptcy case will be forfeited.

Writing Off Uncollectible Accounts

On rare occasions, practices sue individuals to collect the money they are owed. Usually, though, rather than going through the expense of a court case with uncertain results, the practice deems an unpaid balance to be uncollectible and writes it off the expected accounts receivable. A **write-off** is a balance that has been removed from a patient's account.

WARNING!

In the Medicare and Medicaid programs, it is fraudulent to forgive or write off any payments that beneficiaries are responsible for, such as copayments and coinsurance, unless a rigid set of steps has been followed to verify the patient's financial situation. Similarly, it is fraudulent to discount services for other providers or their families, which was formerly a common practice.

EXERCISE 13.7

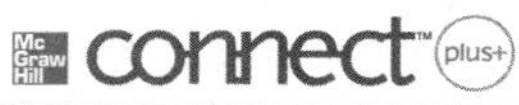

WRITING OFF AN UNCOLLECTIBLE PATIENT BALANCE

The collection agency accepted 50 percent of the amount owed by Ali Mazloum as payment in full. The practice manager has informed you that the remaining balance is to be written off, even though it is a significant amount.

Date: November 30, 2016

1. Verify that Medisoft Network Professional is open and that the Medisoft Program Date is set to November 30, 2016.
2. Open the Transaction Entry dialog box, and select Ali Mazloum's chart number.
3. Verify that Accidental fall is selected in the Case box.
4. In the Payments, Adjustments, And Comments section of the dialog box, click the New button.
5. Verify that the entry in the Date box is 11/30/2016.
6. Click the Pay/Adj Code box twice to display the drop-down list of codes. Key ***W*** to locate WRITEOFF in the list, and then press Tab.
7. Open the drop-down list in the Who Paid box, and select Mazloum, Ali. Press Tab three times.
8. Enter the amount to be written off, ***450.31***, in the Amount box, and press Tab.

9. The Unapplied box reads ($450.31). Click the Apply button.
10. Since WRITEOFF is an adjustment code, the Apply Adjustment to Charges dialog box is displayed.
11. Locate the Balance column. In the This Adjust. column, enter an amount equal to the amount in the Balance column for each outstanding charge, pressing Enter after each entry.
12. When all the charges have been adjusted, the Unapplied amount in the upper-right corner of the dialog box displays 0.00. Click the Close button to close the Apply Adjustment to Charges dialog box.
13. Click the Save Transactions button to save the WRITEOFF adjustment.
14. Confirm that the amount listed under Account Total is now 0.00.
15. Close the Transaction Entry dialog box.

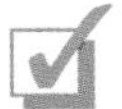 **You have completed Exercise 13.7**

Small Balances

small-balance account overdue patient account in which the amount owed is less than the cost of pursuing payment

Practices also have policies that determine when amounts due are not worth pursuing. The cost of dealing with **small-balance accounts** can exceed the amounts eventually collected, making pursuing collection a poor use of the practice's resources.

In MNP, small-balance accounts can be written off for a single patient, or in batches for multiple patients. When the program writes off the balances, several other features are updated:

- Write-off entries are created and applied to all patient-responsible charges associated with the patient
- The Collection List items associated with the account are updated
- Statements are changed to the status of Done
- A note is added to the write-off entries

Single patient balances are written off in the Apply Charges/Adjustments to Payments dialog box, accessed through the Deposit List dialog box. Multiple patients' write-offs are accomplished using the Small Balance Write-off feature, which is an option on the Activities menu (see Figure 13.20).

When the Small Balance Write-off option is selected on the Activities menu, the Small Balance Write-off dialog box appears (see Figure 13.21).

The Small Balance Write-off dialog box contains two panels: Patient Selection and Write off. The Patient Selection panel, on the left side of the dialog box, lists the criteria required for a balance to be written off.

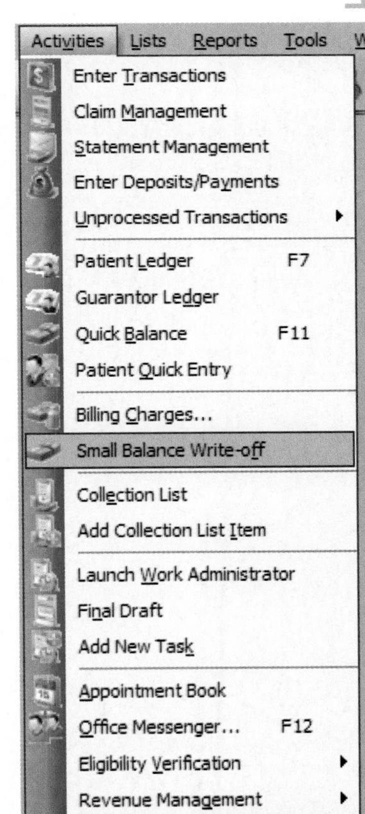

Figure 13.20 Small Balance Write-off Option on the Activities Menu

All or Delinquent Patients Determines whether balances are written off for all patients, or only for patients with overdue accounts. To be

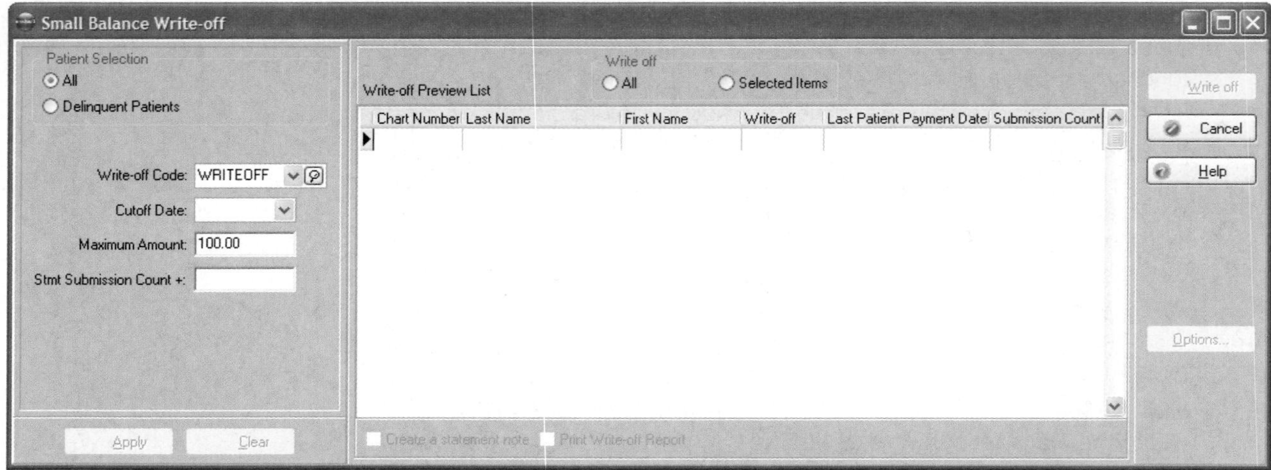

Figure 13.21 Small Balance Write-off Dialog Box

classified as delinquent, a patient must be assigned a payment plan and not have made the required payment.

Write-off Code This field contains the default adjustment code that was set up in Program Options.

Cutoff Date Patients whose last payments were made before this date will be included in the write-off list.

Maximum Amount Lists the maximum amount that will be written off any transaction in the patient's account.

Stmt Submission Count + Lists the number of times a statement must be mailed to the patient before the account can be eligible for small balance write-off.

When the Apply button is clicked, the program searches for accounts that meet the criteria specified in these fields. The results are displayed in the Write off panel on the right side of the dialog box. Patients who met the criteria are listed in the Write-off Preview List, along with the amounts of the proposed write-off.

All or Selected Items Determines whether balances are written off for all patients on the Preview List or just for selected patients. Use the CTRL key to select more than one patient, but fewer than all patients.

Create a Statement Note Adds a note to each write-off that the statement is marked Done.

Print Write-off Report Generates a report that lists the write-offs and the note for each write-off.

Selected Count Displays the number of patient accounts selected in the Preview List.

To write off selected balances, click the Write off button.

connect plus+ EXERCISE 13.8

WRITING OFF SMALL-BALANCE ACCOUNTS

Write off all overdue accounts with a balance of less than $20, a last payment date no later than November 30, 2016, and at least one statement sent.

Date: November 30, 2016

1. Verify that Medisoft Network Professional is open and that the Medisoft Program Date is set to November 30, 2016.
2. Select Small Balance Write-off on the Activities menu. The Small Balance Write-off dialog box is displayed.
3. In the Patient Selection panel on the left, confirm that All is selected.
4. Verify that WRITEOFF is selected as the Write-off Code.
5. Enter ***11/30/2016*** in the Cutoff Date field, and press Tab.
6. Enter ***20*** in the Maximum Amount field, and press Tab.
7. Enter ***1*** in the Stmt Submission Count + field.
8. Click the Apply button. A Confirm dialog box appears with a detailed message about recalculating patient remainder balances and asking if you want to continue. Click OK.
9. The program then recalculates the balances and lists patients who meet the criteria in the Write-off Preview List on the right side of the dialog box. In this instance, one patient, Jo Wong, meets the criteria. Since he has an outstanding amount of $7.47 in two cases (Bronchitis and Increased urination), the total write-off amount is $14.94.
10. Confirm that All is selected in the Write off section above the Preview List.
11. Click the first check box, Create a statement note, located below the Preview List.
12. Leave the second check box, Print Write-off Report, blank.
13. Click the Write off button in the top right of the dialog box. The amount is written off and removed from the Preview List.
14. Close the Small Balance Write-off dialog box.
15. To confirm that the write-off has occurred, open the Transaction Entry dialog box and review Jo Wong's account. Verify that the Increased urination case is selected.
16. Notice that an entry WRITEOFF appears in the Payments, Adjustments, And Comments section, with the description, Small Balance Write-off, in the Description box.
17. Select the Bronchitis case and verify the write-off in that case also. Notice the Account Total at the top of the dialog box is now 0.00.
18. Click the line that lists the write-off to select it. Then click the Note button at the bottom of the Payments, Adjustments, And Comments section.
19. The Transaction Documentation dialog box is displayed. The statement note that the program created as part of the write-off appears in the Documentation/Notes box. Click the Cancel button to close the Transaction Documentation dialog box.
20. Close the Transaction Entry dialog box.

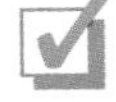

You have completed Exercise 13.8

THINKING IT THROUGH 13.8

Why would a practice write off accounts with small balances? Why not try to collect all monies owed to the practice?

Patient Refunds

patient refund money owed to a patient

The medical office focuses on accounts receivable, but at times the practice may need to issue **patient refunds.** Refunds are made when the practice has overcharged a patient for a service and must return the extra amount, or when a patient has overpaid an account. Note that the balance due must be refunded promptly if the practice has completed the patient's care. However, if the practice is still treating the patient, the credit balance may be carried forward—that is, noted on the patient's statement and account to be applied toward the copayment or other charges for the next visit.

EXERCISE 13.9

connect plus+

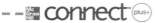

ISSUING A PATIENT REFUND

Process a refund for a patient who has overpaid on his account.

Date: October 3, 2016

1. Verify that Medisoft Network Professional is open and that the Medisoft Program Date is set to October 3, 2016.
2. Open the Transaction Entry dialog box.
3. In the Chart box, key ***SM***, and press Tab to select James L. Smith.
4. Verify that Facial nerve paralysis is displayed in the Case box.
5. Notice that the entry in the Charges section of the window is highlighted in yellow, indicating that this is an overpaid charge. According to the patient's insurance plan, the plan pays 80 percent of charges and the patient pays 20 percent. In this case, 20 percent of the charges ($210) is $42. However, the patient paid $52 and is therefore due a refund of $10. For this reason, the Account Total at the top of the dialog box shows a credit of $10.00.
6. Click the New button in the Payments, Adjustments, And Comments section of the dialog box.
7. Accept the default entry of 10/3/2016 in the Date box.
8. Click the Pay/Adj Code box twice to display the drop-down list, and key ***P*** to locate PTREFUND, the patient refund code. Press Tab.
9. Select Smith, James—Guarantor in the Who Paid box.
10. Enter ***Overpaid—refund*** in the Description box, and press Tab twice to get to the Amount box.
11. Enter ***10*** in the Amount box, and press Tab. Notice that the amount is listed as a positive amount.
12. The Unapplied Amount box should read $10.00.
13. Enter ***4561*** in the Check Number box, and press Tab.

14. Click the Apply button. The Apply Adjustment to Charges dialog box is displayed.
15. Notice that the amount of this refund ($10) is listed in the Unapplied box at the upper-right of the dialog box.
16. Click in the white box in the This Adjust. column. Key ***10***, and press Enter.
17. Click the Close button.
18. Click the Save Transactions button. When a box appears indicating that the statement has been marked done, click OK.
19. Notice that the line listing the procedure charge has changed from yellow (overpaid) to white (fully paid), indicating that the expected amount has been paid. The Account Total at the top of the dialog box is now 0.00.
20. Close the Transaction Entry dialog box.

 **You have completed Exercise 13.9**

chapter 13 summary

LEARNING OUTCOME	KEY CONCEPTS/EXAMPLES
13.1 Explain why it is important to collect overdue balances from patients. Page 636	It is important to collect overdue balances because sums that are not collected are subtracted from income, reducing working capital, meaning that the practice might have to borrow funds and pay interest on those amounts just to pay bills. The average patient is now responsible for paying nearly 35 percent of medical bills, so overdue balances can represent a large part of the practice's income.
13.2 Describe the way in which financial policies help establish payment expectations. Pages 636–637	A financial policy is used to communicate how a practice handles financial matters, such as past-due balances and payments for services not covered by insurance. When patients are aware of and understand a practice's financial policy, they are more likely to pay their accounts on time.
13.3 Describe the procedures followed to identify overdue accounts. Pages 637–647	To identify overdue accounts, create and review a patient aging report. Add the overdue accounts to the collection list, and enter tickler items for them.
13.4 Identify the major federal laws that govern the collection process. Page 647	The Fair Debt Collection Practices Act of 1977 and the Telephone Consumer Protection Act of 1991 regulate debt collections.
13.5 Explain how letters are used in collecting overdue payments. Pages 647–654	A collection letter is most patients' first notice that their bills are past due. (Some practices send a second statement if the first is not paid before they send a collection letter.) Collection letters are generally brief and to the point while preserving a professional and courteous tone. They remind patients of the practice's payment options and their responsibility to pay the debt. Accounts that are further past due receive more aggressive letters.
13.6 Explain payment plans. Pages 654–657	A payment plan is an agreement between a patient and a practice in which the patient agrees to make regular monthly payments over a specified period of time.

LEARNING OUTCOME	KEY CONCEPTS/EXAMPLES
13.7 Discuss the use of collection agencies to pursue patients who have not paid overdue bills. Pages 657–659	A collection agency is an outside firm hired to collect on delinquent accounts. The practice looks for an agency with a reputation for fair and ethical handling of collections. When a patient's account is referred to an agency for collection, the office staff members no longer contact the patient or send statements. The agency provides a statement that shows which patients' accounts have paid and the amounts of the payments. Collection agencies are often paid on the basis of the amount of money they collect.
13.8 Describe the procedures for clearing uncollectible balances and small balances from patients' accounts receivable. Pages 659–665	To clear uncollectible balances, in the Payments, Adjustments, And Comments section of the Transaction Entry dialog box, choose the New button, then fill in and choose the relevant entries, using WRITEOFF—Write off as the Pay/Adj code. To clear small balances, choose Small Balance Write-off in the Activities menu. In Patient Selection, choose All or Delinquent Patients, set the other parameters, and review the resulting list before clearing the accounts.

chapter review

MATCHING QUESTIONS

Match the key terms with their definitions.

_____ 1. ***[LO 13.7]*** collection agency

_____ 2. ***[LO 13.3]*** collection list

_____ 3. ***[LO 13.5]*** collection tracer report

_____ 4. ***[LO 13.6]*** payment plan

_____ 5. ***[LO 13.4]*** Fair Debt Collection Practices Act of 1977 (FDCPA)

_____ 6. ***[LO 13.3]*** tickler

_____ 7. ***[LO 13.8]*** uncollectible account

_____ 8. ***[LO 13.8]*** write-off

_____ 9. ***[LO 13.8]*** patient refund

_____ 10. ***[LO 13.6]*** Truth in Lending Act

a. An agreement between a patient and a practice in which the patient agrees to make regular monthly payments over a specified period of time.

b. A reminder to follow up on an account.

c. An outside firm hired to collect on delinquent accounts.

d. An account that does not respond to collection efforts and is written off the practice's expected accounts receivable.

e. A balance that is removed from a patient's account.

f. A part of the federal Consumer Credit Protection Act that regulates collection practices related to finance charges and late fees.

g. A tool for tracking activities that need to be completed as part of the collection process.

h. A tool for tracking collection letters that were sent.

i. A federal law regulating collection practices.

j. Money that is owed to a patient.

TRUE-FALSE QUESTIONS

Decide whether each statement is true or false.

_____ 1. ***[LO 13.7]*** Accounts that are overdue are treated equally; accounts with small balances are just as likely to be sent for collections as accounts with large balances.

_____ 2. ***[LO 13.4]*** Collection activities regarding patient accounts are considered business collections and are not regulated by federal or state law.

_____ 3. ***[LO 13.6]*** By law, payment plans cannot include finance charges.

_____ 4. ***[LO 13.3]*** Aging reports are used to determine which accounts are overdue.

_____ 5. ***[LO 13.3]*** An account is considered current if it is paid within thirty days.

_____ 6. ***[LO 13.3]*** A tickler item entered on the collection list includes a follow-up date for action.

_____ 7. ***[LO 13.5]*** Accounts that are further past due receive the same letters as accounts that have only recently become past due.

_____ 8. ***[LO 13.6]*** The Equal Credit Opportunity Act (ECOA) prohibits credit discrimination on the basis of race, color, religion, national origin, sex, marital status, or age, or because a person receives public assistance.

_____ 9. ***[LO 13.7]*** A collection agency is an internal part of a medical office that specializes in collecting on delinquent accounts.

_____ 10. ***[LO 13.8]*** A practice sometimes deems an unpaid balance to be uncollectible and writes it off the expected accounts receivable.

MULTIPLE-CHOICE

Select the letter that best completes the statement or answers the question.

1. ***[LO 13.3]*** In the Collection List dialog box, the entry in the Type field, which describes the responsible party, is either *P* for Patient or _____.
   a. *G* for Guarantor
   b. *C* for Child
   c. *I* for Insurance
   d. D for Doctor

2. ***[LO 13.4]*** General regulations for telephone collection practices recommend not calling before 8:00 A.M. or after _____.
   a. 8:00 P.M.
   b. 9:00 P.M.
   c. 5:00 P.M.
   d. 10:00 P.M.

3. ***[LO 13.6]*** An arrangement in which a patient agrees to make a regular monthly payment on an account for a specified period of time is known as a _____.
   a. financial plan
   b. payment plan
   c. payment policy
   d. means test

4. ***[LO 13.8]*** An account that must be written off the practice's expected accounts receivable is _____.
   a. an overdue account
   b. a patient refund account
   c. a tickler account
   d. an uncollectible account

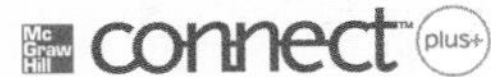

Enhance your learning at **mcgrawhillconnect.com**!
- *Practice Exercises*
- *Worksheets*
- *Activities*
- *Integrated eBook*

5. ***[LO 13.1]*** The average patient is now responsible for paying nearly ________ percent of medical bills.
   a. 10
   b. 25
   c. 35
   d. 50

6. ***[LO 13.3]*** The medical office tracks overdue bills by reviewing the ________.
   a. patient aging report
   b. means test
   c. patient refund report
   d. all of the above

7. ***[LO 13.4]*** Collections from patients are classified as consumer collections and are regulated by ________.
   a. federal laws
   b. state laws
   c. county laws
   d. both a and b

8. ***[LO 13.5]*** For most patients, the collection letter is their ________ notice that their bill is past due.
   a. first
   b. second
   c. third
   d. final

9. ***[LO 13.7]*** After a number of collection attempts that do not produce results, some practices use ________ to pursue large unpaid bills.
   a. patient aging reports
   b. collection agencies
   c. collection tracer reports
   d. bankruptcy

10. ***[LO 13.6]*** If a practice adds finance charges or late fees and the payments are to be made in more than four installments, the arrangement is subject to the ________.
    a. Equal Credit Opportunity Act (ECOA)
    b. Telephone Consumer Protection Act of 1991
    c. Truth in Lending Act
    d. Fair Debt Collection Practices Act of 1977 (FDCPA)

SHORT-ANSWER QUESTIONS

Define the following abbreviations.

1. ***[LO 13.6]*** ECOA ________________________

2. ***[LO 13.4]*** FDCPA ________________________

APPLYING YOUR KNOWLEDGE

Answer the questions below in the space provided.

13.1 ***[LO 13.2]*** What is the purpose of a medical practice's financial policy?

____

____

13.2 ***[LO 13.3]*** What is the first step in the collection process?

____

____

13.3 ***[LO 13.3]*** How is an aging report used to identify accounts for collection?

____

____

13.4 ***[LO 13.5]*** What two steps need to occur before a collection letter can be printed in MNP?

____

____

13.5 ***[LO 13.2]*** Why is it important for a medical practice to share its financial policy with patients?

____

____

13.6 ***[LO 13.7]*** What are the positive and negative factors in using an outside collection agency to pursue overdue patient accounts?

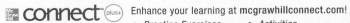

____

____

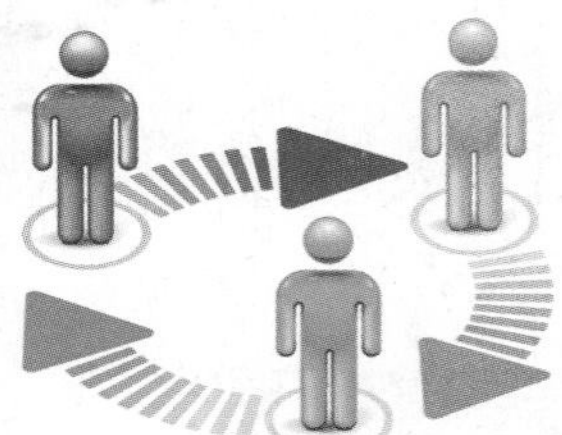

part five

Source Documents

1 source document

FAMILY CARE CLINIC
285 Stephenson Boulevard
Stephenson, OH 60089-4000
614-555-0000

PATIENT INFORMATION FORM

Patient

Last Name	First Name	MI	Sex	Date of Birth
Tanaka	Hiro		__ M X F	2 / 20 / 1981

Address	City	State	Zip
80 Cedar Lane	Stephenson	OH	60089

Home Ph # (614) 555-7373 Cell Ph # (614) 555-0162 Marital Status Single Student Status

SS#	Email	Allergies:
812-73-6000	htanaka@abc.com	penicillin

Employment Status	Employer Name	Work Ph #	Primary Insurance ID#
Full-time	McCray Manufacturing Inc.	(614) 555-1001	812736000 Group HJ31

Employer Address	City	State	Zip
1311 Kings Highway	Stephenson	OH	60089

Referred By: Dr. Bertram Brown Ph # of Referral (614) 567-7896

Responsible Party (Complete this section if the person responsible for the bill is not the patient)

Last Name	First Name	MI	Sex	Date of Birth
			__ M __ F	/ /

Address	City	State	Zip	SS#

Relation to Patient	Employer Name	Work Phone #
__ Spouse __ Parent __ Other		( )

Spouse, or Parent (if minor): Home Phone # ( )

Insurance (If you have multiple coverage, supply information from both carriers)

Primary Carrier Name: OhioCare HMO	Secondary Carrier Name
Name of the Insured (Name on ID Card): Hiro Tanaka	Name of the Insured (Name on ID Card)
Patient's relationship to the insured: X Self __ Spouse __ Child	Patient's relationship to the insured: __ Self __ Spouse __ Child
Insured ID #: 812736000	Insured ID #
Group # or Company Name: Group HJ31	Group # or Company Name
Insurance Address: 147 Central Ave., Haleville, OH 60890	Insurance Address
Phone # 614-555-0101; Copay $ 20; Deductible $	Phone #; Copay $; Deductible $

Other Information

Is patient's condition related to: Reason for visit: Accident - back pain

__ Employment X Auto Accident (if yes, state in which accident occurred: OH) __ Other Accident

Date of Accident: 9/25/2016 Date of First Symptom of Illness: 9/25/2016

Financial Agreement and Authorization for Treatment

I authorize treatment and agree to pay all fees and charges for the person named above. I agree to pay all charges shown by statements, promptly upon their presentation, unless credit arrangements are agreed upon in writing.

I authorize payment directly to FAMILY CARE CLINIC of insurance benefits otherwise payable to me. I hereby authorize the release of any medical information necessary in order to process a claim for payment in my behalf.

Signed: Hiro Tanaka Date: 10/3/2016

source document 2

FAMILY CARE CLINIC
285 Stephenson Boulevard
Stephenson, OH 60089
614-555-0000

KATHERINE YAN, MD
PHYSICIAN'S NOTES

PATIENT NAME: Hiro Tanaka

CHART NUMBER: TANAKHI0

DATE: 10/3/2016

CASE: Accident—Back Pain

NOTES

Condition related to auto accident in Stephenson, Ohio, that occurred on 9/25/2016.

Patient was hospitalized from 9/25/2016 to 9/26/2016.

Patient was totally disabled from 9/25/2016 to 9/26/2016.

Patient was partially disabled from 9/27/2016 to 10/3/2016.

Patient was unable to work from 9/25/2016 to 10/3/2016.

3 source document

FAMILY CARE CLINIC
285 Stephenson Boulevard
Stephenson, OH 60089
614-555-0000

PATIENT NAME: Jorge N. Barrett	**DATE OF BIRTH:** 1/27/1956
CHART NUMBER: BARREJO0	**AGE:** 60
DATE: 10/21/2016	
CASE: Hypertension	

T: 98.6°F P: 88 (reg) R: 14 (unlabored) BP: 184/104 WT: 153 lb

CC: "My wife is worried about my blood pressure."

S: Patient tested his blood pressure at the drug store while picking up a prescription for his wife about a month ago. The reading, he thinks, was about 200/110. His wife, a nurse at Stephenson County Hospital, began checking his blood pressure daily after the initial reading, alternating morning and evening. She has been writing them down and sent a blood pressure log with the patient for this visit. For the last 14 days, his systolic pressure has ranged from a high of 220 to a low of 186. His diastolic pressure has ranged from a high of 110 to a low of 100. The pressures have been taken standing, sitting, and lying down. Because of the readings, his wife encouraged him to seek treatment. He denies symptoms of any kind, and says he feels generally well.

O: Past medical history: Had measles, mumps, and chicken pox as a child; was never immunized for these diseases. Two previous arthroscopic knee surgeries, one in 1986 on the left knee for torn ACL, and one in 1990 on the left knee for removal of bone chips. He reports no problems and a normal recovery following these surgeries. No other major illnesses or hospitalizations. Has migraines, for which he takes Maxalt, 10 mg, PRN. He currently takes a multivitamin daily, and will occasionally take an over-the-counter pain reliever.

Family history: Father deceased at age 81 from complications following a stroke; mother died at 35 (suicide by overdose). Has 3 children, ages 25, 27, and 31, all of whom are alive and well.

Social history: Has never smoked; drinks alcohol socially and estimates consumption at about 3–5 glasses of wine per week. Exercises on a regular basis by working out at a local gym; does about an hour of cardio and aerobic training each workout. He worked as a police officer for 35 years and retired 3 years ago. He now works part-time as a fitness trainer. Has been married for 37 years.

Review of systems: HEENT: Wears glasses for reading. Denies other vision problems. Denies hearing problems. Cardiovascular: Denies chest pain or shortness of breath. GI: No problems with heartburn or elimination. GU: Denies problems with urination or sexual activity. Occasional nocturia. Musculoskeletal: No problems with muscle strength or endurance. Skin: Denies any problems with skin except for occasional dryness during the winter months. Neuro: Denies gait or balance problems. Denies syncopal episodes.

Allergies: Sulfa. Intolerance: Codeine.

Examination: Patient is a well-developed, well-nourished white male in no acute distress. He is alert and oriented in all spheres. HEENT: Normocephalic. Eyes: EOMI. PERRLA. Ears: External ears and auditory canals within normal limits. TMs normal. Oropharynx: Clear. Tongue protrudes in the midline. Throat: Thyroid not palpable. Chest: Clear to auscultation and percussion. Breath sounds full and equal bilaterally. Heart: Normal sinus rhythm without murmurs, gallops, or thrills. Abdomen: Flat and nontender. Extremities: Within normal limits. Deep tendon reflexes 2+ and equal bilaterally. Skin: Within normal limits; survey for nevi is negative. Cranial nerves II through XII intact. Gait normal and unimpaired.

A: Hypertension.

P: Begin lisinopril, 10 mg daily; given 10 days' worth of samples and a prescription sent for #30 to fill as needed.
Patient instructed to avoid alcohol, salt substitutes, or potassium supplements while taking this medication.
Instructed to avoid additional salt in diet.
Asked to check blood pressure daily for the next seven days and continue keeping the blood pressure log.
Return to clinic on 7/19/2016 for recheck and to bring his blood pressure log with him when he returns.
Orders: Hematocrit, calcium, creatinine clearance, fasting glucose, serum potassium, UA, lipid panel, EKG.
Pt. Ed.: Essential hypertension, low-sodium diet.

PATRICIA MCGRATH, MD

4 source document

FAMILY CARE CLINIC
285 Stephenson Boulevard
Stephenson, OH 60089
614-555-0000

PATIENT NAME: Tanaka, Hiro	**DATE OF BIRTH:** 2/20/1981
CHART NUMBER: TANAKHI0	**AGE:** 35
DATE: 10/3/2016	
CASE: Accident—Back Pain	

T: 98.6°F P: 80 (reg) R: 12 (unlabored) BP: 110/70 WT: 98 lb

CC: BACK PAIN

S: Patient is here today on referral from Dr. Bertram Brown. She was involved in a motor vehicle accident on 9/25/2016, hit from behind. She was wearing her seat belt at the time and the car's air bag deployed. The force of the impact caused a brief LOC and she was admitted to the hospital for overnight observation. On release, she was still experiencing stiffness and pain in the lower back with difficulty ambulating. She has been attending physical therapy sessions daily since 9/27/16 and takes ibuprofen, 800 mg t.i.d. for pain. Patient states her pain is now a 2 on a scale of 10, easily managed with the ibuprofen as prescribed.

O: Allergies: Penicillin.
Past medical history: Normal childhood immunizations. Denies surgeries or hospitalizations.
General: Patient is a well-developed, well-nourished 35-year-old Asian woman who appears to be in slight pain, alert and oriented in all spheres.
HEENT: Head: Normocephalic.
Eyes: PERRLA. EOMI.
Neck: Supple; no thyromegaly. No limitation of range of motion.
Back and spine: No spinal tenderness. Lateral bending and forward bending within normal limits with little pain or stiffness. Gait is normal.
Neurological: DTRs are 2+ and equal bilaterally.

A: Low back pain due to motor vehicle accident, resolving.
Allergy to penicillin.

P: Patient is released to return to work 10/4/2016.
Continue with ibuprofen as needed.
May discontinue physical therapy sessions.
Return to clinic if any problems, otherwise for routine preventive care.

KATHERINE YAN, MD

source document 5

ENCOUNTER FORM

DATE: 10/3/2016

TIME: 11:00 am

PATIENT NAME: John Fitzwilliams

CHART #: FITZWJO0

OFFICE VISITS - SYMPTOMATIC		
NEW		
99201	OF--New Patient Minimal	
99202	OF--New Patient Low	
99203	OF--New Patient Detailed	
99204	OF--New Patient Moderate	
99205	OF--New Patient High	
ESTABLISHED		
99211	OF--Established Patient Minimal	
99212	OF--Established Patient Low	X
99213	OF--Established Patient Detailed	
99214	OF--Established Patient Moderate	
99215	OF--Established Patient High	
PREVENTIVE VISITS		
NEW		
99381	Under 1 Year	
99382	1 - 4 Years	
99383	5 - 11 Years	
99384	12 - 17 Years	
99385	18 - 39 Years	
99386	40 - 64 Years	
99387	65 Years & Up	
ESTABLISHED		
99391	Under 1 Year	
99392	1 - 4 Years	
99393	5 - 11 Years	
99394	12 - 17 Years	
99395	18 - 39 Years	
99396	40 - 64 Years	
99397	65 Years & Up	
PROCEDURES		
12011	Simple suture--face--local anes.	
29125	App. of short arm splint; static	
29540	Strapping, ankle	
50390	Aspiration of renal cyst by needle	
71010	Chest x-ray, single view, frontal	

PROCEDURES		
71020	Chest x-ray, two views, frontal & lateral	
71030	Chest x-ray, complete, four views	
73070	Elbow x-ray, AP & lateral views	
73090	Forearm x-ray, AP & lateral views	
73100	Wrist x-ray, AP & lateral views	
73510	Hip x-ray, complete, two views	
73600	Ankle x-ray, AP & lateral views	
LABORATORY		
80019	19 clinical chemistry tests	
80048	Basic metabolic panel	
80061	Lipid panel	
82270	Blood screening, occult; feces	X
82947	Glucose screening--quantitative	
82951	Glucose tolerance test, three specimens	
83718	HDL cholesterol	
84478	Triglycerides test	
85007	Manual differential WBC	
85018	Hemoglobin	
85651	Erythrocyte sedimentation rate--non-auto	
86580	TB Mantoux test	
87072	Culture by commercial kit, nonurine...	
87076	Culture, anerobic isolate	
87077	Bacterial culture, aerobic isolate	
87086	Urine culture and colony count	
87430	Strep test	
87880	Direct streptococcus screen	
INJECTIONS		
90471	Immunization administration	
90703	Tetanus injection	
96372	Injection	
92516	Facial nerve function studies	
93000	Electrocardiogram--ECG with interpretation	
93015	Treadmill stress test, with physician...	
96900	Ultraviolet light treatment	
99070	Supplies and materials provided	

FAMILY CARE CLINIC
285 Stephenson Blvd.
Stephenson, OH 60089
614-555-0000

☐ DANA BANU, MD
☐ ROBERT BEACH, MD
☐ PATRICIA MCGRATH, MD
☐ JESSICA RUDNER, MD
☒ JOHN RUDNER, MD
☐ KATHERINE YAN, MD

NOTES

REFERRING PHYSICIAN	NPI	AUTHORIZATION #

DIAGNOSIS
531.30

PAYMENT AMOUNT
$15 copay, check #456

6 source document

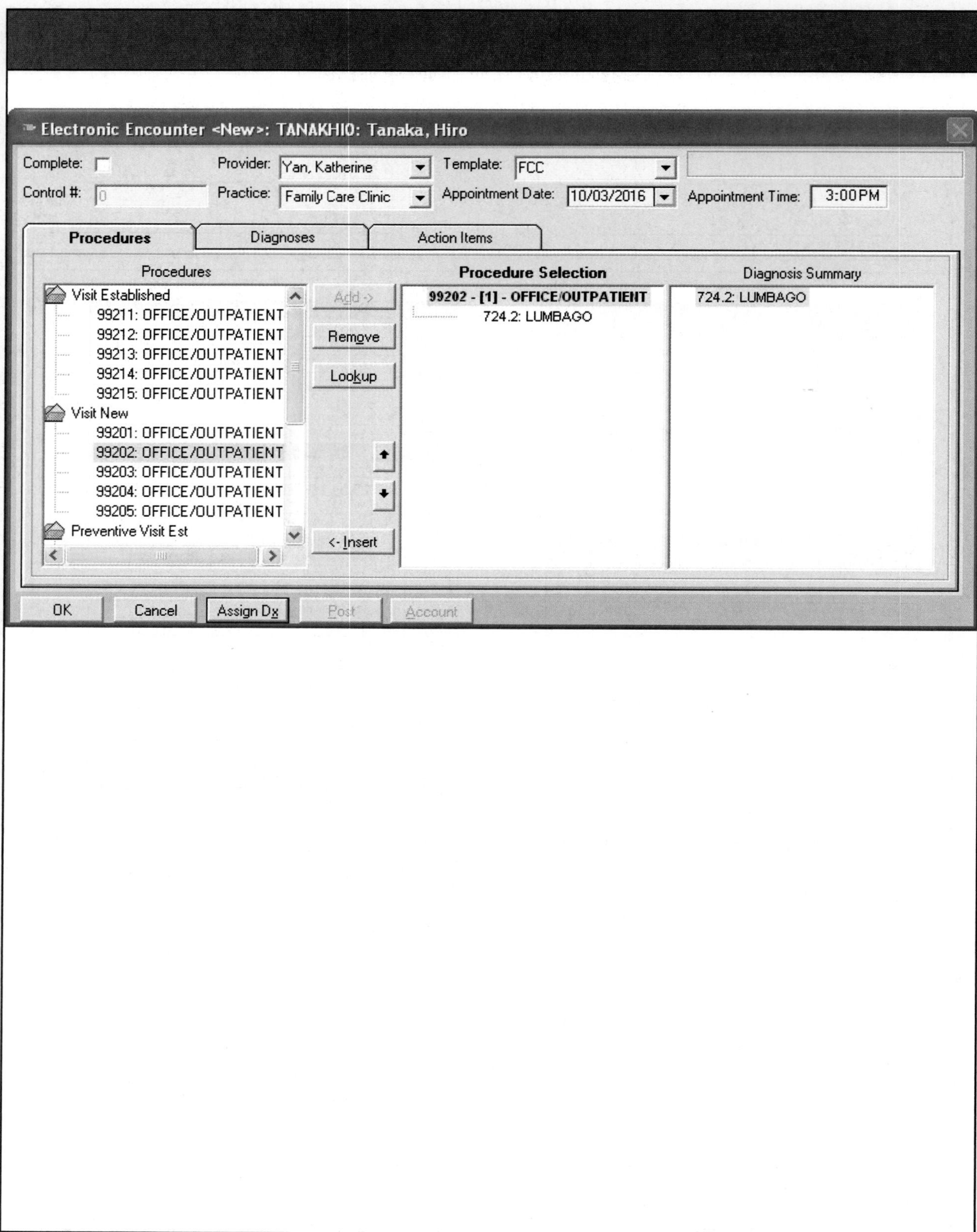
Electronic Encounter <New>: TANAKHI0: Tanaka, Hiro

Complete: [ ] Provider: Yan, Katherine Template: FCC
Control #: 0 Practice: Family Care Clinic Appointment Date: 10/03/2016 Appointment Time: 3:00PM

Procedures | Diagnoses | Action Items

Procedures
- Visit Established
  - 99211: OFFICE/OUTPATIENT
  - 99212: OFFICE/OUTPATIENT
  - 99213: OFFICE/OUTPATIENT
  - 99214: OFFICE/OUTPATIENT
  - 99215: OFFICE/OUTPATIENT
- Visit New
  - 99201: OFFICE/OUTPATIENT
  - 99202: OFFICE/OUTPATIENT
  - 99203: OFFICE/OUTPATIENT
  - 99204: OFFICE/OUTPATIENT
  - 99205: OFFICE/OUTPATIENT
- Preventive Visit Est

Add -> | Remove | Lookup | <- Insert

Procedure Selection
- **99202 - [1] - OFFICE/OUTPATIENT**
  - 724.2: LUMBAGO

Diagnosis Summary
- 724.2: LUMBAGO

OK | Cancel | Assign Dx | Post | Account

source document 7

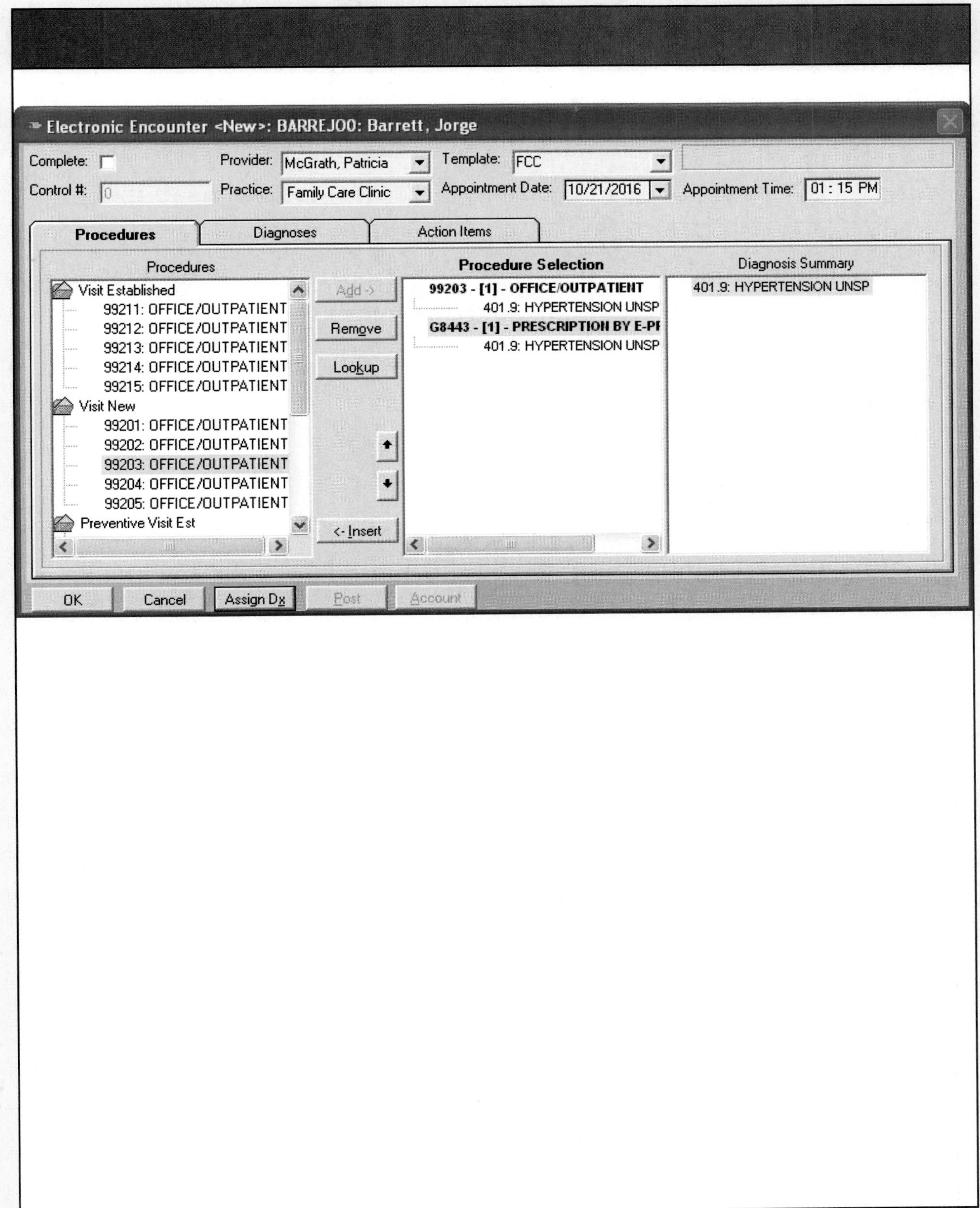

8 source document

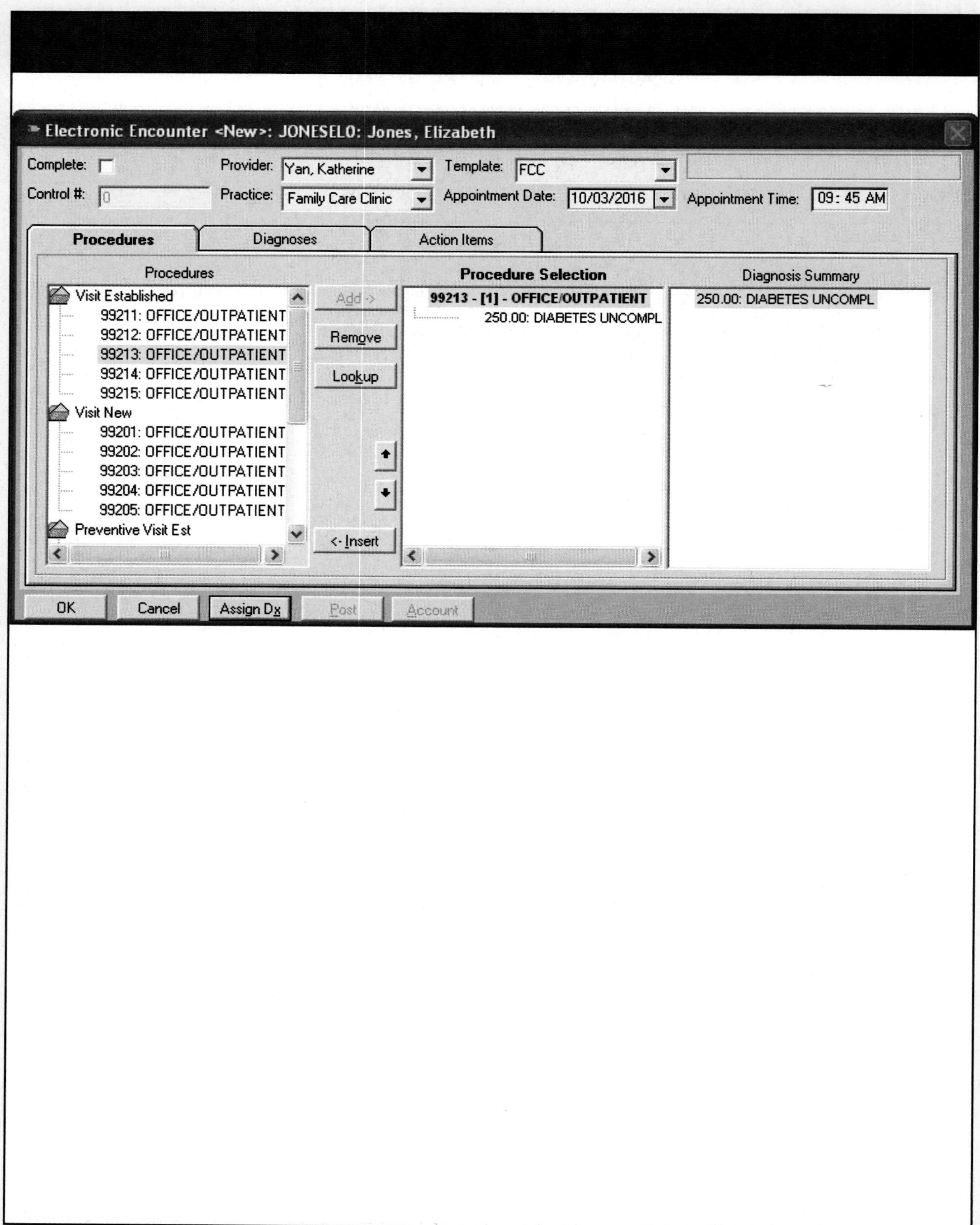

source document 9

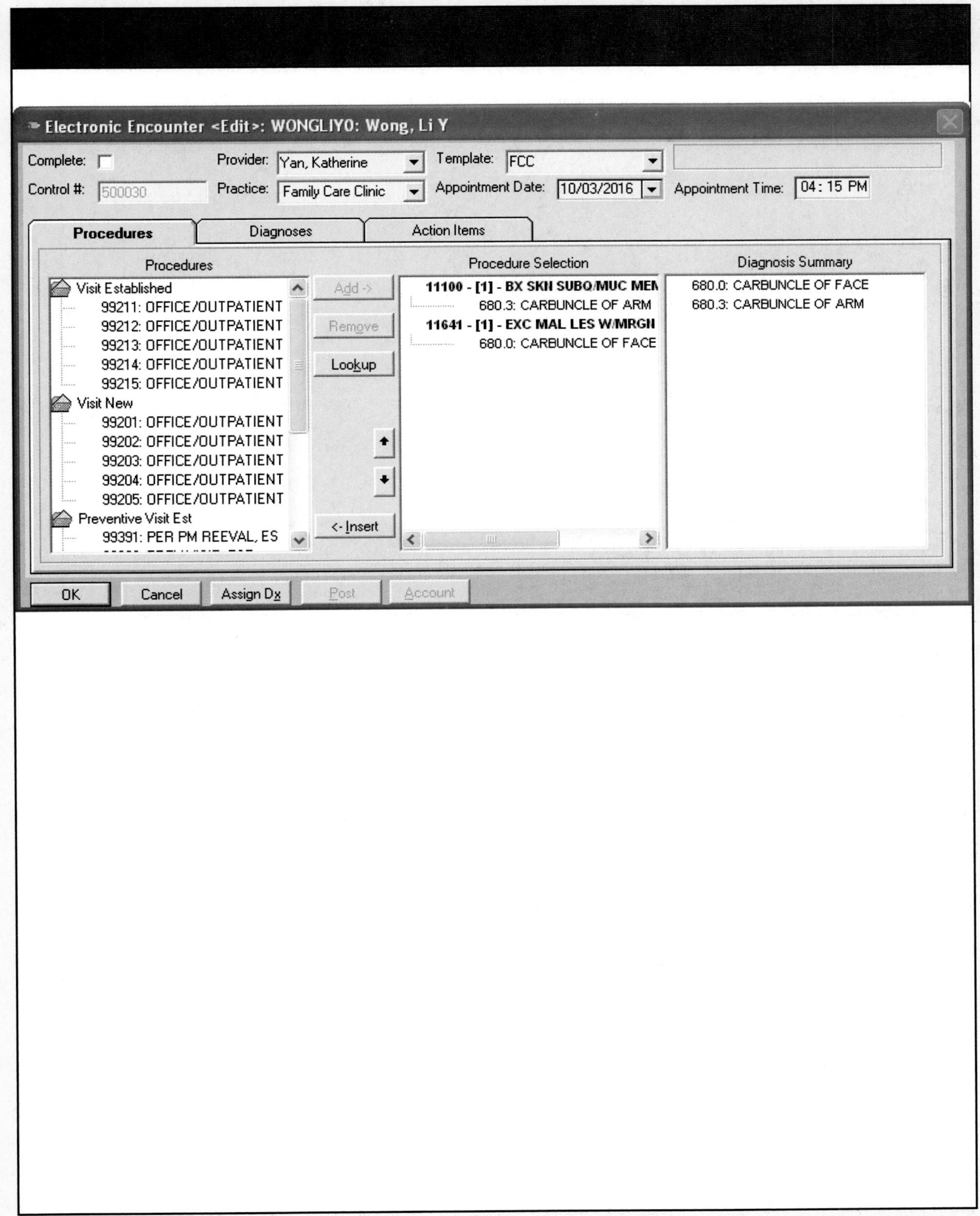

10 source document

CHAMPVA
240 CENTER ST.
COLUMBUS, OH 60220

PROVIDER REMITTANCE
THIS IS NOT A BILL
A PAYMENT SUMMARY AND AN EXPLANATION OF CODES ARE AT THE END OF THIS STATEMENT

FAMILY CARE CLINIC
285 STEPHENSON BLVD.
STEPHENSON, OH 60089-4000

PAGE: 1 OF 1
DATE: 10/03/2016
ID NUMBER: 214778924

PROVIDER: JOHN RUDNER, M.D.

PATIENT: FITZWILLIAMS JOHN CLAIM: 123456789

FROM DATE	THRU DATE	PROC CODE	UNITS	AMOUNT BILLED	AMOUNT ALLOWED	DEDUCT	COPAY/ COINS	PROV PAID	REASON CODE
09/06/16	09/06/16	99211	1	36.00	20.68	.00	15.00	5.68	
09/06/16	09/06/16	84478	1	29.00	8.04	.00	.00	8.04	
	CLAIM TOTALS			64.00	28.72	.00	15.00	13.72	

PROVIDER: KATHERINE YAN, M.D.

PATIENT: FITZWILLIAMS SARAH CLAIM: 234567891

FROM DATE	THRU DATE	PROC CODE	UNITS	AMOUNT BILLED	AMOUNT ALLOWED	DEDUCT	COPAY/ COINS	PROV PAID	REASON CODE
09/06/16	09/06/16	90471	1	15.00	15.00	.00	15.00	.00	
09/06/16	09/06/16	90703	1	29.00	14.30	.00	.00	14.30	
	CLAIM TOTALS			44.00	29.30	.00	15.00	14.30	

******************* CHECK #214778924 IN THE AMOUNT OF $28.02 IS ATTACHED *******************

PAYMENT SUMMARY		TOTAL ALL CLAIMS	
TOTAL AMOUNT PAID	28.02	AMOUNT CHARGED	108.00
PRIOR CREDIT BALANCE	.00	AMOUNT ALLOWED	58.02
CURRENT CREDIT DEFERRED	.00	DEDUCTIBLE	.00
PRIOR CREDIT APPLIED	.00	COPAY	30.00
NEW CREDIT BALANCE	.00	OTHER REDUCTION	.00
NET DISBURSED	28.02		

STATUS CODES:
A - APPROVED AJ - ADJUSTMENT IP - IN PROCESS R - REJECTED V - VOID

source document 11

EAST OHIO PPO
10 CENTRAL AVENUE
HALEVILLE, OH 60890

PROVIDER REMITTANCE
THIS IS NOT A BILL
A PAYMENT SUMMARY AND AN EXPLANATION OF CODES ARE AT THE END OF THIS STATEMENT

FAMILY CARE CLINIC
285 STEPHENSON BLVD.
STEPHENSON, OH 60089-4000

PAGE: 1 OF 2
DATE: 10/03/2016
ID NUMBER: 00146972

PROVIDER: ROBERT BEACH, M.D.

PATIENT: ARLEN SUSAN CLAIM: 123456789

FROM DATE	THRU DATE	PROC CODE	UNITS	AMOUNT BILLED	AMOUNT ALLOWED	DEDUCT	COPAY/ COINS	PROV PAID	REASON CODE
09/05/16	09/05/16	99212	1	54.00	48.60	.00	20.00	28.60	
	CLAIM TOTALS			54.00	48.60	.00	20.00	28.60	

PROVIDER: JOHN RUDNER, M.D.

PATIENT: BELL HERBERT CLAIM: 234567891

FROM DATE	THRU DATE	PROC CODE	UNITS	AMOUNT BILLED	AMOUNT ALLOWED	DEDUCT	COPAY/ COINS	PROV PAID	REASON CODE
09/05/16	09/05/16	99211	1	36.00	32.40	.00	20.00	12.40	
	CLAIM TOTALS			36.00	32.40	.00	20.00	12.40	

PATIENT: BELL SAMUEL CLAIM: 34567891

FROM DATE	THRU DATE	PROC CODE	UNITS	AMOUNT BILLED	AMOUNT ALLOWED	DEDUCT	COPAY/ COINS	PROV PAID	REASON CODE
09/05/16	09/05/16	99212	1	54.00	48.60	.00	20.00	28.60	
	CLAIM TOTALS			54.00	48.60	.00	20.00	28.60	

PROVIDER: KATHERINE YAN, M.D.

PATIENT: BELL JANINE CLAIM: 45678912

FROM DATE	THRU DATE	PROC CODE	UNITS	AMOUNT BILLED	AMOUNT ALLOWED	DEDUCT	COPAY/ COINS	PROV PAID	REASON CODE
09/05/16	09/05/16	99213	1	72.00	64.80	.00	20.00	44.80	
09/05/16	09/05/16	73510	1	124.00	111.60	.00	.00	111.60	
	CLAIM TOTALS			196.00	176.40	.00	20.00	156.40	

PATIENT: BELL JONATHAN CLAIM: 56789123

FROM DATE	THRU DATE	PROC CODE	UNITS	AMOUNT BILLED	AMOUNT ALLOWED	DEDUCT	COPAY/ COINS	PROV PAID	REASON CODE
09/05/16	09/05/16	99394	1	222.00	199.80	.00	20.00	179.80	
	CLAIM TOTALS			222.00	199.80	.00	20.00	179.80	

STATUS CODES:
A - APPROVED AJ - ADJUSTMENT IP - IN PROCESS R - REJECTED V - VOID

EAST OHIO PPO
10 CENTRAL AVENUE
HALEVILLE, OH 60890

PROVIDER REMITTANCE
THIS IS NOT A BILL
A PAYMENT SUMMARY AND AN EXPLANATION OF CODES ARE AT THE END OF THIS STATEMENT

FAMILY CARE CLINIC
285 STEPHENSON BLVD.
STEPHENSON, OH 60089-4000

PAGE: 2 OF 2
DATE: 10/03/2016
ID NUMBER: 00146972

PROVIDER: KATHERINE YAN, M.D.

PATIENT: BELL SARINA CLAIM: 56789123

FROM DATE	THRU DATE	PROC CODE	UNITS	AMOUNT BILLED	AMOUNT ALLOWED	DEDUCT	COPAY/ COINS	PROV PAID	REASON CODE
09/05/16	09/05/16	99213	1	72.00	64.80	.00	20.00	44.80	
	CLAIM TOTALS			72.00	64.80	.00	20.00	44.80	

PAYMENT SUMMARY

TOTAL AMOUNT PAID	450.60
PRIOR CREDIT BALANCE	.00
CURRENT CREDIT DEFERRED	.00
PRIOR CREDIT APPLIED	.00
NEW CREDIT BALANCE	.00
NET DISBURSED	450.60

TOTAL ALL CLAIMS

AMOUNT CHARGED	634.00
AMOUNT ALLOWED	570.60
DEDUCTIBLE	.00
COPAY	120.00
OTHER REDUCTION	.00
AMOUNT APPROVED	450.60

EFT INFORMATION

NUMBER	00146972
DATE	10/03/16
AMOUNT	450.60

STATUS CODES:
A - APPROVED AJ - ADJUSTMENT IP - IN PROCESS R - REJECTED V - VOID

source document 12

BLUE CROSS/BLUE SHIELD
340 BOULEVARD
COLUMBUS, OH 60220

PROVIDER REMITTANCE
THIS IS NOT A BILL
A PAYMENT SUMMARY AND AN EXPLANATION OF CODES ARE AT THE END OF THIS STATEMENT

FAMILY CARE CLINIC
285 STEPHENSON BLVD.
STEPHENSON, OH 60089-4000

PAGE: 1 OF 1
DATE: 11/03/2016
ID NUMBER: 001234

PROVIDER: ROBERT BEACH, M.D.

PATIENT: GILES SHEILA CLAIM: 123456789

FROM DATE	THRU DATE	PROC CODE	UNITS	AMOUNT BILLED	AMOUNT ALLOWED	DEDUCT	COPAY/ COINS	PROV PAID	REASON CODE
10/28/16	10/28/16	99213	1	72.00	72.00	.00	.00	57.60	
10/28/16	10/28/16	71010	1	91.00	91.00	.00	.00	72.80	
10/28/16	10/28/16	87430	1	29.00	.00	.00	.00	.00	R
	CLAIM TOTALS			192.00	163.00	.00	.00	130.40	

R* OUTSIDE LAB WORK NOT BILLABLE BY PROVIDER

PATIENT: SIMMONS JILL CLAIM: 234567891

FROM DATE	THRU DATE	PROC CODE	UNITS	AMOUNT BILLED	AMOUNT ALLOWED	DEDUCT	COPAY/ COINS	PROV PAID	REASON CODE
10/28/16	10/28/16	99212	1	54.00	54.00	.00	.00	43.20	
10/28/16	10/28/16	87086	1	51.00	51.00	.00	.00	40.80	
	CLAIM TOTALS			105.00	105.00	.00	.00	84.00	

PROVIDER: PATRICIA MCGRATH, M.D.

PATIENT: BARRETT JORGE CLAIM: 345678901

FROM DATE	THRU DATE	PROC CODE	UNITS	AMOUNT BILLED	AMOUNT ALLOWED	DEDUCT	COPAY/ COINS	PROV PAID	REASON CODE
10/21/16	10/21/16	G8443	1	.00	.00	.00	.00	.00	
10/21/16	10/21/16	99203	1	120.00	120.00	.00	.00	96.00	
	CLAIM TOTALS			120.00	120.00	.00	.00	96.00	

PAYMENT SUMMARY

TOTAL AMOUNT PAID	310.40
PRIOR CREDIT BALANCE	.00
CURRENT CREDIT DEFERRED	.00
PRIOR CREDIT APPLIED	.00
NEW CREDIT BALANCE	.00
NET DISBURSED	310.40

TOTAL ALL CLAIMS

AMOUNT CHARGED	417.00
AMOUNT ALLOWED	388.00
DEDUCTIBLE	.00
COINSURANCE	.00
OTHER REDUCTION	.00
AMOUNT APPROVED	310.40

EFT INFORMATION

NUMBER	001234
DATE	11/03/16
AMOUNT	310.40

STATUS CODES:
A - APPROVED AJ - ADJUSTMENT IP - IN PROCESS R - REJECTED V - VOID

13 source document

OHIOCARE HMO
147 CENTRAL AVENUE
HALEVILLE, OH 60890

FAMILY CARE CLINIC
285 STEPHENSON BLVD.
STEPHENSON, OH 60089-4000

PAGE:	1 OF 1
DATE:	10/30/2016
ID NUMBER:	001006003

OHIOCARE HMO CAPITATION STATEMENT
MONTH OF OCTOBER 2016

PROVIDERS
BANU DANA
BEACH ROBERT
MCGRATH PATRICIA
RUDNER JESSICA
RUDNER JOHN
YAN KATHERINE

MEMBER NUMBER	MEMBER NAME	CONTRACT NUMBER	CONTRACT STATUS
0003602149	FAMILY CARE CLINIC	YG34906	APPROVED

AMOUNT OF PAYMENT $2,500.00
EFT STATUS: SENT 10/30/16 8:46AM
TRANSACTION #343434

source document 14

FAMILY CARE CLINIC FEE SCHEDULE/PAYMENT SCHEDULE

CPT Code	Provider's Usual Fee	Managed Care Allowed	Medicare Allowed	CPT Code	Provider's Usual Fee	Managed Care Allowed	Medicare Allowed
11100	$148.00	$133.20	$36.72	90703	$29.00	$26.10	$14.30
11641	$204.00	$183.60	$122.23	93000	$84.00	$75.60	$25.72
12011	$202.00	$181.80	$148.70	92516	$210.00	$189.00	$59.32
29125	$99.00	$89.10	$61.21	93015	$401.00	$360.90	$103.31
29540	$121.50	$109.35	$40.50	96372	$40.00	$36.00	$18.74
50390	$551.00	$495.90	$101.47	96900	$39.00	$35.10	$16.42
71010	$91.00	$81.90	$26.77	99201	$66.00	$59.40	$35.58
71020	$112.00	$100.80	$34.71	99202	$88.00	$79.20	$63.28
71030	$153.00	$137.70	$45.25	99203	$120.00	$108.00	$94.28
73070	$102.00	$91.80	$27.06	99204	$178.00	$160.20	$133.56
73090	$99.00	$89.10	$27.44	99205	$229.00	$206.10	$169.28
73100	$93.00	$83.70	$26.37	99211	$36.00	$32.40	$20.68
73510	$124.00	$111.60	$32.56	99212	$54.00	$48.60	$37.36
73600	$96.00	$86.40	$26.37	99213	$72.00	$64.80	$51.03
80048	$50.00	$45.00	$11.20	99214	$105.00	$94.50	$80.15
80061	$90.00	$81.00	$18.72	99215	$163.00	$146.70	$116.96
82270	$19.00	$17.10	$4.54	99381	$210.00	$189.00	$100.27
82947	$25.00	$22.50	$5.48	99382	$218.00	$196.20	$108.13
82951	$63.00	$56.70	$16.12	99383	$224.00	$201.60	$106.00
83718	$43.00	$38.70	$11.44	99384	$262.50	$236.25	$115.30
84478	$29.00	$26.10	$8.04	99385	$247.50	$222.75	$115.30
85007	$21.00	$18.90	$4.81	99386	$267.00	$240.30	$135.69
85018	$13.00	$11.70	$3.31	99387	$298.50	$268.65	$147.13
85025	$13.60	$12.24	$10.79	99391	$165.00	$148.50	$76.39
85651	$24.00	$21.60	$4.96	99392	$184.50	$166.05	$85.69
86580	$25.00	$22.50	$6.86	99393	$192.00	$172.80	$84.63
87076	$75.00	$67.50	$11.29	99394	$222.00	$199.80	$93.56
87077	$60.00	$54.00	$11.29	99395	$204.00	$183.60	$94.63
87086	$51.00	$45.90	$11.28	99396	$222.00	$199.80	$104.64
87430	$29.00	$26.10	$16.01	99397	$236.00	$212.40	$115.37
87880	$24.00	$21.60	$16.01	99444	$30.00	$27.00	$00.00
90471	$15.00	$13.50	$17.82				

Glossary

a

abuse actions that improperly use another person's resources

accept assignment participating physician's agreement to accept the allowed charge as full payment

access levels security option that determines the areas of the program a user can access, and whether the user has rights to enter or edit data

accounts receivable (A/R) monies that are coming into a practice

Acknowledgment of Receipt of Notice of Privacy Practices form accompanying a covered entity's Notice of Privacy Practices; covered entities must make a good-faith effort to have patients sign it

addenda updates to ICD-9-CM

adjudication series of steps that determine whether a claim should be paid

adjustments changes to a patient's account

advance beneficiary notice of noncoverage (ABN) Medicare form used to inform a patient that a service to be provided is not likely to be reimbursed by Medicare

aging classification of accounts receivable by length of time

aging report a report that lists the amount of money owed to the practice, organized by the amount of time the money has been owed

allowed charge maximum charge a plan pays for a service or procedure

Alphabetic Index section of ICD-9-CM alphabetically listing diseases and injuries with corresponding diagnosis codes

American Recovery and Reinvestment Act of 2009 (ARRA) a $787 billion economic stimulus bill passed in 2009 that allocates $19.2 billion to promote the use of health information technology

appeal request for reconsideration of a claim adjudication

appellant person who appeals a claim decision

ASC X12 Version 5010 updated electronic data standard for transmitting HIPAA X12 documents, such as the HIPAA claim (X12 837), that replaces ASC X12 Version 4010 beginning in January 2012

assignment of benefits authorization by a policyholder that allows a health plan to pay benefits directly to a provider

audit formal examination or review, such as a review to determine whether an entity is complying with regulations

Auto Log Off feature of Medisoft that automatically logs a user out of the program after a period of inactivity

autoposting software feature enabling automatic entry of payments from a remittance advice

b

backing up making a copy of data files at a specific point in time that can be used to restore data

balance billing collecting the difference between a provider's usual fee and a payer's lower allowed charge

bankruptcy declaration that a person is unable to pay his or her debts

benefits the amount of money a health plan pays for services covered in an insurance policy

birthday rule guideline that determines which of two parents with medical coverage has the primary insurance for a child; the parent whose day of birth is earlier in the calendar year is considered primary

Blue Cross and Blue Shield Association (BCBS) licensing agency of Blue Cross and Blue Shield plans

breach under the HIPAA Privacy Rule, impermissible use or disclosure that compromises the security or privacy of protected health information that could pose a significant risk of financial, reputational, or other harm to the affected person

breach notification document used by a covered entity to notify individuals of a breach in their protected health information required under the new HITECH breach notification rules

bundled code two or more related procedure codes combined into one

business associate person or organization that requires access to PHI to perform a function or activity on behalf of a covered entity but is not part of its workforce

c

capitated plan insurance plan in which prepayments made to a physician cover the physician's services to a plan member for a specified period of time

capitation a prepayment covering a provider's services for a plan member for a specified period

capitation payments payments made to physicians on a regular basis for providing services to patients in a managed care plan

capitation (cap) rate periodic prepayment to a provider for specified services to each plan member

case grouping of transactions for visits to a physician office organized around a specific medical condition

cash flow the movement of monies into and out of a business

Category I codes procedure codes found in the main body of CPT

Category II codes optional CPT codes that track performance measures

Category III codes temporary codes for emerging technology, services, and procedures

CCI column 1/column 2 code pair edits Medicare code edit in which CPT codes in column 2 will not be paid if reported for same day of service, for the same patient, and by the same provider as the column 1 code

CCI edits CPT code combinations that are used by computers to check Medicare claims

CCI modifier indicator number showing whether the use of a modifier can bypass a CCI edit

CCI mutually exclusive code (MEC) edits edits for codes for services that could not have reasonably been done during one encounter

Centers for Medicare and Medicaid Services (CMS) federal agency in the Department of Health and Human Services that runs Medicare, Medicaid, clinical laboratories, and other government health programs; responsible for enforcing all HIPAA standards other than the privacy and security standards

certification a nationally recognized designation that acknowledges that an individual has mastered a standard body of knowledge and meets certain competencies

charge capture process of recording billable services

charges amount a provider bills for performed health care services

chart folder that contains all records pertaining to a patient

chart number unique alphanumeric code that identifies a patient

chief complaint patient's description of the symptoms or reasons for seeking medical care

Civilian Health and Medical Program of the Department of Veterans Affairs (CHAMPVA) health care plan for families of veterans with 100 percent service-related disabilities and the surviving spouses and children of veterans who die from service-related disabilities

claim adjustment group code (CAGC) used on an RA/EOB to indicate the general type of reason code for an adjustment

claim adjustment reason code (CARC) used on an RA/EOB to explain why a payment does not match the amount billed

claimant person or entity exercising the right to receive benefits

claim control number unique number assigned to a claim by the sender

claim scrubber software that checks claims to permit error correction

claim status category codes used to report the status group for a claim

claim status codes used to provide a detailed answer to a claim status inquiry

claim turnaround time time period in which a health plan must process a claim

clearinghouse company that processes electronic health information and executes electronic transactions such as insurance verification and claim submission for providers

CMS-1500 (08/05) claim the mandated paper insurance claim form

code linkage clinically appropriate connection between a provided service and a patient's condition or illness

code set alphabetic and/or numeric representations for data; a medical code set is a system of medical terms required for HIPAA transactions

coinsurance the portion of charges that an insured person must pay for health care services after payment of the deductible amount; usually stated as a percentage

collection agency outside firm hired to collect on delinquent accounts

collection list tool for tracking activities that need to be completed as part of the collection process

collection tracer report tool for keeping track of collection letters that were sent

companion guide guide published by a payer that lists its own set of claim edits and formatting conventions

compliant billing billing actions that satisfy official requirements

computer-assisted coding assigning preliminary diagnosis and procedure codes using computer software

consumer-driven (directed) health plan (CDHP) medical insurance that combines a high-deductible health plan with one or more tax-preferred savings accounts that the patient directs

continuity of care coordination of care received by a patient over time and across multiple health care providers

coordination of benefits (COB) clause in an insurance policy that explains how the policy will pay if more than one insurance policy applies to the claim

copayment (copay) an amount that a health plan requires a beneficiary to pay at the time of service for each health care encounter

Correct Coding Initiative (CCI) computerized Medicare system that prevents overpayment

covered entity under HIPAA, health plan, clearinghouse, or provider that transmits any health information in electronic form in connection with a HIPAA transaction

covered services medical procedures and treatments that are included as benefits under an insured's health plan

crossover claim claim billed to Medicare and then submitted to Medicaid

***Current Procedural Terminology* (CPT)** the standardized classification system for reporting medical procedures and services

cycle billing type of billing in which statement printing and mailing is staggered throughout the month

d

dashboard a panel in Medisoft that offers providers a convenient view of important information

database a collection of related bits of information

data element smallest unit of information in a HIPAA transaction

data mining the process of analyzing large amounts of data to discover patterns or knowledge

data warehouse a collection of data that includes all areas of an organization's operations

day sheet a report that provides information on practice activities for a twenty-four-hour period

deductible an amount that an insured person must pay, usually on an annual basis, for health care services before a health plan's payment begins

determination payer's decision about the benefits due for a claim

development process of gathering information to adjudicate a claim

diagnosis code a code that represents the physician's determination of a patient's primary illness

dictation the process of recording spoken words that will later be transcribed into written form

digital dictation the process of dictating using a microphone, a headset connected to a computer, a smart phone, or a PDA

disability compensation programs programs that provide partial reimbursement for lost income when a disability prevents an individual from working

disaster recovery plan plan for resuming normal operations after a disaster such as a fire or a computer malfunction

discounted fee-for-service payment schedule for services based on a reduced percentage of usual charges

documentation the record created when a physician provides treatment to a patient

dual-eligible Medicare-Medicaid beneficiary

e

electronic data interchange (EDI) computer-to-computer exchange of routine business information using publicly available electronic standards

electronic encounter form (EEF) an electronic version of the form that lists procedures and charges for a patient's visit

electronic funds transfer (EFT) electronic routing of funds between banks

electronic health record (EHR) a computerized lifelong health care record for an individual that incorporates data from all sources that provide treatment for the individual

electronic medical record (EMR) computerized record of one physician's encounters with a patient over time

electronic prescribing a technology that enables a physician to transmit a prescription electronically to a patient's pharmacy

electronic protected health information (ePHI) PHI that is created, received, maintained, or transmitted in electronic form

electronic remittance advice (ERA) electronic document that lists patients, dates of service, charges, and the amounts paid or denied by the insurance carrier

Employee Retirement Income Security Act of 1974 (ERISA) law providing incentives and protection for companies with employee health and pension plans

encounter the meeting of a patient with a physician or other medical professional for the purpose of providing health care (also known as a visit)

encryption process of converting electronic information into an unreadable format before it is distributed

Equal Credit Opportunity Act (ECOA) law that prohibits credit discrimination on the basis of race, color, religion, national origin, sex, marital status, or age, or because a person receives public assistance

established patient (EP) patient who has received professional services from a provider (or another provider with the same specialty in the same practice) within the past three years

evaluation and management (E/M) codes codes that cover physicians' services performed to determine the optimum course for patient care

explanation of benefits (EOB) document showing how the amount of a benefit was determined

f

Fair Debt Collection Practices Act of 1977 (FDCPA) federal law regulating collection practices

family history (FH) a detailed record of medical events among members of the patient's family, including the ages, living status, and diseases of siblings, children, parents, and grandparents

Federal Employees Health Benefits (FEHB) health care program that covers federal employees

fee-for-service health plan that repays the policyholder for covered medical expenses

fee schedule document that specifies the amount the provider bills for services

filter a condition that data must meet to be selected

financial policy practice's rules governing payment for medical services from patients

flexible savings account (FSA) consumer-driven health plan funding option that has employer and employee contributions

formulary list of a plan's selected drugs and their proper dosages

fraud intentional act of deception to take financial advantage of another person

g

global period days surrounding a surgical procedure when all services relating to the procedure are considered part of the surgical package

group health plan (GHP) plan of an employer or employee organization to provide health care to employees, former employees, and/or their families

guarantor person who is the insurance policyholder for a patient of the practice

h

HCPCS procedure codes for Medicare claims

Health Care Fraud and Abuse Control Program government program to uncover misuse of funds in federal health care programs run by the Office of the Inspector General

health informatics knowledge required to optimize the acquisition, storage, retrieval, and use of information in health and biomedicine

health information exchange (HIE) a network that enables the sharing of health-related information among provider organizations according to nationally recognized standards

health information technology (HIT) the use of computers and electronic communications to manage medical information and its secure exchange

Health Information Technology for Economic and Clinical Health (HITECH) Act provisions in the American Recovery and Reinvestment Act (ARRA) of 2009 that extend and reinforce HIPAA and contain new breach notification requirements for covered entities and business associates, guidance on ways to encrypt or destroy PHI to prevent a breach, requirements for informing individuals when a breach occurs, higher monetary penalties for HIPAA violations, and stronger enforcement of the Privacy and Security Rules

Health Insurance Portability and Accountability Act of 1996 (HIPAA) legislation that protects patient's private health information, ensures health care coverage when workers change or lose jobs, and uncovers fraud and abuse in the health care system

health maintenance organization (HMO) managed health care system in which providers offer health care to members for fixed periodic payments

health plan an individual or group plan that either provides or pays for the cost of medical care; includes group health plans, health insurance issuers, health maintenance organizations, Medicare Part A and B, Medicaid, TRICARE, and other government and nongovernment plans

health reimbursement account (HRA) consumer-driven health plan funding option where an employer sets aside an annual amount for health care costs

health savings account (HSA) consumer driven health plan funding option under which funds are set aside to pay for certain health care costs

high-deductible health plan (HDHP) health plan that combines high-deductible insurance and a funding option to pay for patients' out-of-pocket expenses up to the deductible

HIPAA Electronic Health Care Transactions and Code Sets (TCS) the HIPAA rule governing the electronic exchange of health information

HIPAA National Identifiers HIPAA-mandated identification systems for employers, health care providers, health plans, and patients; national provider system and employer system are in place; health plan and patient systems have not been created

HIPAA Privacy Rule law that regulates the use and disclosure of patients' protected health information

HIPAA Security Rule law that requires covered entities to establish administrative, physical, and technical safeguards to protect the confidentiality, integrity, and availability of health information

HIPAA X12 837 Health Care Claim HIPAA standard format for electronic transmission of the claim to a health plan

HIPAA X12 276/277 Health Care Claim Status Inquiry/Response electronic format used to ask payers about claims

history of present illness (HPI) a description of the course of the present illness, including how and when the problem began, up to the present time

i

ICD-9-CM abbreviated title of *International Classification of Diseases*, Ninth Revision, *Clinical Modification*, the source of the codes used for reporting diagnoses

ICD-9-CM Official Guidelines for Coding and Reporting American Hospital Association publication that provides rules for selecting and sequencing diagnosis codes

ICD-10-CM abbreviated title of *International Classification of Diseases*, Tenth Revision, *Clinical Modification*, which will be used beginning in 2013

indemnity plan type of medical insurance that reimburses a policyholder for medical services under the terms of its schedule of benefits

individual health plan (IHP) medical insurance plan purchased by an individual

insurance aging report a report that lists how long a payer has taken to respond to insurance claims

integrated PM/EHR programs programs that share and exchange demographic information, appointment schedules, and clinical data

k

key components factors documented for various levels of evaluation and management services

knowledge base a collection of up-to-date technical information

m

managed care system that combines the financing and delivery of appropriate, cost-effective health care services to its members

meaningful use the utilization of certified EHR technology to improve quality, efficiency, and patient safety in the health care system

means test process of fairly determining a patient's ability to pay

Medicaid federal and state assistance program that pays for health care services for people who cannot afford them

medical assistant (MA) health care professional who performs both administrative and certain clinical tasks in physician offices

medical biller health care professional who performs administrative tasks throughout the medical billing cycle

medical coder medical office staff member with specialized training who handles the diagnostic and procedural coding of medical records

medical coding the process of applying the HIPAA-mandated code sets to assign codes to diagnoses and procedures

medical documentation and billing cycle a ten-step process that results in timely payment for medical services

medical insurance financial plan that covers the cost of hospital and medical care

medically unlikely edits (MUEs) units of service edits used to lower the Medicare fee-for-service paid claims error rate

medical malpractice the provision of medical services at a less than acceptable level of professional skill that results in injury or harm to a patient

medical necessity treatment that is in accordance with generally accepted medical practice

medical necessity denial refusal by a plan to pay for a procedure that does not meet its medical necessity criteria

medical record a chronological health care record that includes information that the patient provides, such as medical history, as well as the physician's assessment, diagnosis, and treatment plan

Medicare federal health insurance program for people sixty-five or older and some people with disabilities

Medicare Part A, Hospital Insurance (HI) program that pays for hospitalization, care in a skilled nursing facility, home health care, and hospice care

Medicare Part B, Supplementary Medical Insurance (SMI) program that pays for physician services, outpatient hospital services, durable medical equipment, and other services and supplies

Medicare Part C, Medicare Advantage managed care health plans under the Medicare program

Medicare Part D Medicare prescription drug reimbursement plans

Medicare Physician Fee Schedule (MPFS) allowed fees based on the resource-based relative value scale that are the basis for Medicare reimbursements

Medigap plan offered by a private insurance carrier to supplement Medicare coverage

Medi-Medi beneficiary person eligible for both Medicare and Medicaid

Medisoft Clinical Patient Records (MCPR) electronic health record application within Medisoft

Medisoft Network Professional (MNP) practice management application within Medisoft

modifier number appended to a code to report particular facts

MultiLink codes groups of procedure code entries that relate to a single activity

n

National Health Information Network (NHIN) a common platform for health information exchange across the country

National Provider Identifier (NPI) under HIPAA, system for identifying all health care providers using unique ten-digit identifiers

National Uniform Claim Committee (NUCC) organization responsible for claim content

navigator buttons buttons that simplify the task of moving from one entry to another

new patient (NP) a patient who has not received professional services from a provider (or another provider with the same specialty in the same practice) within the past three years

noncovered services medical procedures that are not included in a plan's benefits

nonparticipating (nonPAR) provider a provider who chooses not to join a particular government or other health plan

nonsufficient funds (NSF) check check that is not honored by the bank because the account lacks funds to cover it

Notice of Privacy Practices (NPP) a HIPAA-mandated document stating the privacy policies and procedures of a covered entity

o

Office Hours break a block of time when a physician is unavailable for appointments with patients

Office Hours calendar an interactive calendar that is used to select or change dates in Office Hours

Office Hours patient information the area of the Office Hours window that displays information about the patient who is selected in the provider's daily schedule

once-a-month billing type of billing in which statements are mailed to all patients at the same time each month

Original Medicare Plan Medicare fee-for-service plan

out-of-network a provider that does not have a participation agreement with a plan; using an out-of-network provider is more expensive for the plan's enrollees

out-of-pocket expenses the insured must pay before benefits begin

overpayment improper or excessive amount received by provider from payer

p

package combination of services included in a single procedure code

park privacy and security feature in MCPR that allows a user to leave a workstation for a brief time without having to exit the program

participating (PAR) provider a provider who agrees to provide medical services to a payer's policyholders according to the terms of the plan's contract

password confidential authentication information

past, family, and social history (PFSH) patients' answers to physicians' questions about their personal medical histories, medical events in their families, and factors relating to their social environments

past medical history (PMH) the patient's history of medical problems, including chronic conditions, surgeries, and hospitalizations

patient aging report a report that lists a patient's balance by age, date and amount of the last payment, and telephone number, grouping unpaid bills by the length of time they remain due

patient day sheet a summary of patient activity on a given day

patient examination an examination of a person's body in order to determine his or her state of health

patient flow the progression of patients from the time they enter the office for a visit until they exit the system by leaving the office after a visit

patient information form form that includes a patient's personal, employment, and insurance data needed to complete a health care claim; also known as a registration form

patient ledger a report that lists the financial activity in each patient's account

patient portal secure website that enables communication between patients and health care providers for tasks such as scheduling, completing registration forms, and making payments

patient refund money owed to patient

patient registry method of reporting clinical data to payers using an online service rather than claim-based reporting

patient statement list of the amount of money a patient owes, the procedures performed, and the dates the procedures were performed

patient tracking features function attached to the electronic scheduler that is used during a patient encounter to track where the patient is during the different steps of the encounter

payer health plan or program

pay for performance (P4P) provision of financial incentives to physicians who provide evidence-based treatments to their patients

payment day sheet a report that lists all payments received on a particular day, organized by provider

payment plan agreement between a patient and a practice in which the patient agrees to make regular monthly payments over a specified period of time

payments money paid by patients and health plans

pending claim status in which the payer is waiting for information before making a payment decision

performance measure processes, experience, and/or outcomes of patient care, observations, or treatment that relate to one or more quality aims for health care, such as effective, safe, efficient, patient-centered, equitable, and timely care

personal health record (PHR) private, secure electronic health care files that are created, maintained, and owned by the patient

Physician Quality Reporting Initiative (PQRI) a Medicare program that gives bonuses to physicians when they use treatment plans and clinical guidelines that are based on scientific evidence

place of service (POS) code location where medical services were provided

point-of-service (POS) plan managed care plan that permits patients to receive medical services from nonnetwork providers

policyholder person who buys an insurance plan; the insured, subscriber, or guarantor

postpayment audit review conducted after a claim is adjudicated

practice analysis report a report that analyzes the revenue of a practice for a specified period of time

practice management (PM) program program used to perform administrative and financial functions in a medical office

preauthorization prior authorization from a payer for services to be provided; if preauthorization is not received, the charge is usually not covered

preexisting condition illness or disorder of a beneficiary that existed before the effective date of insurance coverage

preferred provider organization (PPO) managed care network of health care providers who agree to perform services for plan members at discounted fees

premium money the insured pays to a health plan for a health care policy; usually paid monthly

preregistration the process of gathering basic contact, insurance, and reason for visit information before a new patient comes into the office for an encounter

preventive medical services care that is provided to keep patients healthy or to prevent illness, such as routine checkups and screening tests

primary care physician (PCP) physician in a managed care organization who directs all aspects of a patient's care

primary diagnosis the patient's major illness or condition for an encounter

primary insurance carrier the first carrier to whom claims are submitted

primary insurance plan health plan that pays benefits first when a patient is covered by more than one plan

procedure code a code that represents the particular service, treatment, or test provided by a physician

procedure day sheet a report that lists all the procedures performed on a particular day, in numerical order

progress note note documenting the care delivered to a patient, and the medical facts and clinical thinking relevant to diagnosis and treatment

prompt payment laws state laws that mandate a time period within which clean claims must be paid; if they are not, financial penalties are levied against the payer

protected health information (PHI) individually identifiable health information transmitted or maintained by electronic media or in any other form or medium

provider person or entity that supplies medical or health services and bills for or is paid for the services in the normal course of business; may be a professional member of the health care team, such as a physician, or a facility, such as a hospital or skilled nursing home

provider's daily schedule a listing of time slots for a particular day for a specific provider that corresponds to the date selected in the calendar

provider selection box a selection box that determines which provider's schedule is displayed in the provider's daily schedule

q

query request for more information from a provider

r

real-time claim adjudication (RTCA) process used to contact health plans electronically to determine visit charges

record of treatment and progress physician's notes about a patient's condition and diagnosis

records retention schedule a plan for the management of records that lists types of records and indicates how long they should be kept

Recovery Audit Contractor (RAC) entity that audits Medicare claims to determine where there are opportunities to recover incorrect payments from previously paid but noncovered services, erroneous coding, and duplicate services

referral transfer of patient care from one physician to another

referral number authorization number given by a referring physician to the referred physician

referring provider physician who refers the patient to another physician for treatment

regional extension centers (RECs) centers that offer information, guidance, training, and support services to primary care providers who are in the process of making the transition to an EHR system

registration process of gathering personal and insurance information about a patient before an encounter with a provider

relative value scale (RVS) system of assigning unit values to medical services based on their required skill and time

release of information (ROI) process followed by employees of covered entities when releasing patient information

remainder statements statements that list only charges that are not paid in full after all insurance carrier payments have been received

remittance advice (RA) document describing a payment resulting from a claim adjudication

remittance advice remark code (RARC) code that explains a payer's payment decision

resource-based relative value scale (RBRVS) relative value scale for establishing Medicare charges

restoring process of retrieving data from a backup storage device

retention preservation of information on patients' medical conditions and care for possible later use

revenue cycle management (RCM) management of the activities associated with a patient encounter to ensure that the provider receives full payment for services

review of systems (ROS) an inventory of body systems in which the patient reports signs or symptoms he or she is currently having or has had in the past

s

schedule of benefits list of the medical expenses that a health plan covers

secondary insurance plan health plan that pays benefits after the primary plan pays when a patient is covered by more than one plan

selection boxes fields within the Search dialog box that are used to select the data that will be included in a report

self-insured health plans health insurance plans paid for directly by the organization, which sets up a fund from which to pay

self-pay patients patients with no medical insurance

small-balance account overdue patient account in which the amount owed is less than the cost of pursuing payment

SOAP format used to enter progress notes; it stands for *subjective, objective, assessment*, and *plan*

social history (SH) information about the patient's tobacco use, alcohol and drug use, sexual history, relationship status, and other significant social facts that may contribute to the care of the patient

sponsor in TRICARE, the active-duty service member

standards technical specifications for the electronic exchange of information

standard statements statements that show all charges regardless of whether the insurance carrier has paid on the transactions

suspended claim status when the payer is developing the claim

t

Tabular List section of ICD-9-CM listing diagnosis codes numerically

takeback balance that a provider owes a payer following a postpayment audit

Telephone Consumer Protection Act of 1991 federal law regulating collection practices

template preformatted note that contains selections appropriate to the medical condition or type of visit

third-party payer private or government organization that insures or pays for health care on behalf of beneficiaries

tickler reminder to follow up on an account

timely filing health plan's rules specifying the number of days after the date of service that the practice has to file the claim

treatment, payment, and health care operations (TPO) under HIPAA, three conditions under which patients' protected health information may be released without their consent

TRICARE government health program serving dependents of active-duty service members, military retirees and their families, some former spouses, and survivors of deceased military members

Truth in Lending Act part of the federal Consumer Credit Protection Act that regulates collection practices related to finance charges and late fees

u

unbundling incorrect billing practice of breaking a panel or package of services/procedures into component parts

uncollectible account account that does not respond to collection efforts and is written off the practice's expected accounts receivable

upcoding assigning a higher level code than is supported by documentation

user name name that an individual uses for identification purposes when logging onto a computer or an application

usual, customary, and reasonable (UCR) fees set by comparing usual fees, customary fees, and reasonable fees

usual fees normal fees charged by a provider

v

voice recognition software software that recognizes spoken words

w

walkout receipt report that lists the diagnoses, services provided, fees, and payments received and due after an encounter

workers' compensation insurance state or federal plan that covers medical care and other benefits for employees who suffer accidental injury or become ill as a result of employment

write off to deduct an amount from a patient's account

write-off balance that has been removed from a patient's account

x

X12 835 Electronic Remittance Advice (835) electronic transaction for payment explanation

index